AF732916

# *physical science*

## A SEARCH FOR UNDERSTANDING

WALTER R. BROWN

NORMAN D. ANDERSON

J. B. LIPPINCOTT COMPANY

Philadelphia · New York · San Jose

**Dr. Walter R. Brown** has taught junior high school and senior high school science in Missouri, Oklahoma, and Florida, and is now Chairman, Science Department, at Princess Anne Junior High School in Virginia Beach, Virginia. Besides teaching, Dr. Brown has worked as a staff member of the National Science Teacher Association and as a Consultant in Science at the Regional College of Education in Bhubaneswar, India. He has collaborated in the writing of several publications for science students and science teachers. He holds a doctorate in Science Education from The Ohio State University.

**Dr. Norman D. Anderson** has a rich and varied background as a science teacher. He worked for ten years in the public schools of Iowa, where his primary assignment was teaching junior high school science. He has also taught biology, chemistry, physics, and summer courses in science for gifted elementary school pupils. Dr. Anderson holds his doctorate in Science Education from The Ohio State University. Since 1963 he has been a member of the faculty at North Carolina State University at Raleigh, where he teaches prospective science teachers, graduate students in science education, and directs Institutes and Conferences for science teachers. In 1973 he was appointed an Alumni Distinguished Professor at NCSU.

Art work by Alan Young
Cover design and front matter by Sulpizio Associates

Copyright © 1977, 1972 by J. B. LIPPINCOTT COMPANY

All rights reserved. No part of this book may be used or reproduced in any form or by any means, mechanical or electronic, including photocopying, recording or by any information storage and retrieval system, without permission in writing from the publisher.

Printed in the United States of America ISBN-0-397-43744-7 20.791.4

# *preface*

Science plays an important role in your life. Physical science is the branch of science dealing with the study of matter and energy. The knowledge that scientists have gained about matter and energy has been used in developing many new products and machines that have made our lives very different from that of our ancestors. As you study this book, look for ways in which these discoveries by physical scientists affect your life.

*Physical Science: A Search for Understanding* emphasizes how scientists work and how new knowledge is gained. In using this book, you should realize that our understanding of the natural world is continually changing. Therefore, the theories described here should not be considered as final truths. Scientists continue to make investigations and to collect information to test all theories.

Several features have been built into this book to help you learn more easily. The many photographs and diagrams illustrate the ideas described in the text. Study these illustrations and their captions. Use the questions at the end of each numbered section and at the end of each chapter to check your progress.

Learning the meaning of scientific terms is an important part of studying science. Each numbered section begins with a list of some of the terms used in that section. If you are not sure of their meanings, look them up in the glossary at the back of the book or in a dictionary. New terms appear in boldface type, and their pronunciation is given when needed. As you study science, work at building up your scientific vocabulary.

Devising equipment and working with it is an important part of science. Directions for doing many investigations occur throughout the book. Additional investigations are described in the Workshops at the end of the units. You will also notice small activities, which are in color. Investigations and activities will help you to understand the ways in which scientists work as well as to understand the ideas behind them.

# *contents*

## UNIT I

### INTRODUCTION TO THE STUDY OF PHYSICAL SCIENCE



**The items in bold face are activities.**

# UNIT II

## MATTER, MOLECULES, AND MOTION

# UNIT III

## CHEMISTRY: A STUDY OF ATOMS

# UNIT IV

## MAGNETISM AND ELECTRICITY

# UNIT V

## THE ENERGY OF THE NUCLEUS

# UNIT VI

## ENERGY IN WAVES

# UNIT VII

## CAREERS: PUTTING IT TOGETHER

# unit I
# introduction to the study of physical science

John Running/Stock, Boston

# CHAPTER 1

# The Work of the Physical Scientist

IN MANY WAYS science is like a search for a lost object. For the searcher, there is an air of excitement with the possibility of the unexpected just around the corner. For many people this is also true of science.

A search, in addition to the excitement, often involves long periods of hard work with little or no results to show for all the effort. In like manner, science is not just one exciting breakthrough after another. It often takes many months or years of careful work and experimentation before a problem is solved. Often the solution to one problem creates several more, and so the search goes on.

Science and a search also are alike in other ways. Chances for success are increased if a method of going about the job is worked out ahead of time. The use of instruments often helps in both cases. Try to name some things that would help you find an iron nail in a bucket of sand. To find a small jewel from a ring lost in the living room carpet. To learn if the temperature at the bottom of a lake changes as much during the course of a year as does the temperature near the surface.

As you study this chapter, keep asking yourself how you would describe the work of the scientist. How does the work of the physical scientist differ from that of other scientists?

## 1. Staking Out the Territory of Physical Science

**ARE YOU READY?**

Look up the following words if you are not sure of their meanings:

atmosphere; category; migration; science; transmitter; unexplored; volcano.

Imagine for a moment that you have just been placed on an island on which you have never been before. Many questions would probably flash through your mind. Are there other people here? What plants and animals live here? How big is the island? How can I find things to eat and water to drink? Are there things like volcanoes, poisonous snakes, or flesh-eating animals that I need to be afraid of?

Beginning the study of a new subject in some ways is like being placed on an unexplored island. Perhaps it is not quite so exciting, but it does raise a lot of questions.

What is physical science? For that matter, what is science? What kinds of tools do I need in order to study physical science? What does physical science have to do with wanting to be a doctor, a nurse, or a secretary? What does physical science have to do with wanting to be a mechanic, a lawyer, a farmer, or a chemist? What does physical science have to do with any one of the thousands of occupations open to young people today?

Let's take these questions one at a time, beginning with the task of defining the territory of science.

## What Is Science?

**Science** is the search for the explanation of what we observe in nature. Science is also the knowledge about the universe that we believe to be true. In other words, science is a method, a way of trying to find out something, as well as being a body of knowledge—what we already know about the natural universe.

Science includes the study of an enormous variety of things—bacteria and elephants, algae and redwoods, atoms and mountains, and rainbows and the stars. The range of **phenomena** (fə nom′ ə nə), or things that happen in the universe, that is studied by scientists is just as impressive—earthquakes, thunder and lightning, migration of birds, light passing through a prism, and electricity heating the filament of a TV tube, to mention just a few.

Because of the very large territory of the scientist, it is helpful to subdivide science into two or more areas. Perhaps the easiest way to do this is to place things and events in the categories of living and nonliving. **Biology** (bī ol′ ə ji), or life science as it sometimes is called, is the branch of science that deals with living things.

The science of nonliving things is often subdivided into two branches—physical science and earth science. **Physical science**

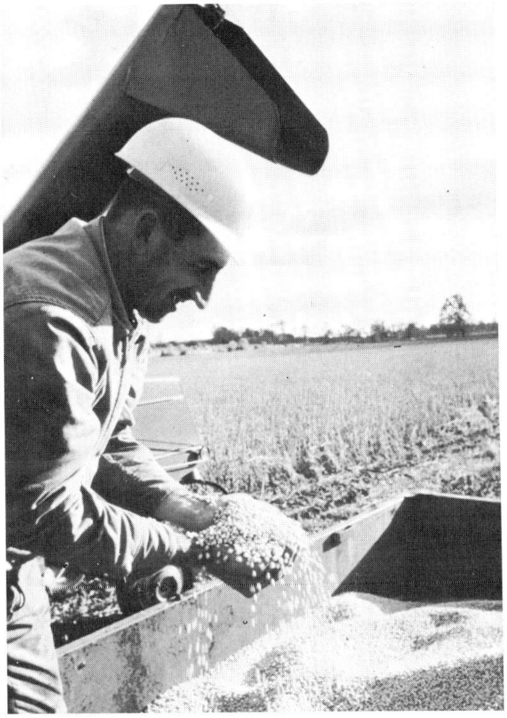

*USDA*

**1.1** Why do these people need to . . .

**1.2** understand something about physical science?

*American Red Cross Photo*

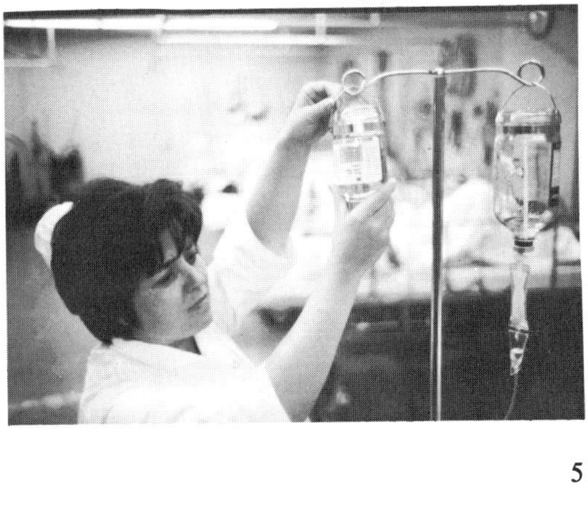

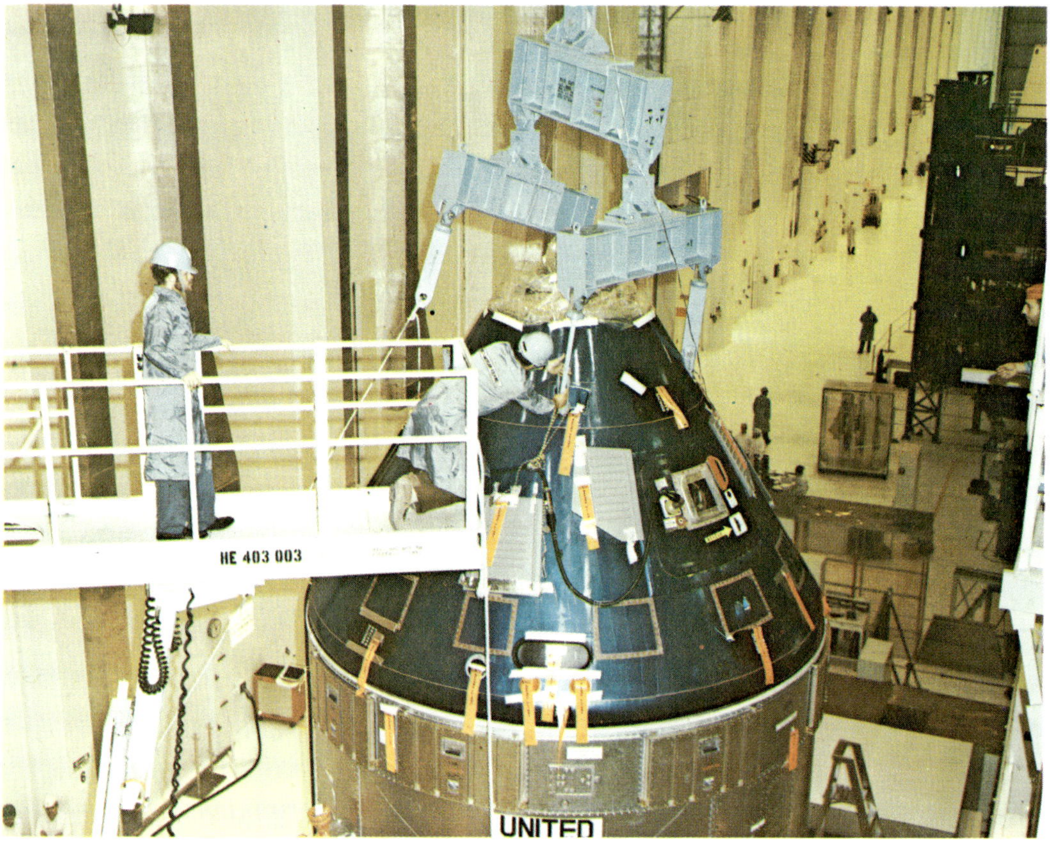


NASA

**1.3** The discoveries of physical scientists have made possible the development of space technology.

includes only the things usually studied in **chemistry** (kem′ is tri) and **physics** (fiz′iks). **Earth science** is defined as the study of the earth, the atmosphere, and the space beyond.

In this book, you will study mainly about matter and energy—the territory of chemistry and physics. By the end of the year you should have a better idea of what these two sciences include. You also will learn that many things scientists study do not fit neatly into the three categories of physical science, earth science and life science. For example, the light of the firefly is studied by both biologists and physical scientists. Physical scientists and earth scientists investigate the energy of waves, of earthquakes, and of the stars.

Some topics, such as the chemical make-up of the atmosphere and the process by which green plants manufacture food, involve ideas from all branches of science. This is especially true at the frontiers of science—attempts to create life in a test tube, to explore the solar system from space vehicles, and to solve the world's food and population problems. As you study physical science, you will encounter many examples of how all the sciences are related to and dependent upon each other.

## Science and Technology

Science is the search for the explanation of natural phenomena and is also the knowledge that we have discovered. **Technology** (tek nol′ ə ji) is the use, or application, of this knowledge by people to make their life easier or better in some way. It is the **technologist** (tek nol′ e jist), working with the discoveries of the physical scientists, who has produced the airplane, the radio and television, and the motion pictures.

It is not always easy to separate science and technology. For example, in the space program knowledge from the science of electronics made possible the development of very small, lightweight radio and TV transmitters. These devices, in addition to their use in space vehicles, have been used to study the bottom of the sea, to follow the migration of animals, and to investigate the changes that occur in the human body during various activities. Thus the technology that grew out of scientific advances in electronics helped generate new scientific knowledge in other fields.

**1.4** How can you make this clock run faster?

*J. W. McDonald*

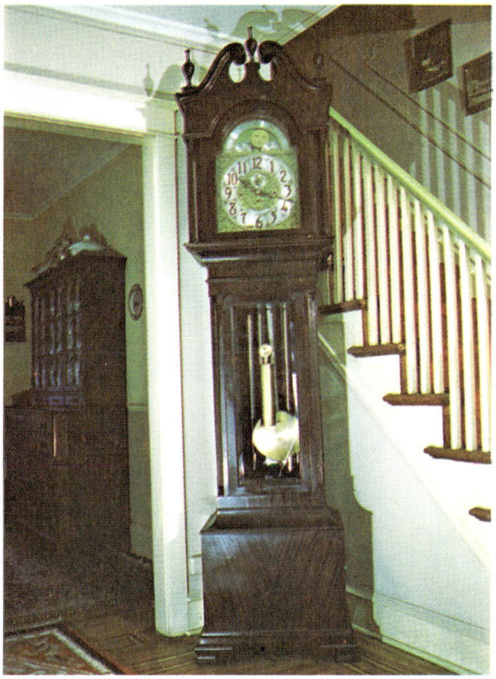


### Have You Learned?

Explain the difference between the pairs of words or phrases listed below. Write your answers briefly, using complete sentences.

1. Biology—Physical Science
2. Physical Science—Earth Science
3. Science—Technology

## 2. Science as a Way of Thinking

**ARE YOU READY?**

Look up the following words if you are not sure of their meanings:

conclusion; critical; curious; experiment; pendulum; reliable; speculate.

Take for example, the problem of finding a small jewel from a ring, lost in the living room carpet. You might begin by walking around the room, hoping that your path might lead you to the lost object. This would be a **trial-and-error** approach. It doesn't involve any reasoning nor does it draw on your knowledge and past experience.

A better way would be to have a plan of action. This might involve going back and forth across the room until each part of the room had been covered. Do you think your plan for finding the jewel would be improved by using a magnet to aid in the search? What knowledge did you use in deciding if it would help to use a magnet?

Would a flashlight be helpful? A vacuum cleaner? What other things would you consider using in trying to find the lost jewel? What plan do you think it would be best to follow in trying to find the object?

## The Scientific Method

Just as there is no magic formula for finding lost objects, there is no magic formula for solving scientific problems. But there are procedures, or a general course of action, that scientists often follow in trying to solve problems. The approach they use is called the **scientific method** and is illustrated by the following example.

Your family receives as a present an old-fashioned clock that has a pendulum and weights on chains to keep it running (Figure 1.4). You set the clock, pull the weights up, start the pendulum swinging, and the clock begins to run. In a few hours you notice that the clock is gaining time. The problem is how to slow the clock down so that it will keep accurate time.

You look for the directions and find none. You check in an encyclopedia and find that the pendulum is what determines how fast this type of clock runs. You speculate that if the pendulum did not swing quite so fast, the clock would not gain time. If this is so, what can be done to slow down the pendulum?

You decide to experiment with a pendulum by using a piece of string and some weights. After thinking about the problem, you decide that there are three things that might affect the rate of the pendulum's swing: the amount of weight on the end of the string, the distance you pull the weight back when setting the pendulum in motion, and the length of the string. Each of these three possible explanations, or **hypotheses** (hī poth′ ə sēz) (plural of **hypothesis**), can be tested by experimenting with a pendulum.

## Experimenting with a Pendulum

**MATERIALS:**

A piece of string, several weights, a ruler, a watch or clock with a second hand

**PROCEDURE:**

From a ring stand or similar support suspend a weight or an object such as a steel nut or several keys as shown opposite. The string should be about 45 centimeters long. Test each hypothesis as directed.

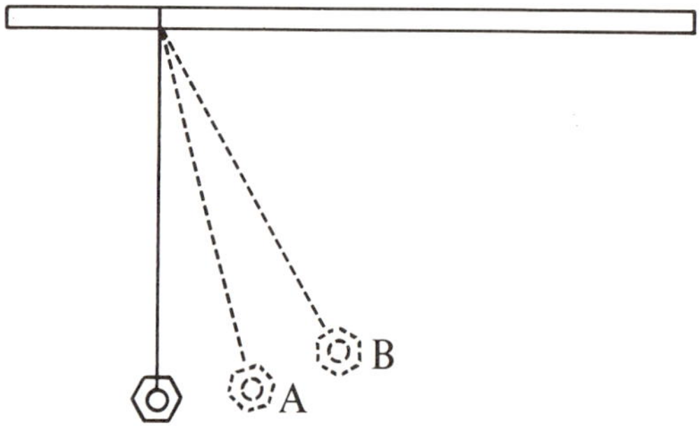


*Hypothesis Number One:* When setting the

pendulum in motion, pulling the weight back farther will make it swing back and forth more times per minute. Directions for testing hypothesis number one: Try pulling the weight back a measured distance, release and count the number of swings per minute. Repeat several times, each time pulling the weight back a different distance. Record your findings, or **data** (dāt′ ə), in a notebook using a table like the one below.

| Trial Number | 1 | 2 | 3 | 4 | 5 |
|---|---|---|---|---|---|
| Distance Weight Pulled Back | | | | | |
| Number of Swings per Minute | | | | | |

*Hypothesis Number Two:* By increasing the weight of the pendulum, the pendulum will swing faster. Directions for testing hypothesis number two: Repeat your experiment, this time varying the weight of the object on the end of the string. Record your data in a table in your notebook.

| Trial Number | 1 | 2 | 3 | 4 | 5 |
|---|---|---|---|---|---|
| Weight of Object Used | | | | | |
| Number of Swings per Minute | | | | | |

*Hypothesis Number Three:* Making the length of the string shorter will make the pendulum swing faster. Directions for testing hypothesis number three: Repeat the experiment again, this time varying the length of the string. Record your data in your notebook.

| Trial Number | 1 | 2 | 3 | 4 | 5 |
|---|---|---|---|---|---|
| Length of String | | | | | |
| Number of Swings per Minute | | | | | |

From your results you should be able to draw a conclusion about which of the factors affects the rate of the pendulum's swing. With this information it should be an easy matter to adjust the clock so that it keeps accurate time. What would you do to make the clock run slower? Faster?

## The Steps of the Scientific Method

In solving the problem of the clock that ran too fast, the procedure followed involved several steps. You found out that the pendulum controls how fast the clock runs. The problem then was to find out how to control the rate of the swing of the pendulum. To do this you looked for things that might affect the rate of the swing. The length of the string, the distance the weight was pulled back, and the amount of weight on the string appeared to be possibilities. Each was stated as a *hypothesis,* and each was *tested by experimentation.* From your results you drew a *conclusion.* Do you see that drawing a conclusion is really deciding whether or not a hypothesis is true?

In summary, the scientific method usually includes identifying the problem, collecting information about the problem, stating a hypothesis, testing the hypothesis by experimentation, and drawing a conclusion.

This book includes many accounts of

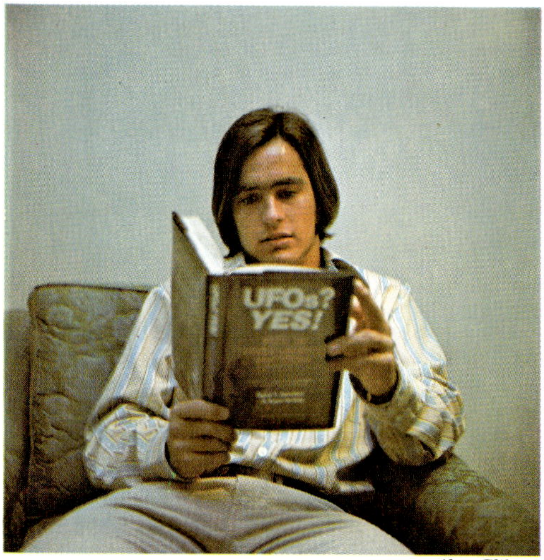


*Alan Cliburn*

**1.5** What evidence do you have for believing something to be true?

how scientists have used the scientific method in solving problems. As you study this book, try to learn more about how this method works. Meanwhile, try your hand at using the scientific method in solving one of the problems suggested below.

## Practicing the Scientific Method

Listed below are three problems. See if you can solve one of these problems by devising a way to test the suggested hypothesis or a hypothesis that you state.

After conducting your experiments, draw a conclusion about the hypothesis you tested. Does your experiment provide you with enough information to solve the problem? Or does your experiment simply eliminate a possible answer and leave the problem unsolved?

PROBLEM 1: What can be done to lower the temperature at which water freezes?
*Possible Hypothesis:* Water with salt dissolved in it freezes at a lower temperature than pure water.

PROBLEM 2: Does an object's weight affect how fast it falls?
*Possible Hypothesis:* If dropped at the same time, a heavy metal ball, such as a shot used at track meets, will strike the ground sooner than a lighter ball the same size.

PROBLEM 3: Does light or sound travel faster?
*Possible Hypothesis:* If a bass drum is hit, an observer some distance away will see it being hit before he hears the resulting noise.

## Scientific Attitudes

Some people argue that science can best be described by considering scientists' **attitudes** (at′ ə tüd). Scientists are usually very curious. They like to try new things, to tackle new problems and ideas.

Scientists are expected to be *open-minded.* They collect all the evidence they can, even though some of the evidence may prove that their ideas are wrong. They also *withold judgment* on a question until they have all the evidence they can obtain. If new evidence is later found, scientists must be *willing to change their minds.*

Scientists are described as being *critical-minded.* They are always asking questions. What evidence do you have for believing something to be true? Did you read it in a book? If so, was it a reliable book—a book written by a person considered to be an expert on the subject of the book?

Which of these scientific attitudes do you have? Are you curious? Open-minded? Do you withhold judgment until you have enough information to reach a decision? Are you willing to change your mind?

Do you think that all people should try to have scientific attitudes? Would the world be a better place to live if they did?

### Have You Learned?

Below are five steps usually used by scientists when solving a problem. Together they make up the *scientific method.* Place them in their correct order.

1. State a hypothesis.
2. Draw a conclusion.
3. Identify a problem.
4. Experiment.
5. Collect information.

## 3. The Tools of the Physical Scientist

**ARE YOU READY?**

Look up the following words if you are not sure of their meanings:

alcohol; chemicals; goggles; laboratory; methods (of science).

The most important tools used by scientists are their minds and the methods of science, which were described in Section 2. In order to help them use these mental tools more exactly, physical scientists have developed a great number of physical tools. Your school probably will have

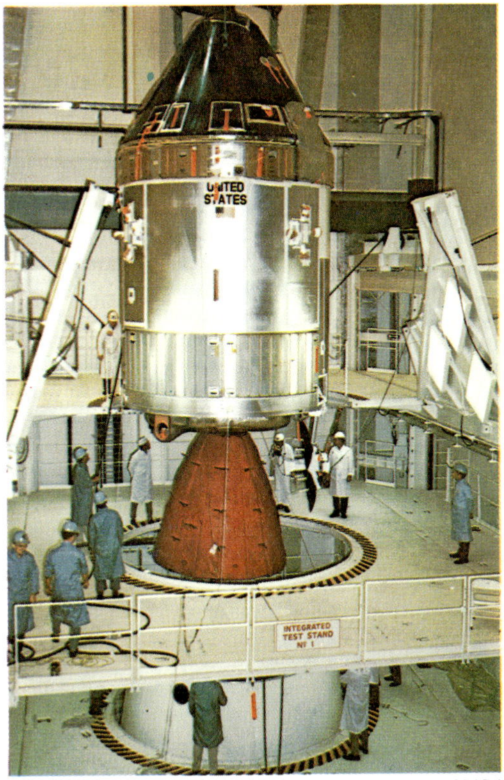


NASA

**1.6** Mental and physical tools have combined to make this module possible.

some of these for you to work with, and you will learn about many more while studying this book. Using equipment and reading about how scientists use tools will help you to understand how the scientist does research.

Many pieces of equipment commonly used in physical science are shown in Figure 1.7 (pages 12-13). Study the illustrations, noting the name of each item with which you are not familiar.

### Safety—an Important Factor

When you use scientific equipment, *safety* is a very important thing to remem-

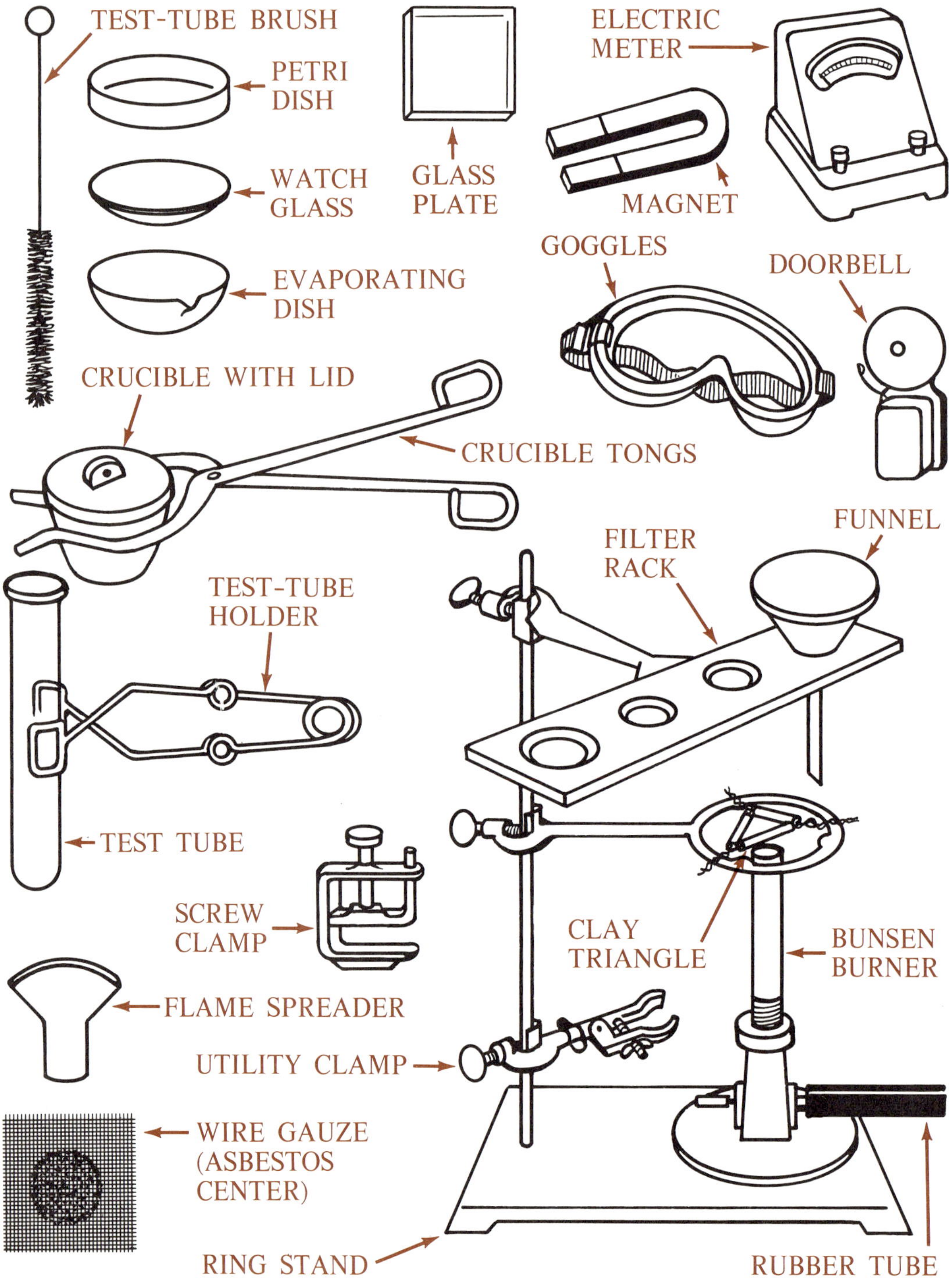


**1.7** Common laboratory equipment

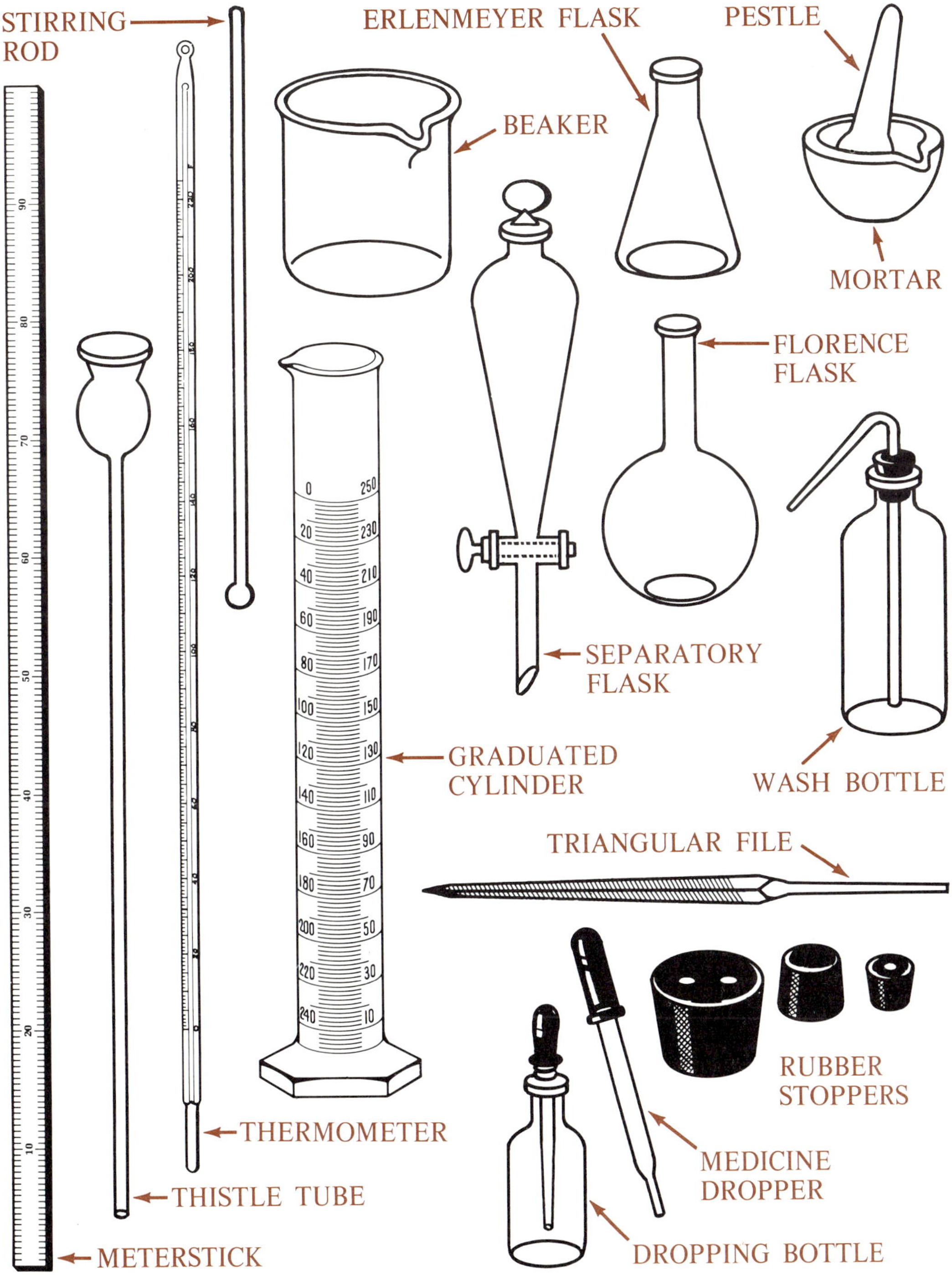

STIRRING ROD
ERLENMEYER FLASK
PESTLE
BEAKER
MORTAR
FLORENCE FLASK
SEPARATORY FLASK
GRADUATED CYLINDER
WASH BOTTLE
TRIANGULAR FILE
RUBBER STOPPERS
THERMOMETER
MEDICINE DROPPER
THISTLE TUBE
DROPPING BOTTLE
METERSTICK

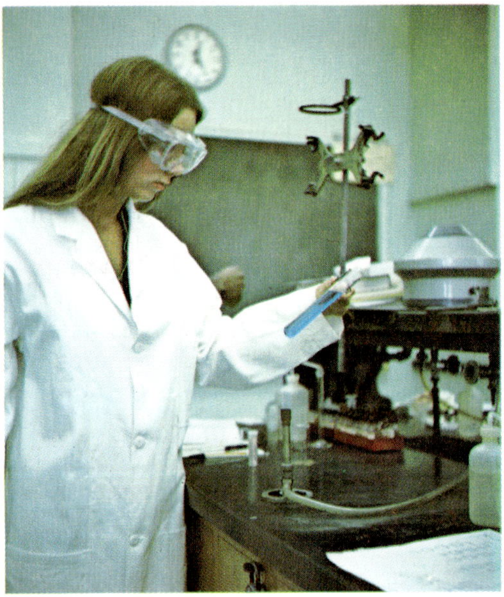

*Alan Cliburn*

**1.8** When heating a test tube, hold the top away from you.

ber. You should always follow directions carefully in order to avoid accidents. It is a good idea to wear safety goggles and a plastic apron in order to protect your eyes and clothing. In some states there are laws about safety in school laboratories.

Working in a laboratory is in many ways similar to working in a kitchen. You often need a source of heat, which is usually provided by a **Bunsen** (bun′ sən) **burner.** If natural or bottled gas is not available or if an open flame is not desirable, heat may be obtained by using an electric hot plate. As in the kitchen, you must always be careful to avoid being burned or setting your clothing on fire.

Liquids are usually heated in either a **beaker** (bēk′ ər) or a **test tube.** Beakers may be held above the flame by placing them on a **ring stand,** and a test tube may be held above the flame by use of a test-tube holder. Special precautions should always be taken in heating certain chemicals, such as alcohol, that might catch fire or explode. Remember that any piece of equipment that has been near a source of heat may be extremely hot and should not be touched until you are certain that it has cooled.

When heating a liquid in a test tube, care should be taken not to point the top of the tube toward anyone. If the liquid is heated too rapidly, bubbles may form at the bottom of the tube. When this happens, the hot liquid may be expelled from the tube with a great deal of force.

Each of the chemicals that you will want to work with has certain characteristics or **properties** (prop′ ər ti). Some of these properties make these chemicals very dangerous to work with unless you know how to handle them. Alcohol, for example, is very **flammable** (flam′ ə bəl), which means that it will catch fire very easily. Probably the alcohol that you will be working with is also poisonous and should never be tasted. Therefore, no work in chemistry should be done unless a teacher is nearby to supervise.

Many of the tools that scientists work with might be called toys, because many children play with them in one form or another. These toys include those with motors of many kinds. An electric train or racing-car set can be used to study several important scientific principles.

Electricity is an important field of physical science, and you will want to learn a great deal about it. Doorbells and all of the other electrical appliances in your home and school will provide equipment for observation and experiment. But, as you already know, electricity can be dangerous as well as interesting. No one

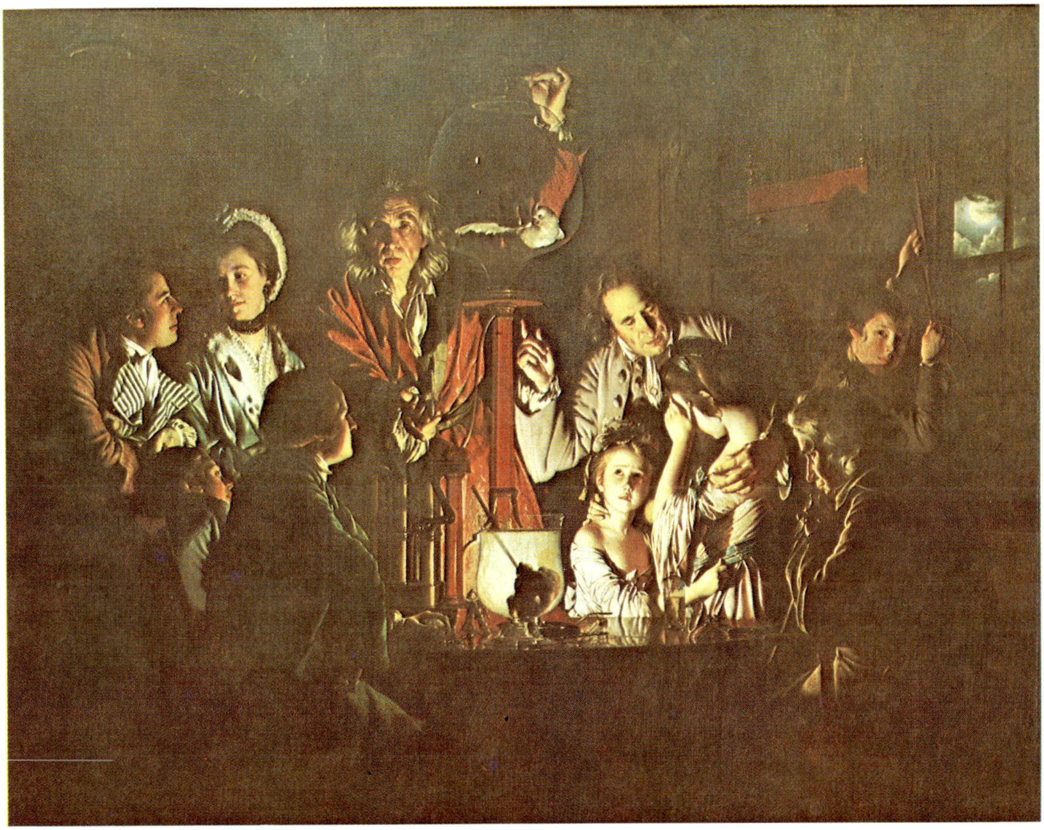

The Tate Gallery—London

**1.9** This painting, called the *Experiment with the Air Pump*, was painted in the second half of the eighteenth century. At that time there was great popular interest in science and scientific equipment. Do you recognize any of the laboratory equipment?

should attempt to work with electrical equipment unless he is certain that he understands what he is doing.

If your school does not have all of the equipment pictured in Figure 1.7 (pages 12-13), or if you wish to set up a laboratory at home and cannot afford to buy this equipment, you can often find ways to **improvise** much of it. As heat source you can use a candle, an alcohol lamp, or an electric burner. Measuring cups and spoons can be used as measuring instruments. But, when using improvised equipment even more than when using real scientific tools, safety must always be kept in mind. Be especially careful in heating or cooling glass jars and bottles. They are not made of the special glass used in chemistry glassware, such as Pyrex, and will break if rapidly heated or cooled.

Several pieces of equipment and procedures used in the laboratory are described in the Workshop at the end of this chapter.

## Have You Learned?

1. On a sheet of paper draw a picture of each of the following pieces of equipment, and explain how it is used.
   a. Bunsen burner
   b. beaker
   c. ring stand
   d. test tube
2. Explain the safety precautions that one should take in connection with the following.
   a. protection of eyes and clothing while working in the laboratory
   b. heating a liquid in a test tube
   c. heating a flammable liquid such as alcohol
   d. using improvised containers such as glass jars and bottles

## 4. Measurement—an Important Tool

**ARE YOU READY?**

Look up the following words if you are not sure of their meanings:

average; compare; convert; decimal; fraction; measurement; universal; volume.

Physical scientists use many tools to help them observe nature more carefully. A few of these tools were discussed in the last section, and many others will be described later in this book. But simply observing is not enough. Scientists must always compare their observations with those made by other scientists. Therefore, they must be able to describe *exactly* what they saw.

How would you describe the height of your best friend? A possible answer is "My best friend is about average in height." This answer does not tell us very much. Average when compared to what? To your friend's classmates? To all the boys and girls in the school? To the boys on the school basketball team?

Although the reply that your friend is about average height is not very useful, it does illustrate an important characteristic of measurement. *Measurement involves comparisons.* The length of an object may be measured by comparing its length with that of another object—a pencil, your foot, or the cover of this book. What are the disadvantages in using these objects to make the comparisons of length?

There are advantages to using **standard units** of length in making measurements. In the United States, the *inch*, *foot*, *yard*, and *mile* are common standard units used in measuring length or distance. Using these units, you might describe your best friend as being 5 feet, 2 inches tall. Since we are all familiar with the units *feet* and *inches*, we would have a better idea of

**1.10** This advertising card (on the opposite page) of an eighteenth-century London maker of scientific instruments shows a bust of Sir Isaac Newton and various instruments. How many of the instruments can you identify?

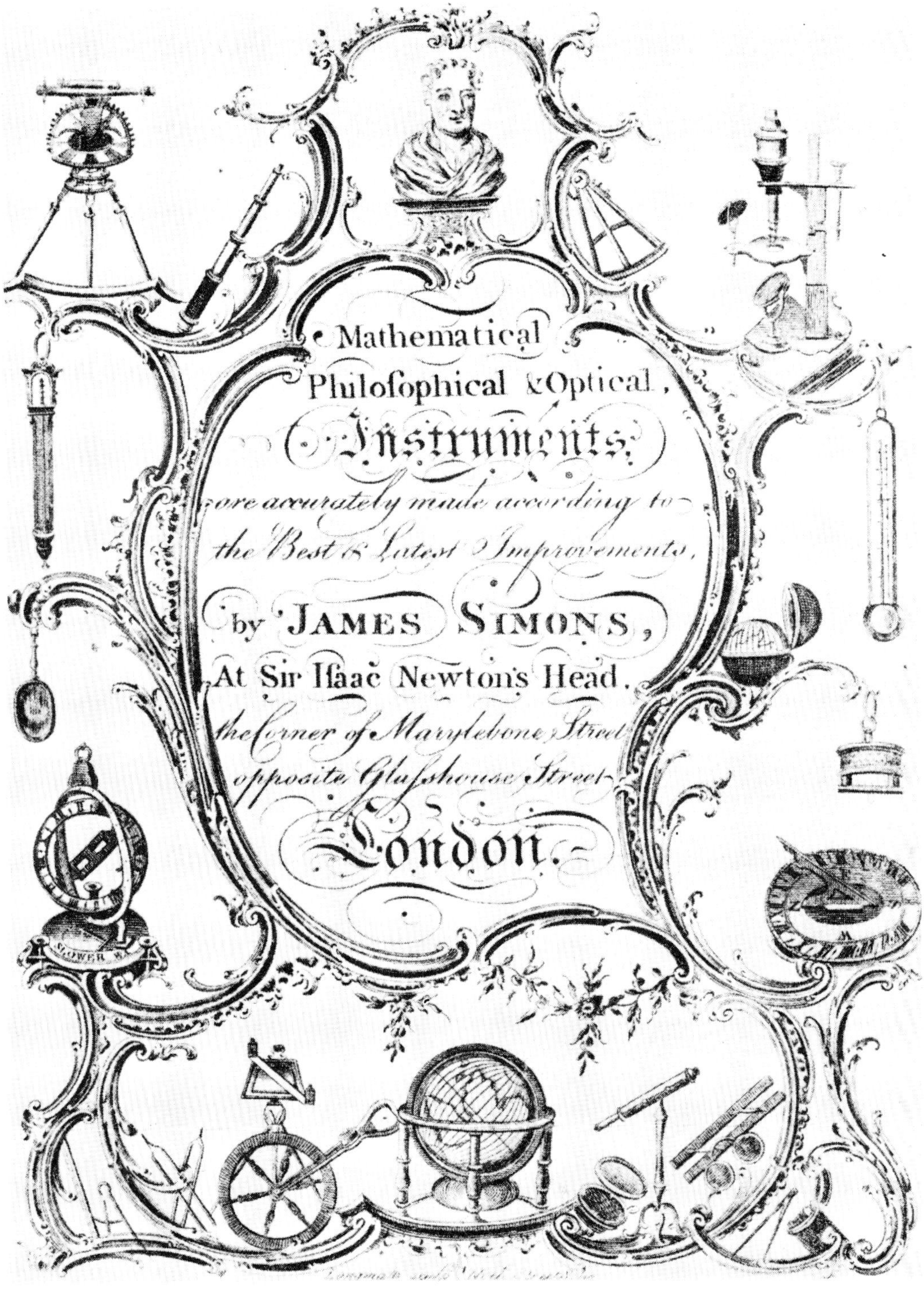
Mathematical
Philosophical & Optical,
Instruments;
are accurately made according to
the Best & Latest Improvements,
by JAMES SIMONS,
At Sir Isaac Newton's Head,
the Corner of Marylebone Street
opposite Glasshouse Street
London.

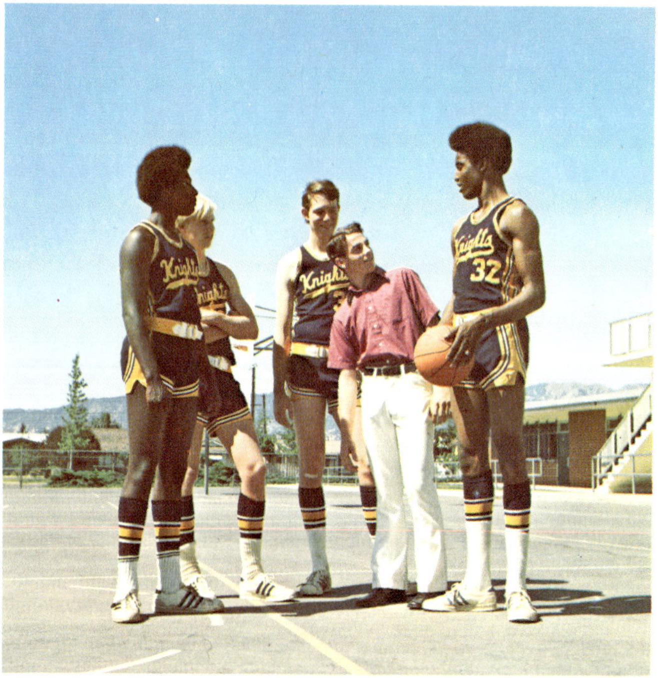


**1.11** Just what is "average" height?

*Alan Cliburn*

your friend's height than we did when the reply was "about average in height."

## The Metric System

Scientists generally use the **metric** (met′ rik) **system** in making their measurements. In addition to widespread scientific usage, this system of weights and measures is used in many foreign countries. India, China, Japan, and the U.S.S.R. have recently converted or are converting to the metric system. Even the United Kingdom, home of the English system of weights and measures that we use, has decided to make the change to the metric system.

Making measurements using the metric system is essentially the same as using our English system. The only difference is that different units are used. Distance is measured in **meters** (mē′ tər) instead of yards. Weight is measured in **grams** (gram) instead of ounces, and volume is often measured in **liters** (lē′ tər) instead of quarts.

## Measuring Length in Meters

The standard unit of length in the metric system is the meter (abbreviated m), which is 39.37 inches long. The meter is divided into smaller units, the ones most commonly used being the **centimeter** (sen′ tə mē′ tər) (cm) and the **millimeter** (mil′ ə me′ tər) (mm). The centimeter is $^{1}/_{100}$ of a meter, or about $^{2}/_{5}$ of an inch. The millimeter, which is $^{1}/_{1,000}$ of a meter, is about the thickness of 5 pages of this book.

The most commonly used unit larger than a meter is the **kilometer** (kil′ ə me′ tər) (km). Equal to 1,000 meters, the kilometer is $^{6}/_{10}$ of a mile. In countries using the metric system, the distances between cities are expressed in kilometers.

As you may have guessed, prefixes used in the metric system indicate how much smaller or larger the unit is than its basic unit, such as meter and gram. The three commonly used prefixes are *milli-* ($^{1}/_{1,000}$), *centi-* ($^{1}/_{100}$), and *kilo-* (1,000). Would you guess a *milligram* to be smaller or larger than a *gram*?

## Measuring Weight in Grams

The gram (g) is the metric unit used in measuring weight. A gram is equal to 0.035 of an ounce, or 28.35 grams equals one ounce. A dime weighs about 2.5 grams.

A gram is divided into smaller units, the most frequently used being the **milligram** (mg). The milligram is equal to $^{1}/_{1,000}$ of a gram, which is about the weight of one small grain of sand. A **kilogram** (kg) is 1,000 grams, or equal to 2.2 pounds.

## Measuring Volume Using Metric Units

As in the English System, there are two ways to express the volume of an object using metric units. Volume is often measured in *cubic* units, such as cubic inches and cubic feet. The **cubic centimeter** (abbreviated *cc* or *cm*$^{3}$), which is equal to the volume of a cube one centimeter on a side, is one of the frequently used metric

**1.12** (*Left*) The speedometers of some imported automobiles show measurements in kilometers per hour and in miles per hour. You get quite a shock when you see the needle pointing to 110. (*Right*) How far to Morristown, New Jersey? Gradually the metric system is coming into use in the United States. You will see more and more signs like this one. And further in the future you will see signs only in metric.

*Lansing Wagner*

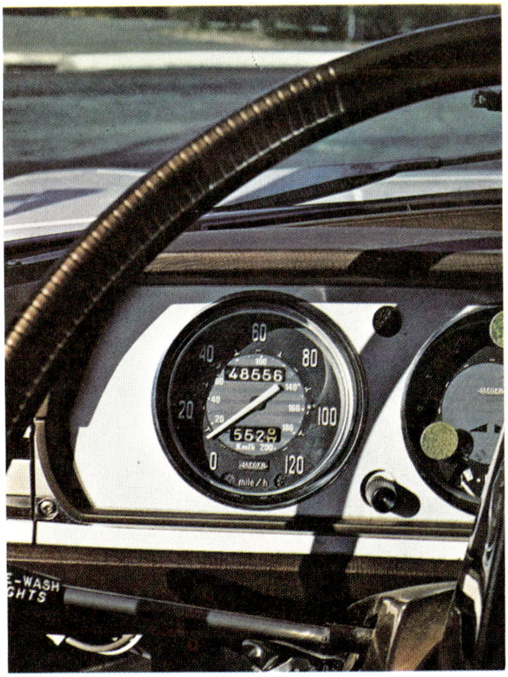


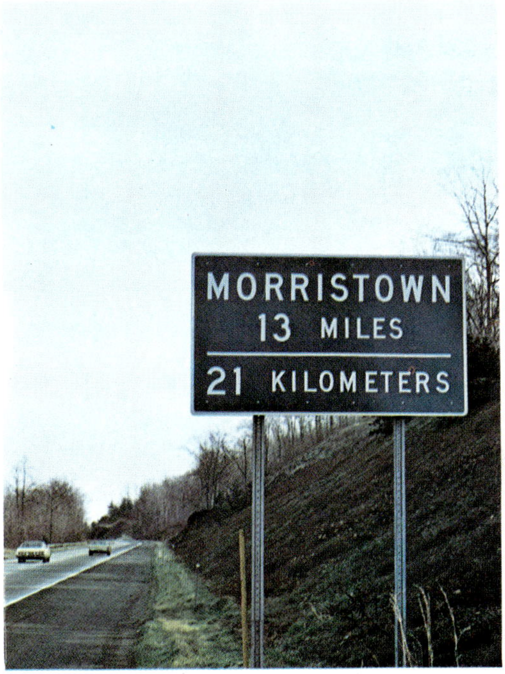

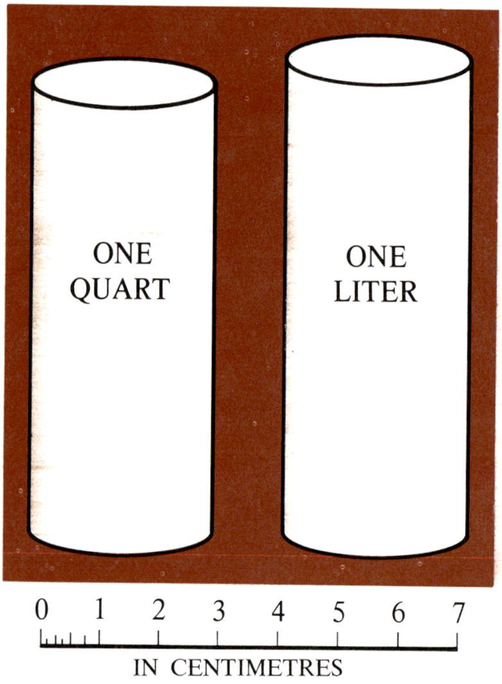


**1.13** A quart compared with a liter

units of volume. The cubic centimeter or "cc" is the unit used by physicians when giving a "shot."

In the English System, volume also is expressed in pints, quarts, and gallons. The *liter* (l), which is equal to 1.06 quarts, is the unit used in the metric system. The *milliliter* (ml), which is ${}^{1}/_{1,000}$ of a liter, is used in measuring smaller quantities. *One milliliter is equal to one cubic centimeter*, thus "cc" and "ml" are units that can be used interchangeably.

## Why Use the Metric System?

Scientists use the metric system because it has many advantages over our system of feet, pounds, and quarts. Because all metric units are related to each other by a factor of ten (ten, hundred, thousand, etc.), it is relatively easy to change a measurement from one unit to another. Measurement in the metric system involves the use of decimals. Measurements in English units often result in fractions that are difficult to work with.

### Using the Metric System

PROBLEM: Change the measurement of the width of a dollar bill from centimeters to meters and from inches to yards.

Width of Dollar Bill = 6.6 cm = $2\ {}^{19}/_{32}$ inches

Since 100 cm = 1 meter, 6.6 cm ÷ 100 = number of meters, or = .066 of a meter

Since 36 inches = 1 yard $2\ {}^{19}/_{32} \div 36$ = number of yards $= {}^{83}/_{32} \div {}^{36}/_{1} = {}^{83}/_{32} \times {}^{1}/_{36} = {}^{83}/_{1,152}$ of a yard.

Is it easier to convert centimeters to meters, or inches to yards? Which answer is easier to work with—.066 of a meter or ${}^{83}/_{1,152}$ yards?

Because of the almost universal usage of the metric system, it is easier for scientists around the world to share the results of their investigations. Can you explain why this is so? The system of weights and measures used by a country also affects its trade with other countries. Since a majority of the countries are either using the metric system or changing to it, many people think that the United States should also make the change. Legislation already has been introduced into Congress that, if passed, would result in our buying meat by the kilogram, gasoline by the liter, and cloth by the meter.

### Have You Learned?

Match up the phrase in the right-hand column that defines each of the words in the column to the left.

| | |
|---|---|
| 1. Centimeter | a. 1/1,000 of a liter |
| 2. Milligram | b. 1,000 meters |
| 3. Meter | c. 1,000 liters |
| 4. Milliliter | d. 1/100 of a meter |
| 5. Kilometer | e. 1/1,000 of a gram |
| 6. Cubic Centimeter | f. a little more than a quart |
| 7. Liter | g. 1/1,000 of a meter |
| 8. Millimeter | h. 1,000 grams |
| 9. Kiloliter | i. 100 centimeters |
| 10. Kilogram | j. equal to one milliliter |

## 5. Physical Scientists Use Mathematics

**ARE YOU READY?**

Look up the following words if you are not sure of their meanings:

abbreviate; average; data; decimal point; equation; experiment; graph; horizontal; kilogram; pendulum; plot (on a graph); predict; quantity; vertical.

Mathematics is a very useful tool for helping scientists figure out the meaning of information they have collected. For example, in the pendulum experiment you collected data on how fast it swung back and forth under certain conditions. By looking at your data you could see that shortening the string made the pendulum swing faster. But what if you wanted to figure out how long to make the string in order to have a pendulum that would swing back and forth once every 2 seconds? The easiest way would be to use mathematics.

### Using Graphs to Analyze and Predict

A student was interested in finding an easy way to predict the weight of BBs by counting them. He weighed some BBs and obtained the data in Table I.

TABLE I

| *Number of BBs* | *Weight* |
|---|---|
| 4 | 1.4 grams |
| 6 | 2.1 grams |
| 9 | 3.2 grams |
| 11 | 3.9 grams |
| 18 | 6.3 grams |
| 27 | 9.5 grams |

One way to study the relationship between two quantities, such as number of the BBs and their weight, is to draw a graph. The data in Table I are shown plotted on a graph in Figure 1.14. Notice that the bottom scale signifies the number of BBs and starts with zero at the left. The vertical scale signifies weight, and each unit represents one half a gram. In plotting a graph you have to experiment with making the scale so that all the data will fit on the graph.

To illustrate how the points are placed on the graph, look at the first pair of numbers in Table I. It shows that 4 BBs

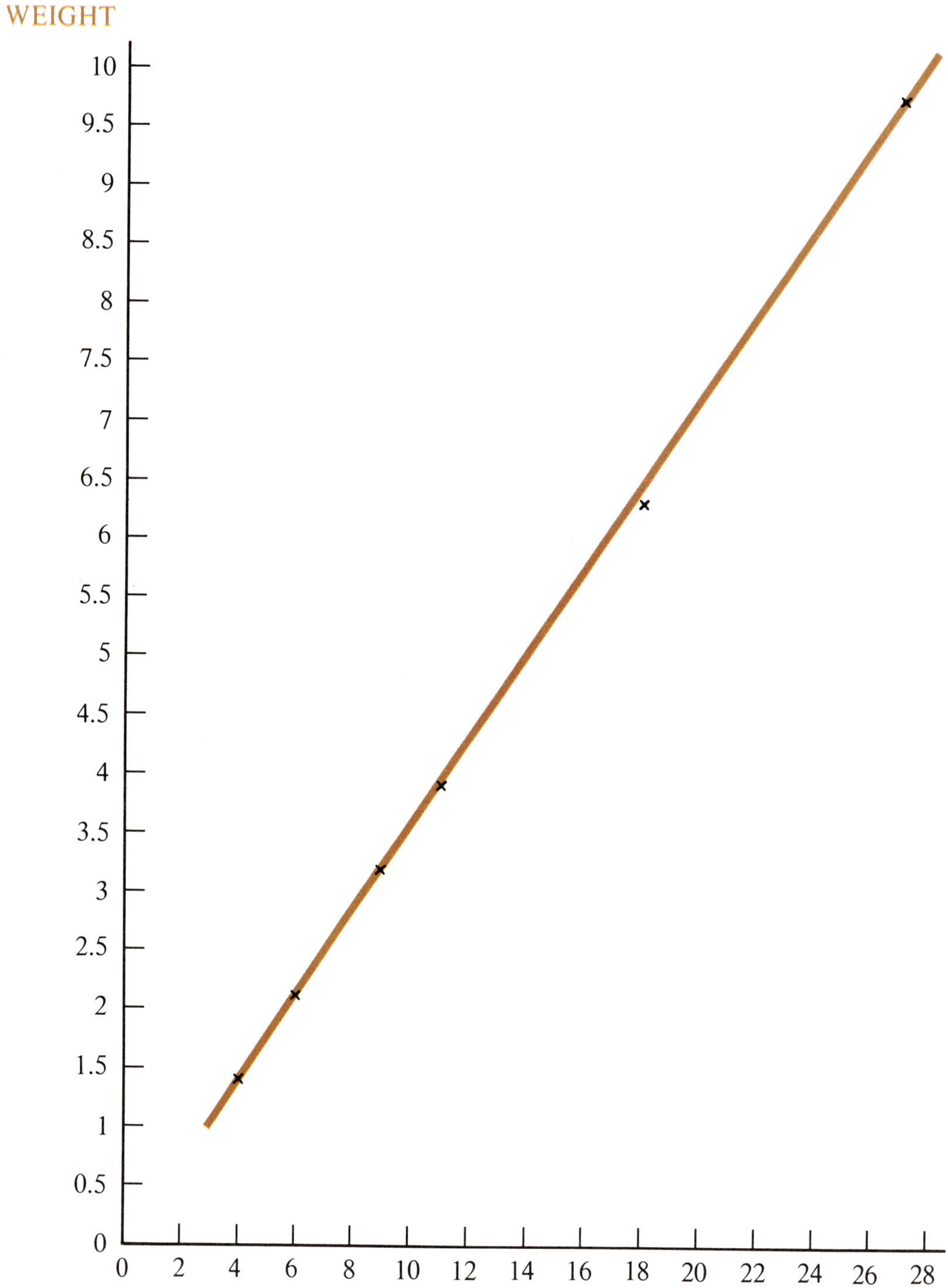


**1.14** A graph showing number of BBs versus the weight of the BBs

weighed 1.4 grams. Now look at the graph. The leftmost point on the graph is above the "4" on the bottom scale and across from "1.4" on the vertical scale. Once the points were plotted, they were connected by a line. A word of caution—not all graphs have a nice straight line like the one in Figure 1.14.

Now comes the beauty of using a graph. Look at the graph in Figure 1.14, and see if you can figure out how much 15 BBs would weigh. Go across the bottom scale to 15 and up until you reach the line. Now go straight across to the left scale where you can read weight. That's right—about 5.3 grams! Try making other predictions, say finding the weight of 1 BB, 12 BBs, and 25 BBs. Can you also predict how many BBs would weigh 1 gram? 8 grams?

However, there are some disadvantages to using a graph. It is not always convenient to carry a graph around. If you wished to predict the weight of 10,000 BBs, you would have to have a very large graph. Also if the BBs had been weighed to the nearest thousandth of a gram, it would have been difficult to show these weights accurately on a graph.

## Using Formulas to Solve Problems

One kind of **formula** (fôr′ mū lə) is a mathematical equation that tells us what to do to solve a certain problem. Take for example the problem of finding the weight of a large number of BBs. The total weight of several BBs must equal the number of BBs times the weight of one BB. Do you see why this is so?

There are several ways we can find the weight of one BB. We could weigh one BB of course. However, since BBs may vary slightly in weight, perhaps it would be better to find the average weight of all the BBs. Look at Table I again, and notice that 27 BBs weigh 9.5 grams. If we divide 9.5 grams by 27 we find that one BB weighs about 0.4 of a gram. Using data from Table I, find the average weight of a BB by dividing the other weights by the corresponding number of BBs. For example, divide 6.3 grams by 18. Can you explain why you don't get exactly the same answer for each pair of data?

In order to show how we can write a formula, let's assume that our answer of 0.4 of a gram is the correct weight of one BB. We have already said that total weight equals the weight of one BB times the number of BBs. If we let $W$ stand for total weight and $N$ stand for the number of BBs, we can write the formula in the form of an equation.

$$W = (0.4)(N) \text{ or } W = 0.4N$$

If we wish to know the weight of 10,000 BBs, we put the 10,000 in the place of the $N$ in the formula and do the multiplication to find the answer.

$$W = (0.4)(10{,}000) = 4{,}000 \text{ grams}$$

Practice using the formula to find the weight of 72 BBs; 1,500 BBs; 4,000 BBs. Can you suggest ways the formula can be improved to make the predicted weights more accurate? Can you devise a way of testing your answer?

## Writing Very Small and Very Large Numbers

Physical scientists describe large objects and distances in the universe and they also work with the smallest. In doing so they must use both very, very large numbers and very, very small numbers. To do this, they often use a system of abbreviations that saves time and makes writing the number easier.

For example, the weight of the earth is estimated to be about 6,000,000,000,000,000,000,000,000 kilograms. This figure is not only difficult to write without making a mistake, but it is almost impossible to remember. So the scientist abbreviates it as $6 \times 10^{24}$ kg., which is read "six times ten to the twenty-fourth power." It means that the number 10 is multiplied times itself 24 times, and this number is then multiplied by 6.

Table II shows the multiples of ten from 10 to one million written in this method.

**TABLE II**

| | |
|---|---|
| $10 = 10^1$ | 10 times one is 10 |
| $100 = 10^2$ | $10 \times 10$ equals 100 |
| $1,000 = 10^3$ | $10 \times 10 \times 10$ equals 1,000 |
| $10,000 = 10^4$ | $10 \times 10 \times 10 \times 10$ equals 10,000 |
| $100,000 = 10^5$ | $10 \times 10 \times 10 \times 10 \times 10$ equals 100,000 |
| $1,000,000 = 10^6$ | $10 \times 10 \times 10 \times 10 \times 10 \times 10$ equals 1,000,000 |

60,000 is equal to 6 times 10,000, so this figure would be written as $6 \times 10^4$. Can you write the following figures in abbreviated form? 200; 300; 5 million (5,000,000).

This system of abbreviation is very easy to use with large numbers because the **exponent** (eks pō′ nənt), the small number that indicates how many times the ten is multiplied by itself, shows us *directly* how far the decimal point is moved to the right. The number 6 can be written as 6.000 . . . and as many other zeros as you want, since they are to the right of the decimal point. The figure 600 is abbreviated as $6 \times 10^2$, which can be read as "six followed by two zeros." $6 \times 10^6$ is written as a six followed by 6 zeros or 6,000,000. How many zeros are there in $3 \times 10^3$? $7 \times 10^{15}$? $2 \times 10^1$? Can you write each of these numbers?

Just as these exponents show how many places to the right the decimal point is to be moved, a *negative* exponent shows how many points to the left the decimal point is moved. Since the figure 1 can be written as . . . 00001.0 with any number of zeros preceding it, the figure $10^{-1}$ indicates that the decimal is moved one place to the left. Thus, $10^{-1}$ equals 0.1. Table III shows several common small decimal numbers, from $^1/_{10}$ (0.1) to $^1/_{10,000,000}$ (0.0000001).

**TABLE III**

| |
|---|
| $0.1 = 10^{-1}$ |
| $0.01 = 10^{-2}$ |
| $0.001 = 10^{-3}$ |
| $0.0001 = 10^{-4}$ |
| $0.00001 = 10^{-5}$ |
| $0.000001 = 10^{-6}$ |
| $0.0000001 = 10^{-7}$ |

Can you write $3 \times 10^{-2}$ as a decimal

number? Your answer was correct if you wrote $3 \times 10^{-2} = 3 \times 0.01 = 0.03$. Also try $6 \times 10^{-5}$; $2 \times 10^{-8}$; $1 \times 10^{-3}$.

Table IV contains some large and small numbers used by scientists. Can you write each in the long form?

**TABLE IV**

| *Measurement* | *Number* |
|---|---|
| Speed of light | $3.0 \times 10^{10}$ centimeters per second<br>$1.86 \times 10^{5}$ miles per second |
| Distance from earth to sun | $9.3 \times 10^{7}$ miles |
| Weight of an electron | $9.1 \times 10^{-31}$ of a kilogram |
| Diameter of a bacterium | $3 \times 10^{-6}$ of a meter |

### Have You Learned?

Discuss each of the following questions briefly. Use complete sentences.

1. What are the advantages and disadvantages of using graphs?
2. How are averages found mathematically? What formula would show how to find an average of three numbers?
3. How do scientists abbreviate very large or very small numbers? What are the advantages of this method?

## 6. Tips for Studying Physical Science

**ARE YOU READY?**

Look up the following words if you are not sure of their meanings:

application; data; engineer; experiment; gem; glossary; ham radio; hypothesis; prefix; reference (book); suffix.

Just as the physical scientist uses certain approaches and instruments in studying the mysteries of nature, there are methods and aids that a student can use in learning about physical science. In science, identifying the problem to be investigated is of the utmost importance. In like manner, in studying science it is important to understand why something is being learned.

### Reasons for Studying Physical Science

1. *We live in an age of science.* Can you imagine what it would be like to live in a foreign country and not be able to speak or understand the language? Not knowing something about atomic energy, electricity, rockets, and color TV is somewhat like that. If you don't believe it, try reading a newspaper or listening to a news program on radio or TV without using your knowledge of science. A knowledge of the big ideas of science and their application is needed for understanding many of the things going on in the Space Age.

2. *Many jobs require a knowledge of science.* The number of scientists and

engineers increases each year. In fact, it is estimated that over ninety percent of the scientists who have ever lived are alive today! But perhaps more important is the fact that workers in almost every field of work use science. How many ways can you suggest that a farmer might use science? A housewife? A mechanic? A nurse? Can you name an occupation that doesn't require any knowledge of science? Debate your answer with your classmates.

3. *Studying science should help you to ask questions and to be a better thinker.* It is good that you question why you should learn about science. The questioning mind is an important characteristic of scientists. In studying science you should ask many questions. You will also learn that we don't have answers to all of the questions—at least not yet. Besides asking questions, you will get a chance to try to solve problems and to experiment to see if your hypothesis was true. This should be good preparation for solving some of the problems that you now face and will face throughout life.

4. *Hobbies and recreation often involve science.* Your great-grandparents probably didn't have as much time for hobbies and recreation as you do. Because of advances made by science and technology, we now work fewer hours per week and have more leisure time to enjoy. And science, which played a big role in making this leisure time possible, is also involved in many of our hobbies and other recreational activities. Hobbies in which scientific knowledge is used include photography, gardening, fishing, building and flying model airplanes, gem collecting, and building and operating ham radio stations.

These reasons for studying science are very general. They don't explain why a student should learn a certain piece of scientific information. Or maybe your question is why *you,* one student in millions, should know these things. These are two important points that teachers and other educators struggle with every day. And what complicates the problem is that no one knows what you will be doing, or will need to know, 20 or 30 or 40 years from now. We do know that the world is changing very rapidly, and many of the jobs of the future, say in the year A.D. 2000, don't even exist today!

## Principles, Methods, and Learning

How can schools help you get ready to live in an age that we know so little about? In answer to this key question, we think there are three important things to remember.

1. Although science is continually changing, the big ideas change more slowly than do the details or facts. One big idea is that you can't get more work out of a machine than you put in. We continue to accept this idea while we go about making all kinds of changes in the kinds of machines we use, in the way they are built, and the kinds of work they do. As another example, consider the progress that has been made since the Wright brothers flew their first airplane in December 1903. Although there have been many changes in the design of airplanes since then, the basic principles of why an airplane flies remain unchanged.

*Point:* As you learn science, ask yourself what are the big ideas involved in an experiment or phenomena? These

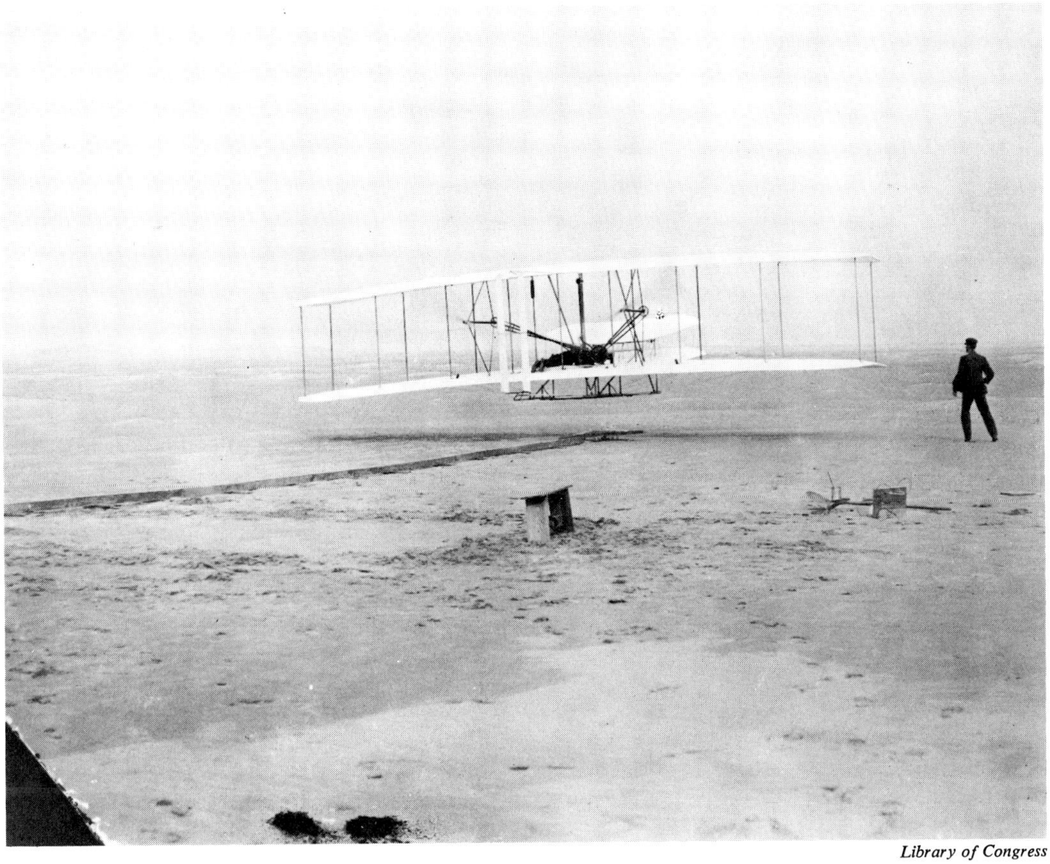

Library of Congress

**1.15** The first flight of the Wright brothers at Kitty Hawk, North Carolina, December 17, 1908

big ideas are what you will remember and find useful 20 or 30 years from now.

2. Science is defined as a *way* of searching for answers as well as a body of knowledge about the universe. It is believed that the *methods* of science and scientific attitudes are useful in solving many kinds of problems.

*Point:* Concentrate on *how* scientists know as well as on *what* they know. Also look for opportunities to use a scientific approach and scientific attitudes in your work.

3. Since we are so uncertain about the nature of the future in this rapidly changing world, the emphasis is placed on learning how to learn. It has been predicted that people in your generation will have to be trained for 3 or 4 different jobs in their lifetimes. Can you suggest a job that existed 50 years ago that no longer exists? Even if you keep the same job, advances will make it necessary for you to continue to learn if you want to keep up. Can you name a job that is done exactly the same way as it was done 50 or 100 years ago?

*Point:* Try to find ways you learn best, and work on improving your study habits. You'll be surprised how much difference a little extra effort can make.

## Learning the Language of Science

As in the case of other subjects, you will need to learn the language if you are to understand science. You have already encountered some of these words in this first chapter—*chemistry*, *meter*, *hypothesis*, *pendulum*, and *Bunsen burner*. Did you notice how these words are printed in **boldface** type the first time they are used? As you study this book, watch for the new words, and learn their meaning and their pronunciation.

If you come to a word you don't know, check the *glossary* at the back of the book. The glossary is a special dictionary of scientific words used in this book. If a word is not listed in the glossary, look up its meaning in a dictionary.

Many words used in science have built-in clues that can help you learn their meanings. If you know that *tele* means *distant* or *far off* and *scope* means to *examine* or *see*, you will realize that a **telescope** is used to see distant objects.

### Determining the Meanings of Words

Listed below are several prefixes and suffixes that are parts of words commonly used in physical science.

| *Prefixes* | *Meanings* |
|---|---|
| anti- | against |
| chromo- | color |
| bi- or di- | two |
| hydro- | water or hydrogen |
| poly- | many |
| mono- | single, one |
| micro- | small or one-millionth |
| photo- | light |
| tele- | distant, far off |
| therm- | heat |
| ultra- | more than, beyond |
| infra- | below, within |
| mega- | great, 1,000,000 |
| sub- | below, under |
| super- | above, beyond |

| *Suffixes* | *Meanings* |
|---|---|
| -lysis | loosen, come apart |
| -saccharide | sugar |
| -synthesis | a building up |
| -scope | examine, see |
| -logy | study of |
| -cide | kill |
| -gram | written, drawn |
| -meter | measure |
| -graph | drawn, recorded |
| -gen | produced |
| -mer | part |
| -plast | molded, formed |

Determine the meaning of the words in the list below. Check your accuracy by consulting the glossary or a dictionary.

microscope
polymer
insecticide
thermometer
photometer
subzero
micrometer
photosynthesis
disaccharide
electrolysis
chromoplast
geology

## Keeping Records

Scientists know the importance of keeping complete and accurate records. If they wish to figure out what happened in an experiment or to repeat it, they consult their notebooks for notes, drawings, and other data they may have recorded. Good record-keeping is an important part of their work.

It is also important to keep good records in studying physical science. Even though it may not be required, it is a good idea to keep a separate notebook, or section in your notebook, for physical science. Record the data for the investigations and experiments that you do as part of your class work. In a few cases the data you collect in an experiment may be needed in a later section of the book.

Write the answers to questions at the end of the sections and chapters in your notebook. Also include notes you make when studying a section in your textbook, or when reading about the topic in a reference book, such as an encyclopedia, or in another textbook. This information will then be easily available when it comes time to review or when you need it for some other purpose.

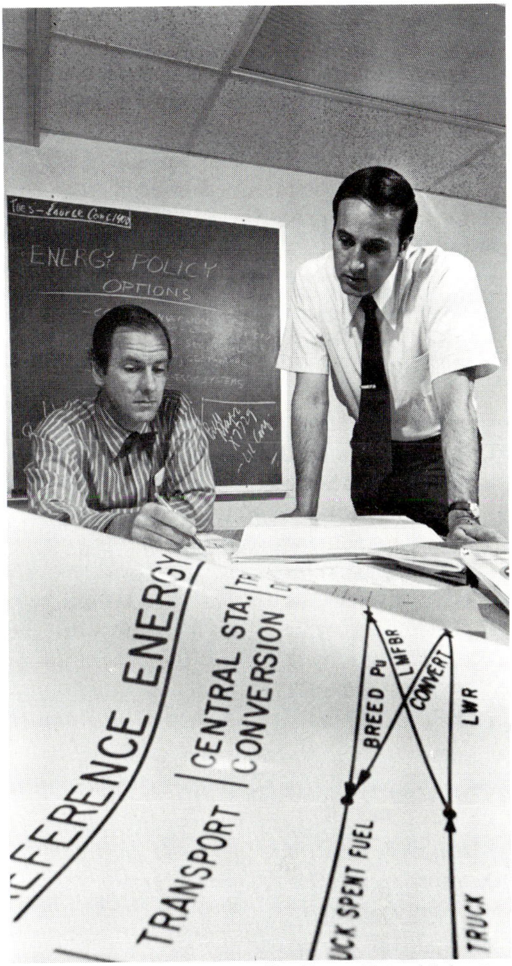


*Brookhaven National Laboratory*

**1.16** Keeping good records helps good planning.

### Have You Learned?

Match the prefixes or suffixes in the columns on the right with the correct meanings, listed on the left.

| | | | |
|---|---|---|---|
| 1. Measure | 6. Above, beyond | a. anti- | f. super- |
| 2. Below, under | 7. Written, drawn | b. hydro- | g. sub- |
| 3. Kill | 8. Water or hydrogen | c. photo- | h. -cide |
| 4. Against | 9. More than, beyond | d. therm- | i. -gram |
| 5. Heat | 10. Light | e. ultra- | j. -meter |

## REVIEW QUESTIONS

1. Define the terms *science* and *technology*. What do they have in common, and how are they different?
2. Name several branches of science, and explain what is included in each.
3. Describe the procedures generally followed by scientists in solving problems.
4. What are several important scientific attitudes?
5. Name the basic units of length, volume, and weight in the metric system. How do they compare in size with the foot, quart, and pound?
6. Explain how to draw a graph showing the relationship between the number of pennies and their total weight.
7. What are some reasons for studying physical science?
8. Give five examples of words used in science for which the meanings can be figured out by knowing the meanings of prefixes and suffixes.

## CAN YOU FIND OUT?

*It may be necessary to use an encyclopedia or other reference book in answering the following questions.*

1. What is the difference between the sciences of physics and chemistry?
2. How do scientists use the developments of the science of electronics to study the migration of birds and of fish?
3. How is a pendulum in a clock adjusted in order to speed up or slow down the clock?
4. What is the difference between test tubes made of Pyrex and those made of ordinary glass?
5. Why does a cold drinking-glass often break when boiling water is poured into it?
6. How were the units of the English System of measurement, such as the foot, yard, rod, etc., first developed?
7. What are the *disadvantages* of having the U. S. change to the metric system of measurement?
8. What are the different shapes used for graphs, other than the one shown in Section 5? What are the advantages and disadvantages of each?
9. From what languages did each of the prefixes and suffixes listed on page 28 come?
10. Many predictions have been made about how we will live during the twenty-first century. Can you find one of these predictions and write a report about it?

## REFERENCES FOR ADDITIONAL STUDY

BLACK PIONEERS AND INVENTION by Louis Haber. Harcourt Brace Jovanovich, Inc.
Contains short biographical sketches of fourteen black American scientists, engineers, and inventors

BUILD-IT-YOURSELF SCIENCE LABORATORY by Raymond Barrett. Doubleday & Company, Inc.
Tells how a laboratory can be set up at home or in a school that does not have a regular science laboratory

CHANGING TOOLS OF SCIENCE: FROM YARDSTICK TO CYCLOTRON (Revised Edition) by Irving Adler.
The John Day Company, Inc.
Describes many modern science tools

DISCOVERING SCIENTIFIC METHOD by Hy Ruchlis. Harper & Row, Publishers.
Describes the methods of science with many examples of how scientists use these methods

THE ENCYCLOPEDIA OF CAREERS AND VOCATIONAL GUIDANCE (Volume I: Planning Your Career; Volume II: Careers and Occupations), William Hopke (Editor-in-Chief). J. G. Ferguson
Probably the best reference on choosing a career and the various aspects of hundreds of different kinds of jobs, including many in science and technology

MR. WIZARD'S SCIENCE SECRETS (Second Edition) by Don Hurbet. Hawthorn Books, Inc.
A collection of over 150 experiments done at home using simple equipment

SCIENCE AND SERENDIPITY: GREAT DISCOVERIES BY ACCIDENT by D. S. Halacy, Jr. Macrae Smith Co.
Describes 11 examples of chance discoveries, such as Goodyear's discovery of how to vulcanize rubber, and the background of each of these discoveries

THE SCIENTIST by Henry Margeneau and the Editors of Time-Life Books, A Division of Time Inc.
Describes with essays and color photographs the work of the scientist

THINK METRIC by Franklin M. Branley. Thomas Y. Crowell Company.
Deals with the history of measurement, metric conversions, and activities helpful in learning how to use the metric system

# *Workshop... Unit I*

Directions for using several pieces of common laboratory equipment are given in this section. Procedures frequently used in the laboratory also are described. You may need to practice using some of these procedures now. Also refer to this section when doing experiments in the following chapters.

**Lighting a Bunsen Burner.** Connect the hose of the burner to a gas supply. Open the valve on the gas supply part of the way and hold a lighted match to the edge of the top of the burner. (See Figure W1.1.)

The size of the flame can be changed by opening and closing the valve on the gas supply. A yellow flame indicates that more air is needed, and the burner tube can be turned to accomplish this. If the flame goes out, the air supply should be reduced by turning the burner tube in the opposite direction. The hottest part of the flame is just above the tip of the inner cone of the flame.

**Cutting Glass Tubing and Rods.** Short pieces of glass tubing and rods are often needed in science experiments. To cut a piece of glass tubing, lay it on a table. Make a scratch by drawing the edge of a triangular file across the tubing where you want the cut to be. Hold the tubing as shown in Figure W1.2 with your thumbs opposite the scratch. Press your thumbs against the glass tubing and pull outward at the same time. If the tubing does not

**W1.1** Be careful how you light your Bunsen burner.

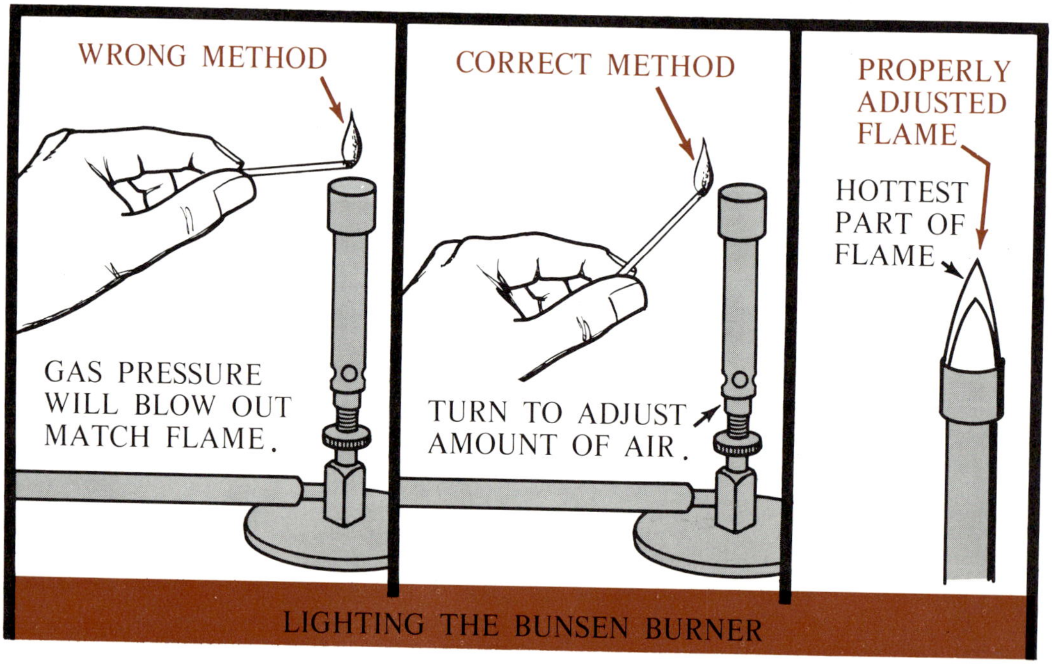

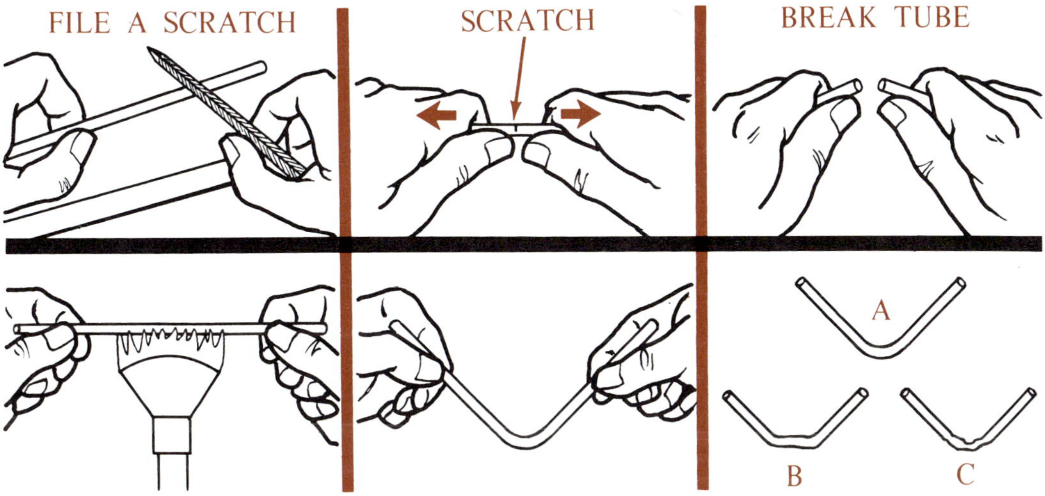


**W1.2** Cutting or bending glass tubing is easy—but be careful!

break easily, make the scratch deeper with the edge of the file.

For safety, wrap the tubing in a towel when you break it, making sure your thumbs are exactly opposite the scratch.

**Bending Glass Tubing.** Place a *flame spreader*, often called a *wing top*, on the burner. Place the tubing in the flame and slowly turn it until it becomes soft. (See Figure W1.2.) Remove the tubing from the flame and bend it by raising the ends as shown in the diagram. After the glass has hardened, lay the bent tubing on something to cool.

*A* in Figure W1.2 illustrates a good bend. It has a gradual bend and will allow gases or liquids to pass through it easily. *B* is the result of holding the tubing too low in the flame. *C* is what happens when a flame spreader is not used or not enough of the glass is heated. Practice bending tubing until you can make bends like *A* in Figure W1.2.

**Polishing the Ends of Glass Tubing and Rods.** The ends of glass tubing or rods have sharp edges. These edges can be made smooth by *fire-polishing* the ends in a flame. Slowly rotate the end of the tube or rod in the flame. If a piece of tubing is left in the flame too long, the ends will be sealed. It is always a good idea to lay hot glass on a piece of asbestos or wire gauze while it cools. This will prevent damage to the tabletop and serves as a reminder that the glass is hot! (Figure W1.3)

**Placing Glass Tubing in a Stopper.** This can be a very dangerous procedure if you are not careful. Check the size of the holes

**W1.3** Polishing glass tubing

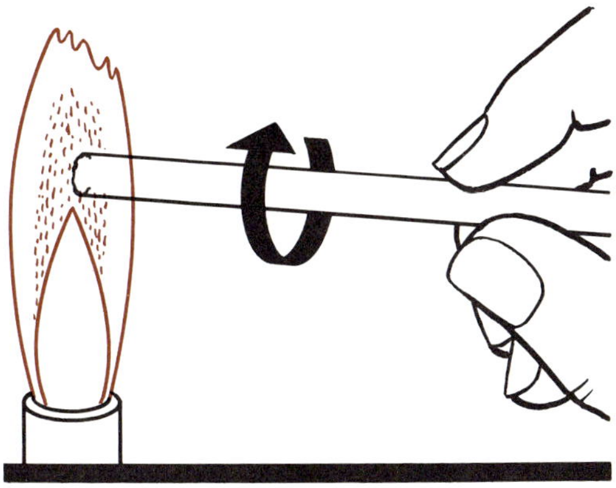

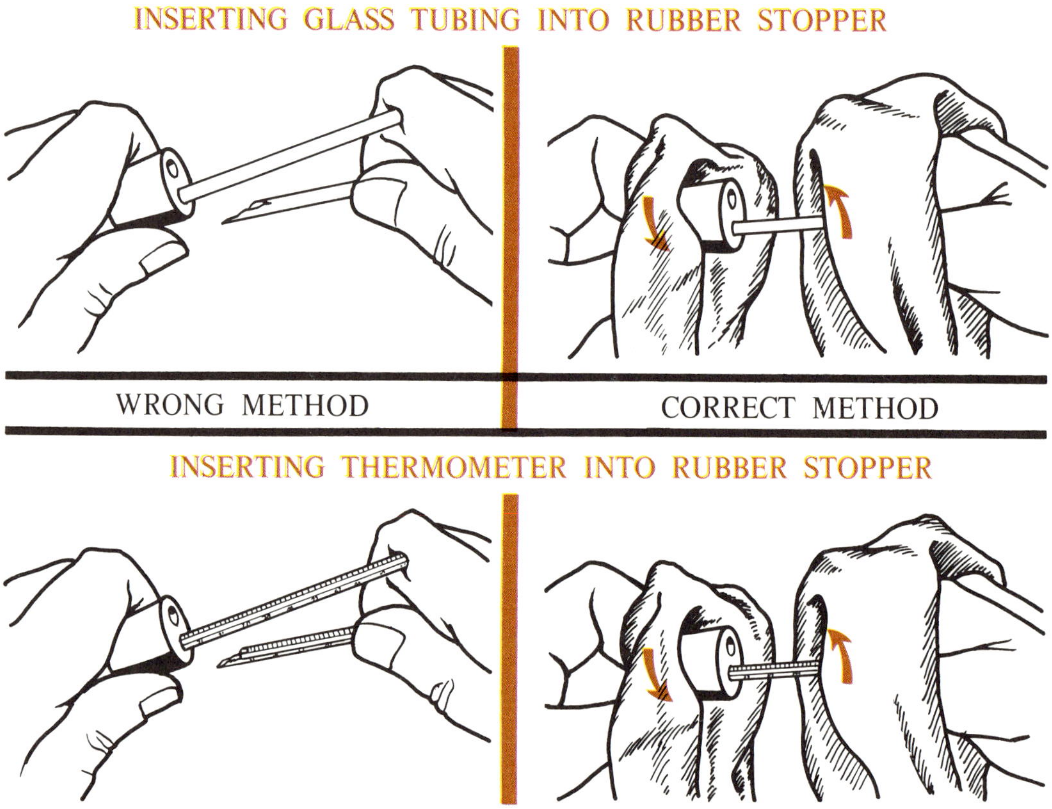


**W1.4** Make sure you know the correct way of putting glass tubing or a thermometer into a rubber stopper. Work with your two hands very close together. Take time to study these diagrams.

in the rubber stopper to see if they are just a little smaller than the glass tubing. The rubber stopper should stretch just enough to hold the tubing firmly. If the holes in the rubber stopper are too small, select a stopper with larger holes.

Place a drop of glycerine or some water on the end of the glass tubing. This will help make the tubing go through the stopper more easily. Wrap the glass tubing and the stopper in a towel. Then push the tubing through the stopper by using a gentle force and a twisting motion (Figure W1.4).

**Caution: Your hands should not be more than a centimeter apart. Never hold the tubing or stopper in such a way that the end of the tubing is pointed toward or pushing against the palm of your hand. If the tubing breaks, it may be rammed into your palm if it is held this way.**

This procedure also is used in inserting thermometers in rubber stoppers, and equal caution should be taken.

**Weighing with a Balance.** The two kinds of balances most frequently used in the laboratory are shown in Figure W1.5. The balance at the right in Figure W1.5 is called a *double platform balance*; the other is a *triple beam balance*.

To weigh an object on the double platform balance, the object is placed on the left platform. Weights are then placed on the right platform to balance the weight of the object. The rider on the front of the balance is used to add the small amount of weight needed to make the indicator point toward zero on the scale. Rather than waiting for the balance to stop swinging to see if the indicator is on zero, watch to see if it moves to either side of zero the same distance. This will save time in weighing things. The weight of the object is found by adding the weights on the right platform and the weight indicated by the rider.

In the case of the triple beam balance, the three riders are moved until the indicator points to zero on the scale or swings to either side of zero an equal distance. The rider that represents the heaviest weight is moved first (the middle one on the balance in the diagram). The candle in the diagram weighs more than 30 grams but less than 40 grams. The rider on the middle beam that is marked off in 10-gram intervals is placed on 30. The back rider is moved next. The candle weighs more than 35 grams and less than 36 grams. The back rider is placed on 5. The front rider is moved last, and the candle is found to weigh 35.30 (30 + 5 + .30) grams.

**Filtering.** Figure W1.6 shows how filter paper is folded to make a cone that will fit in a funnel. The cone is formed by separating three of the thicknesses of the paper from the fourth after the paper has been folded in quarters. Press the cone of

**W1.5** With a little practice, you will quickly learn how to use these balances.

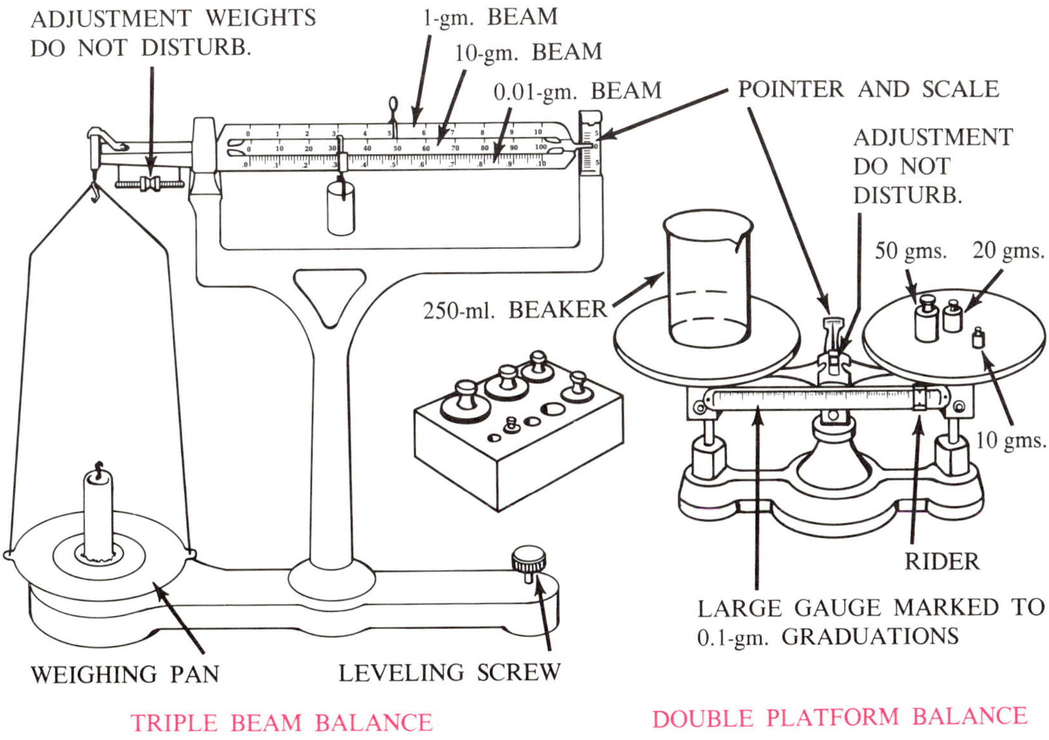

**W1.6** Folding filter paper and pouring

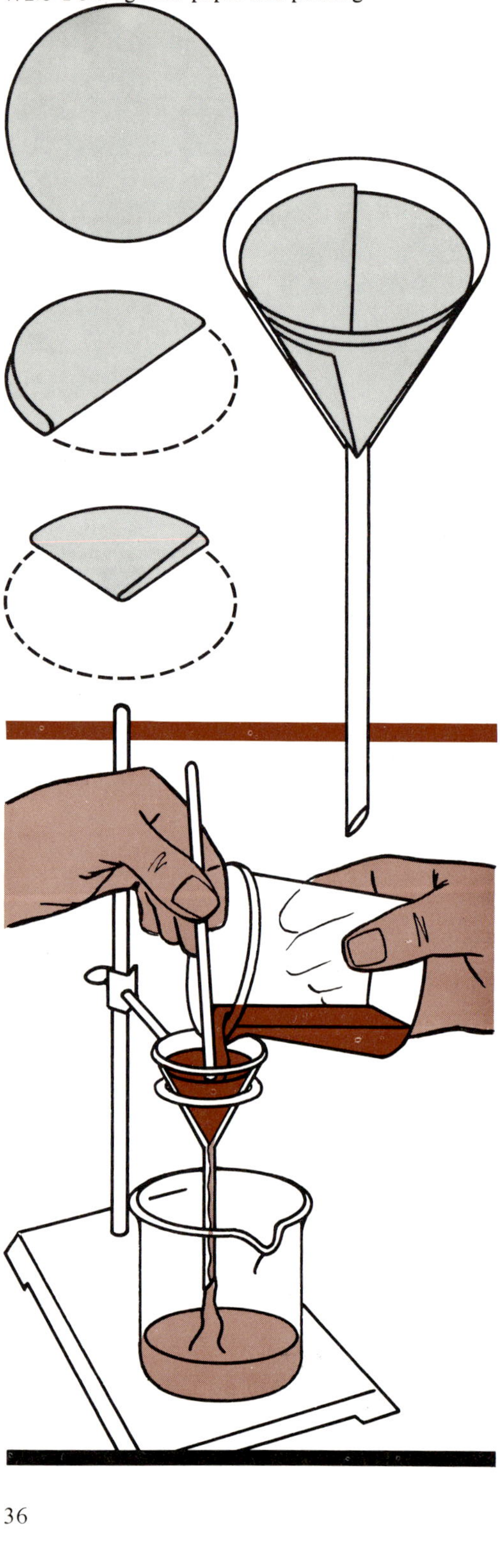

filter paper against the funnel, and wet it so that it keeps the shape of the funnel. Figure W1.6 shows how a glass stirring rod can be used in pouring liquids. The liquid will probably filter faster if the stem of the funnel is against the side of the beaker as shown.

**Smelling Chemicals.** Figure W1.7 shows the correct way to smell a substance. *Do not* place your nose directly over the container. *Do not* inhale deeply as some odors are very unpleasant—you need only a sniff for most observations.

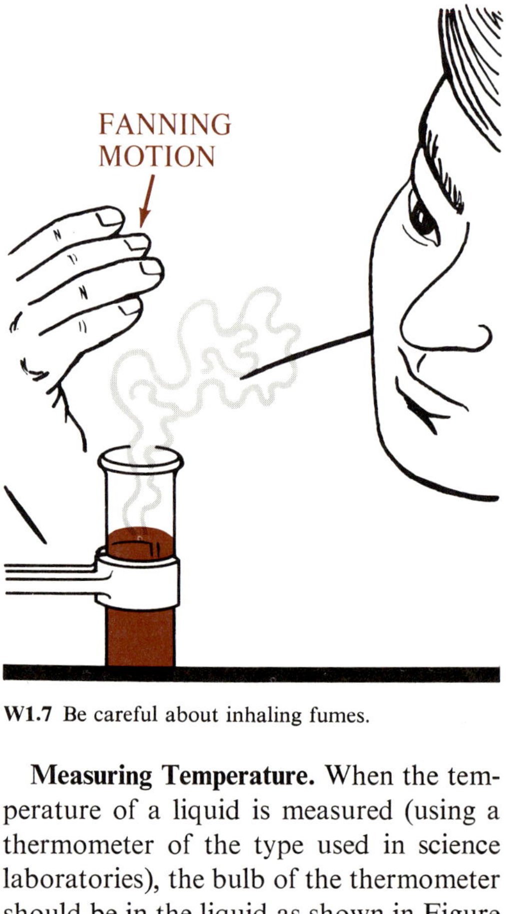


**W1.7** Be careful about inhaling fumes.

**Measuring Temperature.** When the temperature of a liquid is measured (using a thermometer of the type used in science laboratories), the bulb of the thermometer should be in the liquid as shown in Figure W1.8. When the thermometer is removed

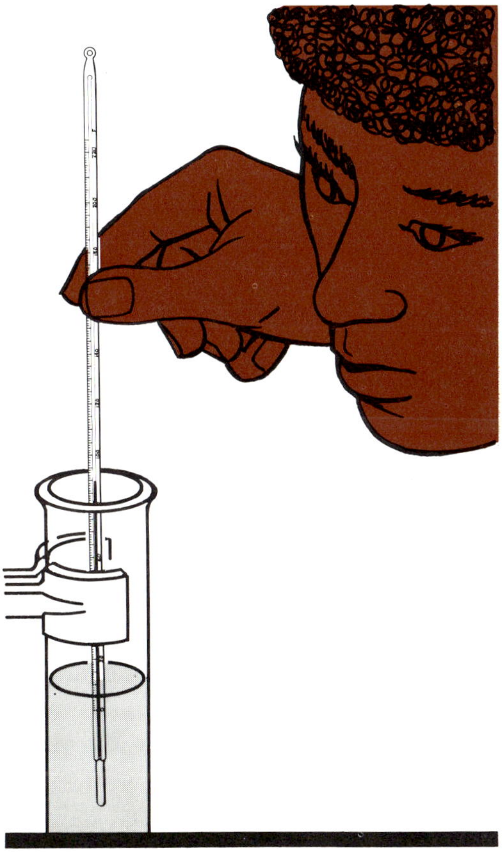

**W1.8** Read the temperature with bulb in liquid.

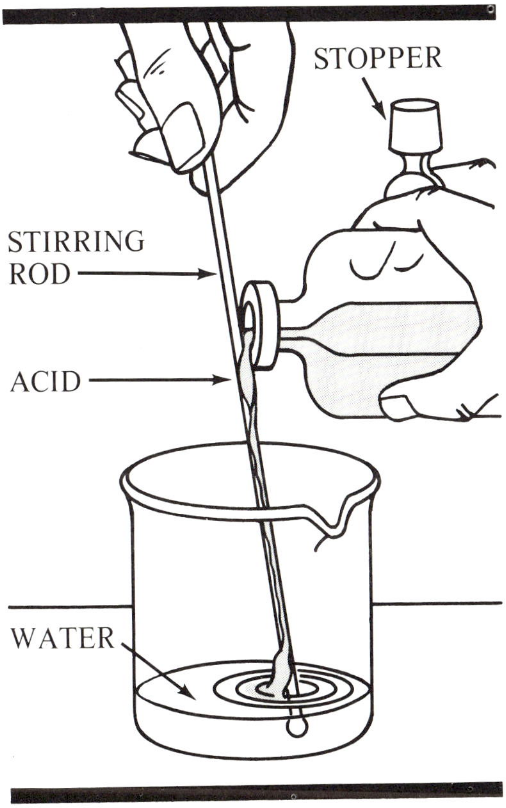


**W1.9** Follow this method for diluting an acid.

from the liquid, the column of mercury or alcohol in the thermometer soon shows the temperature of the air. Thermometers used to measure the body temperature of humans are of a different type and can be removed without affecting the temperature they indicate.

**Diluting Acids.** Solutions are diluted by mixing them with water. When you wish to dilute an acid, it should be done as shown in Figure W1.9. *The acid is added to the water*, and never the other way around. The acid should be *slowly* poured down the stirring rod and the solution continually stirred. When acids are added to water, heat is produced and this is why it is important to add the acid slowly and to stir the solution.

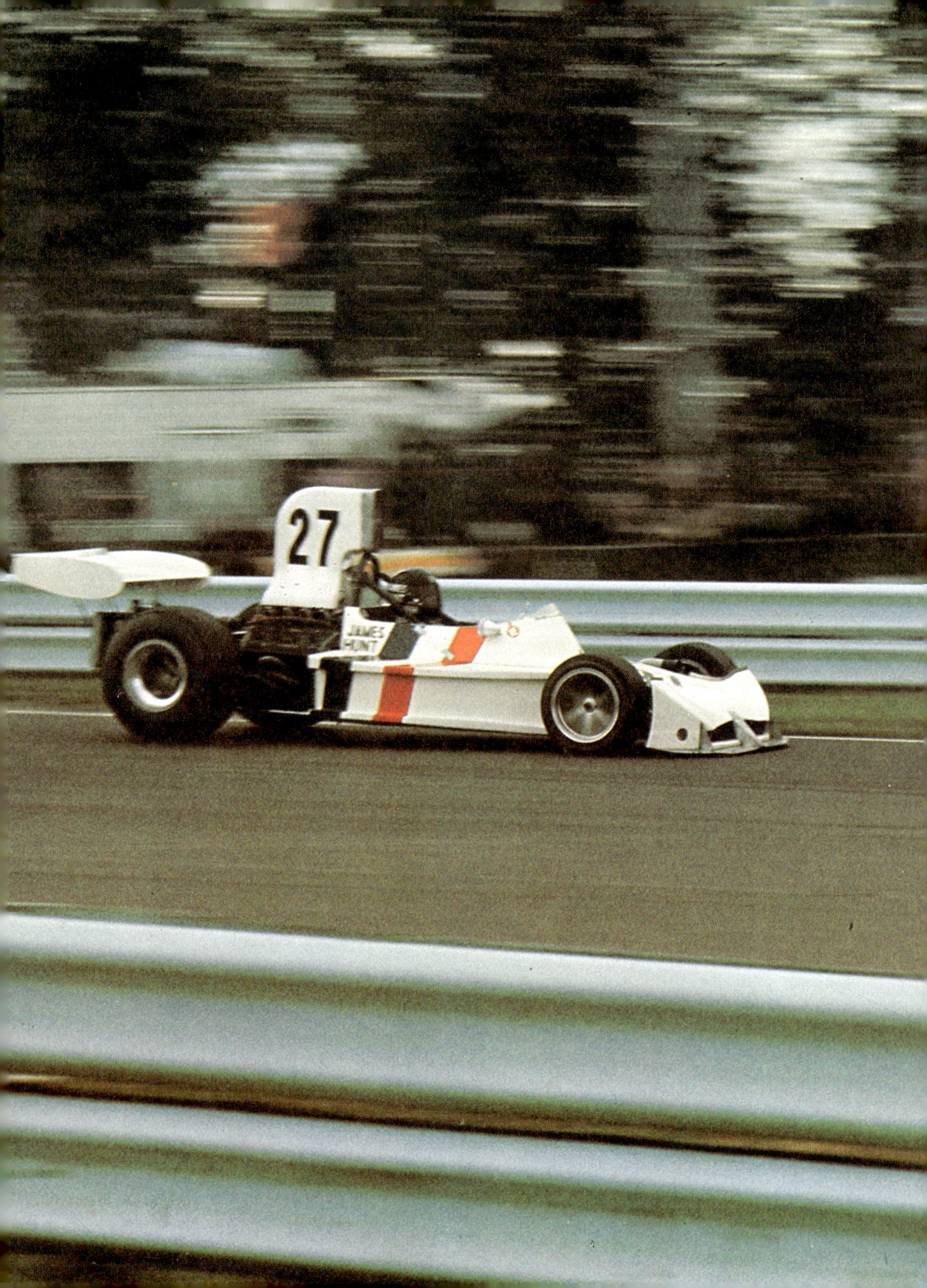
27
JAMES
HUNT

# *unit II*

# *matter, molecules, and motion*

*Olivier Rebbot/Stock, Boston*

CHAPTER 2

# Matter and Energy

EARLY PEOPLE DISCOVER FIRE, and science begins. The study of falling rain, of flying through the air or in outer space, and of exploring the oceans—all these are the jobs of the physical scientist.

The entire universe is the laboratory of the physical scientist. What is the universe made of? How does it behave? What makes it move?

## 1. What Is the Universe Made of?

**ARE YOU READY?**

Look up the following words if you are not sure of their meanings:

characteristic; comparison; kilogram; liquid; quantity; solid; standard; weight.

Look around you. Everything that you see is called **matter** by the scientist. Your pencil, a glass of water, a rock—all these objects are examples of matter. All these bits of matter have two *characteristics* in common. The most apparent of these characteristics is *weight.*

It is not difficult to see that solids such as rocks, and liquids such as water, have weight. But what about gases such as air? Do gases have weight? This question can be answered by doing an experiment.

### Determining if Air Has Weight

If your school has a balance that can be used to weigh very light objects, the only other equipment you will need is a toy balloon.

First weigh the balloon empty and record the weight. Next blow the balloon up and tie the open end. Weigh the inflated balloon, and record the weight. Does the inflated balloon weigh more than the balloon before it was blown up? How do you explain what you found out?

You may wish to repeat the experiment using a football or other object that you can inflate. Do your conclusions agree with those obtained using the balloon?

A second characteristic of matter is that it takes up space. That is, each bit of matter occupies a certain amount of the universe, and no other bit of matter can occupy the same space at the same time.

## Investigating Matter in Space

**MATERIALS:**

A pencil, a glass of water, a large container of water such as a small aquarium, a handkerchief or similar piece of cloth

**PROCEDURE:**

First, look at the pencil. Feel it. Tap it on the table. Does it take up space? Can any other piece of matter occupy the same space at the same time?

Now look carefully at the water in the glass. Does the water occupy the space inside the glass? Place the pencil in the glass. Does the level of the water rise slightly as the pencil is placed in the water? Can you explain this observation?

Pour the water from the glass and dry the glass with a towel. Look carefully at the glass. Is it empty or is it full of matter? Place the handkerchief in the glass so that it will not fall out when the glass is turned upside down. Slowly push the glass, open mouth down, into the large container of water, as shown in Figure 2.1. Slowly remove the glass from the water, being careful to keep the mouth pointed down. The handkerchief should be completely dry. Can you explain why? What type of matter occupied the space inside the glass and kept the water out? Did the water go up into the glass a little distance? How can this be explained?

In summary, all matter has weight and occupies space. We have also seen that two bits of matter cannot occupy the same space at the same time.

**2.1** Why doesn't the handkerchief inside the glass get wet?

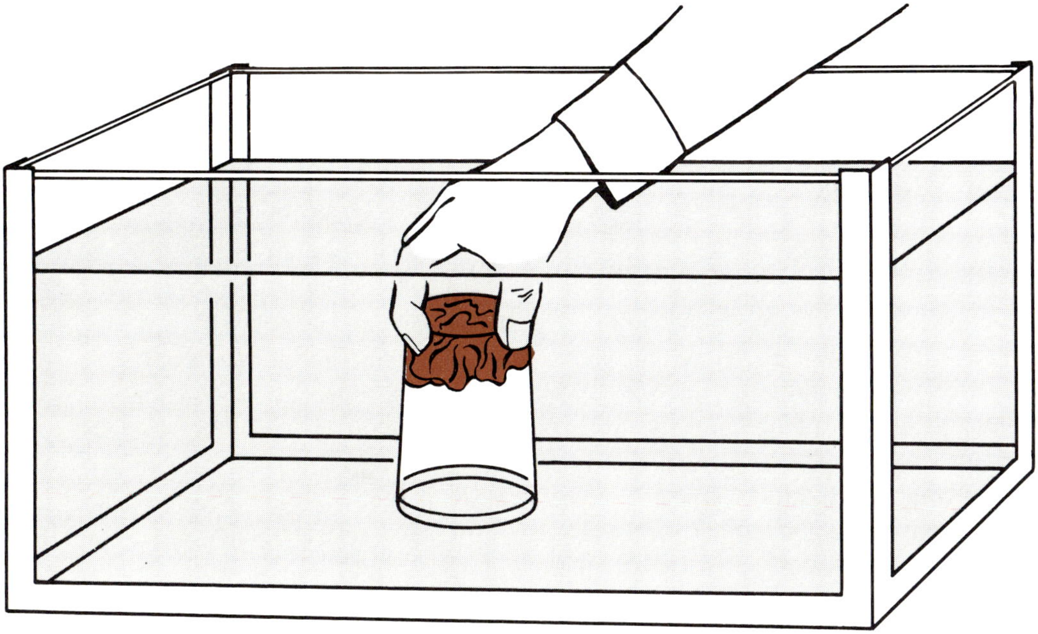

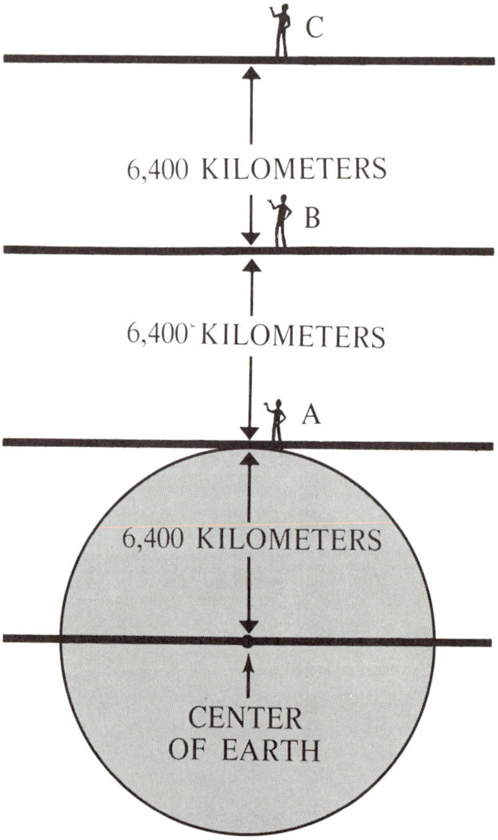


**2.2** The weight of an object on earth changes with its distance from the center of the earth.

## Why Not Use Weight to Measure the Amount of Matter?

You probably already know that some objects contain more matter than do other objects. How can we measure the amount of matter contained in an object? A single large pencil may contain more matter than several small ones. Therefore counting the number of objects that you have is not a good measure of the amount of matter. But then, size alone is not a good indicator of the amount of matter in an object either. A cubic centimeter of iron contains more matter than a cubic centimeter of wood. Also, a certain quantity of matter may increase in size with an increase in temperature. But the amount of matter present in the object remains the same.

During the seventeenth century, Sir Isaac Newton, an English physical scientist, suggested that every bit of matter attracts every other bit of matter. He also believed that the greater the amount of matter in the objects, the greater is the attraction between them.

According to this idea there is a **gravitational** (grav′ ə tā′ shən əl) **attraction** between the earth and every other object in the universe. We can measure this force or pull, which we call **weight.** An object that contains more matter will weigh more than an object that has less matter in it. The attraction between the earth and a boy weighing 80 kilograms is twice as strong as the attraction between the earth and a boy who weighs 40 kilograms. The reason for this is that the larger boy contains twice as much matter as the smaller boy.

We also know that the weight of an object varies with its distance away from other bodies of matter. Thus, you weigh a little less on top of a mountain than you do when you are standing at sea level, because you are father away from the center of the earth when you are on top of the mountain. At sea level, you are about 6,400 kilometers from the center of the earth. If you moved 6,400 kilometers out into space, you would weigh only ¼ as much as you do at sea level (Figure 2.2).

In other words, if you double the distance between two attracting bodies, you decrease the gravitational pull between them to one-fourth. If you were to move

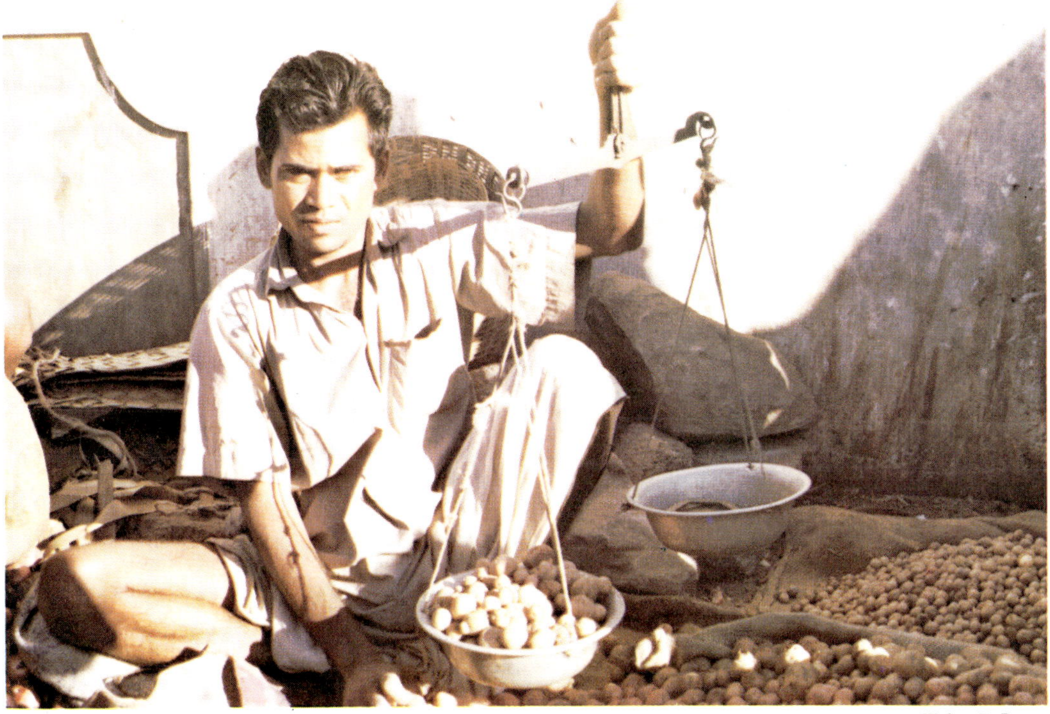

*Walter R. Brown*

**2.3** A vendor in India weighs potatoes by comparing their mass with a known mass, which is in the other pan of the balance.

another 6,400 kilometers out into space, you would be three times farther away from the center of the earth than you were when you were at sea level. At this point, the pull of gravity would be only $^1/_9$ as great.

Can you see the pattern in the way in which the gravitational attraction between two bodies decreases as the distance between them increases? If you weight 50 kilograms at sea level (6,400 kilometers from the center of the earth), how much will you weigh 19,200 kilometers above the earth (25,600 kilometers from the center of the earth)? At 25,600 kilometers out in space?

Since the moon contains considerably less matter than the earth, you would weight only about $^1/_6$ as much there as you do on earth. But whether you are at sea level on the earth, or on a high mountain, or on the moon, you still contain the same amount of matter. So weight, while it depends upon the amount of matter in an object, varies with the location of the object and is therefore not a very satisfactory measure of the amount of matter.

## Mass of an Object

Because of the difficulty in using weight to describe the amount of matter in an object, scientists talk instead about the **mass** (mas) of an object. The quantity or amount of matter in an object is known as its mass, and the mass of an object is always the same, regardless of the location or position of the body.

One way to measure the mass of an object is simply to compare the pull of gravity on the object with the pull of gravity of another object of known mass. Perhaps you remember from Chapter 1 that measurement always involves comparing something with a *standard.*

The man in the photograph on page 43 is using a balance to compare the mass of vegetables with a standard mass. The standard normally used to calculate mass is the kilogram. By balancing the vegetables with pieces of metal of known masses, this man calculates the mass of the vegetables. He would probably tell you that the vegetables *weigh* "so many kilograms," but what he has actually calculated is the mass.

### Have You Learned?

On a sheet of paper list the numbers for the questions below. By each number write *T* if the statement is true and *F* if false.

1. Everything in the universe is made of matter.
2. Liquids and gases can occupy the same space at the same time.
3. All forms of matter have weight.
4. The size of an object is a measure of the amount of matter in it.
5. The weight of a piece of iron always remains the same, regardless of its location.
6. If you were on the moon, you would have the same mass as you did on earth.
7. A pan balance will always give the same results, regardless of its location.
8. Weight is the same as mass.
9. Weight is caused by the gravitational attraction between two bodies.
10. Mass is caused by the gravitational attraction between two bodies.

## 2. Physical Properties of Matter

**ARE YOU READY?**

Look up the following words if you are not sure of their meanings:

chemical change; container; evaporate; hypothesis; mass; matter; pores (in your skin); property; volume.

We use two characteristics in deciding whether or not something is matter. In addition to taking up space and having weight or mass, matter has several other characteristics that can be easily observed. Characteristics of a piece of matter that do not involve chemical changes are called **physical properties.** Several physical properties of matter are discussed in this section.

### Three States of Matter

A pencil, a glass of water, and some air represent the three forms or **states of matter.** Your pencil is an example of matter in its **solid** state. It has a definite shape and a definite volume. A solid piece of matter does not need support to help hold its shape. If it is placed in a container, a solid will retain its original shape regardless of the shape of the container.

Water is a **liquid.** The following activity shows the properties of a liquid.

## Checking the Properties of Liquid Matter

**MATERIALS:**

A liter jar completely full of water, several other containers of various sizes and shapes

**PROCEDURE:**

Note the shape of the water in the liter jar. Pour the water into one of the other containers. Did the water take on a different shape? Repeat with each of the other containers and note the shape of the water in each. Now carefully pour the water back into the liter jar. What is the volume of the water? Did it change?

**2.4** A liquid takes the shape of its container, and it has a definite volume.

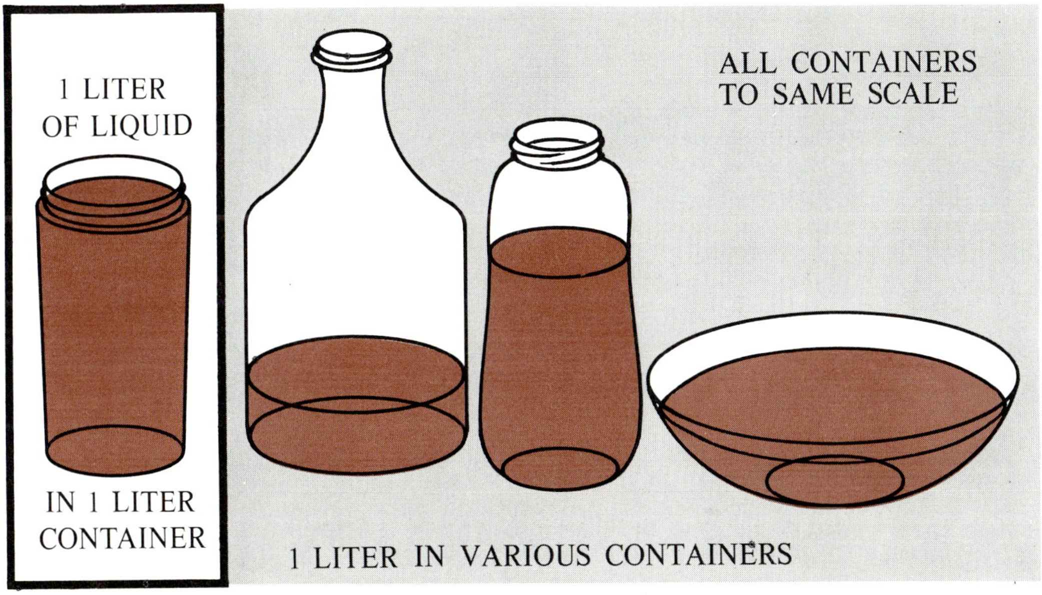


Liquids, like solids, always fill a definite amount of space. That is, their volume remains the same. If you did not spill any of the water while doing the above activity, the volume of the water remained one liter. If you pour the liter of water in a 4-liter jar, only part of the jar is filled. But, unlike a solid, the liquid assumed the shape of the container into which it was put.

**Gas** is the third form that matter can exist in. If you break a bottle of perfume in one corner of the room, it evaporates, and you can soon smell it in any part of the room. This indicates that the gas has completely filled the space. Thus, we can say that gases have neither definite shapes nor definite volumes.

### Two Objects in the Space of One

But, if matter takes up space, and air is matter, how is it possible for the perfume gas to fill up the room completely? This observation illustrates another physical property of matter, called **porosity** (pô ros′ ə ti). You should be able to remember this word without difficulty, because the small openings in your skin are called **pores** (pôr).

Gases, like all forms of matter, have a great deal of space between the particles that make them up. One gas can easily pass through another gas by moving into the empty spaces.

---

### Examining the Porosity of a Liquid

**MATERIALS:**

100 ml of alcohol, 100 ml of water, a graduated cylinder that is large enough to measure at least 200 ml of liquid

**PROCEDURE:**

Pour the 100 ml of water into the large graduated cylinder. Slowly pour the alcohol into the water, and stir the mixture carefully. How much liquid do you have in the cylinder? Remember that an aim of science is to explain things that happen in nature. Before reading the next paragraph, try to explain your observations.

---

Water and alcohol are both **porous** (pô′ rəs). When the two are mixed together, some of the alcohol particles occupy the space between the particles of water, and vice versa. Not all liquids behave the same way as alcohol and water. For example, try adding cooking oil to water and see what happens.

Solids are generally less porous than liquids. However, many are easily penetrated by some types of matter. Perhaps you have seen water seeping through a cement wall or have read about layers of rocks in the earth that contain water or petroleum.

### Dissolving One Substance in Another

**Solubility** (sol′ ū bil′ ə ti) is another physical property of matter. It is a measure of how much of a substance will **dissolve** (di zolv′) in another substance.

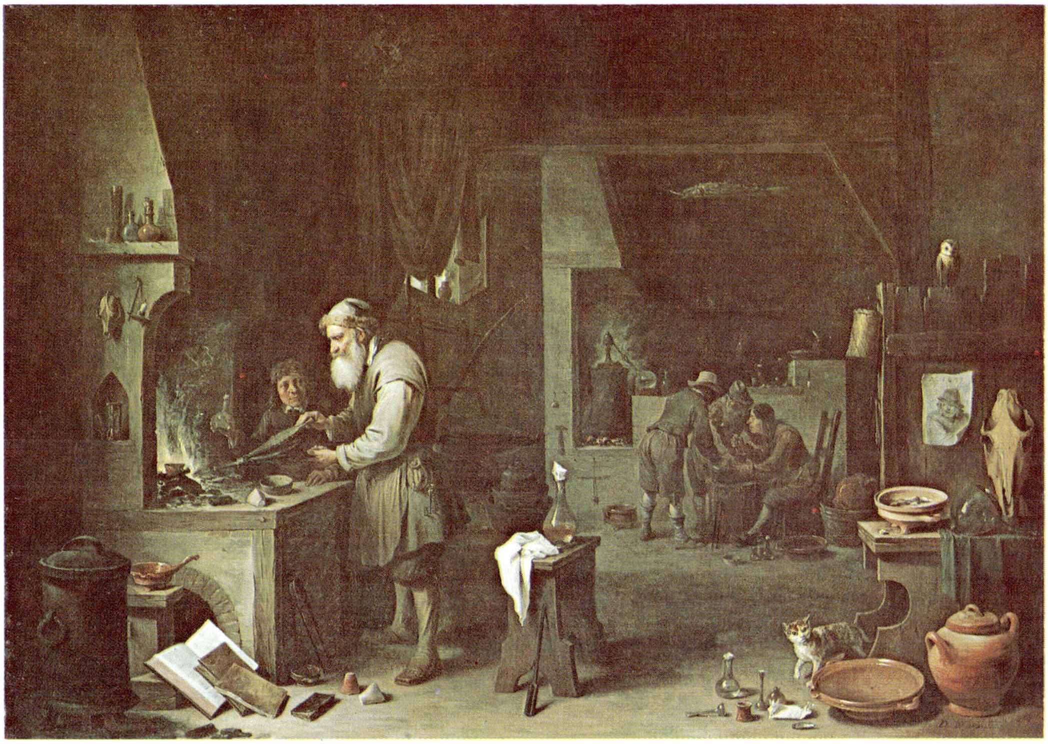

*Courtesy, John G. Johnson Collection, Philadelphia*

**2.5** This seventeenth-century alchemist's laboratory is very different from the laboratories used by the scientists of the twentieth century. What differences can you find?

## Determining Solubility

**MATERIALS:**

Beakers, balance, thermometer, glass rod, table sugar, table salt, sand, hypo (chemical used in photographic darkrooms), copper sulfate

**PROCEDURE:**

Place exactly 50 ml of tap water in a beaker, and record the temperature of the water. The temperature of the water should be within a degree or two of room temperature. If it is not, allow the water to stand until it reaches room temperature.

Weigh the beaker containing the water, and record the weight in your notebook. Slowly add table salt to the water, stirring with a glass rod. Continue adding table salt until no more will dissolve. Weigh the beaker containing the **solution** (sə lü′ shən) of salt-water, and record the weight. The difference between the two weights is the weight of the table salt that was dissolved.

Repeat the experiment with other substances such as sugar, sand, hypo, and copper sulfate. Be sure to record the two weights for each substance.

Make a list of the substances you dissolved, placing the one that dissolved the most at the top of the list, the one that dissolved the least at the bottom, and the others arranged accordingly. Compare your results with your classmates'.

What do you think would happen if the water were warmer than room temperature? Can you devise an experiment to test your hypothesis?

In this activity, you should have observed that salt dissolves in water, and sand does not. Therefore, we say that salt is **soluble** (sol′ u bəl) in water, and sand is **insoluble** (in sol′ ū bəl). The amount of a substance that will dissolve is a physical property that can be used in identifying it. For example, if you used hypo, you should have found that more of it dissolves in 50 ml of water than does either sugar or salt.

## Density

In addition to the fact that all matter takes up space, all matter has weight. But you may have observed that a brick is considerably heavier than a block of wood of the same size. In this case, we say that the brick is more **dense** (dens) than the wood. **Density** (den′ sə ti) is another physical property of matter.

### Calculating the Density of Matter

You may have measured and weighed several rectangular objects while studying Chapter 1. Use these measurements to calculate the volume and density of each object. If you did not have these data begin by measuring the length, width, and height of three rectangular objects and weigh each of them.

The volume can be found by multiplying the length times the width times the height. These directions for finding the volume can be stated as a **equation:** $V = L \times W \times H$ or simply $V = LWH$. Find the volume of each object in cubic centimeters, and record your answer in a table like Table I.

To find the density of each object, divide its weight by its volume. The formula is $D = \frac{W}{V}$. Your answer will be in grams per cubic centimeter. Record your answers in the table below.

TABLE I

| *Name or Number of Object* | *Volume in Cubic Centimeters* | *Weight in Grams* | *Density g/cc* |
|---|---|---|---|
| | | | |

As you can see from this activity, density is a measure of *weight per unit volume.* By comparing the densities, you can easily see how much more dense brick is than wood, even if the samples you used were of different sizes. The densities of several common materials are shown in Table II.

**TABLE II**
*Densities of Some Common Metals*

| *Metal* | *Density (Grams/cc)* |
|---|---|
| Aluminum | 2.7 |
| Brass | 8.2-8.7 |
| Gold | 19.3 |
| Iron, cast | 7.0-7.7 |
| Lead | 11.3 |
| Magnesium | 1.7 |
| Mercury | 13.6 |
| Steel | 7.6-7.8 |
| Zinc | 7.1 |

In order to calculate density you must be able to find the volume of an object. With a rectangular piece of solid material this is an easy job. But can you find the volume of something that is not rectangular, such as a rock or a piece of chalk?

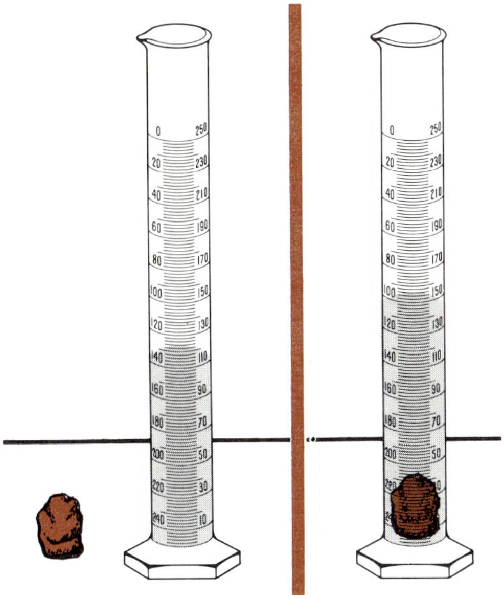

**2.6** Finding the volume of an irregular object

## Finding the Density of an Irregular Object

**MATERIALS:**

A large graduated cylinder, a small, irregularly shaped solid object that is small enough to fit into the cylinder, enough water to fill the cylinder about half full

**PROCEDURE:**

Pour the water into the graduated cylinder and read the volume. Drop the irregularly shaped object into the water, being careful not to splash out any water. Notice that the level of the water rises. Read the volume of the water now. The difference between the two readings is the volume of the object. Can you see why this is true? Using this method, find the volume of a small stone, weigh it, and then calculate its density.

Can you suggest a way of using this method to find the volume of an irregularly shaped piece of matter that is light enough to float? Can you experiment to check the accuracy of your method?

### Other Physical Properties

In addition to the physical properties of matter described in this section, there are several other properties that can be used to identify a substance. Color is often useful. Some solids can be described in terms of their hardness and how easily they can be broken. Can you name other physical properties of matter?

**Have You Learned?**

From the list at the right, select the word that most accurately completes each statement below. (Do not write in your book.)

| | |
|---|---|
| 1, 2, 3. The three common states of matter are _____, _____, and _____. | a. mass<br>b. shape |
| 4. The _____ of solids and liquids always remains the same. | c. gas |
| 5. Two gases can fill the same container at the same time because gases are _____. | d. insoluble<br>e. liquid |
| 6. Multiplying the length times the width times the height of a solid object is a measure of the _____. | f. volume<br>g. density |
| 7. Weight per unit volume is _____. | h. weight |
| 8. _____ is the measure of how much of a substance will dissolve in a certain liquid. | i. solubility<br>j. temperature |
| 9. A substance that will not dissolve in a liquid is said to be _____. | k. solid |
| 10. Generally, increasing the _____ of a liquid will increase the amount of a solid that can dissolve in it. | l. porous |

## 3. What Moves Matter?

**ARE YOU READY?**

Look up the following words if you are not sure of their meanings:

centimeter; energy; English system (of measurement); gram; kilo-; matter; metric system (of measurement); unit (of measurement); vertical.

A book falls from the table to the floor. A baseball flies through the air when hit with a bat. A model rocket soars high into the air so long as its motor burns, then falls back to earth. And a space probe moves from the earth to the moon and beyond. In studying matter, we often find ourselves talking about objects that are in motion.

**Energy** (en′ ər ji)—the cause of all motion—is defined as *the ability to do work.* If we observe work being done on an object, we know that energy is present. But the scientist has a special definition for the word work. You may define work as mowing the grass, washing the car, or taking a test. To the scientist, **work** means that a stationary object is moved from one place to another, or that the direction or speed of a moving object is changed.

In order to do work a **force** must be applied to some matter. Suppose you wish to move a desk from one side of the room to another. You will either have to *push* or *pull* the desk, in order to get it to move. This is all that a force is—*a push or a pull.*

When you apply a force against matter, you need energy. This energy comes from the food you eat, and a constant supply is necessary since you constantly use forces. Walking, running, throwing a baseball are all examples of forces being used to do work. And each of these requires a supply of energy.

Machines also require a supply of energy when they do their work. A bulldozer pushes a pile of dirt, using the energy contained in the diesel fuel. The energy stored in an automobile battery is used to start the engine. Electric energy is used to turn a fan that pushes air away from it. In each case, a force is applied that results in the movement of matter.

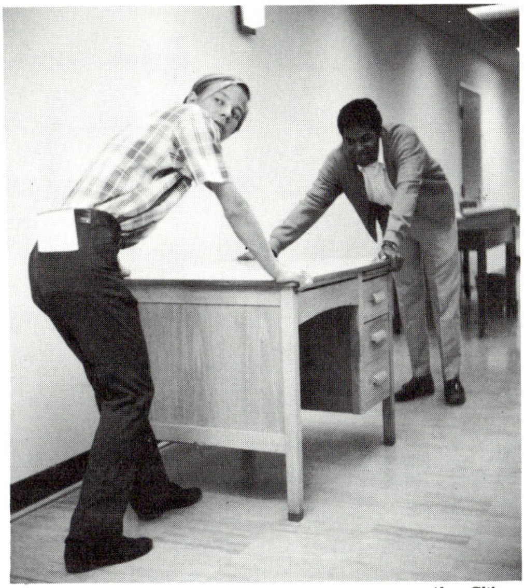

*Alan Cliburn*

**2.7** Force is either a *push* or a *pull.*

## Measuring the Amount of Work Done

It is a simple matter to measure the amount of work done on an object. Work is done when a force moves something a certain distance. Therefore, to calculate the work done, all we need to do is to multiply the amount of force times the distance the matter was moved.

If you lift an object that weighs 1,000 grams, you must exert a force of more than 1,000 grams on that object. This is because you are lifting the object against the pull of gravity, and the force you apply must more than balance the weight of the object if it is to move it. If you apply less force than this, what will happen? Will the object move?

## Calculating Work

**MATERIALS:**

A spring scale, a small weight (also called a mass) and a meterstick

**PROCEDURE:**

Attach the weight to the scale, and lift it straight up to the top of the stick. Multiply the force necessary to lift the weight, as shown by the scale, times the distance you moved the weight. The equation for this is: WORK = FORCE × DISTANCE or $W = FD$.

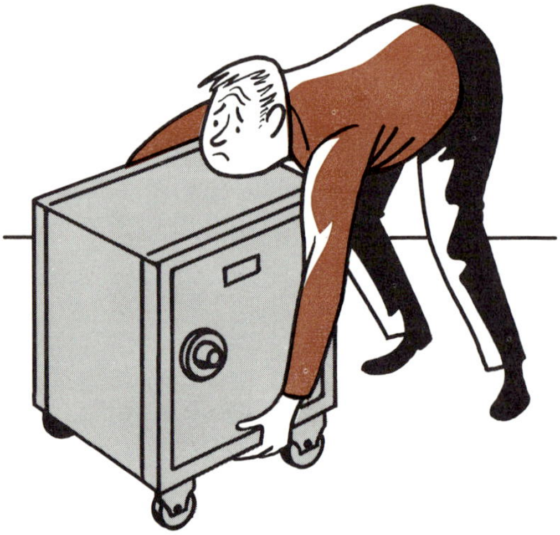

If you used the English-System units, you will have measured *pounds* of force times *feet* of distance. In this case, your answer will be called **foot-pounds** *of work.* For example, if you use 100 lbs. of force to move an object 20 ft., how much work did you do?

*100* lbs. × *20* ft. = *2,000* ft.-lbs. of work.

In the metric system, you would have measured force in units of kilograms and distance in meters. Therefore, the work done would be calculated in units of kilogram-meters. For example if you use 100 kilograms of force to move an object 10 meters, how much work did you do?

*100* kg × *10* m = *1,000* kg-m of work

In the metric system energy and work are measured in **joules** or in **kilogram-meters.** One foot-pound equals 1.35 joules or 0.14 kilogram-meter.

## Units of Power

The amount of work accomplished in moving a desk from one side of the room to the other is the same regardless of *how long* it took you to do it. But scientists, engineers, and others are often interested in knowing how fast a certain amount of work is done. The rate at which work is done is called **power** (pou′ ər). To do a given amount of work quickly requires more power than doing the same amount of work more slowly.

To calculate power, we divide the amount of work done by the time it took to do it. To see how this works, let's take an example using English System units. This way you will be better able to compare the power of your body with that of a motorcycle or automobile.

If you move a 100-pound weight 5 feet you have done 100 lbs. × 5 ft. = 500 foot-pounds of work. If it took you 10 seconds to do this work, the power involved would

**2.8** The work done equals the weight (mass) of the desk times the distance it is pushed.

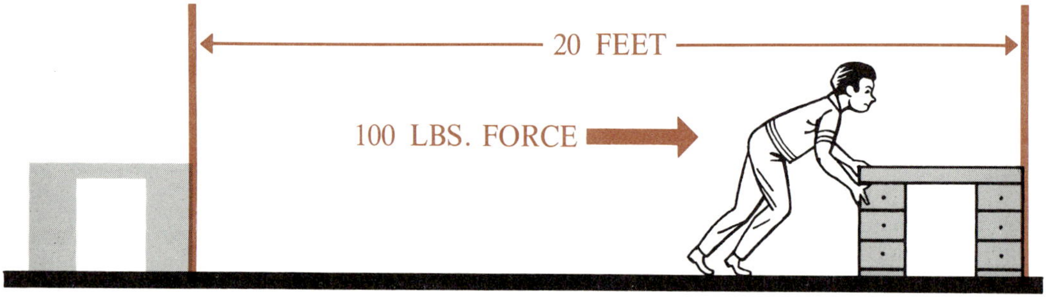

be $\frac{500 \text{ ft.-lbs.}}{10 \text{ secs.}} = 50$ ft.-lbs. per second. If you did this amount of work in 100 seconds, the power would equal 5 ft.-lbs. per second.

You have probably heard of the basic unit of power, called the **horsepower** (hôrs′ pou′ ər). One horsepower is equal to 550 ft.-lbs. of work per second. Early investigators thought that this was the amount of work that an average horse could do. How much work per second could be done by an automobile engine that is rated at 220 horsepower?

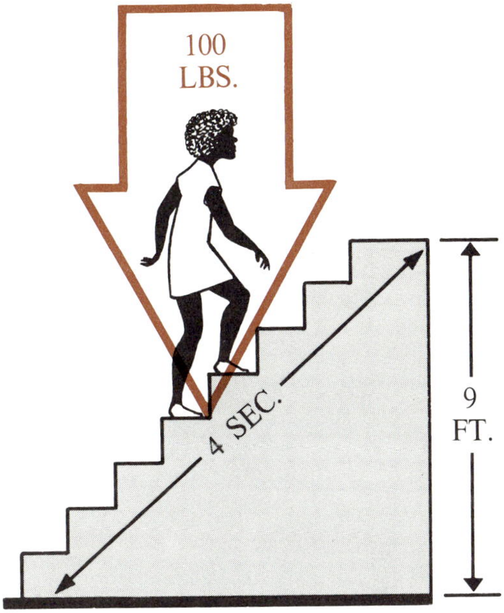


**2.9** Find the horsepower using the English units.

## Determining Your Horsepower

You can determine your horsepower by timing how long it takes you to run up a flight of stairs. Your weight times the vertical height of the stairs is the amount of work done. The work divided by the time required in seconds tells you how much power you exerted in foot-pounds per second. To convert to horsepower, divide by 550. The formula:

$$\text{H.P.} = \frac{(\text{Weight})\,(\text{Height})}{(\text{Time required})\,(550)}$$

If for some reason you cannot do this yourself, calculate the horsepower being developed by the girl in Figure 2.9. Your class also may wish to experiment with other methods of measuring horsepower, such as climbing a rope or lifting objects from the floor to a table.

Another unit of power is commonly used in rating electrical machines. This is called the **watt** (wot), and is equal to about ¾ ft.-lb. per second. The watt is a very small unit, so most large electrical machines are rated in **kilowatts** (kil′ ə wot′), which is a unit equal to 1,000 watts. A kilowatt, then, equals about 750 ft.-lbs. per second or about $1^1/_3$ horsepower. Or turning it around the other way, one horsepower is about ¾ of a kilowatt.

## Have You Learned?

Select the phrase from Column B that best defines each word in Column A. (Do not write in your book.)

| *Column A* | *Column B* |
|---|---|
| 1. Energy | a. the basic unit of power |
| 2. Force | b. how fast a certain amount of work is done |
| 3. Power | c. a push or a pull |
| 4. Horsepower | d. 1,000 watts |
| 5. Kilowatt | e. ability to do work |

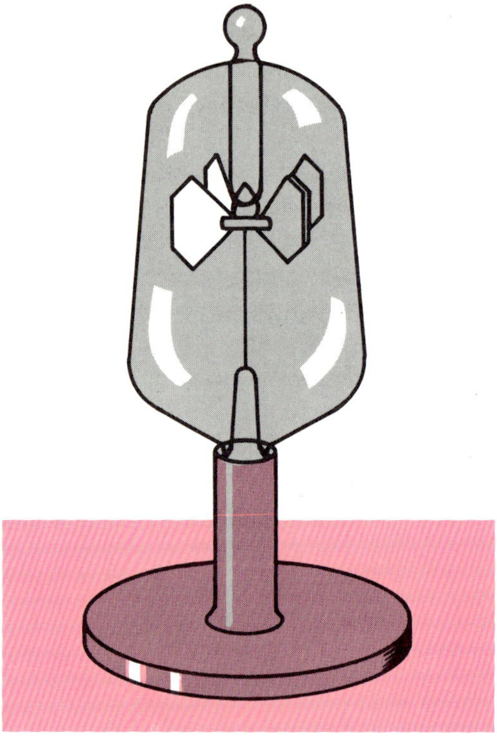

**2.10** The vanes of a radiometer will turn when it is placed in direct sunlight.

## 4. Forms of Energy

> **ARE YOU READY?**
>
> Look up the following words if you are not sure of their meanings:
>
> atom; chemical; electric current; potential; work.

Although we cannot see energy, we can see the effects of energy. We can observe the work that a moving marble does on another marble when the two collide. We can observe steam being forced from the mouth of a teakettle when it is filled with water and placed over a source of heat. The little motor shown in Figure 2.10 will turn when it is placed in direct sunlight. You can observe what happens when two chemicals, such as baking soda and vinegar, are combined. We can observe the movement of a fan blade, caused by the electric current flowing through the motor.

### Different Forms of Energy

These examples show that there are several forms or sources of energy. The form of energy that perhaps you are best acquainted with, and the one that early scientists first identified, is the energy of a moving object. When you shoot a marble, throw a ball, or pedal a bicycle, you are putting an object into motion. If these objects hit something, the energy they possess becomes apparent in the work they do! The energy of moving objects and that found in machines is called **mechanical** (me kan′ ə kəl) **energy.**

Another form of energy is **heat.** Heat causes air to move, changes water to steam that can be used to make a steam engine run, and it is often produced when other forms of energy are used up. Chapter 4 describes this important form of energy and some of the ways it is used.

The ability of light to do work does not seem very important, perhaps, until we consider that all of the growth of all of the green plants in the world is due to this form of energy. Closely related to light are the waves of energy from the sun that cause painful sunburn. The waves that cause our radios and televisions to work are also very much like light in many ways. Generally all of these forms of energy are grouped together and called **radiant** (rā′ di ənt) **energy.**

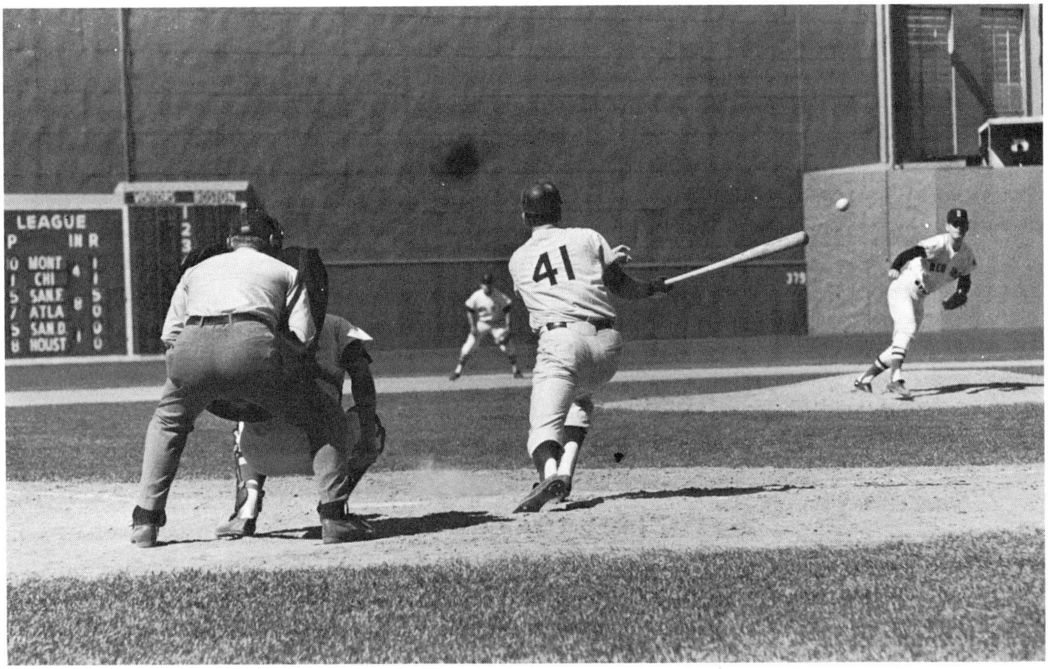

*Mike Mazzaschi/Stock, Boston*

**2.11** We all have a natural feeling for mechanical energy. Every time we move any part of our bodies the movement is an example of mechanical energy.

**2.12** Most experimental solar houses use panels on the roof. These convert light energy (solar energy) to heat. Just how heat is stored and put to use are the big problems that scientists and engineers must solve.

*Robert Perron*

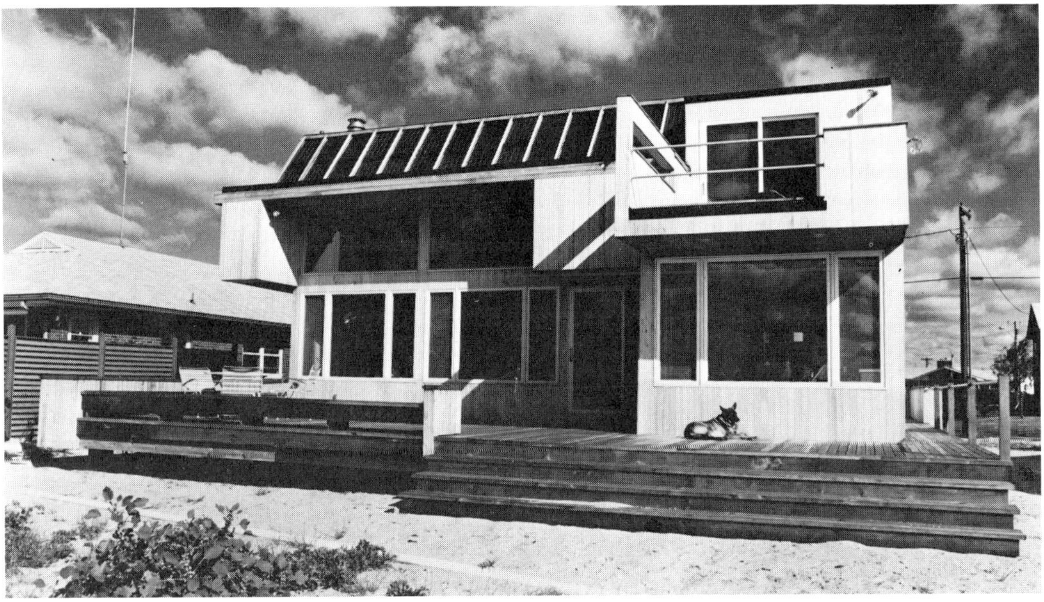

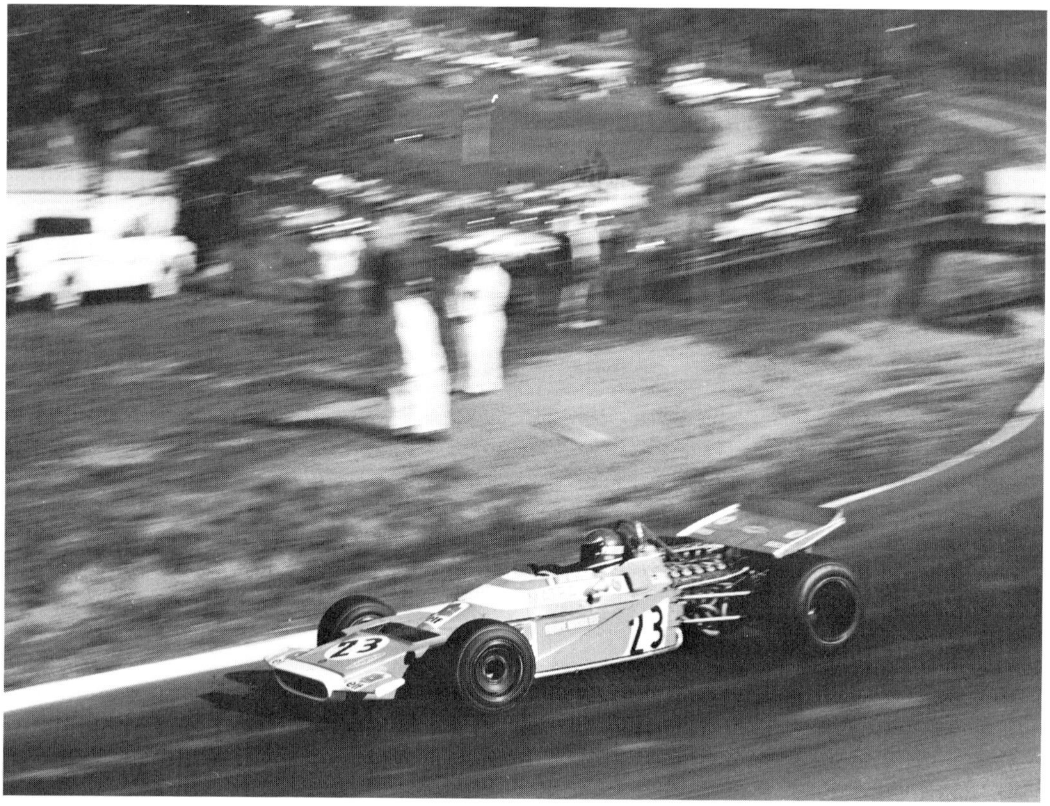


Steven Potter/Stock, Boston

**2.13** What kinds of energy are being demonstrated here? You know there is movement, so there must be mechanical energy. Chemical energy stored in the gasoline produced mechanical energy.

**Chemical** (kem′ ə kəl) **energy** is a fourth form of energy. The energy that you use to run, to breathe, and to circulate your blood comes from the chemical energy stored in the food that you eat. Energy stored in fuels, such as coal and gasoline, is another example of chemical energy. Energy is stored in an automobile battery as chemical energy and is used to start the engine, sound the horn, and burn the lights.

You often use the energy of an electric current to do work for you. This form of energy can be used to run the motors of fans, refrigerators, air-conditioners, and other large appliances. The work that an electric current does on these motors is easy to observe. **Electrical energy** also does work when it passes through an electric toaster or iron, even though the work is not so apparent to us. Electrical energy is also used to produce both heat and light in an electric light or flashlight.

One of the outstanding accomplishments of modern science has been the releasing of the energy of the *atom.* The energy of an atomic bomb blast comes from atoms splitting into two or more parts. When **nuclear** (nü′ kli ər) **energy** is released, a tremendous amount of work can be done

—as much or even more than is sometimes done by a hurricane or an earthquake.

### Another Way of Classifying Energy

In addition to describing energy as being of different forms, depending on its source, energy also is classified as being **potential** (pə ten′ shəl) energy or **kinetic** (ki net′ ik) energy. Energy that is stored is called *potential energy*. Take for example a large rock that is resting on the top of a mountain. It has potential energy since energy was required to place it there. If the rock falls to the bottom of the mountain, it loses some of its energy.

As the rock falls, it is said to have *kinetic energy*. Kinetic energy is the energy of moving objects or energy being used. A moving car, water running down a hill, and a sailboat being pushed along by the wind are all examples of kinetic energy.

#### Have You Learned?

Match the forms of energy in Column B with the examples in Column A.

| *Column A* | *Column B* |
|---|---|
| 1. Energy used to start automobiles | a. chemical |
| 2. Energy obtained from food | b. electrical |
| 3. Energy of a falling rock | c. heat |
| 4. Atomic energy | d. mechanical |
| 5. Produced by friction | e. nuclear |
| 6. Form that reaches us from the sun | f. radiant |

Match examples in Column A with best description in Column B.

| *Column A* | *Column B* |
|---|---|
| 7. Energy in storage battery of car | g. kinetic energy |
| 8. Energy of falling rock | h. potential energy |
| 9. Energy contained in coal | |
| 10. Energy in a spring of a watch | |

## 5. Energy Changes

**ARE YOU READY?**

Look up the following words if you are not sure of their meanings:

conservation; elevation; kinetic energy; mechanical energy; potential energy; radiant energy.

### Changes in Form

If a book rests on the top of a table, all of its energy is potential. That is, as long as the book remains on the table, it is not doing any work. If, however, you push the book from the table, it falls and may do work on an object on the floor below the table's edge. The following experiment will demonstrate this.

## Observing the Energy of a Falling Book

**MATERIALS:**

A book, a table, a meter-stick, a short narrow strip of wood (preferably wedge-shaped), a paper cup, a thumbtack, a light weight ball such as a Ping Pong ball

**PROCEDURE:**

Place the paper cup on the end of the meter-stick, securing it with the thumbtack. Place the wedge of wood under the meterstick, approximately $^2/_3$ of the distance from the paper cup to the opposite end, as shown in Figure 2.14. Place the ball in the cup, and place the entire apparatus in such a way that the higher end of the meterstick is under the edge of the table. Place the book on the table, and push it off so that it will strike the higher end of the meterstick. What happens to the ball? Where did the energy that made the ball move come from?

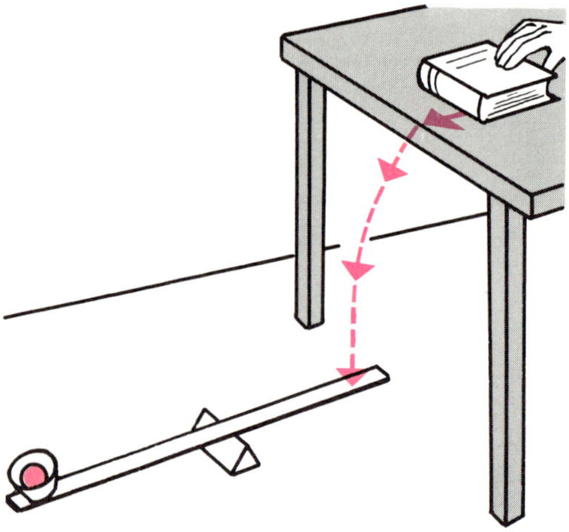

**2.14** What will happen to the ball in the cup when the book strikes the other end of the stick?

At the moment the falling book hit the ground, all of its energy was kinetic energy—the energy of motion. Yet when the book was on the table top, all of its energy was considered to be potential or stored energy. As the book fell, its potential energy was changed into kinetic energy.

Try to think of some other examples of changes of potential energy to kinetic energy. They are all around you.

## Changes from One Form to Another

You have learned that energy is continuously changing from potential to kinetic and back again. The changes of energy from one form to another are also common and easily observed. Let us consider the examples diagrammed on page 59.

Radiant energy from the sun **evaporates** (i vap′ ə rāt) water in the ocean, changing it into a gas called **water vapor.** As the water vapor loses its heat energy to the surrounding air, it forms clouds and eventually may fall as rain into a lake behind a high dam. The potential energy of the water behind the dam is changed into kinetic energy by allowing it to fall through a long tube. It passes through a **turbine** (tėr bən), a machine much like a fan, which turns when the water strikes the blades. The shaft of the turbine turns an electric **generator** (jen′ ər ā′ tər) that produces an electric current. The electric current travels through wires to houses. There it can be changed into light energy, into heat energy, or used to make electric motors run.

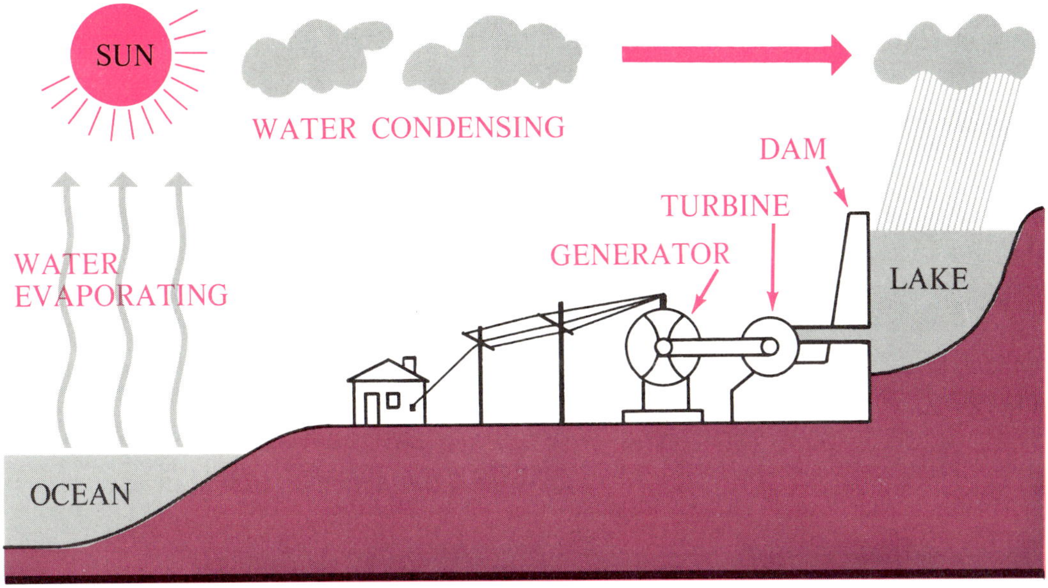


**2.15** Light energy, heat energy, mechanical energy, and electrical energy are all important factors in the cycle shown in this diagram.

In this example, the *radiant* energy from the sun was changed to *heat* energy when it struck water in the ocean. This heat energy caused the water to evaporate, and the water vapor was lifted to a high elevation behind the dam. The mechanical energy of the falling water was changed into the mechanical energy of the turning turbine, which in turn was changed into *electrical* energy by the generator. This electrical energy could then be changed into *light*, *heat*, and *mechanical* energy.

The important point to learn from this example is that energy can be changed from one form to another. The energy is not used up anywhere in the process, but it is changed from one form to another over and over again.

The idea that energy is not used up is one of the most important principles of science. This idea is called the **Conservation of Energy,** and may be summarized by saying that energy can neither be created nor destroyed.

This principle was first stated over one hundred years ago. Only a few years ago an exception to this idea was discovered, when it was found that during the release of atomic energy some of the matter of the atom was changed to energy. However, for changes of energy from one form to another that we observe in our daily lives, the principle of the Conservation of Energy is still true.

## Devices for Changing Energy from One Kind to Another

Scientists and engineers are constantly trying to discover easier and cheaper ways to change energy from one form to another. For example, a way has been worked out by which heat can be changed directly into electrical current. This dis-

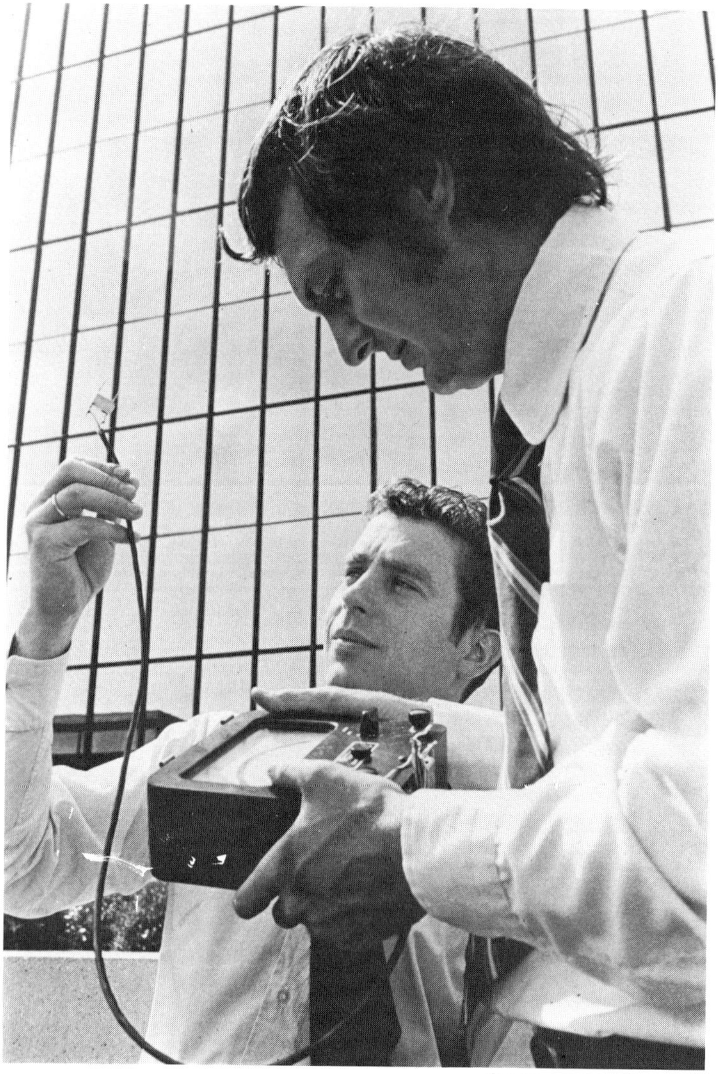

*Courtesy of Bell Laboratories*

**2.16** Solar batteries used to power telephone lines

covery resulted in the development of a thermometer that can measure very high temperatures inside machines where ordinary thermometers would be destroyed. Another example is the discovery of how to change light directly into electrical current. At the present time, a few telephone systems are powered by solar cells that produce electrical energy from sunlight.

However efficient these changes of energy from one form to another, it is important to remember that we can never get more energy out of a system than we put into it. If we could, we would be creating energy. When you lift a 3-kilogram book from the floor and place it on a table that is 1 meter high, *you* have used up energy in doing 3 kilogram-meters of work on the book. This energy is now in the form of potential energy because of the book's position on the table. If the book falls, its 3 kilograms of mass will again move 1 meter, and 3 kilogram-meters of work will again be done.

In the next chapter you will learn that some energy is changed to heat and other kinds of energy in machines.

## Have You Learned?

Explain in brief, complete sentences what changes of energy take place in the following situations.

1. A rock falls from the top of a mountain into the valley below.
2. Water evaporates and falls as rain.
3. Wood is burned to boil water, which then evaporates.
4. Gasoline is burned in a truck motor and the truck is driven to the top of a hill.
5. Water runs through a waterwheel, which is connected to a millstone that grinds grain.

## REVIEW QUESTIONS

*From the list of words at the right select the one that best completes each sentence below. Each answer may be used more than once, if necessary. (Do not write in your book.)*

1, 2. All bits of matter have two characteristics. They have _____ and they take up _____.

3. A cubic meter of iron will contain more _____ than a cubic meter of wood.

4. Weight is a measure of the pull of _____ on an object.

5. While weight may vary with the location of an object, its _____ always remains the same.

6. A _____ has a definite shape and a definite volume.

7. A substance that dissolves in a liquid is said to be _____.

8. If you divide the weight of an object by its volume, you find the _____ of the object.

9. Water will soak into a sponge because the sponge is _____.

10. _____ is the ability to do work.

11. If you multiply the distance an object is moved times the amount of force used to move the object, you have calculated the amount of _____ done.

12. A basic unit of power, equal to 550 ft.-lbs. of work, is the _____.

13. A unit of power used in rating electrical motors is the _____.

14. A _____ may be either a push or a pull.

15. Light waves and radio waves are both examples of a kind of energy called _____ energy.

16. The battery of a car has _____ energy stored in it.

17. The form of energy that comes from the splitting of atoms is called _____ energy.

18. As a car rolls down a hill, its potential energy changes into _____ energy.

19. An important principle of science known as the _____ of Energy states that energy can neither be created nor destroyed.

20. During the release of _____ energy, some matter is changed into energy.

a. atomic
b. chemical
c. conservation
d. density
e. energy
f. force
g. gas
h. gravity
i. horsepower
j. insoluble
k. kilowatt
l. kinetic
m. liquid
n. mass
o. matter
p. nuclear
q. porous
r. radiant
s. solid
t. soluble
u. space
v. weight
w. work

## CAN YOU FIND OUT?

*It may be necessary to use an encyclopedia or other reference books in answering these questions.*

1. How much does the air above a square inch of your desk weigh? How much would the air above a square foot weigh? What is the weight of the air above the entire desk top?
2. What are some of the observations that prove that some solids are porous?
3. What is the liquid with the highest density? What are some liquids that are less dense than water?
4. How many horsepower can horses actually develop?
5. How does the energy of earthquakes and hurricanes compare with the energy of atomic bombs?
6. What is a thermocouple? How do thermocouples work and where are they used?
7. What are the sources of energy used in weather and communication satellites?

## REFERENCES FOR ADDITIONAL STUDY


ENERGY by Mitchell Wilson and the Editors of Time-Life Books, A Division of Time Inc. (Distributed by Silver Burdett Company.)
A well-illustrated book that contains descriptions of various kinds of energy and their uses

EXPERIMENTS WITH WATER by Harry Sootin. Grosset & Dunlap, Inc.
Twenty simple experiments involving water, including fluid pressure, freezing and boiling, surface tension, and Archimedes' principle

MATTER by Ralph Lapp and the Editors of Time-Life Books, A Division of Time Inc. (Distributed by Silver Burdett Company.)
A combination of beautiful illustrations and interesting essays on the different states of matter and other characteristics

SCIENCE EXPERIMENTS WITH WATER by Sam Rosenfeld. Harvey House, Inc., Publishers.
A collection of experiments and explanations using water, including topics such as floating, adhesion and cohesion, and the nature of solutions

THE WONDERS OF PHYSICS: AN INTRODUCTION TO THE PHYSICAL WORLD by Irving Adler. Golden Press.
An interesting survey of the subject matter of physics; begins with 25 questions that a good observer might ask at the beach

# CHAPTER 3

# Energy and Motion

MANY OF THE OBJECTS in the universe are in motion. Automobiles start and stop, airplanes move rapidly around the world, rockets blast off and push their capsules into orbits around Mars or into space beyond. The planets revolve around the sun, and moons orbit several of the planets.

Moving objects and the causes of their motion are among the things studied in the science of physics.

## 1. Moving Matter

> **ARE YOU READY?**
>
> Look up the following words if you are not sure of their meanings:
>
> energy; force; gravity; mass; Newton (Sir Isaac); work.

As you learned in the last chapter, energy is the ability to do work. Work was defined as the movement of an object, or *mass*, from one place to another. When an object is in the process of being moved, we say that it is in **motion.**

We have all seen objects in motion—a falling rock, a batted ball, a train. In each of these examples, it is easy to understand that a force causes the motion. Gravity pulls the rock downward. A bat pushes

**3.1** Motion is produced by unbalanced forces.

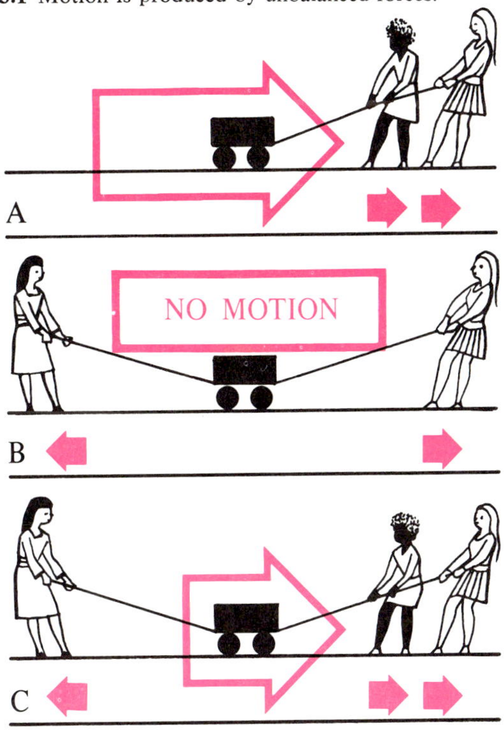

the ball. The engine of the train pulls the cars along after it.

But many forces other than these also act on these objects, and these forces affect the motion that we see. The direction and the speed of the moving object depends upon the *total* effect of all of the forces acting on it. Suppose, for example, that two girls were pulling on ropes tied to a wagon. If they both pulled in the same direction, the wagon would move along behind them. If they each pulled in an opposite direction but with the same amount of force, the wagon would not move at all. If a third girl joined in pulling the wagon in one direction, the movement would be toward the *two* girls, but it would be slower than it was when only two girls pulled in the *same* direction. (See Figure 3.1.)

## Experimenting with Force and Motion

**MATERIALS:**

Two spring scales, a heavy weight, a piece of string

**PROCEDURE:**

Attach one spring scale to the weight with the string, and slowly pull it across the desk or floor. Try to pull the weight along at a steady speed. Read and record the amount of force shown by the spring scale.

Attach the second spring scale to the weight, and pull it across the desk by pulling on both scales together, as shown in the diagram. Read and record the amount of force shown by each balance.

The sum of the two forces may be slightly larger than the force used to pull the weight with only one scale. Can you explain this observation? An experiment that may help you to answer this question may be performed by repeating this activity several times, increasing the angle between the scales (angle *A* in Figure 3.2).

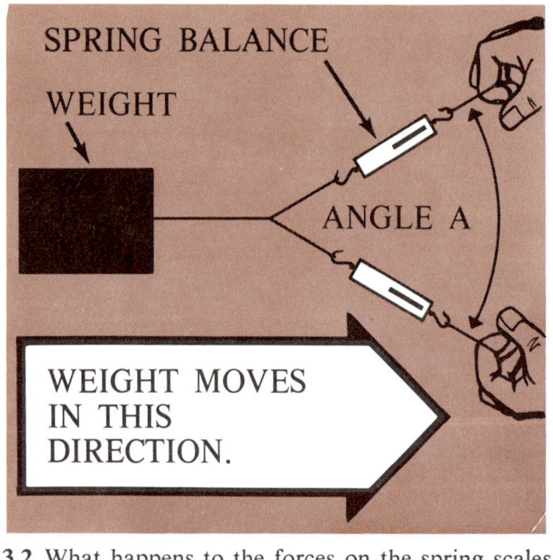


**3.2** What happens to the forces on the spring scales when angle A is increased or decreased?

The strength and the direction of the forces applied to an object are not the only factors that determine the motion. The mass of the object also is important.

## Experimenting with Mass and Motion

**MATERIALS:**

Heavy object (such as large bolt or 500-gram weight), pulley, string, weights of assorted sizes, ring stand or support, brick or books to keep ring stand from moving

**PROCEDURE:**

Set up the apparatus as shown in Figure 3.3. Hang weights at point *B* until the total weight is equal to, or just balances the object *A*. Then add more weight to *B* and observe the rate at which the object *A* moves upward.

The weight on the end of the string (*B* in Figure 3.3) produces a downward force. By means of the pulley and string, this force is applied in an upward direction on the object (*A* in Figure 3.3). What happens to object *A* if the upward force is exactly equal to the weight of object *A*? No movement takes place. If more weight is added to weight *B*, more upward forces will be applied to object *A*, and it will move upward. How does the amount of weight *B* affect the rate at which object *A* moves upward?

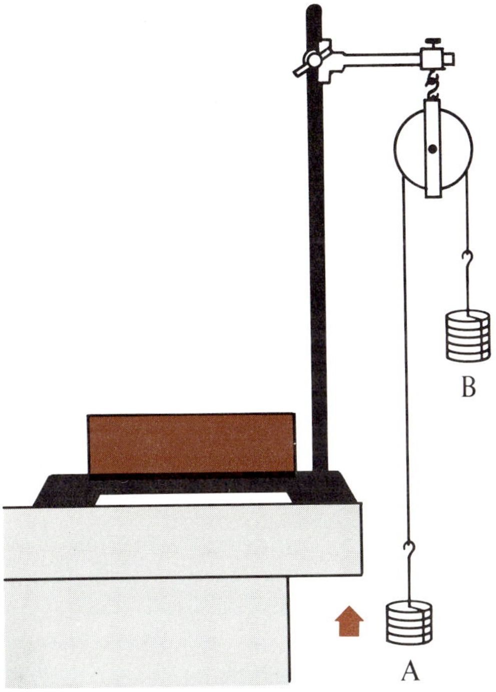


**3.3** What will happen if more weight is added to B?

As long as the weight of object *A* and the upward force are equal, object *A* remains stationary. The tendency for a body to remain stationary is called **inertia** (in ėr′ shə).

As the results of your experiment should indicate, objects with large masses have more inertia than objects with smaller masses. In other words it takes more force to speed up the motion of a large mass than it does to speed up the motion of a small mass.

## Feeling Inertia

**MATERIALS:**

Five coins of the same value, a playing card or piece of cardboard of a similar size, a drinking-glass

**PROCEDURE:**

Place the cardboard over the mouth of the drinking-glass with one of the coins on top, directly over the center of the glass, as shown in Figure 3.4a. Quickly flick the card forward with your forefinger so that the card is moved out from under the coin. If done properly, the coin should fall into the glass.

Stack up four coins, one on top of the other. Again using your forefinger, flick a fifth coin sharply against the bottom coin in the stack. The struck coin should move out from under the stack, leaving the other three coins in place. (Figure 3.4b)

**3.4a** Where will the coin land?

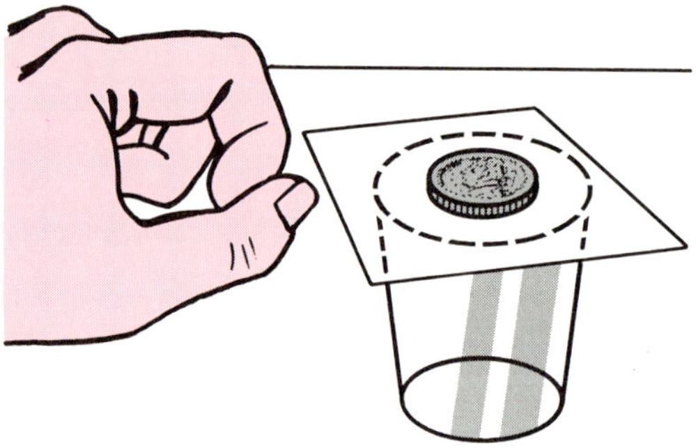

**3.4b** How many coins in the stack will move?

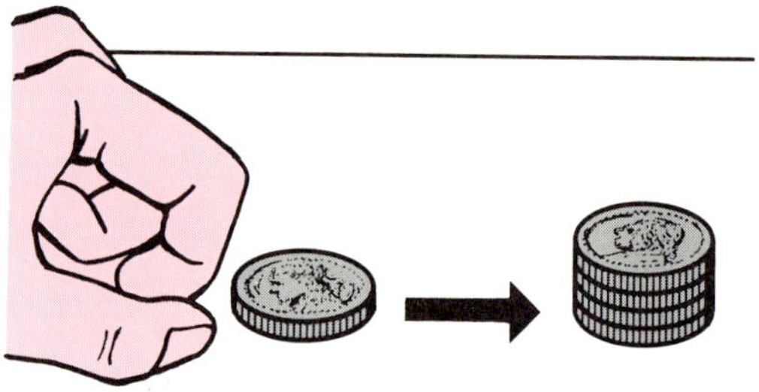

**3.5** An object in motion will continue to move until it is acted upon by an outside force.

*Alan Cliburn*

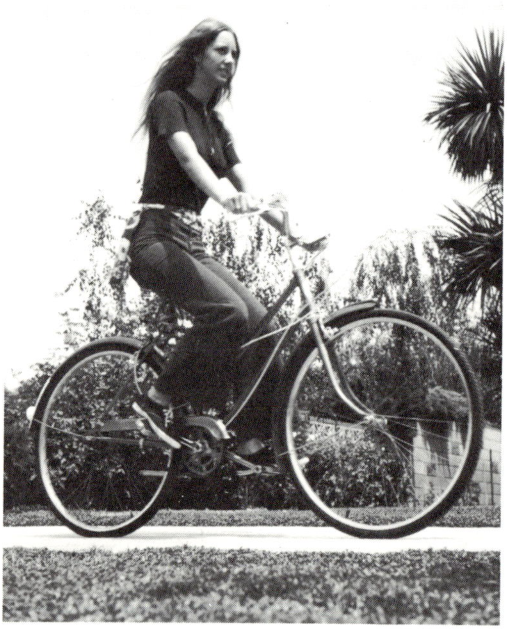

The cardboard in Figure 3.4a moved because a force was applied to it. Because of its inertia, the coin did not move forward but fell into the glass because of the force of gravity. Can you explain why the stack of coins in Figure 3.4b did not move forward?

Imagine a spaceship far out in space. If all of the forces acting on the ship are equal, the ship will continue to move in a straight line and at a constant speed. At blast-off, a large force was needed to overcome the inertia of the ship and to overcome the pull of gravity. However, once this has been done, the rocket motors can be shut off, and the ship will drift on without changing speed or direction.

If we wish to **accelerate** (ak sel′ ər āt) the ship—either slow it down or speed it up or change its direction—we must apply a force to it. The tendency of the spaceship

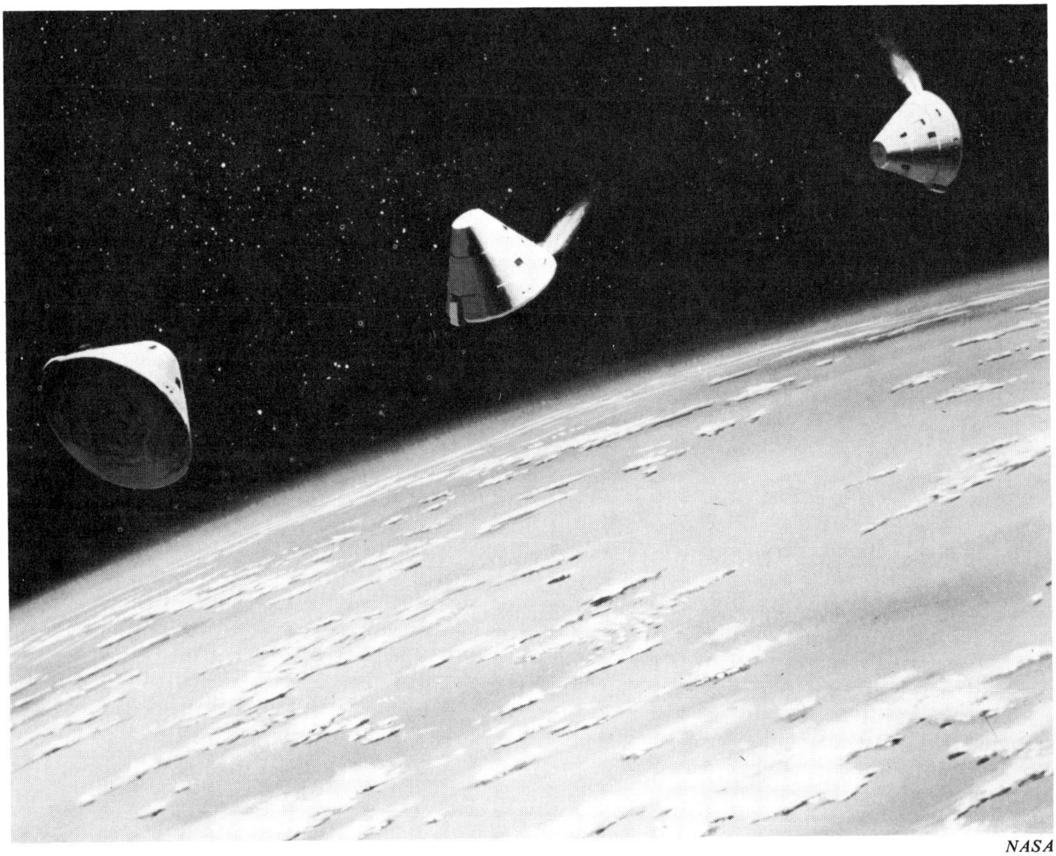

NASA

3.6 Drawing of the Command Module being oriented by the pilot so that the base heat shield takes the friction heat. To change the position, it is necessary that force provide the "push."

to remain in motion is also called *inertia.* Here on the earth, a bicycle continues to move after the rider stops pedaling because of inertia. In summary, inertia is the tendency for an object at rest to remain at rest and for an object in motion to continue its motion.

The idea of the inertia of all matter was first stated by Sir Isaac Newton, the same English scientist who worked with the laws of gravitation. Newton's so-called **First Law of Motion** may be stated thus: *Any matter that is in motion will continue to move at a constant speed and in the same direction until it is acted upon by an outside force. A body at rest will remain at rest until acted upon by an outside force.* In other words, all acceleration is caused by *outside* forces.

Inertia depends upon the *mass* of the body, since it does not increase or decrease if the object moves far out into space. An object on the moon would have the same amount of inertia as it does on the earth, even though its weight would be less on the moon. Therefore, the measurement of the inertia of an object is also a measure of the body's mass.

**Have You Learned?**

Newton's First Law of Motion states that "any matter that is in motion will continue to move at a constant speed and in the same direction until it is acted upon by an outside force." Identify in each of the following situations the "outside forces" that cause either a change in speed or in direction.

1. A boy is coasting downhill on a bicycle, and his speed is increasing.
2. A slowly moving car hits a tree and stops.
3 A ball is thrown upward into the air. It slows down, stops, and then speeds up as it falls back to Earth.
4. An airplane taxies down a runway, gaining speed as it goes. Then, it takes off and flies away.
5. A train moves at a steady speed around a curve in its tracks.

## 2. Making Work Easier

**ARE YOU READY?**

Look up the following words if you are not sure of their meanings:

advantage; clockwise; counterclockwise; effort; lever; work.

In order to move matter we must apply a force to it. People have invented many **machines** that they use in doing the work involved in moving matter.

Many machines are used because they allow us to move a heavy object with little effort. For example, suppose that you want to lift a box weighing 40 kilograms. If you simply pick up the box without the help of a machine, you will have to apply a force that is equal to the weight of the box—40 kg. However, with a machine you might be able to raise the box by applying a force of only 10 kg. Thus, by using a machine, it is easier for you to do the work.

If the weight of the object is divided by the effort of force actually used, a number is obtained that is called the **mechanical advantage** of the machine. In the example above, the mechanical advantage of the machine used to lift the box is 4 (40 kg ÷ 10 kg).

### Finding the Mechanical Advantage of a Lever

**MATERIALS:**

A meterstick, a weight (mass) or other heavy object, a spring scale, a small block of wood, preferably triangular

**PROCEDURE:**

Place the small block of wood under the exact middle of the stick. Place the weight about halfway between the end of the stick and the block of wood (see Figure 3.7). Hook the spring scale over the other end of the stick and lift the weight off the table by pulling *down* on the spring scale. Read the force as shown on the spring scale, and record on a piece of paper or in your notebook. The **force** is shown on the spring scale. This is called the **effort** *E*.

If you do not know the weight of the object *W* being lifted, hang it from the spring scale and record its weight.

Divide the weight of the object *W* by the effort *E*. The result is the mechanical advantage of the lever. What happens to the mechanical advantage if you move the object toward the center of the stick? What happens to the mechanical advantage if you move the object away from the center of the stick?

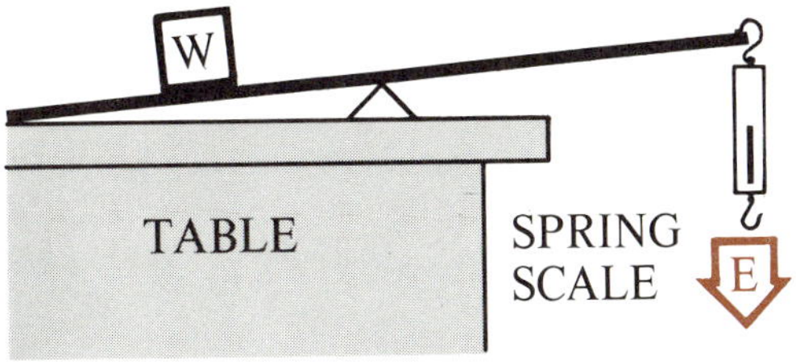


**3.7** Will more, or less, effort (force) be required if the weight (mass) is moved closer to the fulcrum?

A lever such as this one accomplishes two things. First, it changes the *amount* of the force needed to lift the weight, as shown by the mechanical advantage figure. It also changes the *direction* of the application of the force, allowing you to lift the weight *upward* by pulling *downward.*

You might use a lever such as this if you wanted to move a heavy rock. A crowbar, a claw hammer, and a seesaw are examples of this type of lever. Each has a **fulcrum** (ful′ krəm) over which it turns.

Each of these levers has two forces acting on it. One pulls in such a way that the lever tends to rotate in a clockwise direction around the fulcrum. The other force pulls the lever in a counterclockwise direction. (See Figure 3.9 page 70.)

Perhaps you have noticed that a lightweight boy on a seesaw can balance a heavier boy by moving as far away from the fulcrum as he can. If you were to make careful measurements of this, you would find that a boy weighing 70 kilograms and sitting 1 meter from the fulcrum could be balanced by a boy weighing only 35 kilograms if the lighter boy sat at a distance of 2 meters from the fulcrum. The product of the force and the distance from the fulcrum is called the **torque** (tork). In this

**3.8** It is fun to investigate levers using a seesaw.

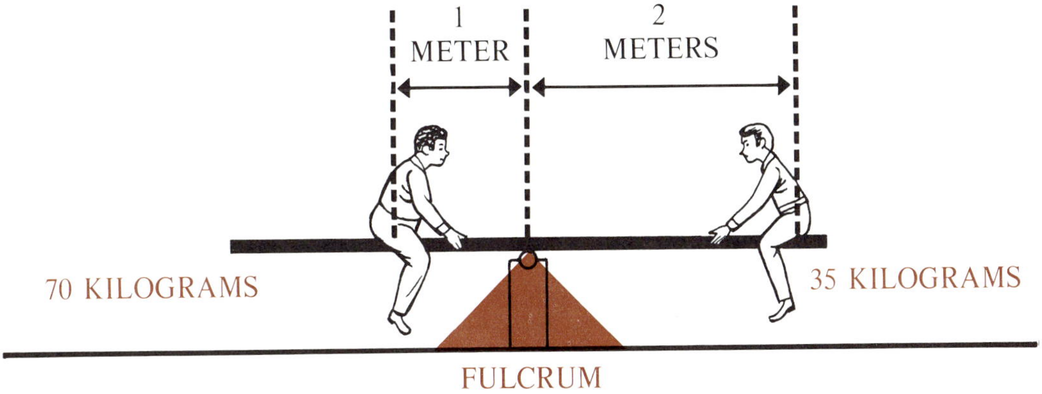

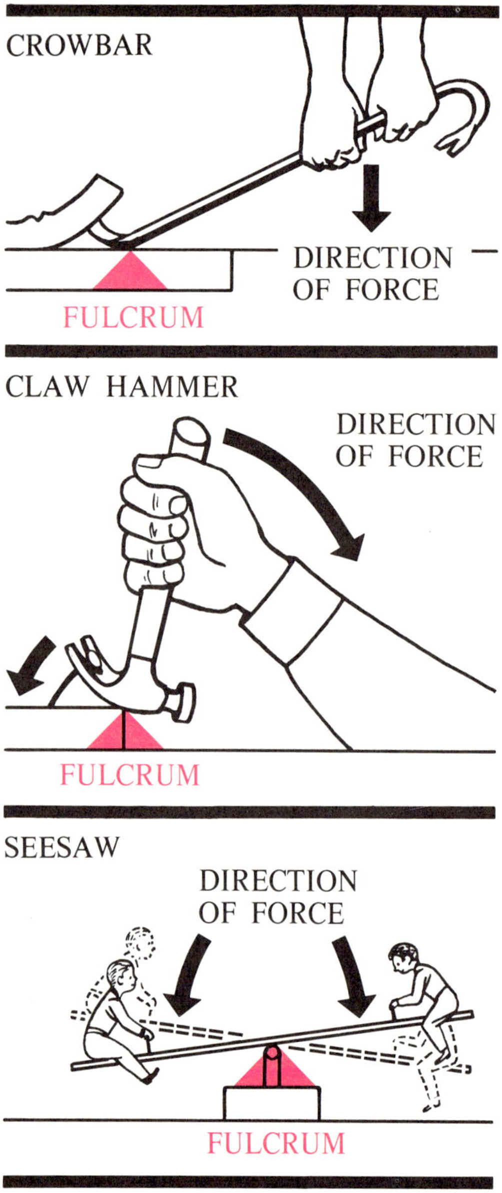


**3.9** Examples of common levers

example, the torque on one side of the lever is 70 kilograms × 1 meter = 70 kilogram-meters. The torque on the other side is 35 kilograms × 2 meters = 70 kilogram-meters, and it is in the opposite direction. From this you can see that the seesaw will balance. (See Figure 3.8 page 69.)

Not all levers are of the type with the fulcrum between the two forces. A wheelbarrow is a lever with the weight placed *between* the fulcrum (the axle) and the point at which the force is applied. The fisherman shown in the photograph below is using a third type of lever. He is applying an upward force to the lever at a point *between* the fulcrum and the force exerted by the fish.

**3.10** In what direction is the force applied here?

*Norman D. Anderson*

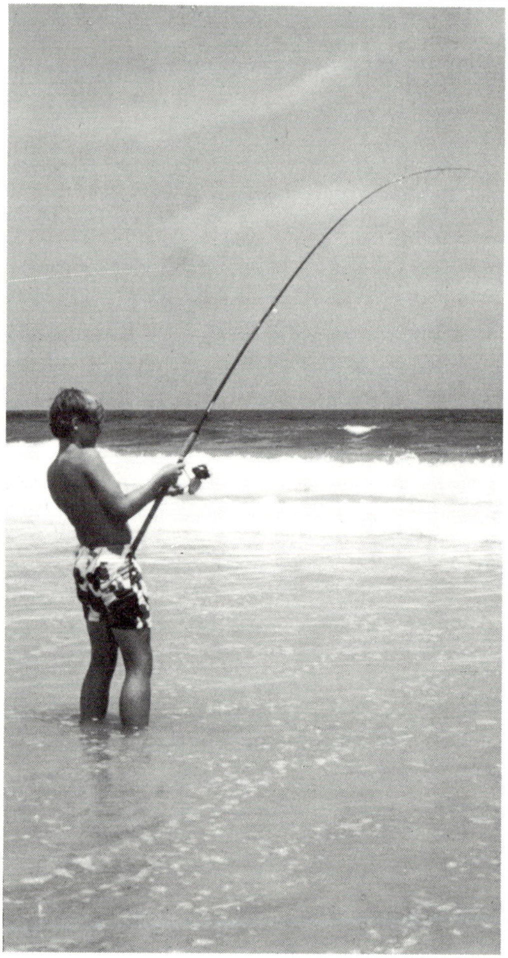

## Experimenting with Levers

**MATERIALS:**

A meterstick, a weight (mass), a spring scale

**PROCEDURE:**

First, arrange the lever as if it were a wheelbarrow, with the weight between the fulcrum (the floor) and the upper end of the stick. Lift the weight off the floor by lifting up on the spring scale attached to the free end of the stick. How much effort is required to lift the weight? What is the mechanical advantage of this lever? What happens to the mechanical advantage if the weight is moved closer to the fulcrum? What happens if the weight is moved closer to the force?

Next, place the stick flat on the floor. Place the weight near one end and attach the spring scale to the stick about ⅔ of the length of the stick away from the weight. Hold one end of the stick down with your hand as shown in the drawing below. Lift the weight by lifting up on the spring scale. What is the mechanical advantage of this lever? What happens to the mechanical advantage if the force is moved closer to the fulcrum? What happens if the force is moved away from the fulcrum?

What are the advantages and disadvantages of using these two types of levers? How do these two types compare with the type that has the fulcrum between the load, or weight, and the effort?

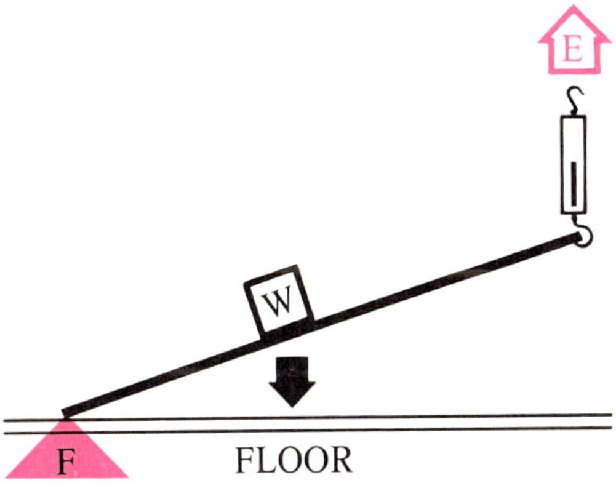


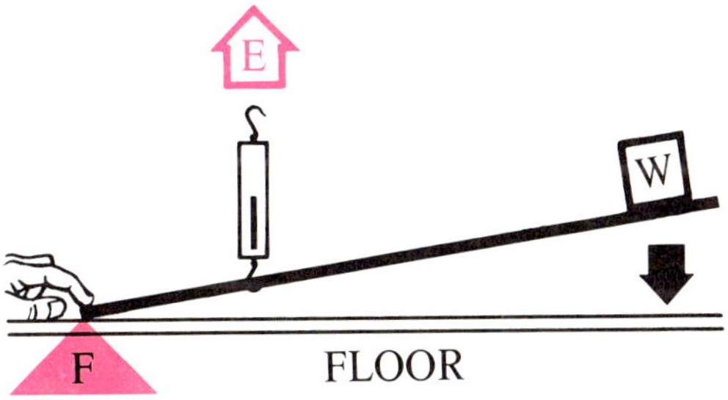


Calculating the torque forces of these types of levers is just as easy as with the first type. The distance from the object being moved to the fulcrum is multiplied by the weight of this object. This figure represents the torque forcing the lever in one direction around the fulcrum. The force exerted upward is measured by the scales. If this force is multiplied by the distance the scales are from the fulcrum, the result is that the torque turns the lever against the weight of the lifted object.

If you are concerned with taking very accurate measurements, as scientists always are, you may have had some difficulty deciding where to measure the position of the object being lifted by these levers. Is the distance from the fulcrum to the weight measured from the front face of the weight, from the back, or from the middle? This problem is especially important in the case of a wheelbarrow, where the weight is spread over a large area.

To solve this problem we have to suppose that all of the weight of an object acts as if it were concentrated at a single point. This point is known as the **center of gravity** of the object. For an object that is uniform in weight throughout, the center of gravity will be at the *geometric* center. Can you estimate where the center of gravity of a meterstick will be? You can easily test your answer, because the stick should balance if it is supported directly under its center of gravity. Consider the drawing below.

**3.11** Can you estimate where the geometric center of these forms will be?

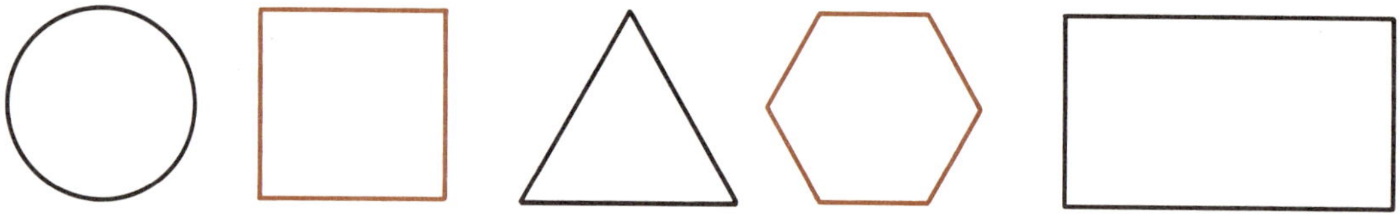

## Summary

The use of machines, such as the lever, to move an object has several advantages. Some machines change the *direction* of a force. For example, an object can be lifted by pulling down. Other machines change the *distance* the object is moved. The fisherman moves the pole a small distance and the fish is moved a greater distance. Still other machines change the amount of *force* required. A great weight can be lifted by a small force.

### Have You Learned?

1. Three types of levers are diagramed below. In each, identify the fulcrum *F*, the effort *E*, and the weight *W*.

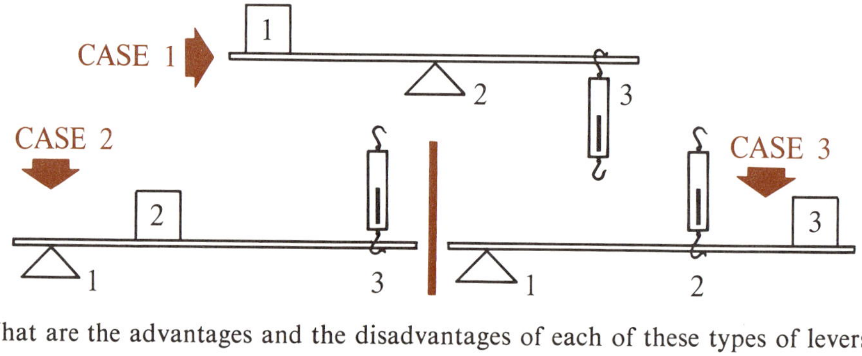


2. What are the advantages and the disadvantages of each of these types of levers?

## 3. Other Types of Machines

> **ARE YOU READY?**
>
> Look up the following words if you are not sure of their meanings:
>
> lever; machine; mechanical advantage; pulley; work.

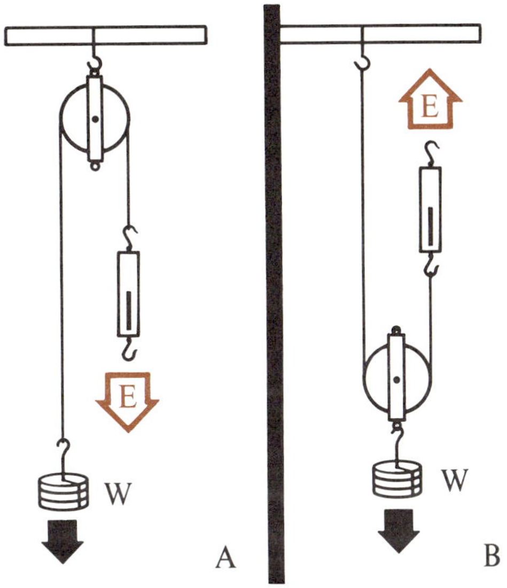


Levers are not the only types of simple machines available to help man do his work more easily. Pulleys are commonly used to move objects when the use of a lever would be impractical.

### Making Two Types of Pulleys

**MATERIALS:**

A pulley (or an empty thread spool with a piece of coat-hanger wire to hold it with), a length of string, a weight, a spring scale

**PROCEDURE:**

Place the string over the pulley with the weight on one side and the spring scale on the other, as shown in the Figure A. Read the spring scale and calculate the mechanical advantage. (See *A* above.) Next, tie one end of the string to an overhead support, or have someone hold it. Attach the weight to the pulley, and lift it with the spring scale, which is attached to the free end of the string as shown in the Figure B. Calculate the mechanical advantage of this pulley system. (*B* above)

In what ways do these machines change the force needed to lift the weight?

In the first part of this activity, using the stationary pulley, you should have found a mechanical advantage of about 1. In other words, you gained no advantage in effort by using this machine. What did you gain?

In the second part of this activity when you used a traveling block pulley, a mechanical advantage of approximately 2 was found. With this machine, you could lift a 100-gram weight with an effort of only a little more than 50 grams. To understand how this can be so, look again at your pulley. The total downward pull is the weight of the object being lifted plus the weight of the pulley. Assume that this total is 100 grams. To balance this downward pull of 100 grams, there must be a

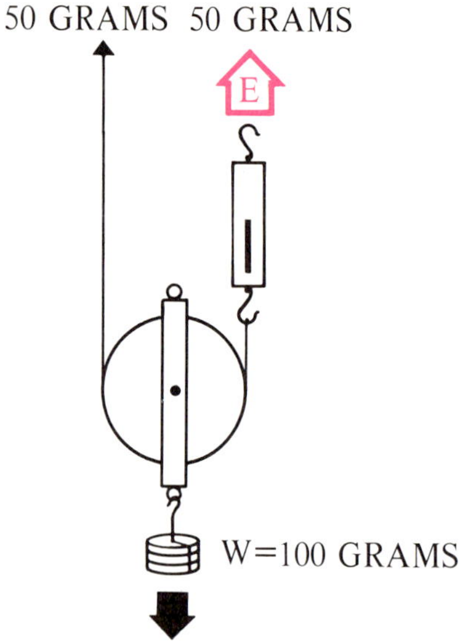


**3.12** Each string supports only a portion of the total weight.

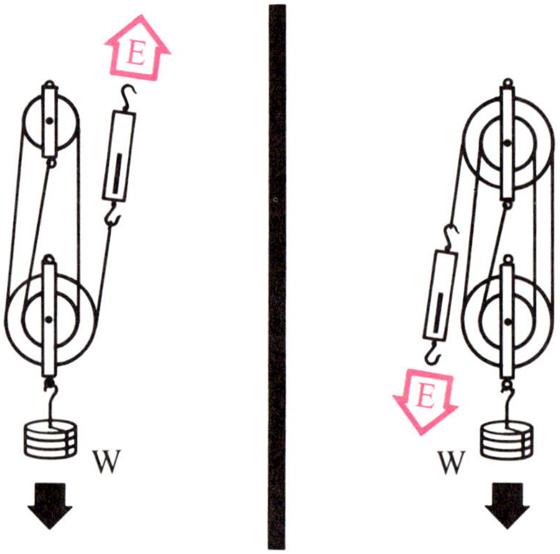


**3.13a,b** The mechanical advantage of both pulley systems is four.

total upward pull of 100 grams by the two strings. Your spring scale shows that one string supports 50 grams, so you can easily see that the other string supports the other 50 grams.

Figure 3.13a above shows a combination of several of these pulleys. The weight of the object being lifted plus the weight of the traveling block pulley is supported by four ropes. Thus, each rope bears ¼ of the total weight. Since the effort is put into one of these weight-bearing ropes, the effort will be only ¼ of the total weight being raised. The mechanical advantage of this **block and tackle** is about 4. Notice that this mechanical advantage is equal to the number of *weight-bearing ropes* involved.

Figure 3.13b shows a more normal arrangement for a block and tackle, with the effort being exerted in a *downward* direction. In this arrangement, we would again find a mechanical advantage of 4. Can you explain why this is so?

Another simple machine is the **inclined (in klīn′) plane.** Two common examples of inclined planes are the planks used in loading trucks and the ramps in hospitals for patients using wheelchairs.

## Working With an Inclined Plane

**MATERIALS:**

A board several centimeters wide and at least one meter long, a toy car, a weight that can be set into or on the car, a spring scale, a stack of books about 30 centimeters high

**PROCEDURE:**

Place the board so that it forms a ramp from the floor to the top of the stack of books. Pull the car, carrying the weight, up the inclined plane by use of the spring scale as shown in Figure 3.14. Try to pull the car at a steady speed.

Calculate the mechanical advantage of this machine by dividing the weight of the car by the force required to pull it up the inclined plane. How can you change the mechanical advantage of the inclined plane?

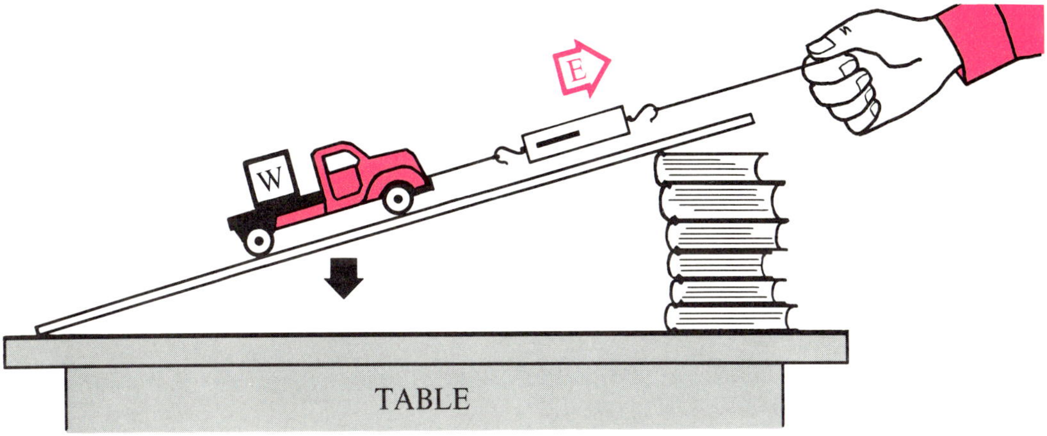


**3.14** What happens to the effort (E) required to pull the truck if the inclined plane is made steeper?

The **wedge** (wej) used to split logs, and the sharp edge of a knife blade are other examples of inclined planes (Figure 3.15). A **screw** (skrü) is an inclined plane placed **spirally** (spī′ rəl i), like a corkscrew.

## The Amount of Work Done

At first, it might appear to you as though the use of machines such as the crowbar, the wheelbarrow, the pulley that moves upward with the weight, and the inclined plane all save work. However, work is measured by multiplying the weight raised times the distance that it is moved. As the following activity will show, machines are *not* capable of saving work. These machines simply make work *easier*.

**3.15** Examples of common inclined planes

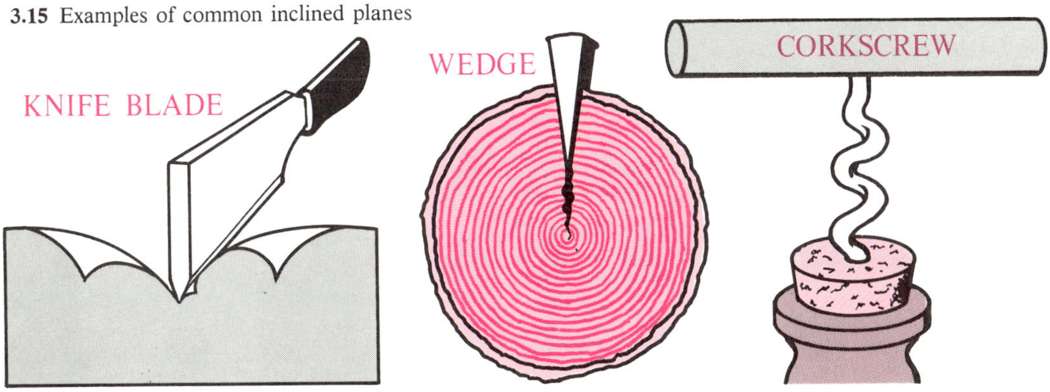

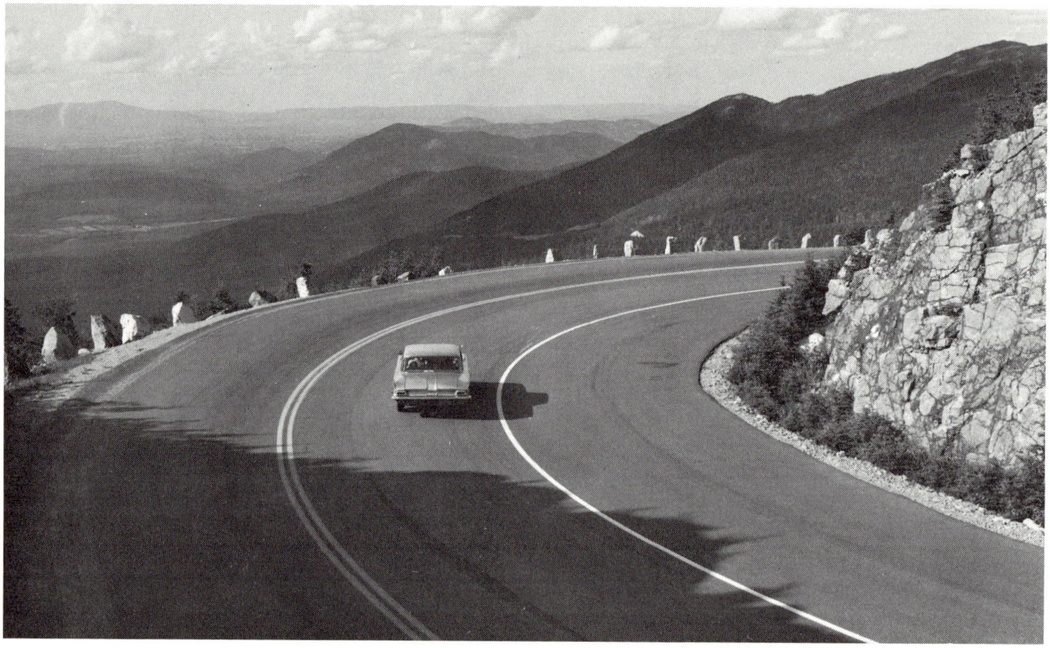

New York State Department of Commerce photo

**3.16** A mountain road is a type of inclined plane.

## Calculating the Work Done by a Machine

**MATERIALS:**

A meterstick or yardstick, a heavy weight, a spring scale, a small block of wood (preferably triangular), a pulley, a length of string, a board several centimeters wide and one meter long, a toy car, a stack of books about 60 centimeters high

**PROCEDURE:**

Set up the lever as you did in the activity on page 68. Move the weight upward by pulling on the spring scale. Measure the height moved by the weight, and calculate the work done (weight × distance). Measure the distance moved by the spring scale and calculate the work put into the machine (effort × distance). How does the work put into the lever compare with the work done by the lever? Set up each of the other activities (pages 71, 73, and 74) and calculate the work put into the machine and the work obtained. To calculate the work done by the inclined plane, a slightly different set of data is needed. The final effect of using this machine was to move the car and weight to the top of the stack of books. Therefore, the work done by the machine is equal to the total weight raised times the height of the books. The work put into the machine is equal to the force as shown by the spring scale times the distance the spring scale actually moved—the length of the board.

*Save the data from this activity for use in the next section.*

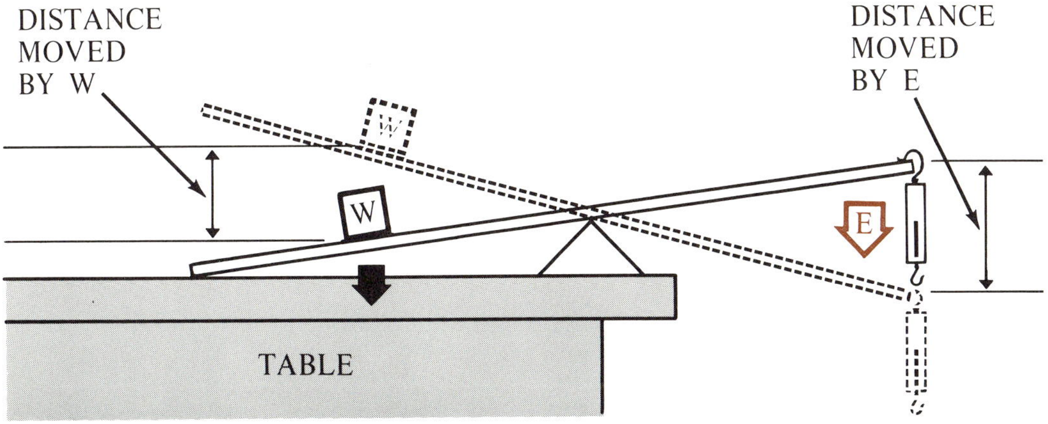


**3.17** The distance moved by W and the distance moved by E are used on page 79 to calculate the ideal mechanical advantage.

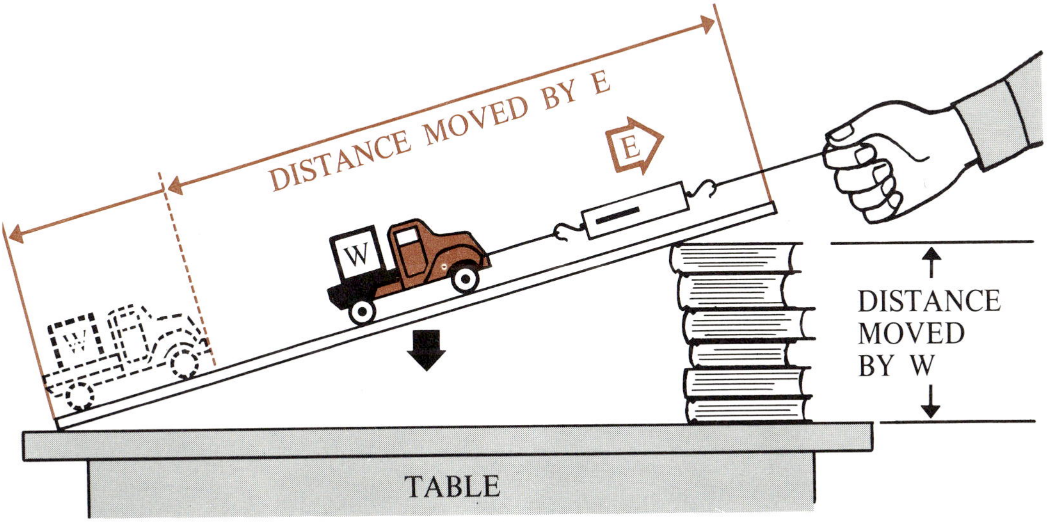


**3.18** The vertical distance moved by W and the length of the board moved by E are used on page 79 to calculate the ideal mechanical advantage.

These three machines—the lever, the pulley, and the inclined plane—are called **simple machines.** Many common tools are examples of these machines. For example, a screwdriver and a brace and bit are both types of levers.

Can you explain how to calculate the distances between the fulcrum and the resistance, and the fulcrum and the effort involved in these tools?

**Complex machines,** however complicated they may seem, are merely combinations of various simple machines. Look at some complex machines. Can you see any parts that are levers, or pulleys, or inclined planes in Figure 3.19 on the next page?

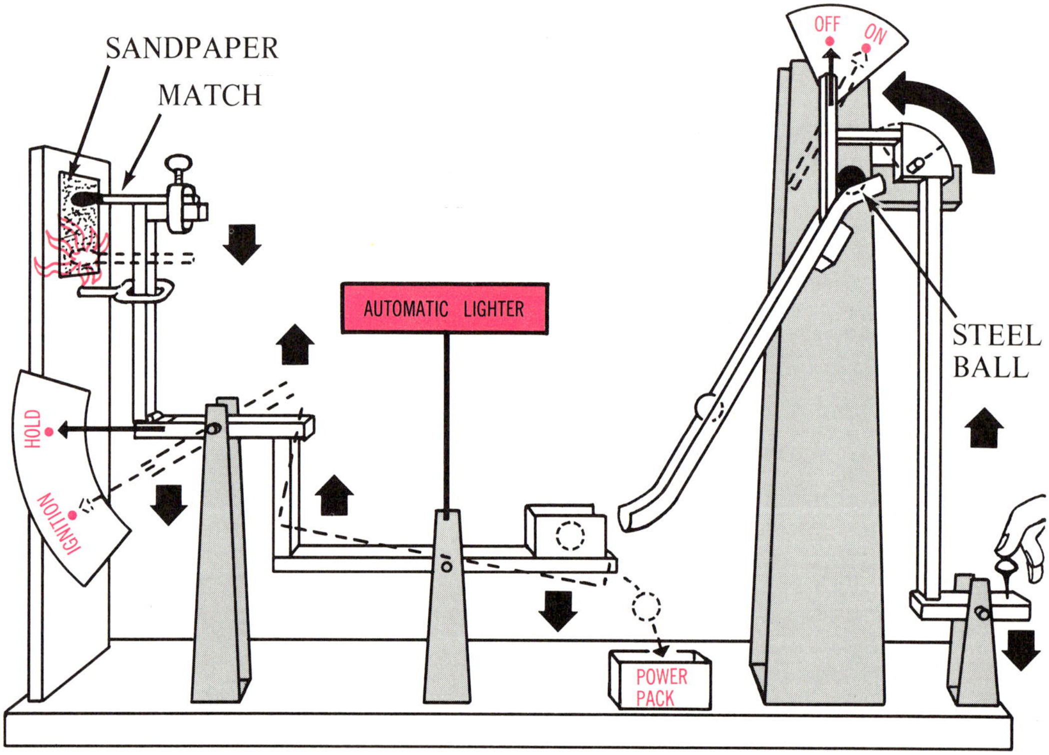


**3.19** Can you follow the mechanical forces as this "Automatic Lighter" goes into action?

## Have You Learned?

Calculate the answers for the following problems:

1. Using a block and tackle, a man lifts one ton (1,000 kg) by pulling on the rope with a force of 50 kg. What is the mechanical advantage of this pulley system?

2. If a block and tackle has five weight-bearing ropes, approximately how much effort will be required to lift a 50 kg weight (mass)?

3. If you push on the end of a lever with an effort of 25 kg and move it 2 meters, how much work did you put into the machine?

4. A tractor pulls a trailer to the top of a hill that is 50 meters high. If the weight of the tractor plus the weight of the trailer plus the weight of the load totals 20,000 kilograms and the tractor exerts a pull of 2,000 kilograms, how much work is done? If the road up which the tractor moved is 1,000 meters long, how much work is put into the job?

## 4. Overcoming and Using Friction

> **ARE YOU READY?**
>
> Look up the following words if you are not sure of their meanings:
>
> actual; efficient; friction; ideal; inclined plane; mechanical advantage; projection.

In the last section, you learned how to calculate the mechanical advantage of a machine. By using the *actual* weight of the object moved and dividing this by the *actual* effort that it took to move the object, you obtained the *actual* mechanical advantage.

You also saw that when the effort that it took to move an object was less than the weight of the object, you had to move the force over a longer distance than the object actually moved. If the distance the force moves is divided by the distance the weight moves, an *ideal* mechanical advantage is calculated. Because of friction, the actual mechanical advantage is not as large as the ideal mechanical advantage.

### Noticing Ideal Versus Actual Mechanical Advantage

**MATERIALS:**

The data obtained while doing the activity on page 76, pencil and paper

**PROCEDURE:**

For each of the simple machines studied so far, calculate the actual mechanical advantage (weight ÷ effort). Calculate the ideal mechanical advantage by dividing the distance the spring scale moved by the distance the weight moved. (For example, see Figure 3.17.) Remember that in the case of the inclined plane, the useful distance the weight is moved is the height of the stack of books. (See Figure 3.18.) Compare the figures for each machine. Is the actual mechanical advantage (AMA) less than the ideal mechanical advantage (IMA) in each case?

If the actual mechanical advantage is divided by the ideal mechanical advantage, a fraction is obtained. This fraction indicates the **efficiency** of the machine. The efficiency of any machine is always less than 100%.

The **ratio** (rā′ shi ō) that shows the efficiency of a machine is a comparison of the work obtained from the machine compared with the work put into the machine. Therefore, another way to compute the efficiency of a machine is to divide the

$$\frac{\text{AMA}}{\text{IMA}} = \text{EFFICIENCY} = \frac{\text{WORK DONE ON WEIGHT}}{\text{WORK DONE BY EFFORT}}$$

work done on the weight (weight × distance moved) by the work done by the effort (effort × distance moved). This ratio is the same as that calculated by using the actual and the ideal mechanical advantages.

Since a certain amount of energy is needed to perform a certain amount of work, we can say that machines actually waste energy. Yet energy cannot be destroyed by these machines. The loss in energy shown by the efficiency ratios must have been changed in form. Generally, this change means a conversion to heat energy.

One of the main causes of this loss of energy is **friction.** Heat is produced as a result of friction. Rub your hands together very rapidly, and you can feel the heat generated.

## Observing Friction

**MATERIALS:**

A weight, a board several centimeters wide and one meter long, a length of string, a spring scale, a piece of sandpaper, 4 thumb-tacks, a small piece of cotton

**PROCEDURE:**

Tack the sandpaper to the board. Pull the weight by means of the spring scale across the sandpaper and onto the board. Record the effort necessary to pull the weight along at a steady speed while it is moving across the sandpaper and while it is moving across the bare board.

Rub the cotton across the board and across the sandpaper. Explain the observations that you make.

**3.20** The rough surface of this board increases friction.

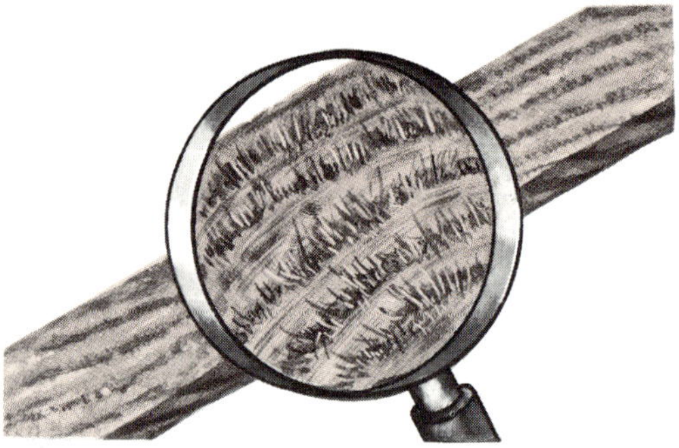

One explanation for the cause of friction is that the surfaces of the two objects being rubbed together have projections that catch on each other. Thus, the movement of an object is slowed down somewhat, and a greater effort is needed to move it over rougher surfaces.

Any time two surfaces move against each other, we can expect to find friction. Can you find the spots of possible friction in each of the machines you used in Sections 2 and 3?

Since the presence of friction in a machine wastes energy, it would be useful if a way could be found to eliminate friction or at least reduce it as much as possible. Making the two surfaces that touch each other as smooth as possible is one way of doing this. If you were to sandpaper the board used in the last activity so that it was very, very smooth, you would find that the weight would move with less effort. **Lubrication** (lü′ brə kā′ shən) is another method of reducing friction. Oil and grease are often placed on the moving parts of machines for this purpose.

The friction caused by sliding an object over another is much greater than the friction caused by rolling one object over another. The Egyptians and other ancient peoples probably knew this, and placed rollers under the huge stones that they used in their buildings. We use wheels for the same purpose. In a heavy machine, the axle is generally supported by a steel **bearing** (bãr′ ing). The rollers or balls of these bearings hold the axle in one position, yet allow it to touch only a rolling surface.

**3.21** The ancient Egyptians used logs as rollers. The stone blocks for the pyramids were placed on wooden sledges, and these were pulled up earthen ramps, which had been put up against the face of the pyramid. The rollers reduced the friction between the sledge and the earthen ramp. Each block weighed about 2,250 kilograms.

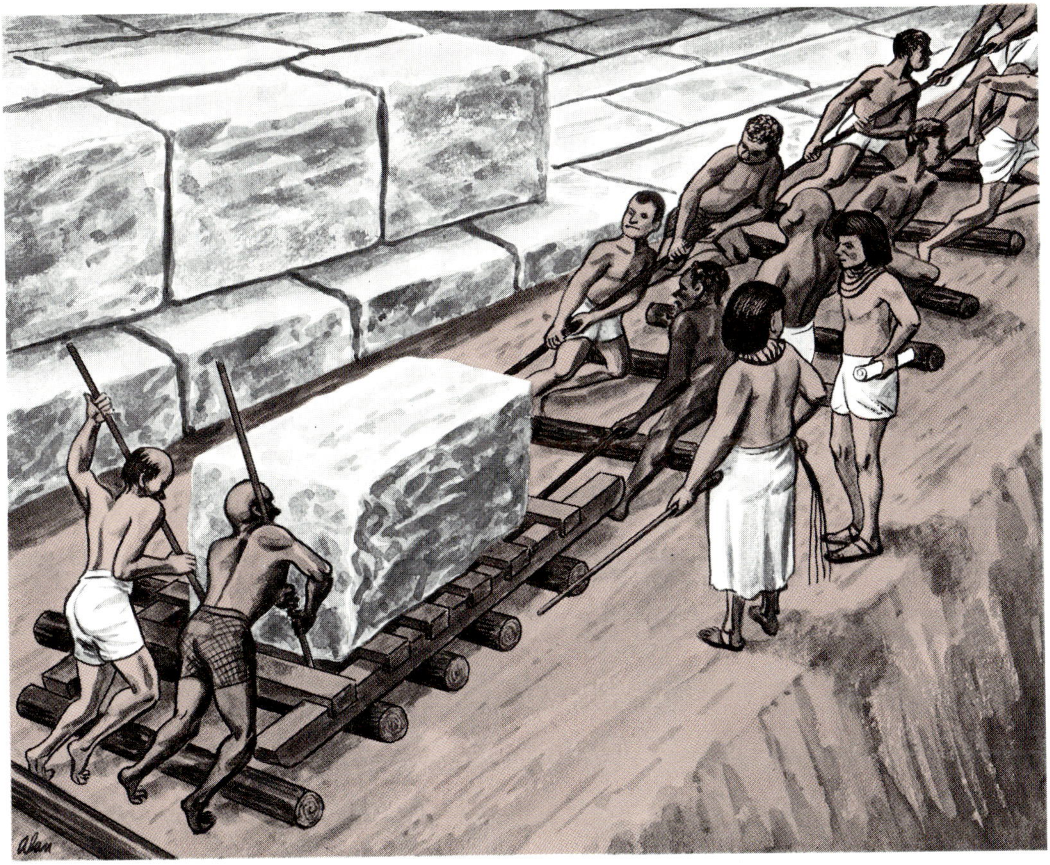

But friction is not all bad. Have you ever fallen from a bicycle because its wheels slid on some loose rocks? Or have you ever fallen because you slipped on ice on the sidewalk? Friction between the

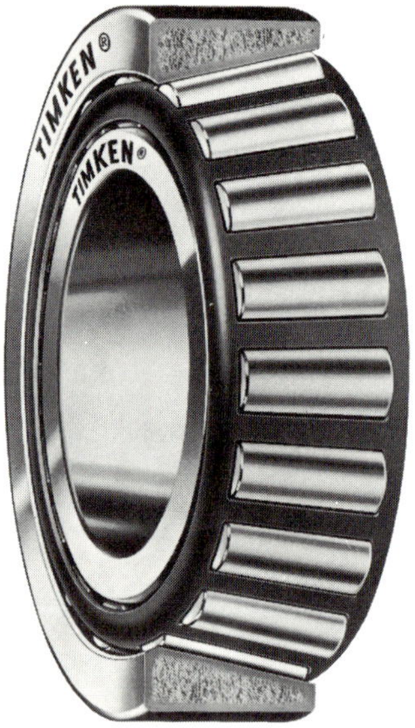


*The Timken Company*

**3.22** The rollers of these bearings hold the axle in one position, yet allow it to touch only a rolling surface.

bottoms of our shoes and the ground allows us to walk without slipping. Without friction we could not move as we do now.

Because of this it is necessary for us to increase friction at certain times. We make ice less slippery by putting sand or ashes on it. We increase the friction between the tires of a car or bicycle and the road by putting deep grooves in the rubber of the tire. When a car is stuck in the snow or mud, the driver will often try to increase the friction by putting some type of rough material between the tire and the ground.

Imagine that suddenly friction were to disappear for a time. Can you describe how you would act? What would happen to the dishes on the breakfast table? How would you get to school? What would happen to objects that are held together by nails and screws? Could you write on a piece of paper with a pencil?

## Have You Learned?

Answer the following questions, using as few words as possible.

While lifting a weight of 1,000 grams with a block and tackle, a boy exerted an effort of 100 grams. He noticed that in order to lift the weight 1 meter, he had to pull the end of the rope 12 meters.

1. Calculate the actual mechanical advantage (AMA) of the pulleys.
2. Calculate the ideal mechanical advantage (IMA) of the pulleys.
3. Using the AMA and the IMA, calculate the efficiency of the machine.
4. Calculate the efficiency of the machine *without* using the AMA and the IMA.
5. Explain why the AMA was smaller than the IMA.

**3.23** The tread or grooves of a rubber tire

*The Goodyear Tire & Rubber Company*

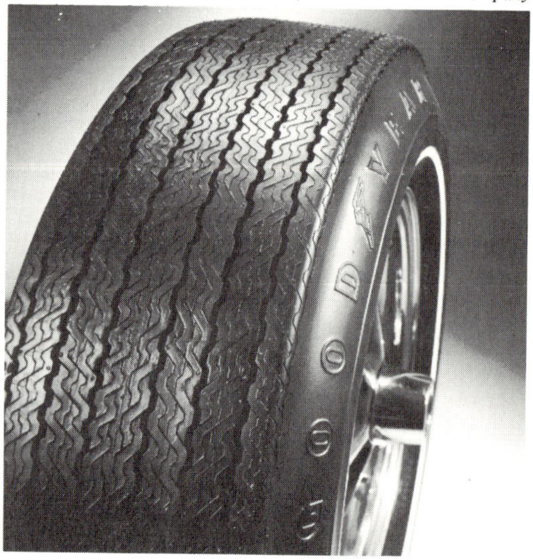

## 5. Behavior of Fluids

> **ARE YOU READY?**
>
> Look up the following words if you are not sure of their meanings:
>
> force; liquid; matter; mercury; resistance.

So far we have considered the effects of forces on only solid objects. **Fluids** (flü′ id), forms of matter that will flow, have a few special properties that should be understood. Both gases and liquids are fluids.

Perhaps you have felt the resistance of air when you rode on a bicycle or in an open car. You may know how difficult it is to row a boat because of the resistance of water. If so, you already realize that some fluids offer more resistance to the objects passing through them than do other fluids. We recognize that some fluids do not pour so easily as others. Heavy motor oil and syrup are examples of **viscous** (vis′ kəs) fluids.

Perhaps you have noticed that certain liquids can be poured into a container until they rise above the rim, yet do not spill over. Or perhaps you have seen a water bug walk on the surface of the water of a pond. Or you may have seen a steel sewing needle floating on the surface of a glass of water. In each case, the surface of the water acted as if it were a sheet of film, thicker than the other portions of the liquid. This effect is known as **surface tension.**

All matter is apparently composed of tiny particles, called **molecules** (mol′ ə kūl). Each molecule in a substance attracts every other molecule near it. This attraction between molecules of the same type is known as **cohesion** (kō hē′ zhən).

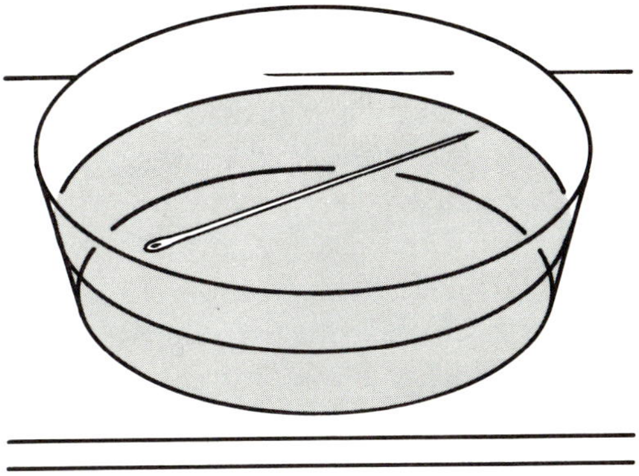

3.24 Can you do this?

At the surface of a liquid, almost all of the pull on a molecule is from molecules on its sides and from the molecules below it. As a result of these unbalanced cohesive forces, the molecules on the surface of a liquid are pulled very closely together. This packing forms the surface film that is so surprisingly strong. Water dropped on a piece of waxed paper or mercury spilled onto a tabletop illustrates one effect of this cohesive force (Figure 6.9 page 193). These liquids tend to form balls due to the attraction of the molecules for each other. As you might guess, the cohesive forces within solids are much stronger than they are in liquids.

3.25 At the surface of a liquid, almost all of the pull on a molecule is from molecules on its sides and from the molecules below it.

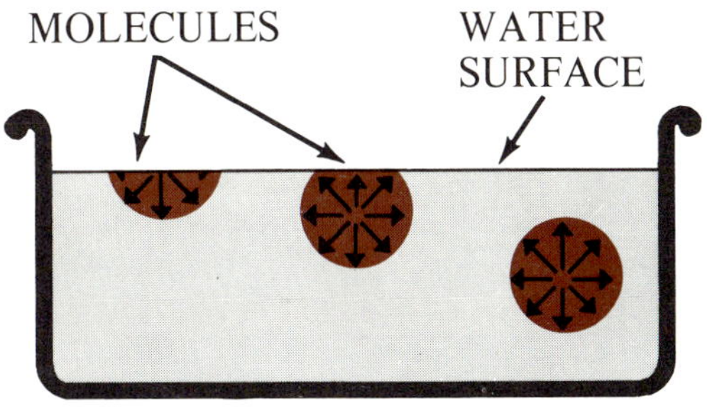

The opposite property is **adhesion** (ad hē′ zhən), which accounts for some other interesting phenomena of liquids. Adhesion is the attraction between *unlike* molecules. Examples of adhesion are the sticking of glue, paste, or adhesive tape to various objects. If an object is made wet when it is dipped into a liquid, we know that the adhesive forces between the molecules of the liquid and the molecules of the object are stronger than the cohesive forces between the molecules of the liquid.

### Water Rises up Tiny Tubes

Perhaps you have seen cases in which liquids were able to move through small openings in solids, apparently rising against the pull of gravity. This phenomenon is known as **capillary** (kap′ ə ler′ i) **action.** It is caused by a combination of cohesive and adhesive forces.

## Observing Capillary Action

**MATERIALS:**

A container of water, a bottle of ink, a facial tissue, a paper towel, two small plates of glass, two rubber bands

**PROCEDURE:**

Tear a narrow strip from the facial tissue. Place one end in the container of water. Observe what happens.

Place a drop of ink on a piece of scrap paper. Dip the end of the paper towel into the drop of ink. Observe what happens.

Place one of the rubber bands over the end of one of the small glass plates. The rubber band should remain as near to the edge of the plate as possible. Lay the other glass plate over the first. The rubber band should act as a block, holding the two plates of glass slightly apart at one edge while allowing the opposite edges to touch each other. Place the second rubber band around both plates, at right angles to the first rubber band, to hold them tightly in place.

Stand the two pieces of glass on edge in such a way that the narrow edge of the wedge is to your left and the broader edge, formed by the rubber band block, is to your right. Keeping the plates in this position, stand them up in the water. Observe carefully. Does the water seem to rise up between the plates of glass? Does it rise higher where the two plates are close together?

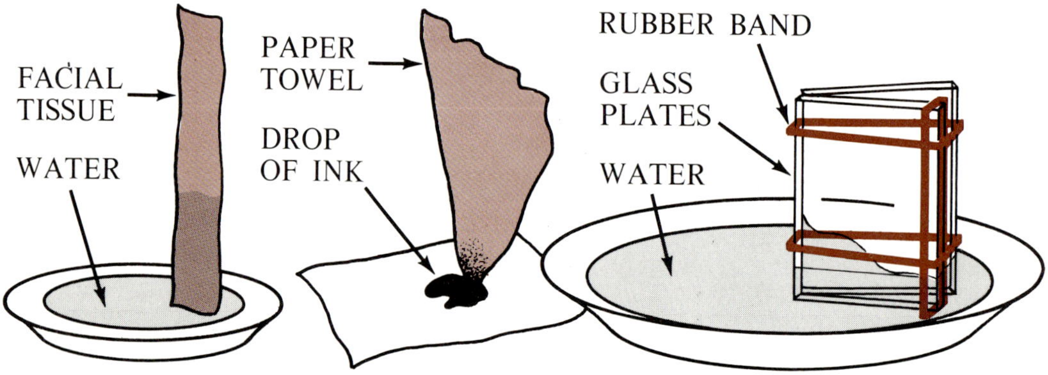

The word *capillary* means "hairlike," and capillary action occurs only in small, "hairsized" spaces. If your school owns some capillary tubes, you may be able to make several interesting observations. You will notice that the surface of the water within the capillary tube is curved *downward*, as shown in Figure 3.26. The strong adhesive force between the water molecules and the glass molecules pulls the edges of the water column up the tube. The fairly strong surface tension, or cohesive force, of the water forces the water in the center of the tube to follow, but to a slightly lesser height. As a result the water rises in the tube. The smaller the diameter of the tube, the higher the water will rise. This is because the surface tension does not have to act over such a large area in the smaller tube.

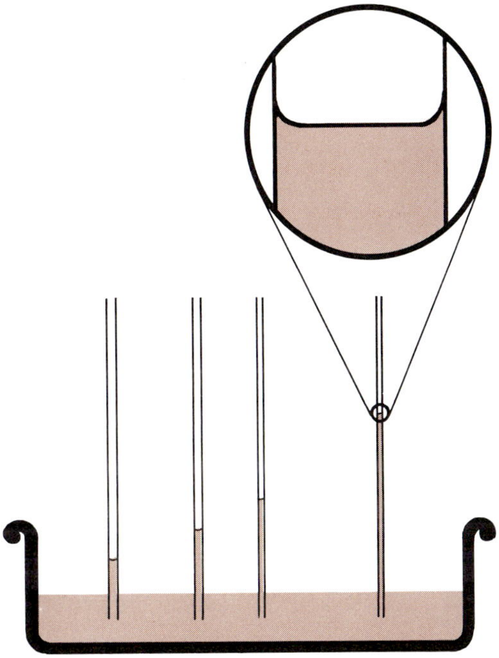

**3.26** Notice the various water levels in the tubes.

Mercury is an example of a liquid that does not rise in a capillary tube. Neither will mercury wet a glass tube, as water does. Both of these phenomena occur for the same reason. In the case of mercury, the cohesive forces are stronger than the adhesive forces. The attraction between the molecules of mercury are greater than the attraction between the molecules of glass and those of mercury. As a result, when a capillary tube is placed in mercury, the liquid is actually forced *down* the tube, as shown on page 86.

## Have You Learned?

From the list at the right select the word that best completes each sentence below. Each answer may be used more than once, if necessary. (Do not write in your book.)

1. Matter that will flow is known as ____.
2. ____ causes the surface of a liquid to act as if it were thicker than the rest of the liquid.
3. Motor oil and syrup are examples of ____ liquids.
4. Attraction between molecules of the same type is known as ____.
5. Liquids move through small, hairlike spaces by ____.
6. Attraction between molecules of different types is known as ____.
7. All matter is composed of tiny particles called ____.

a. cohesion
b. capillary action
c. surface tension
d. adhesion
e. molecules
f. fluid
g. viscous

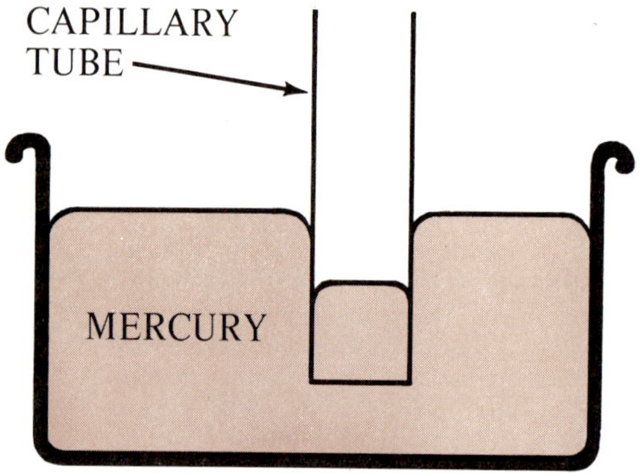


**3.27** Capillary tube in mercury

## 6. Pressure in Fluids

> **ARE YOU READY?**
>
> Look up the following words if you are not sure of their meanings:
>
> apparent; compressed air; density; fluid; force; piston; unit; weight.

Since both liquids and gases are matter, they have weight. They, like solids, exert a force against the objects on which they rest. This force is called **pressure** when it is calculated as the amount of force acting on a unit of surface area.

For example, a cubic meter of water weighs 1,000 kilograms. If we place this water in a tall container that has a bottom with an area of one square meter, the water will exert a pressure of 1,000 kilograms per square meter on the bottom of the container. If we add a second cubic meter of water to the container, the water will push on the bottom of the container with a force of 2,000 kilograms (1,000 × 2). The pressure at the bottom of the container will be 2,000 kilograms per square meter (Figure 3.28).

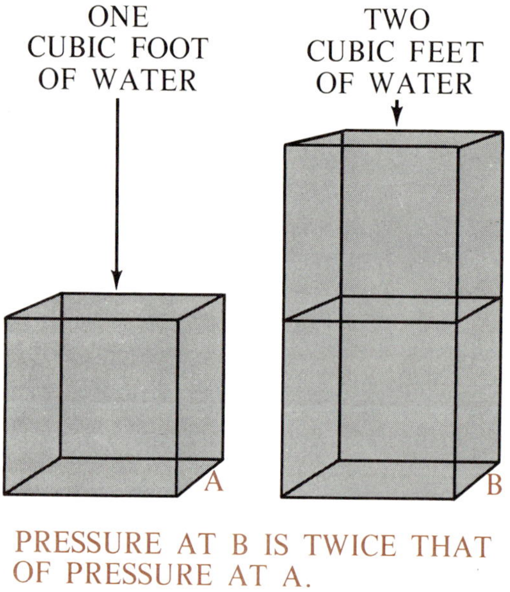


**3.28** If a second cubic meter of water is placed on top of the first, the pressure will be doubled.

The pressure at the bottom of two containers of differing shapes is the same if the height of the water is the same in each. To calculate the pressure at the bottom of a lake, all we need to know is the depth of the water at the point we are interested in. If the water is 10 meters deep, it exerts a pressure of 10,000 kilograms per square meter. It makes no difference how the lake is shaped or what volume of water is in the lake.

Naturally, the density of the substance is important in calculating pressure. The heavier a fluid is per unit volume, the greater its pressure will be at a certain depth. All that one needs to do to calculate the pressure of a fluid is to multiply the density of the fluid times the depth of the fluid. For example, the pressure of a column of mercury 1 meter high is 1,360 grams per square centimeter!

The pressure of a fluid is exerted in *all* directions—downward, upward, and to all sides. You can demonstrate the sideward pressure by punching a few small holes in the side of a tall juice can. When the can is filled, the water will be forced out through the holes. Near the bottom of the can, where the pressure is the greatest, the water will spurt out with more force.

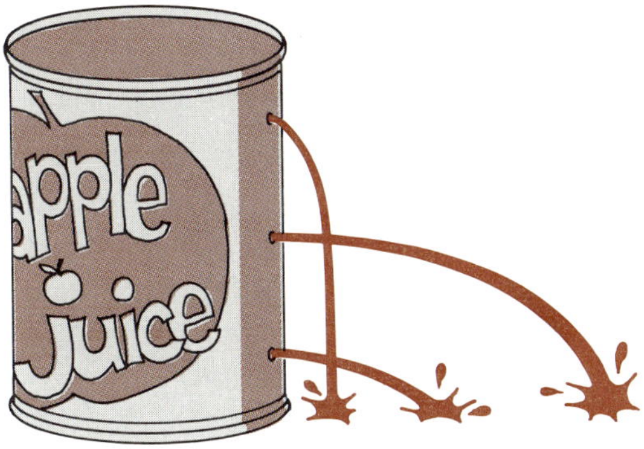


**3.29** If the pressure is greatest at the bottom, why doesn't the lowest stream go as far out as the stream near the middle of the can? The distance each stream travels away from the can depends on two things—the force with which the water spurts out and the distance it has to fall. Try increasing the distance the water has to fall. How does this change the horizontal distance away from the can of each spurt of water?

The idea that pressure applied to an enclosed fluid acts equally in all directions was first stated by a French scientist named Pascal (pas kal′), and is now known as **Pascal's Law.** Figure 3.30 shows what can happen if you exert pressure on the liquid in a glass jug by sharply hitting the cork stopper. Perhaps you have done this same "experiment" accidentally when you tried to force the stopper into an overfull Thermos bottle.

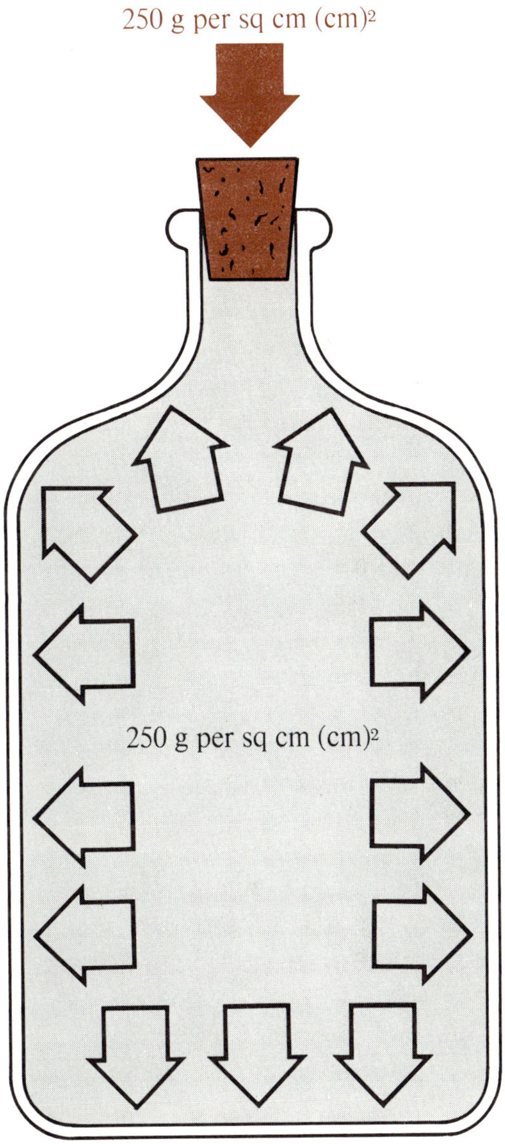


**3.30** Cork pressure equals pressure on inside walls.

Technologists have invented many machines that apply Pascal's Law. Those that use the pressure of a liquid are called **hydraulic** (hī drô′ lik) devices. Those that use gases are known as **pneumatic** (nü mat′ ik) devices. Regardless of which fluid is used, all of these machines work in much the same way. Since the pressure throughout the machine is the same, a small force applied to a small area will result in a large total force being exerted in all parts of the fluid.

The Figure 3.31 shows how such a machine might work. Suppose that the small piston *A* has a surface area of 1 sq. centimeter, and the large piston *B* has a surface area of 1,000 sq. centimeters. A force of 5 kilograms applied to the small piston will increase the pressure of the fluid within the machine by 5 kilograms per square centimeter. The total increase in force against the large piston will then be 5,000 kilograms! Remember that Pascal's Law states that the pressure in enclosed liquids acts equally in all directions. In the case of the machine in Figure 3.31, the force on the large piston is equal to 5 kilograms per square centimeter × 1,000 square centimeters (area of large piston), or 5,000 kilograms.

As you already have learned, we cannot obtain more work from a machine than we put in. If the large piston moves one cm, how far will the smaller piston travel?

## Floating Objects

The force in fluids that is exerted in an upward direction causes certain objects to float in them. This force is called **buoyancy** (boi′ ən si).

**3.31** This hydraulic lift can raise 5,000 kilograms when a 5-kilogram mass are put on the small piston.

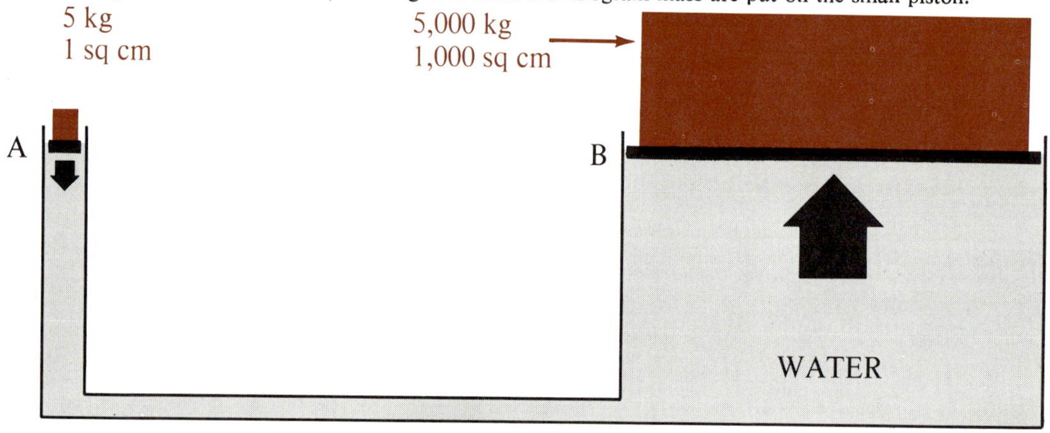


## Investigating Buoyancy

**MATERIALS:**

A tin can about the size of a beaker, enough water to fill this can, a large, flat pan (such as a cake pan), a sensitive spring scale, a small tin can that can be attached to the spring scale, a small, very dense object (such as a piece of lead or iron), a short piece of string

**PROCEDURE:**

Set the larger tin can in the shallow pan. Completely fill the larger can with water, until its surface tension allows the water to be heaped up over the top of the can. Tie the dense object to the spring scale with a piece of string, and record its weight. Then carefully lower the weight into the can of water. Water should pour over the rim of the can and into the shallow pan below. Record the weight of the object while it is under water. Calculate the difference between the weight of the object out of water and its weight while under water. The apparent loss of weight is due to the buoyant force of the water (Figure 3.33).

Remove the object and the large tin can from the shallow pan. Into the smaller tin can carefully pour the water that overflowed and was caught. Calculate the water weight.

The weight of the water that was pushed out by the object should be the same as the apparent loss of weight of the object while it was under water. How does the volume of this amount of water compare with the volume of the object?

You have just observed a phenomenon discovered by the Greek Archimedes (är′ kə mē′ dēz) more than 2,000 years ago. He discovered that an object in a fluid is pushed upward by buoyancy that is equal to the weight of the fluid displaced (or pushed out of the way) by the object.

This principle of Archimedes explains why some objects float and others do not. Suppose we have an object one cubic meter in size weighing 500 kilograms. When placed in water, it sinks until it displaces 500 kilograms, or ½ cubic meter of water. Since the weight of the water displaced is equal to the weight of the object, it floats. How much of the object would be under water? If the weight of the object were more than 1,000 kilograms, what would happen when placed in water?

A submarine is made heavier by taking seawater into its ballast tanks, and is made

**3.32** How does this craft sink or float?

*Official U. S. Navy Photograph*

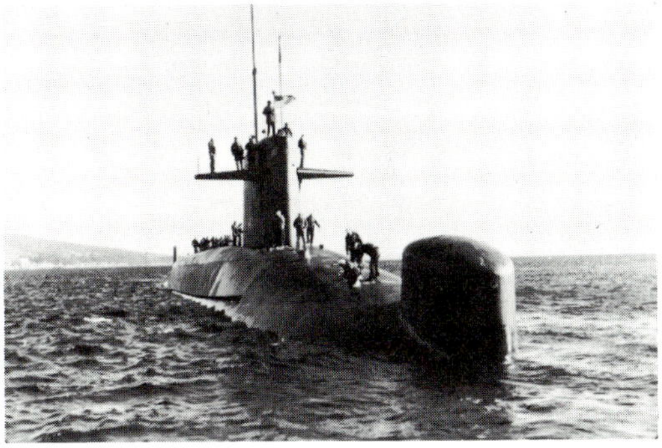

**3.33** Objects in water weigh less than in air.

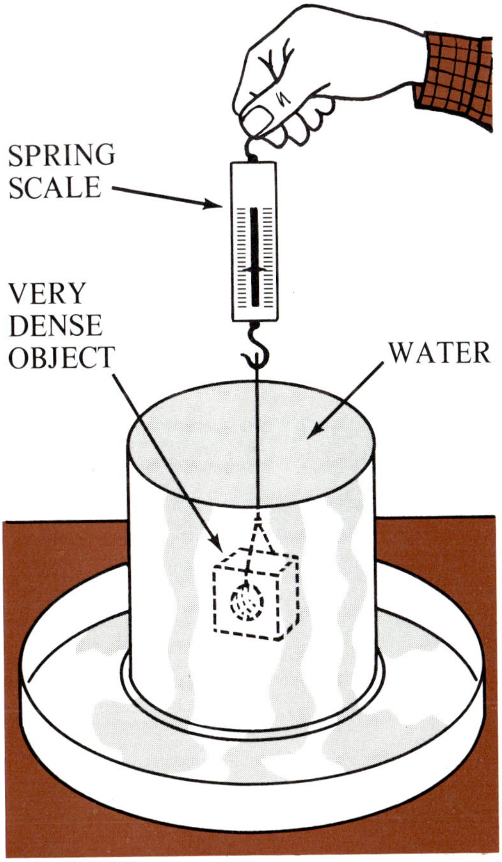

lighter by blowing the water out with compressed air. Can you explain why these actions make the submarine sink or float?

## Have You Learned?

On a sheet of paper list the numbers for the questions below. By each number write *T* if the statement is true and *F* if false.

1. The pressure of a liquid is equal to its total downward force.
2. Pressure is measured by multiplying the depth of the liquid times the density of the liquid.
3. The pressure of a liquid is exerted only downward on the bottom of the container and upward on any floating object.
4. A hydraulic device is a machine that applies Pascal's Law.
5. A pneumatic device is one that uses liquids like water and oil.
6. An object in a liquid is pushed upward with a force that is equal to the weight of the fluid displaced by the object.
7. Archimedes was a Greek who discovered the principle of buoyancy.
8. A cubic foot of water weighs 1,000 kg. At a depth of 3 meters the pressure of the water in a lake is 3,000 kg per square meter (3 × 1,000), regardless of the volume of the water in the lake.
9. An object that has a volume of one cubic meter will float in water if its weight is *less* than 1,000 kg (one cubic meter of water weighs 1,000 kg).
10. A hydraulic device will produce more work than is put into it.

## 7. Science of Falling Bodies

**ARE YOU READY?**

Look up the following words if you are not sure of their meanings:

accelerate; average; maximum; resistance; skydive.

Suppose that we were to drop a heavy rock from a tall building or an airplane. If we were able to observe it carefully, we would discover that it moved faster and faster as it fell. If we were to measure the speed of this falling rock, we would find that at the end of the first second, it was moving at a rate of 9.8 meters per second. At the end of the second second, the speed of the falling rock would be about 19.6 meters per second. And, at the end of the third second, its speed would be 29.4 meters per second. Notice that the rock fell about 9.8 meters per second faster each second.

Can you figure out how far the rock would have fallen at the end of the first second? Since the speed of the rock at the time it was dropped was zero, and its speed at the end of the first second was 9.8 meters per second, its *average* speed during this second was 4.9 meters per second. When an object is increasing its speed at a uniform or even rate, the average speed can be found by adding the speed at the beginning (0) to the speed at the end (9.8 meters/second) and dividing by 2 ($0 + 9.8 = 9.8$; $9.8 \div 2 = 4.9$ meters/second).

If the rock's average speed was 4.9 meters per second and it fell for one second, it must have fallen 4.9 meters.

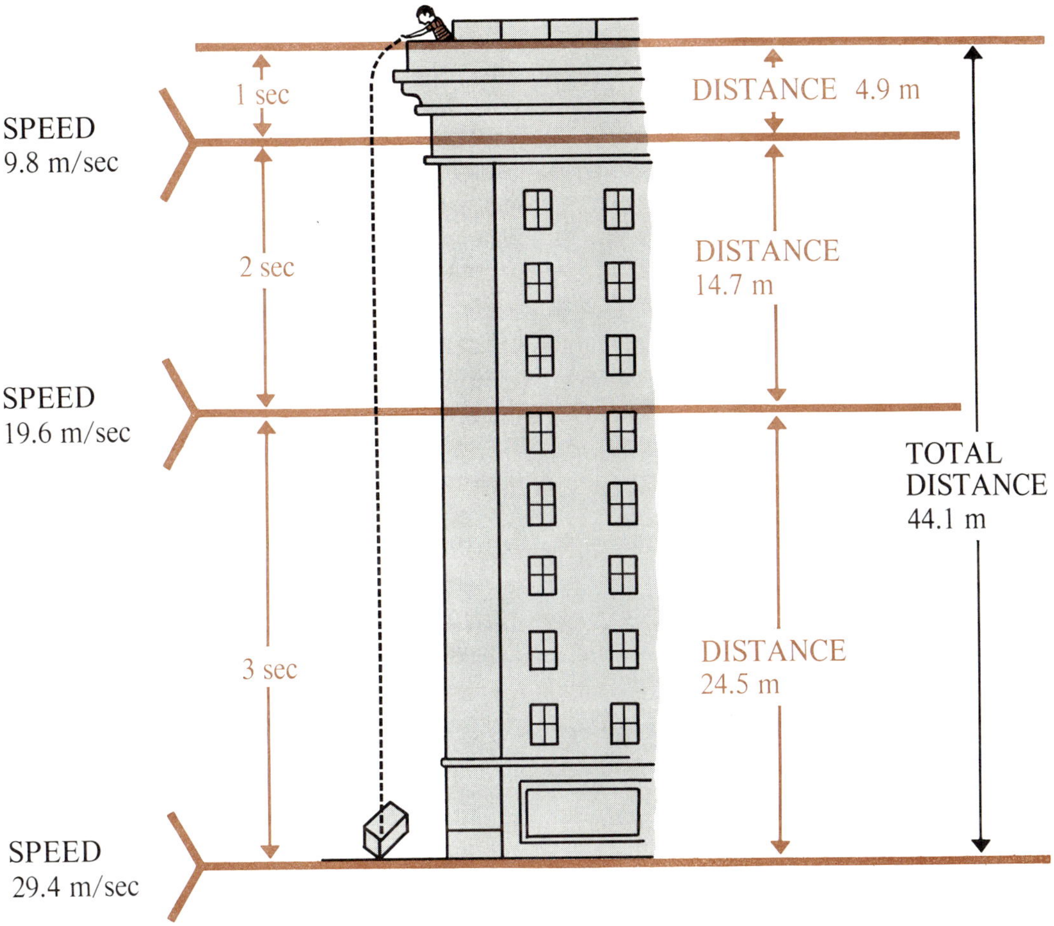


**3.34** Notice that the speed of the box increased as it fell.

Can you calculate how far the rock would fall during each of the next two seconds and how far it would fall during the entire three seconds? Check your answers by comparing them with those in Figure 3.34.

The force that causes this increase in speed is the gravitational pull of the earth. The increase in speed of a freely falling body due to the gravitational pull of the earth is known as **g.** In most parts of the world, one g is approximately 9.8 meters per second for each second the object falls.

To calculate the final speed of a falling body, you multiply 9.8 meters times the number of seconds the object falls. From this answer, the average speed and the distance covered also can be calculated. Do you see how this can be done?

Of course, the rock is falling through the air, and the push of the air against the rock slows it down. The figures given above would be exact only if the rock were falling in a **vacuum** (vak′ u əm), a place where there is no air. As the speed of the falling rock increases, the upward push of the air also increases. Eventually a maximum speed is reached, and no further increase in speed takes place.

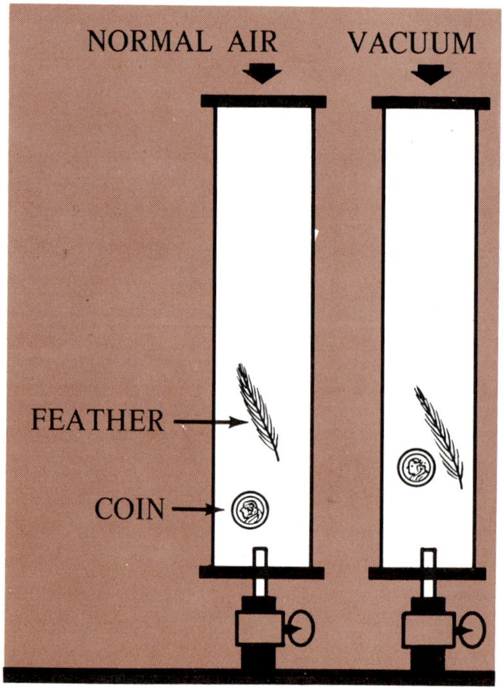


**3.35** When the air is removed from this tube, the coin and the feather will fall at the same speed.

When a skydiver jumps from an airplane, his downward speed increases very much like the rock described above. When his speed reaches about 240 kilometers per hour, the resistance of the air balances the pull of gravity, and his speed does not increase. When he opens his parachute, the air pushes against a larger surface, his speed decreases, and he lands safely.

An increase in the speed of an object is known as **acceleration** (ak sel′ ər ā′ shən). You may have learned this word in speaking of automobiles. When a car's speed is increased, we say that it is *accelerating*.

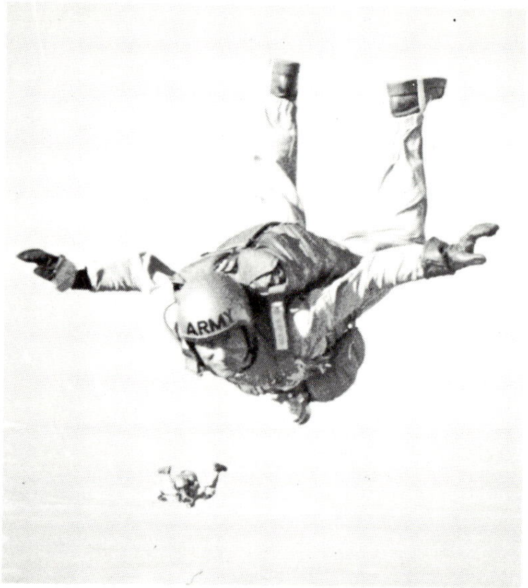


*Office of Secretary of Defense*

**3.36** Even without his parachute the speed of a skydiver will not increase beyond about 240 kilometers per hour. Can you explain why?

The gas pedal that is pushed down by the driver to increase the speed of a car is called the *accelerator*.

The speed of an object does not always increase, of course. A ball batted vertically into the air will *decrease* in speed. In this case, three forces are acting on the ball. The first is the force with which it is batted upward. Second is the pull of gravity. The third is the resistance of the air that the ball passes through. The result of all these forces is to slow the speed of the ball down until it eventually stops. Then the ball begins to fall toward the earth, in the same way the freely falling rock did (Figure 3.34).

If you can accurately measure the time it takes an object that is thrown upward into the air to reach its highest point, you can easily calculate its speed when it left the earth. The method is the *same* as that used for the falling body, since the forces

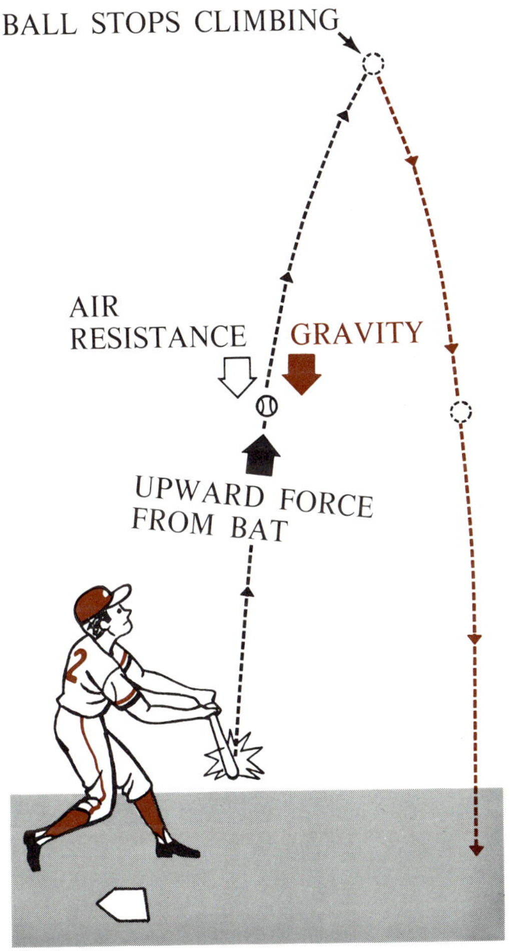


**3.37** What forces act upon the pop fly to cause the ball to slow down, stop, and then speed up again?

are the same. By multiplying the number of seconds times the decrease in speed due to the pull of gravity (9.8 meters for each second of flight), you will find the original speed of the object. For example, if an object is thrown upward and reaches its peak in 3 seconds, its starting speed was 29.4 meters per second. ($9.8 \times 3 = 29.4$). Using these figures, can you calculate how high the object went? (See Figure 3.37 above.)

## Investigating Falling Bodies

You can use a water rocket, which can be purchased at many hobby and toy stores, to investigate the motion of falling bodies. Follow the directions that come with the water rocket in filling it with water and air. Shoot the rocket off on a playground or other level place out of doors. Use a stopwatch to measure the time between when it reaches its highest point and when it strikes the ground.

The formula, $S = \frac{1}{2}at^2$, can be used to calculate how high the rocket went. $S$ equals distance in meters, $a$ equals the acceleration of gravity (9.8 meters per second per second), and $t$ equals time in seconds. For example, if it takes 2½ seconds for the rocket to reach the ground from its highest point, it went 30.6 meters high ($\frac{1}{2} \times 9.8 \times 2\frac{1}{2} \times 2\frac{1}{2} = 30.6$).

You can check the accuracy of your results by also measuring the height the rocket reached. This can be done by observing the position of the rocket's shadow when it is at its highest point. Another method involves having an observer stand a certain distance from the launching site and measuring the angle at which the rocket is above the ground at its highest point. Figure 3.38 shows how you can make a sighting instrument to measure the angle. Fasten a protractor to a meterstick. Hang a weight from a string that is thumbtacked to the meterstick as shown in the figure. Sight along the meterstick toward the highest point the rocket reaches. Have a friend read the angle indicated by where the string crosses the protractor.

Can you figure out how high the rocket went by making a scale drawing like Figure

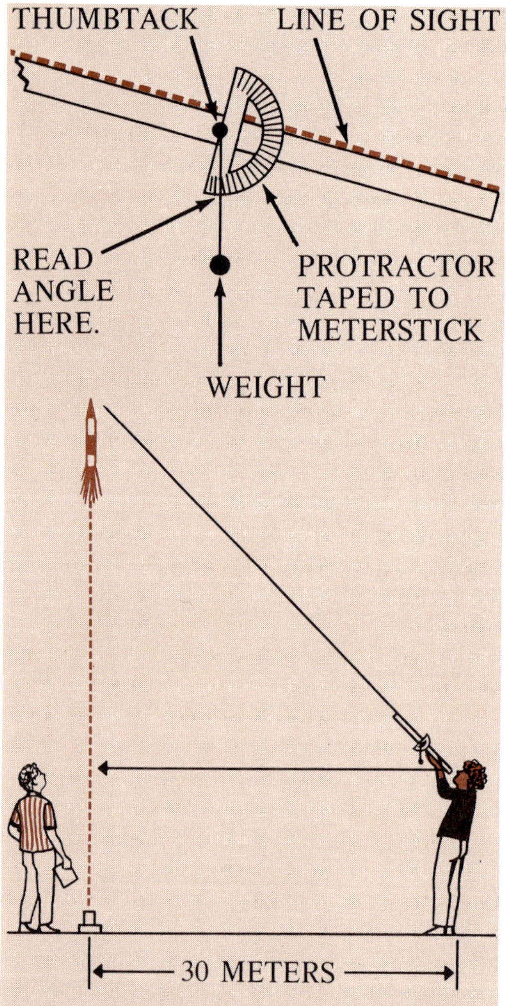


**3.38** How to measure the height of a rocket

3.38 on graph paper? How do your results using either of these methods compare with those obtained by measuring the length of time it takes for the rocket to fall back to the earth? Can you calculate its speed as it strikes the ground?

To the scientist, this *slowing down* of the speed of a moving object is also acceleration. Thus, acceleration is *any* change in the speed of an object.

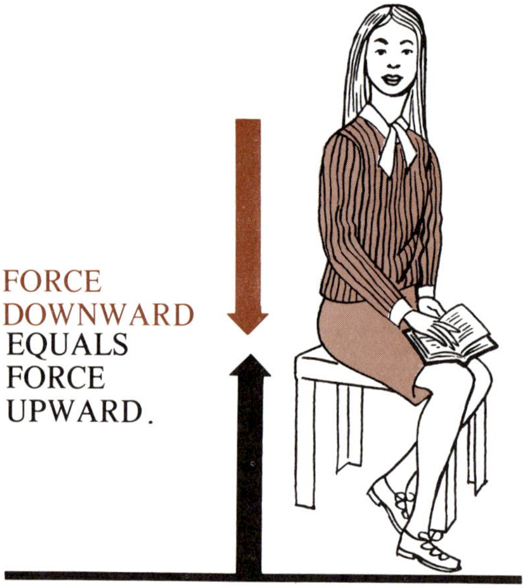


**3.39** Force downward = force upward
How do you know that this true?

Now imagine a train that is moving along the tracks at a constant speed. The force pulling the cars along balances all of the other forces acting on the train. However, the train comes to a curve in the tracks. The curved rails force the train to change its direction. The physicist considers this *change in direction* also to be acceleration. Can you now state a complete definition for the term acceleration? (Figure 3.40)

While it is true that all acceleration is caused by a force, not all forces cause acceleration. When you sit in a chair, you are exerting a force downward on the chair. This force is due to the pull of gravity and is equal to your weight. However, no motion takes place, because the chair is exerting a force *upward* on you that is equal to your weight. What would happen if the upward force of the chair were less than the downward force of your weight? (Figure 3.39 above)

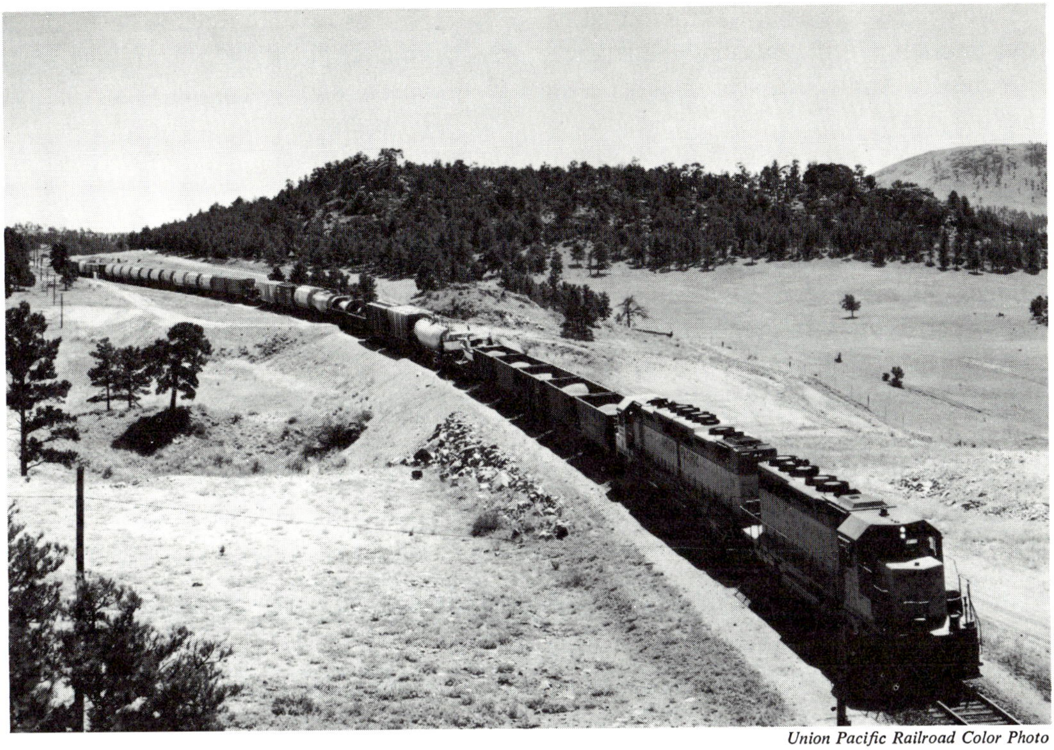

Union Pacific Railroad Color Photo

**3.40** Is this train accelerating?

## Have You Learned?

Calculate the answers to the following problems. For these use **g** + 9.8 meters per second per second.

1. What is the speed of a freely falling object after it has been falling for 4 seconds?
2. How far will a freely falling object fall in 3 seconds?
3. If an object is thrown upward at a speed of 19.6 meters per second, what is the *total* length of time it takes to reach its greatest height and fall back to earth?
4. In question 3 above, how high will the object go?
5. How far will a freely falling object fall during its second second?

# 8. Speed, Velocity, and Momentum

**ARE YOU READY?**

Look up the following words if you are not sure of their meanings:

average (speed); geometry; impact; mass; mathematics; parallelogram; protractor.

Speed is an idea with which you are already acquainted. It is the rate at which an object is moving. If we know the speed of a moving object, we can calculate how far it will move in a given length of time. For example, if we know that an airplane flies at an average speed of 1,200 kilometers per hour, we can estimate that in four hours it will fly 4,800 kilometers.

You also know from your experience that the greater the force that is applied to an object, the faster the object will move. If one boy is pulling a loaded wagon, and he is able to move it 30 meters in 10 seconds, its speed would be 3 meters per second (30 meters ÷ 10 seconds = 3 meters per second). If a second boy comes to help, perhaps the loaded wagon can be moved 30 meters in only 5 seconds. The added force increased the speed of the wagon by how many meters per second?

Speed tells us only how fast something is moving. If you start out walking from your house, and you walk at a speed of six kilometers per hour for two hours, where will you be? The answer to this question will depend upon the *direction* you walk. If you walk in a circle, you may be back home again.

Scientists use the term **velocity** (və los′ ə ti) to describe the speed of an object in a certain direction. Thus, the velocity of an airplane might be described as being 1,000 kilometers per hour in a southwesterly direction.

## Calculating Location Using Velocity

**MATERIALS:**

A ruler, a pencil, a road map

**PROCEDURE:**

Find the scale of the map. (English units are used here because most road maps available to students have distances measured in miles.) It will look something like the photograph shown here (Figure 3.41). Select any spot near the center of your map, and mark it with an *X*.

Assume that an airplane left this spot near the center of the map and flew south (toward the bottom of the map) at an average velocity of 200 miles per hour for one hour. Draw a line to show the path of its flight, and place a 0 at this point. If it then turned east and flew for two hours at an average velocity of 100 miles per hour in this direction, where would it be? Draw a line to mark this path.

**3.41** Read the scale for distance for map use.

*Hammond Incorporated*

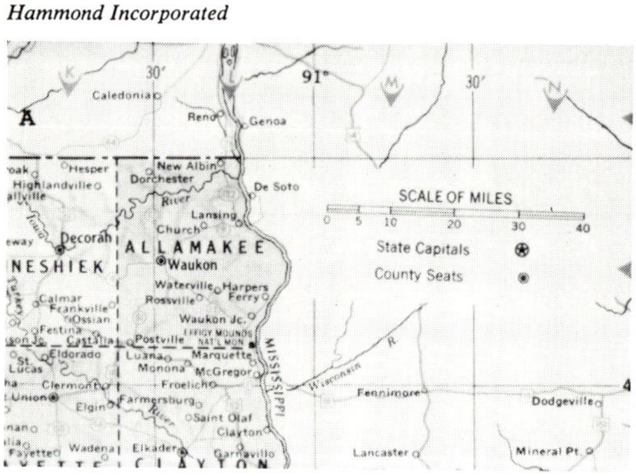


The lines that you drew in the activity above are called **vectors** (vek′ tər). Vectors show both the speed of the moving object and its direction. Therefore, vectors may be used to diagram velocities.

The push of the jet engine of an airplane causes it to move at a certain speed and in a certain direction. If a wind is blowing in the same direction that the plane is moving (a tailwind), the airplane will move even

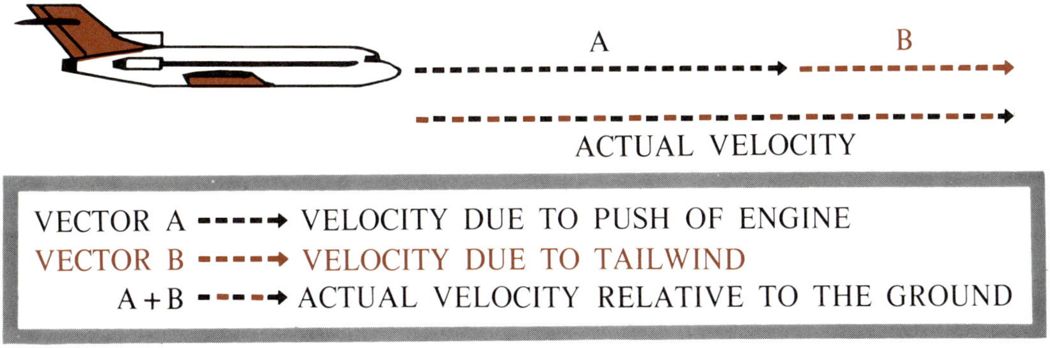


**3.42** Plane in a tailwind

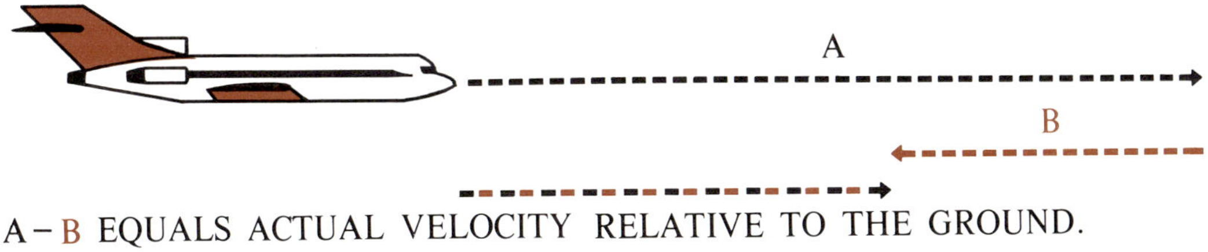


**3.43** Plane in a headwind

faster. In cases such as this, we simply add the vector of the plane's velocity to the vector of the wind's velocity. (See Figure 3.42 above.)

If the wind is blowing in a direction opposite to that of the movement of the airplane, we again add the vectors. However, this addition is done *geometrically.* That is, the velocity of one force is considered to be in a negative direction.

Suppose, however, that the wind is blowing at right angles to the direction the airplane's engine is pushing. What will be the velocity of the airplane? Again we can use the mathematics of geometry to get an answer.

## Diagraming Vectors

**MATERIALS:**

A meterstick, a pencil, a piece of paper, a protractor

**PROCEDURE:**

Place *X* an near the upper left-hand corner of the paper. This represents the present location of the airplane. Draw a vector representing the push of the plane's engine that would move it to the right at 200 kilometers per hour. For this, use a scale of one centimeter equals 20 kilometers per hour. Now draw a vector representing the velocity of a wind of 50 kilometers per hour blowing at right angles (90°) to the direction of the airplane's flight, toward the bottom of the page.

You should have a drawing that looks like Figure 3.44 on page 98.

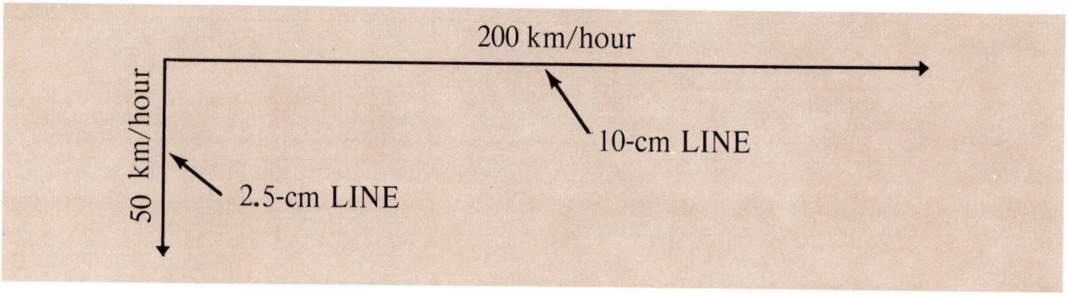


**3.44** The first step is to draw lines representing the velocity of the airplane and that of the wind.

To diagram the actual velocity of the airplane, complete the parallelogram. A vector drawn from the *X* to the opposite corner of the parallelogram represents the velocity of the airplane (See Figure 3.45).

Can you describe the velocity of the airplane in words? Remember that the velocity includes both speed and direction.

Change the velocity of the wind in the above problem by changing its direction.

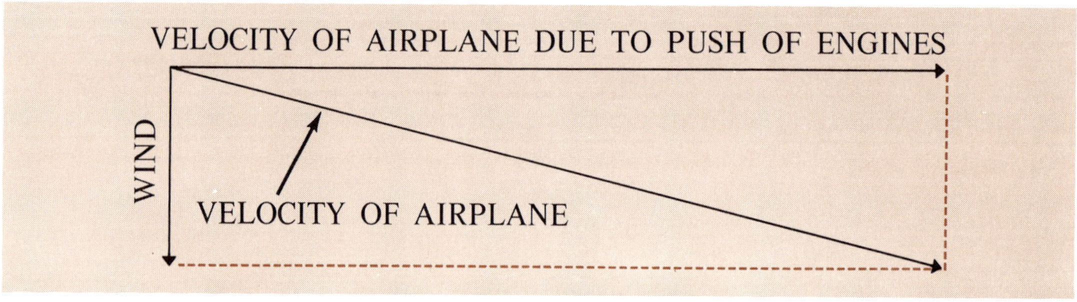


**3.45** The diagonal line represents the actual velocity (speed and direction) of the airplane.

Can you still calculate the velocity?

Again place an *X* near the left-hand side of the page. Now draw a vector to the right, representing a velocity of 200 kilometers per hour in that direction. Suppose that this is the velocity that you want the airplane to fly, but there is a wind blowing at 75 kilometers per hour in a direction at right angles to this line of flight, toward the bottom of the page. Can you construct a parallelogram that will show the direction that the pilot must head the plane and the force that he must have the engine apply to it if he is to have his plane travel on your flight plan?

---

Vectors also can be used to represent forces. As an example, let's consider the problem of the girls pulling on the wagon that was described on page 64. Suppose that two boys each pull with a force of 30 kilograms at a 45° angle to the forward direction of the wagon. Using a scale of 10 kilograms = ¼ cm, the forward force on the wagon can be found by making a drawing as shown in Figure 3.46 on page 99.

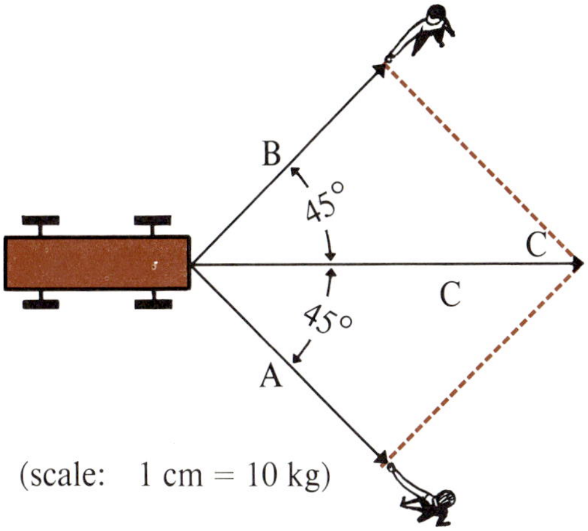


**3.46** Try this with two spring scales.

Line *A* represents the force being applied by one boy, and line *B* the force of the other boy. Line *C* represents the forward force on the wagon. It is about 4.5 centimeters long. Based on the scale of 10 kilograms = 1 cm, the forward force is about 45 kilograms. How does this answer compare with the one you found experimentally in section one?

The idea of velocity is related to several other important ideas in science. For example, if two weights are dropped from the top of a building, you know that at the end of the first second of fall they will both have a velocity of 9.8 meters per second in a downward direction. Even if one of these weights weighed 1 kg and the other weighed 100 kg, both would have the same velocity (if we ignore the resistance of the air). But would you be willing to catch both of these objects? Your common sense tells you that the heavier object, the one with the greater mass, would hit you much harder than the lighter one would.

The impact of a moving object is caused by what is called the **momentum** (mō men′ təm) of the object. To calculate momentum, multiply the mass of the object times its velocity. The momentum of the smaller weight would be 1 kg × 9.8 m per second downward = 9.8 kg-m per second downward. The momentum of the larger weight is 100 kg-m/sec. downward. The momentum of the larger weight is 100 times as great as the smaller object, because of its greater mass.

If we imagine two people standing on a frictionless surface and pushing against each other, we might predict that both would move, but in opposite directions. If both of these people weighed the same, the speeds with which they would move away from each other would be equal. If one weighed twice as much as the other, the heavier person would be pushed away at a speed only *one-half* as great as that of the lighter person (Figure 3.47).

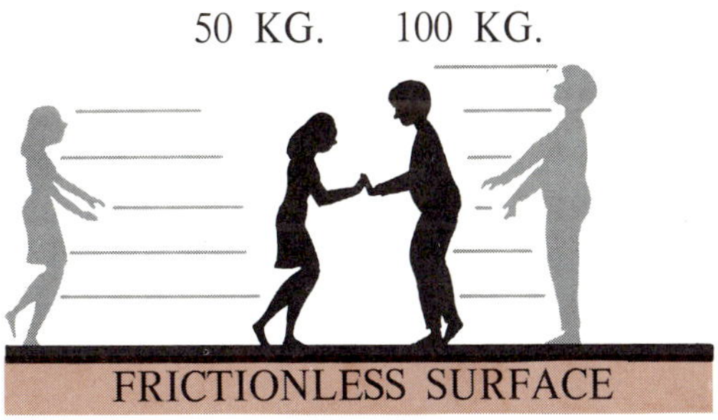


**3.47** Compare the weight and speed of each.

For example, suppose that one person weighs 100 kg and reaches a speed of ½ meter per second. The other person, weighing 50 kg will reach a speed of 1 meter per second. The momentum of each will be *equal*, except for direction (100 kg × ½ m/sec. = 50 kg × 1 m/sec.). Thus, you can see that momentum, like energy, is conserved.

**Have You Learned?**

Match up the proper definition from the list to the right with each word in the column on the left.

1. Vector
2. Momentum
3. Velocity
4. Parallelogram
5. Speed

a. a 4-sided figure in which opposite sides are parallel to each other
b. the distance something travels in a given amount of time
c. the impact of a moving object
d. speed in a certain direction
e. lines used to show both speed and direction of a moving object

## 9. Action and Reaction

**ARE YOU READY?**

Look up the following words if you are not sure of their meanings:

accelerate; exhaust; friction; orbit; reaction; satellite; unbalanced (force).

In many varied situations motion is produced by forces. Always, in each case, *two* bodies are pushing against each other. In Figure 3.48 opposite, both the girl and the boat are pushing against each other. Even though you may consider a task as play, the scientists will define the result of forces as "work."

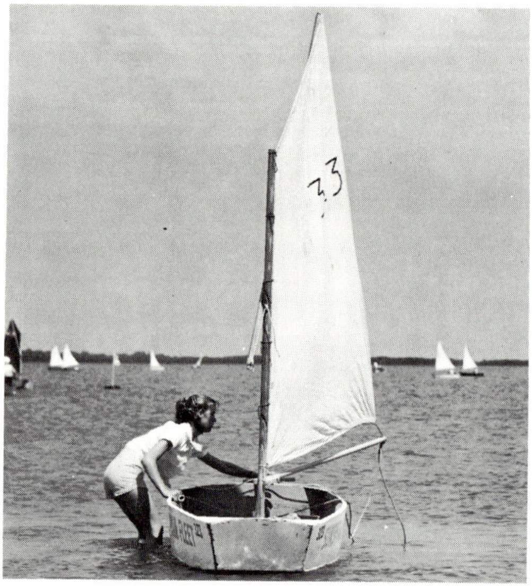


*Florida State News Bureau*

**3.48** A scientist could define this action as "work."

### Playing with Action and Reaction

**MATERIALS:**

A toy car with a spring or battery-powered motor, a piece of stiff cardboard, several round pencils, a smooth tabletop

**PROCEDURE:**

Place the pencils under the cardboard so as to form rollers, as shown in Figure 3.49. Place the car on the cardboard and start the motor. Describe the motions that you observe.

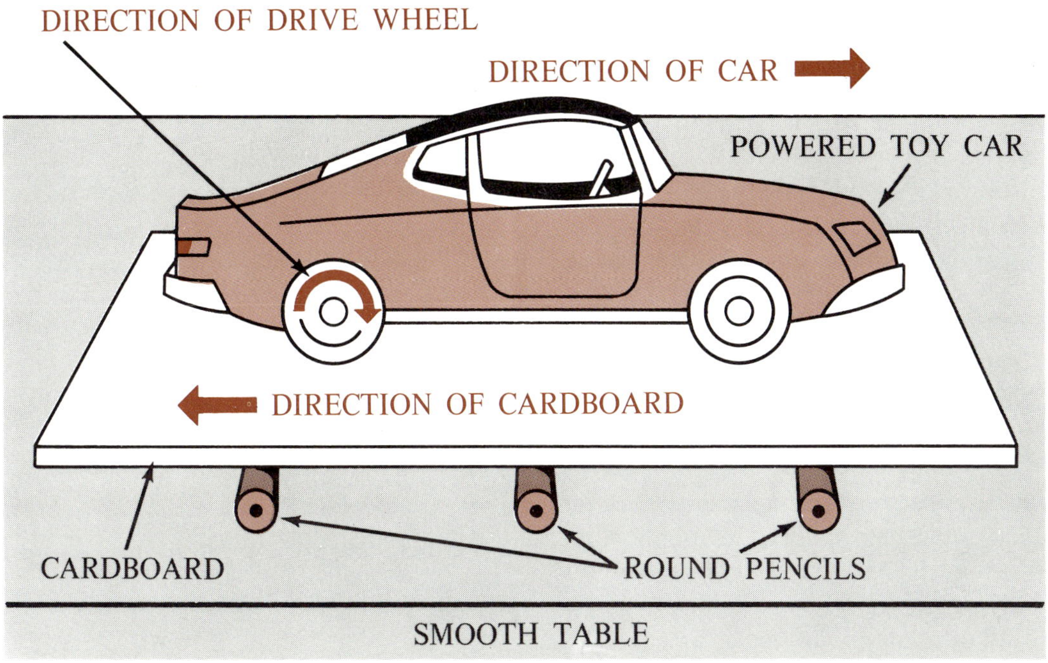


**3.49** Why does the cardboard move in the direction shown in this diagram?

The motor of the car applied a force to the wheels of the car. This caused the wheels to turn, and due to the friction between the wheels and the cardboard, this force was transferred to the cardboard. If the car had been resting on a stationary surface, the only motion you would have observed would have been the car moving forward. In this case, however, the cardboard was accelerated too, and in a direction opposite to that of the car. (See Figure 3.49 above.)

## Skateboarding with Action and Reaction

**MATERIALS:**

A skateboard or pair of roller skates

**PROCEDURE:**

Stand on the skateboard with your back to the wall. Without moving your feet, move away from the wall while still standing on the skateboard. How did you do it?

Again stand on the skateboard, but this time away from the wall. Quickly step off the skateboard. Describe what happens to the skateboard.

In order to move away from the wall, you had to apply a force against the wall. But the wall did not move. Therefore, another force must have been applied against you, which caused you to move away from the wall.

Both of these forces acted when you stood away from the wall and tried to step off of the skateboard. You applied a force on the skateboard with the bottom of your shoe, similar to the one you apply to the floor when you walk. But instead of your forward motion being the only motion, the skateboard moved too. Its direction was opposite to yours.

These phenomena demonstrate an important idea in physics, called Newton's "Third Law of Motion," which states that "for every action [motion] there is an equal and opposite reaction." In other words, when one body exerts a force on a second body, the second body exerts a force on the first. These two forces are equal to each other, but in opposite directions.

When the wheels of an automobile apply a force on the ground, the car accelerates. This acceleration of the automobile is due to a force being applied to the wheels by the earth in a direction opposite to that applied to the earth by the wheels. Can you explain why the earth does not move in a direction opposite to that of the car, as the cardboard did in the activity on page 100?

An understanding of the principles of action and reaction is needed every day by scientists and engineers who are concerned with controlling the motion of any object. Perhaps the most exciting use of these scientific principles is their application to space travel.

You have probably blown up a balloon and then released it and watched it push itself through the air. In the blownup balloon, the **compressed** (kəm prest′) air is pushing in all directions. When the balloon is released, the forces become unbalanced, as shown in Figure 3.50, and the balloon moves. The force here is exerted against the front wall of the balloon, and the balloon moves because of the *lack* of equal pressure against the back wall.

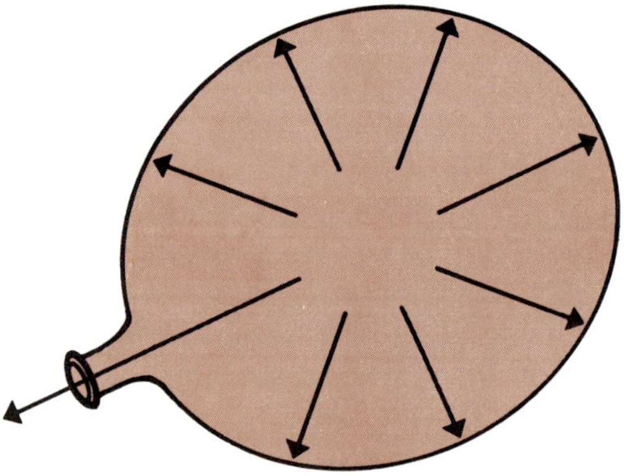

**3.50** Try to explain why the balloon would move toward the upper right. This illustrates Newton's Third Law of Motion.

The rocket engines used to put satellites into orbit around the earth or to send capsules on trips through space use this same principle. Gases are exhausted through the back of the rocket at very high speeds, and the unbalanced force against the front of the rocket moves it. This forward force is known as the **thrust** of the rocket. It is the force that propels the rocket.

In the past, some people said that a rocket would not work in outer space because there was no air for it to push against. Since rocket flights now occur almost daily, this comment is no longer often heard. Can you think of what you would tell a person who still believes rockets must have air to push against?

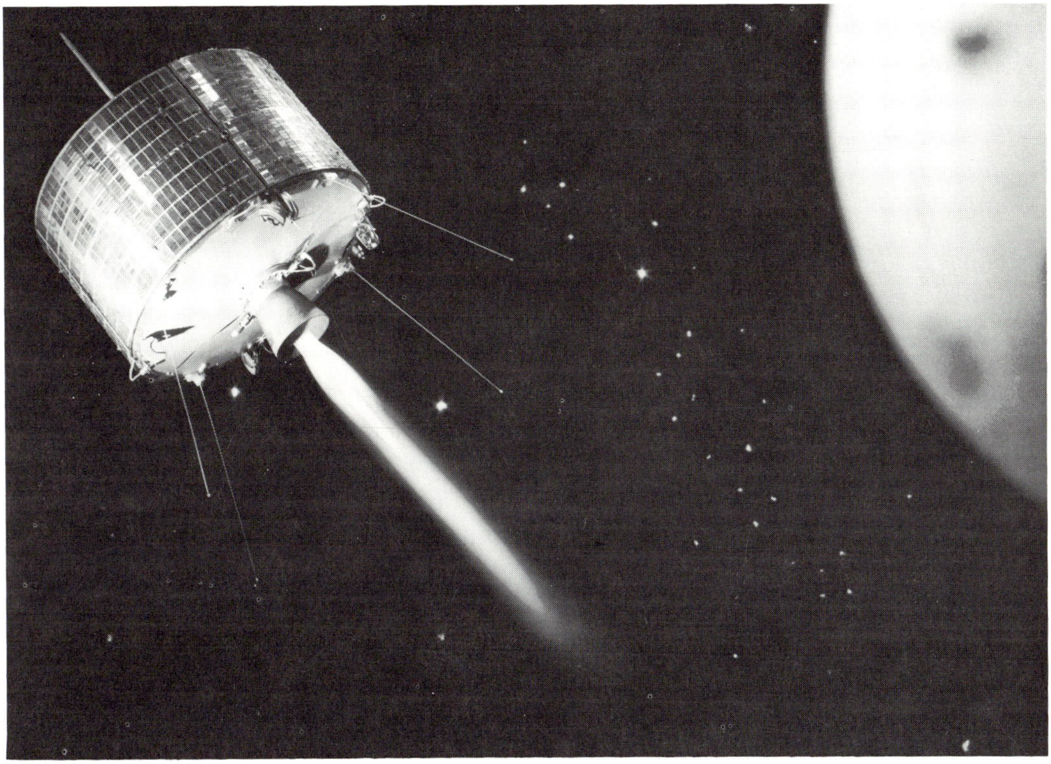

NASA

**3.51** If there is no atmosphere, how can this Syncom spacecraft work?

### Have You Learned?

Answer the following questions with as few words as possible.

1. State Newton's "Third Law of Motion."
2. Explain what causes an airplane to move forward when its propellers are turning.
3. Explain how a rocket uses Newton's Third Law.
4. Explain why, if you step out of a boat, the boat moves away from you in the opposite direction.
5. Explain why the earth does not apparently move in the opposite direction from a rapidly accelerating automobile.

## 10. Observing Motion

**ARE YOU READY?**

Look up the following words if you are not sure of their meanings:

apparent; axis (of earth); Mars; orbit; planet; velocity.

If you were to observe the planet Mars at the same time each night for several weeks, you would find that the planet generally seems to move eastward against the background of stars. However, sometimes its direction and speed suddenly seem to change, and for the next few weeks it seems to move toward the west. Then its path again changes, and the planet seems to move again in an eastward direction. (See Figure 3.52.)

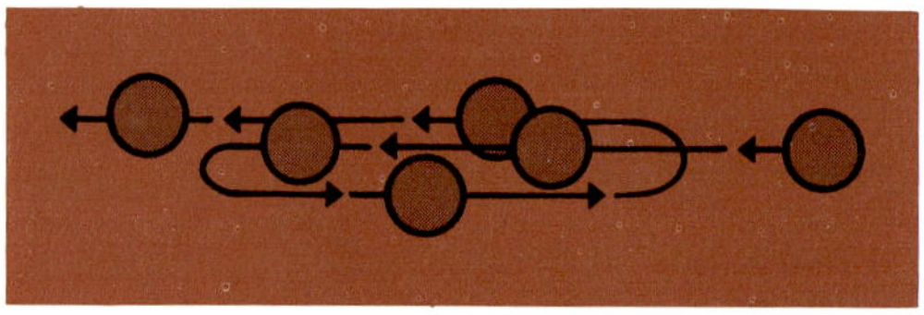

**3.52** The retrograde movement of Mars

You probably already know that Mars, like the earth, moves in an orbit around the sun. The explanation for the apparent change of the planet's path is that *you* are also moving around the sun, at a faster speed than Mars. As the earth catches up with Mars and passes it, the direction of movement of Mars against the background of stars seems to change.

While studying the motion of an object, it is always necessary to consider the motion of you, the observer. The difference between *observed* motion and *actual* motion is often difficult to determine. Have you had an experience of sitting in a car or train and looking out the side window at another vehicle? The other vehicle slowly begins to move ahead, and for an instant you feel as if the car or train in which you are riding is moving *backward.* Until you can see some stationary object—the ground or a telephone pole—you cannot be certain which vehicle is actually moving.

## Observing Falling Bodies

MATERIALS:

A bicycle, a ball, a piece of string about 1.5 meters long, a pencil, two friends

**PROCEDURE:**

Stick the pencil into the ground, tie the string to it, and have one person hold the string tightly in a straight line upward above the pencil. This will mark the location of the pencil.

A second person should ride the bicycle slowly past the string and drop the ball at the exact instant that he passes over the pencil. The third person should stand to the side, so that he can describe the path of the ball as it falls and note where it hits the ground. See Figure 3.53 on page 105.

To the bicycle rider, the ball seems to fall straight down, hitting the ground directly under the hand from which it was dropped. To the observer standing to one side, the path of the ball seems to be at an angle, hitting the ground considerably ahead of the point above which it was dropped. The difference in the observation of these two people is that one observer is stationary while the other observer is in motion.

Try pitching a ball at a post as you ride by on a bicycle. If you are to hit the post, you must throw the ball *before* you reach

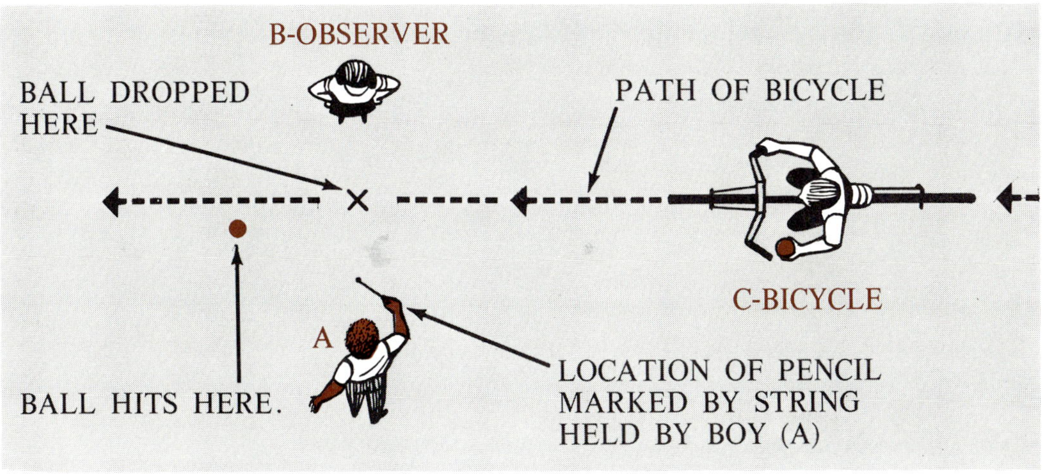


**3.53** All you need to do this experiment is a bicycle, a ball, and two friends.

a point alongside the post. However, to you the ball may seem to travel in a path at right angles to the bicycle (Figure 3.54).

Describing the path of a falling or thrown object such as these may seem like a simple matter, since it is easy for you to stand to one side and watch the motion. However, the motion that you observe is not the *actual* motion of the object. You cannot observe the actual motion in these cases because *you are in motion yourself*, even when standing to one side. The earth on which you are standing is turning on its axis. In addition to this rotational motion, it is going around the sun, and the sun and its planets are rushing through space. Where would you stand in order to observe the *actual* movement of an object?

All motion you observe then, is **relative** (rel′ ə tiv). This means that what you see depends upon the motion of other objects. Whenever we describe motion, we must compare it with other objects, all of which are also in motion.

**3.54** Have you ever tried this? How good is your aim from a moving bicycle?

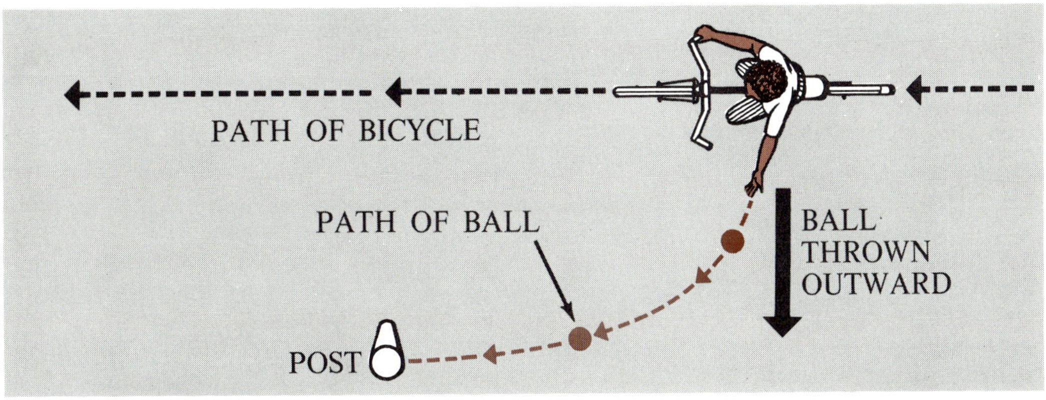

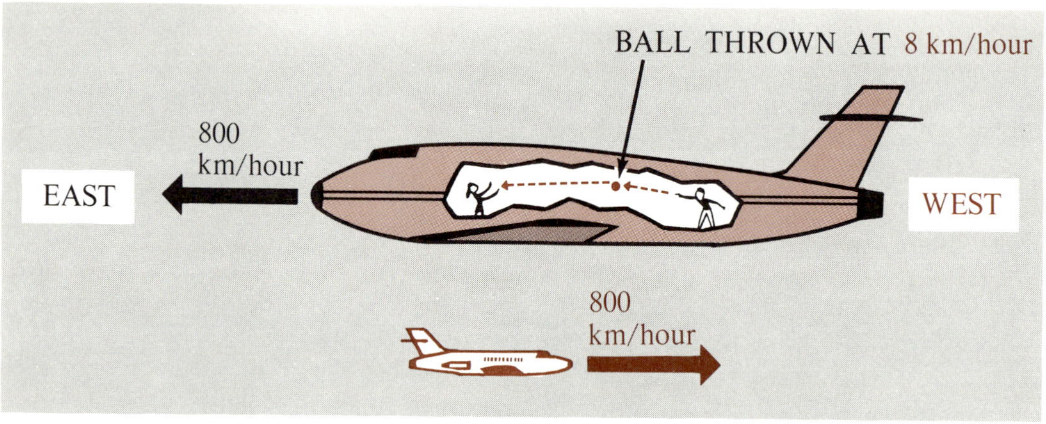


**3.55** Would you be afraid to catch a ball that is thrown in a moving airplane?

To illustrate this idea, suppose that you are standing in the back of the cabin of an airplane that is traveling eastward at a speed of 800 kilometers per hour. You throw a ball to a friend who is standing in the front part of the plane. The velocity of the ball, *relative* to you both, was a movement in an eastward direction at, say, 8 kilometers per hour. *Relative* to an observer on the ground, the velocity of the ball would be 808 kilometers per hour in an easterly direction (the 800 kilometers-per-hour speed of the plane plus the 8 kilometers-per-hour speed of the ball). *Relative* to the pilot of a plane flying west at 800 kilometers per hour, the velocity of the ball would be 1,608 kilometers per hour eastward. What would be the velocity of the ball relative to a plane flying east at 400 kilometers per hour? To a plane flying east at 1,000 kilometer per hour? Consider Figure 3.55 above.

## Have You Learned?

On a sheet of paper list the numbers for the questions below. By each number write *T* if the statement is true and *F* if false.

1. The velocity of Mars changes twice each year.
2. If you are sitting in a chair, you can observe the actual motion of things around you.
3. When we describe motions, we must compare them with the motion of other objects.
4. It is difficult to describe the motion of planets because the earth is moving.
5. All motion that you observe is relative.

## REVIEW QUESTIONS

1. Describe three types of acceleration that can take place in a single moving object such as an airplane.
2. Newton's First Law of Motion deals with inertia. State this law, and explain what it means, giving several examples.
3. Draw as many types of simple machines as you can. Explain the advantages and disadvantages of each type.
4. Explain the difference between the *actual* and the *ideal* mechanical advantage of a machine. Explain why they rarely are equal in the same machine.
5. What is the difference between *cohesion* and *adhesion*? Give examples of each.
6. How does Archimedes's discovery of buoyancy explain why some objects float in water while others sink?
7. State Pascal's Law, and give examples of how it may be used.
8. Explain the difference between *speed* and *velocity*; between *acceleration* and *momentum*.
9. Newton's Third Law of Motion deals with action and reaction. State this law, and explain what it means, giving several examples.
10. What is meant by the statement "all motion that you observe is relative"? Give some examples of relative motion.

## CAN YOU FIND OUT?

*It may be necessary to use an encyclopedia or other reference books in answering these questions.*

1. Is the pull of gravity the same for every place on the surface of the earth? Explain your answer.
2. Rapid acceleration increases the weight of an object. How much is this increase in airplanes and in rocket capsules?
3. How can scientists show that the inertia of an object depends upon its mass and not upon its weight?
4. When an unmanned satellite is in an orbit around the earth, it constantly changes its forward direction. What outside forces cause these changes?
5. Lubrication and the use of round bearings have been mentioned as techniques used to overcome friction. What other methods have been used?
6. An automobile mechanic may use a tool called a "torque wrench." How does this tool work, and what is it used for?
7. What are the efficiencies of various types of engines? Which seem to be the most efficient?
8. Most automobiles have hydraulic braking systems. Try to find out how they work.
9. Capillary action is very important to plants. Try to find out how.
10. Archimedes has been called "The Father of Experimental Science." Try to find out why. What else did he do besides discover the principle of buoyancy?
11. Using both the concepts of buoyancy and of density, can you explain why some liquids will float on water and others will sink?
12. Galileo experimented with the acceleration of falling bodies. What did he discover?
13. What is the amount of $g$ at different places on earth?
14. What is the relationship between *momentum* and *kinetic energy*? Between *kinetic energy* and *impact*?
15. Explain how a rocket engine produces thrust in outer space. Some people believe that it must have air to push against. Why is this idea not true?

## REFERENCES FOR ADDITIONAL STUDY

BASEBALL-ISTICS: THE BASIC PHYSICS OF BASEBALL by Robert Froman.

G. P. Putnam's Sons.

A humorous book using baseball to illustrate many of the basic principles of physics

CAREERS AND OPPORTUNITIES IN PHYSICS by Phillip Pollack. E. P. Dutton & Co., Inc. Describes specialties in physics and the educational requirements in each field

HOW WILL WE MEET THE ENERGY CRISIS?: POWER FOR TOMORROW'S WORLD by Millard Reed and others. Julian Messner. A survey of our energy needs and resources with an examination of future sources—solar cells, controlled thermonuclear fusion, tides, and geothermal energy

MACHINES by Robert O'Brien and the Editors of Time-Life Books, A Division of Time Inc. (Distributed by Silver Burdett Company.) A beautifully illustrated series of accounts about the scientific principles of machines with many examples included

MOTION by Evans Valens. The World Publishing Company. Discusses the laws of motion against a background of everyday experience

ORBIT—A PICTURE STORY OF FORCE AND MOTION by Hy Ruchlis. Harper & Row, Publishers. Describes the physics of orbiting bodies—acceleration, gravity, inertia, momentum, etc.

RELATIVITY FOR THE MILLIONS by Martin Gardner. The Macmillan Company. Explains Einstein's Theory of Relativity and the implications

WHEELS by Wilfred Owen, Ezra Bowe, and the Editors of Time-Life Books, A Division of Time Inc. (Distributed by Silver Burdett Company.) Made up of eight picture-essays ranging from the invention of the wheel to the forthcoming automation in transportation

CHAPTER 4

# Heat Energy

THE IMPORTANCE OF HEAT ENERGY was recognized by the ancient Greeks, who, over 2,000 years ago, listed fire as one of the four elements of which they believed everything was made. The other three were water, air, and earth.

The effects of heat energy on matter are easily observed. Heat causes ice to melt and liquid water to change to a gaseous form. There are many sources of heat. Rub your hands together, and feel the heat produced by friction. Use a magnifying glass to focus the rays of the sun, and start a fire. The flame of a candle produces heat energy as do many electrical appliances such as toasters and irons. But what is heat, and how can we explain the effects it has on matter?

## 1. Measuring Temperature

**ARE YOU READY?**

Look up the following words if you are not sure of their meanings:

estimate; evaporation; senses; temperature; thermometer; unreliable.

One of the first steps toward understanding the nature of heat was the development of instruments capable of measuring temperature. It is difficult for us to realize that the first thermometer was made only about 350 years ago. Before that time people had only their own senses to tell them when one object was hotter than another. As the following activity will show, a person's ability to estimate temperature is really not at all very accurate.

**4.1** Sixteenth-century thermometer by Galileo

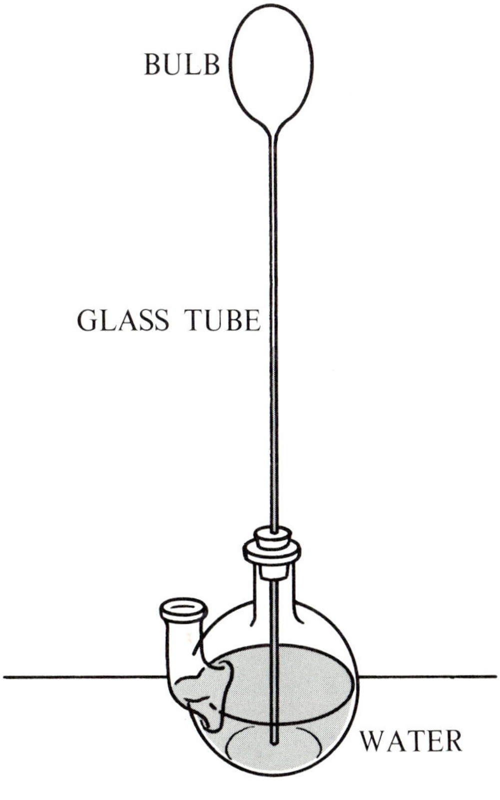

## Estimating Temperature

**MATERIALS:**

Four containers, one containing hot water, two lukewarm water, and the fourth cold water

**PROCEDURE:**

Place the four containers in a line on the table before you. Have a fellow student place one hand in pan *A* and the other hand in pan *B* for about thirty seconds. Have him remove his hands and immediately place one hand in pan *C* and the other in pan *D*. Ask him if the water in pan *C* is warmer or colder than that in pan *D*. Can you explain the reason for his answer? Repeat the experiment with other people. Do you always get the same results?

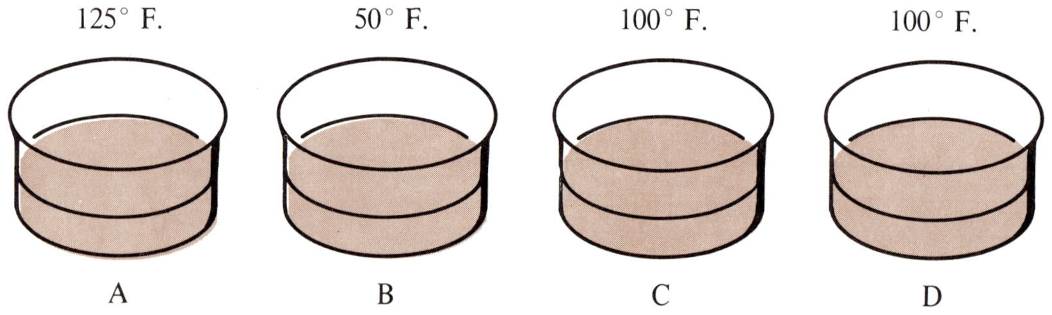


The first attempt to build a thermometer was probably made during the last half of the sixteenth century by an Italian named Galileo (gal′ ə lē′ ō). Not many details are known about Galileo's experiments with measuring temperature, but his first thermometer probably looked much like the drawing on page 109.

## Building a Simple Thermometer

**MATERIALS:**

A container of water, a small, thin-walled flask, a one-holed stopper, a piece of glass tubing several centimeters long, a cube of ice

**PROCEDURE:**

Carefully insert the glass tubing through the stopper, and place the stopper tightly in the top of the flask. Place the open end of the glass tube in the water, as shown in Figure 4.2 on page 111. Place both of your hands around the flask until a number of bubbles of air leave the mouth of the tube. Remove your hands, but leave the end of the glass tubing under water, holding the flask by using only two fingers near the stopper. Observe the water inside the tube. Run cool water over the flask, or place an ice cube on top to cool it still further. Describe what happens to the water level within the tube.

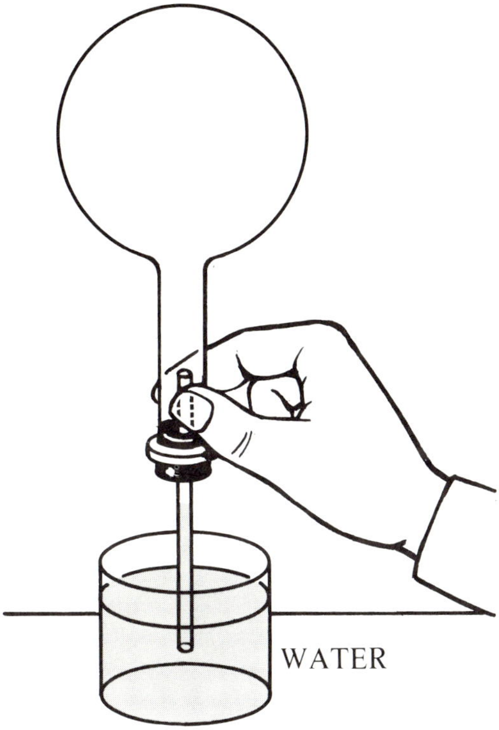


**4.2** Galileo's air thermometer

By measuring the height of the column of water within the tube, Galileo could estimate the difference in the temperature of the air in the bulb of the thermometer at one time compared with another time. After this crude beginning, it was a simple matter to discover that the equipment could be turned upside down and the liquid placed inside the bulb, as shown in Figure 4.3 opposite. In this thermometer, the liquid itself expands as it becomes heated, and its height is a crude measure of its temperature. Since the evaporation of the water and changes in the pressure of the air made the instrument unreliable over a period of time, scientists soon developed a thermometer that was sealed at both ends to prevent evaporation. Alcohol or mercury was used to avoid

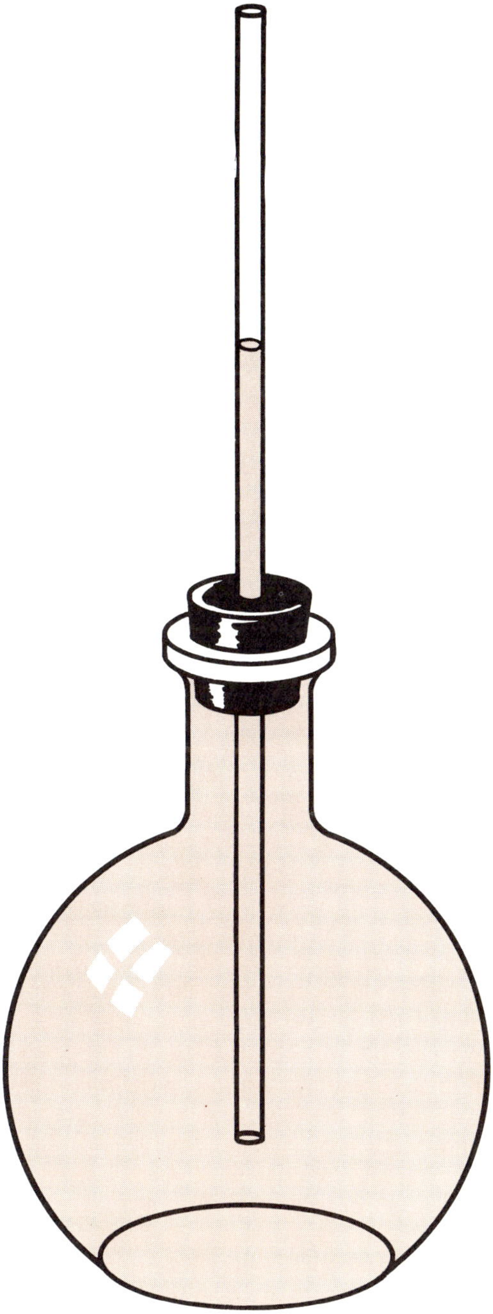

**4.3** A water thermometer is like Galileo's thermometer but upside down.

freezing. This is very similar to the thermometers that we use today.

The problem of measuring temperature was not yet solved, however. Now each scientist could easily construct his own thermometer, but the growth of science depends largely upon the ability of scientists to describe to each other the details of their experiments. In this way, each experiment can be repeated and checked, over and over again. A method had to be found that would allow any scientist, anywhere in the world, to mark his thermometer so that it was exactly like the thermometers of other scientists.

In the early 1700s, about 120 years after Galileo built his first thermometer, a usable system of **calibrating** (kal′ ə brāt ing) was developed. A German scientist named Fahrenheit (far′ ən hīt) mixed salt with ice and called the temperature of this mixture zero degrees (0°). As another temperature, he took that of his own body, which he called 96 degrees. The distance between these two set temperatures was then divided into 96 equal spaces, each called one degree. (Other scientists could, of course, follow the same procedure, since 96° is close to the average temperature of the healthy human body.)

Temperature is often measured with a **Fahrenheit thermometer,** on which 32° indicates the freezing point of water and 212° the boiling point. Normal body temperature of humans is 98.6° F, and we feel most comfortable when air temperatures are in the seventies.

Scientists frequently use a **Celsius** (sel′ sē əs) **thermometer** on which zero is the freezing point of water, and 100 is the boiling point. The Celsius temperature scale is frequently referred to as the **Centigrade** (sen′ tə grād) scale. Since these scales are the same, these names can be used interchangeably. Normal body temperature is 37° C (read "thirty-seven degrees Celsius" or "thirty-seven degrees Centigrade"), and a room temperature of 72° F is equal to about 22° C.

Many of the thermometers you may use in the laboratory will be calibrated in Celsius degrees. Practice using a Celsius thermometer by determining the temperature of the air in your classroom, of tap water, and of a beaker of ice water.

### Have You Learned?

On a sheet of paper list the numbers for the questions below. By each number write *T* if the statement is true and *F* if false.

1. A person's estimate of temperature is usually quite accurate.
2. The first real thermometer was probably built by Galileo.
3. The first calibration of a thermometer was made by Galileo.
4. On the Celsius temperature scale, water freezes at approximately 100°.
5. On the Centigrade temperature scale, water boils at approximately 100°.
6. The first thermometer depended upon the expansion of a liquid.
7. Mercury is used in today's thermometers partly because it freezes at a lower temperature than water.
8. Zero degrees on the Fahrenheit scale was the temperature of a mixture of ice and salt.
9. Galileo was the first scientist to use the Centigrade temperature scale.

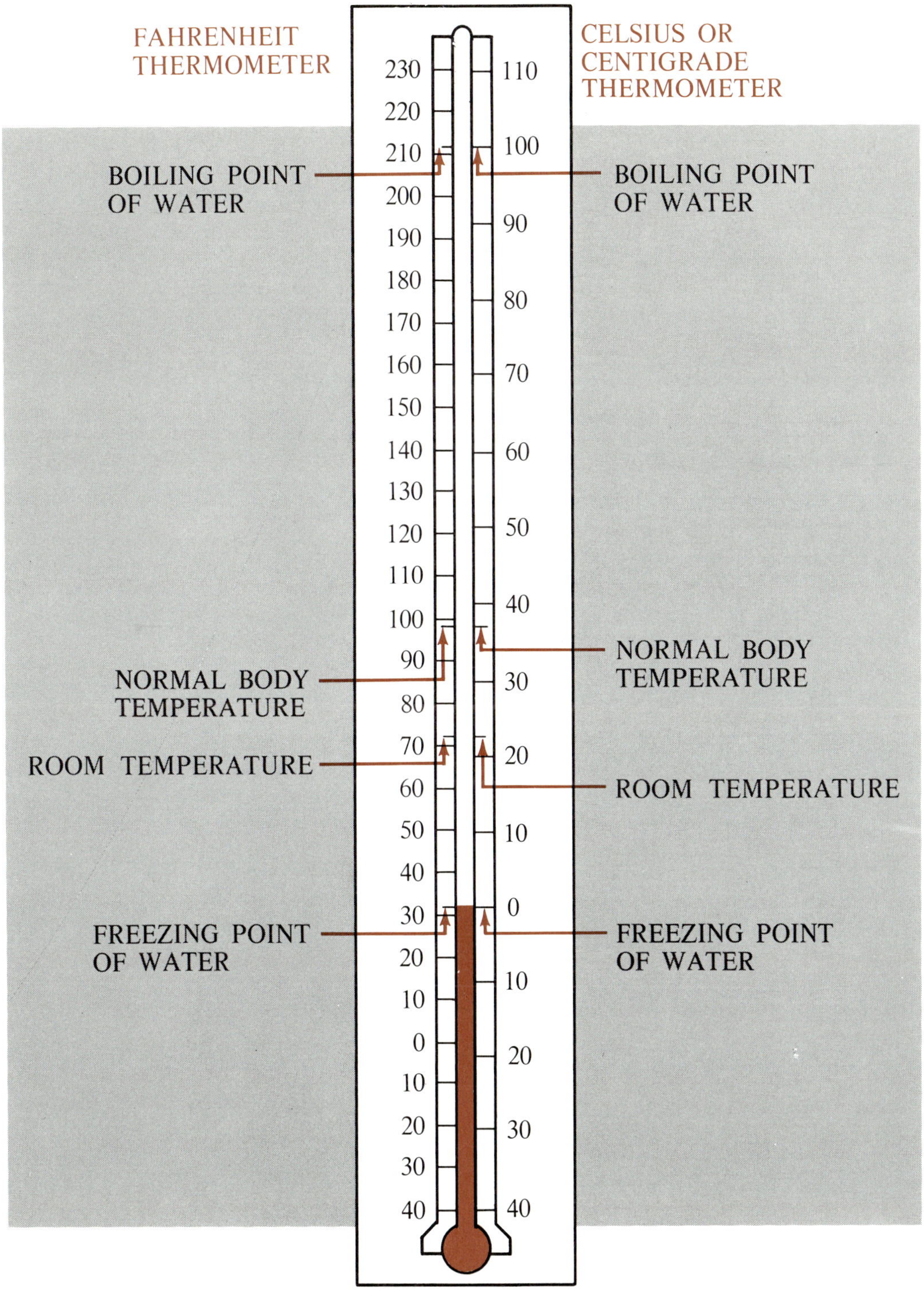


**4.4** As a means of helping you learn the Celsius temperature scale, most of the temperatures are given in Celsius degrees.

## 2. Effects of Heat on Matter

> **ARE YOU READY?**
>
> Look up the following words if you are not sure of their meanings:
>
> alloy; form (of matter); heat; molecule; volume.

We have all observed the effects of heat energy when matter changes from one form to another. Liquid water begins to boil and changes to a gas when we add heat to it. If, however, we remove heat from liquid water, it soon freezes into solid ice. By adding heat to an ice cube, we can change it into a liquid; by cooling steam we can also change it to a liquid.

---

### Observing a Change of State

**MATERIALS:**

2 metal containers, a source of heat, several ice cubes, a thermometer

**PROCEDURE:**

Place a few ice cubes in one of the metal containers, and place it over the heat source, observing it as it melts. Before the ice has completely melted, measure the temperature of the water with the thermometer.

Continue heating the water until it begins to boil. Measure the temperature of the boiling water.

Place the extra ice cubes in the second metal container, and when it is cool, hold it over the steam coming from the boiling water. What happens to the steam as it touches the cold metal?

---

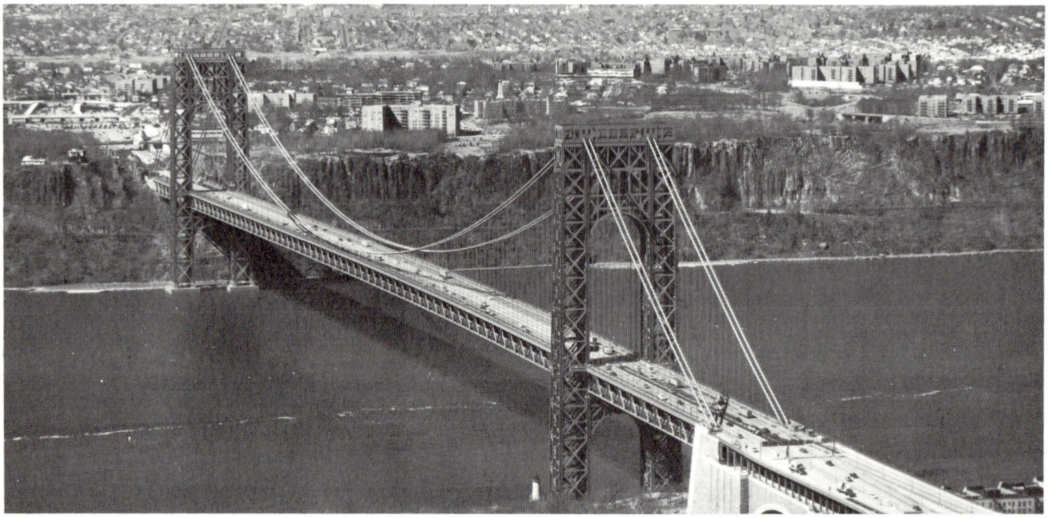

*The Port of New York Authority*

**4.5** Bridges such as this one are built so that they can expand or contract without danger.

Another effect of heat on matter, which is not so apparent, is the change in the size of the matter as the temperature of the matter changes. Railroad tracks and concrete bridges and sidewalks are made with a gap at the end of each section so that, as their temperature increases, the solid materials can increase in size, or **expand** (eks pand′), without breaking (Figure 4.6).

Most liquids and gases also expand when they are heated and **contract** (kən trakt′), or get smaller, when cooled.

## Making a Gas Expand

**MATERIALS:**

A heat-resistant test tube, a balloon, a metal container that can be tightly sealed with a cork, a source of heat

**PROCEDURE:**

Place the balloon over the mouth of the test tube, as shown in Figure 4.7 on page 116. Carefully heat the bottom of the tube and observe the action of the balloon.

Dent the side of the metal container slightly. Be careful not to break through the metal. Place the cork securely in the opening in the top of the can, trapping the air inside. **Caution: Do not force the cork into the opening too tightly.** Place the container on the source of heat. Stand safely out of the way as the air in the can is heated. Observe the action of the dented surface and of the cork.

## Volume and Linear Expansion

One effect of adding heat to a substance is usually an increase in the volume of the matter. Even raising the temperature by one degree will result in a small increase in volume. If this small increase is shown as a fraction of the original volume, we have what is known as the **coefficient** (kō′ ə fish′ ənt) **of volume expansion.** The coefficient of expansion for water, for example, is approximately 0.0002. This figure indicates that a liter of water will expand at the rate of 0.0002 of a liter for each degree Celsius of temperature increase.

To find the increase in the volume of 50 liters of water when the temperature is increased 30° C, the volume of the water is multiplied times the coefficient of volume expansion times the number of degrees the temperature has increased (50 × 0.0002

**4.6** Expansion joint

*Walter R. Brown*

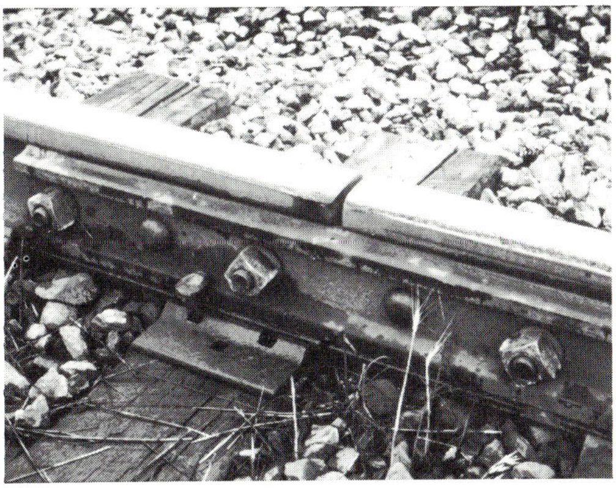

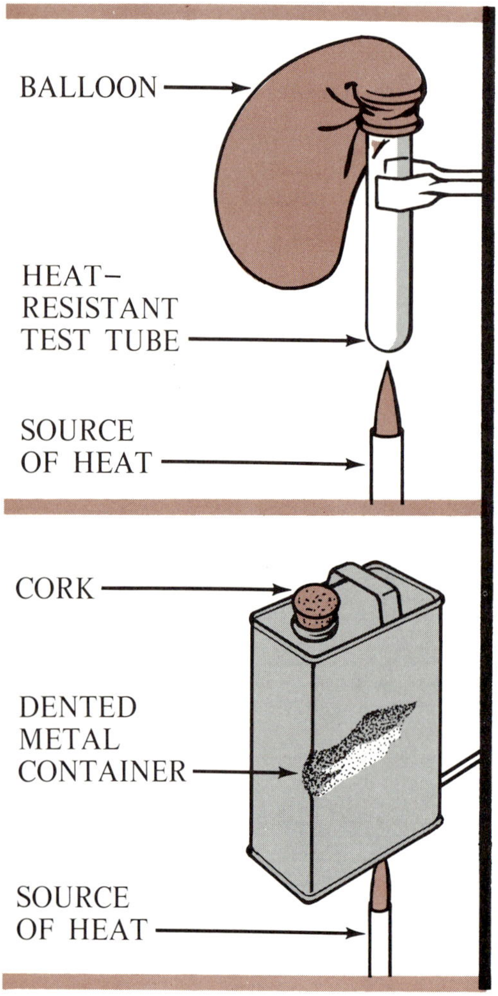


**4.7** Procedure for Expansion of Gases on page 115

$\times$ 30 = 0.3 of a liter). Perhaps 0.3 of a liter does not seem like a very large increase. But consider how important this might be if a sealed container full of water were being heated. Boilers and radiators of cars are designed to allow for this expansion of water.

Engineers, who are concerned with the building of bridges and buildings out of solid materials, often use **coefficients of linear expansion.** The coefficients given in the chart below show the change per unit length for each Celsius degree of temperature change. This means a meter-long bar of Invar, which is an alloy of iron and nickel, will expand 0.0000009 ($9.0 \times 10^{-7}$) of a meter if its temperature is increased 1° C. Which material listed in the table will expand the most? The least? Which two materials will expand at the same rate?

The metal bar, shown in the photograph (Figure 4.8) on page 117, demonstrates the unequal expansion rates of two metals. A strip of brass and a strip of Invar have been tightly bonded together. When heated, the bimetal bar bends because the two metals do not expand at the same rate. From the table of coefficients following, can you figure out which way the bar will bend?

COEFFICIENT OF LINEAR EXPANSION
*(Per Degree Celsius)*

| | |
|---|---|
| Invar | 0.0000009 |
| Pyrex | 0.000003 |
| Glass | 0.000009 |
| Iron | 0.000011 |
| Steel | 0.000013 |
| Gold | 0.000014 |
| Copper | 0.000017 |
| Brass | 0.000019 |
| Silver | 0.000019 |
| Aluminum | 0.000023 |

## The Molecule

As you have seen, gases expand also. But, unlike solids and liquids, the coefficients of volume expansion of all gases are nearly equal. The coefficient is approximately 0.0037 ($3.7 \times 10^{-3}$) at temperatures

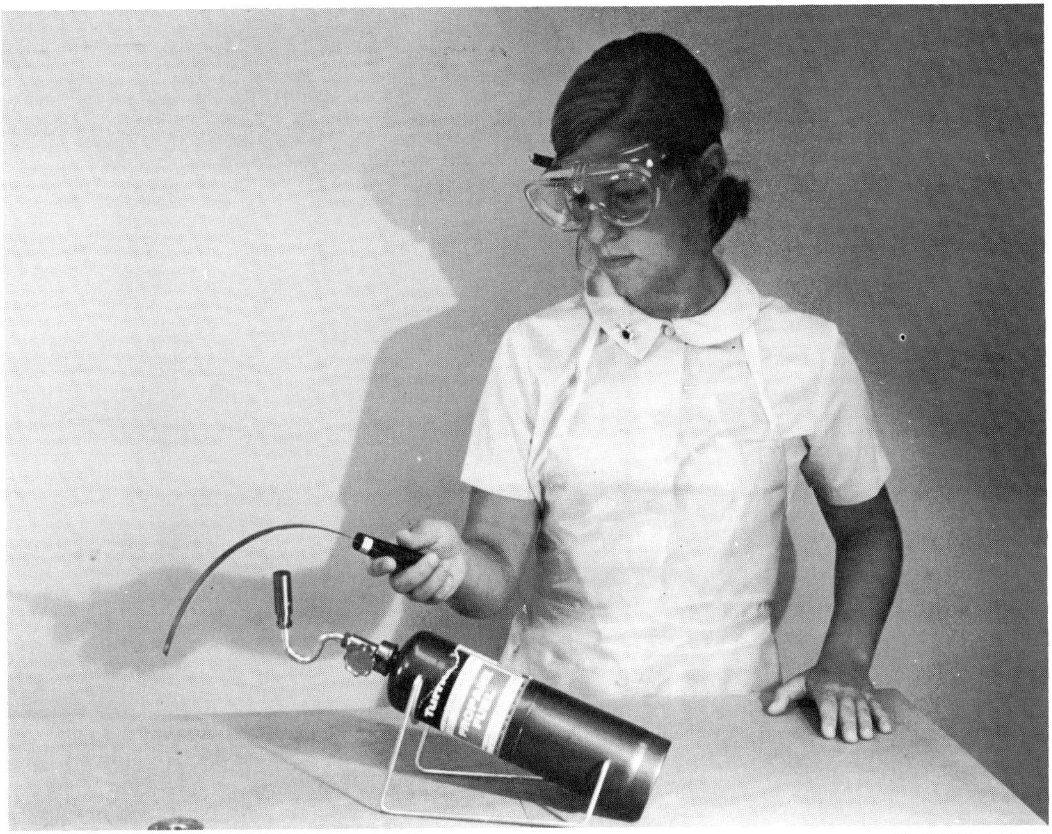

Norman D. Anderson

**4.8** When heated, the bimetal bar bends because the two metals do not expand at the same rate.

near 0° C. It is not important that you remember this number, but compare it with the coefficient for water previously given. The expansion of gases is much greater than the expansion of other forms of matter, either solids or liquids.

How can we explain these observations? Why does matter expand at a definite rate? Why do gases expand more than solids and liquids when their temperature is increased 1° C? And why, at a certain temperature, does matter change form?

In order to answer these questions, we first must understand more about the nature of matter itself. We can easily divide a container of water into two equal parts. Each of these halves can be divided again, and we can continue this process until the water particles become too small to work with. Yet the smallest particle produced in this way would still be water.

What do you think would happen if we could continue to divide these water particles still further? Could we continue the process indefinitely? Scientists say that this is not the case. Instead they suggest that eventually we must reach a point at which we have the smallest particle of water possible, a molecule. When heat is added to a substance, work is done on the molecules. In some way, the heat energy forces the molecules apart. And at a certain distance from each other, the attraction between the molecules is broken and a change of state takes place.

## Have You Learned?

On a sheet of paper list the numbers for the questions below. By each number write *T* if the statement is true and *F* if false.

1. Most types of matter expand when they are cooled.
2. When we say that matter changes state, we mean that it has contracted.
3. Solid structures, such as those made of concrete, are built with spaces in their surfaces so that they can expand without breaking.
4. The term "coefficient of linear expansion" refers to the change in volume of a substance when it is heated.
5. All gases expand at approximately the same rate.
6. If the temperature of 100 liters of water is raised by 10° C, the volume of the water will increase by 2 liters. (The coefficient of volume expansion of water is 0.0002.)
7. The rate of expansion of all liquids is nearly equal.
8. When heat is added to a substance, its molecules are made to move farther apart.
9. The rate of expansion of the gas oxygen is much greater than the rate of expansion of solid brass.
10. If two metals having different expansion rates are bonded together and then heated, they will both expand at the same rate.

## 3. What Is Heat?

**ARE YOU READY?**

Look up the following words if you are not sure of their meanings:

absorb; attract; calibrate; fluid; pressure; theory.

After the invention of a thermometer that could be calibrated by any scientist, a careful study of the nature of heat could begin. At first, it was thought that the thermometer actually measured the heat of the object. However, experiments with the thermometer easily disproved this idea. It was found that if a certain amount of heat is applied to two different substances, the rise in temperature of the two substances is not the same. For example, if a block of iron weighing 100 grams and 100 grams of water are both placed over a fire for the same length of time, the temperature of the iron will increase much more rapidly than the temperature of the water.

This ability of a substance to absorb heat is now called **specific heat**, and is found to be different for each substance. Almost every substance has a lower specific heat than does water. In other words, it takes more heat to warm a given amount of water 10° C than it takes to increase the temperature 10° C of the same amount of air, iron, and other materials. As a result, water warms up more slowly and releases heat more slowly than do other substances. This explains why the temperature of a large body of water is usually cooler than that of the surrounding land during the day and warmer during the night. Do you see why this is so?

## Water Boils at Different Temperatures

Experiments with carefully calibrated thermometers also showed that water does not always boil at the same temperature. These experiments with the thermometers determined that the boiling point of water depends upon the pressure of the air.

### Changing the Boiling Point of Water

**MATERIALS:**

A heat-resistant, round-bottomed flask, a small quantity of water, a source of heat, a stopper for the flask, ice cubes

**PROCEDURE:**

Place the water in the open flask, and heat it until the water boils. *Remove the flask from the fire*, and quickly place the stopper in the mouth of the flask, sealing it securely.

The flask is now full of steam, which is water in a gaseous form. It contains very little air. As the steam cools, it **condenses** (kən dens′) back into water. Since water takes up much less space than the steam did, the pressure inside the flask is reduced to a very low point—much less than normal air pressure. To hurry the condensation process, place the ice cubes against the wall of the flask or pour cool water over the flask. **Caution: There is some danger that if the flask is cracked or has a weak spot in it, the pressure of the air may cause it to collapse. Be certain that you wear goggles and hold the flask in such a way that you are protected from flying glass.** The lower the temperature within the flask, the lower will be the air pressure. If you can get the air pressure low enough, the water remaining in the flask should begin to boil again. How is it possible for water to boil without adding heat?

**4.9** Does it seem strange that a bag of ice cubes can make water boil?

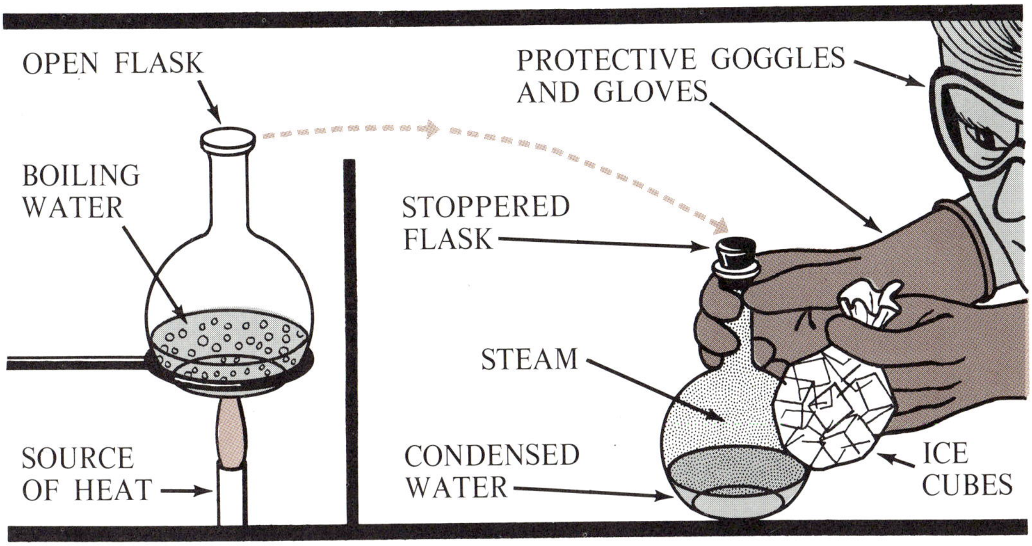

Air pressure is due to the weight of the air above the surface of the boiling water. As you climb a mountain, the amount of air above you becomes less and less. So the pressure at high **altitudes** is less than it is at sea level. Water will boil at 100° C at sea level. High in the Rocky Mountains water will boil at about 93° C, and atop Mount Everest, almost 9,000 meters above sea level, it will boil at about 71° C.

It was also discovered that once water or any other liquid reaches the boiling point, the addition of more heat does not change the temperature of the liquid.

## Working with Boiling and Freezing Temperatures

**MATERIALS:**

Several ice cubes, a container, a source of heat, a thermometer

**PROCEDURE:**

Place the ice cubes in the container, and heat it. As the ice begins to melt, measure

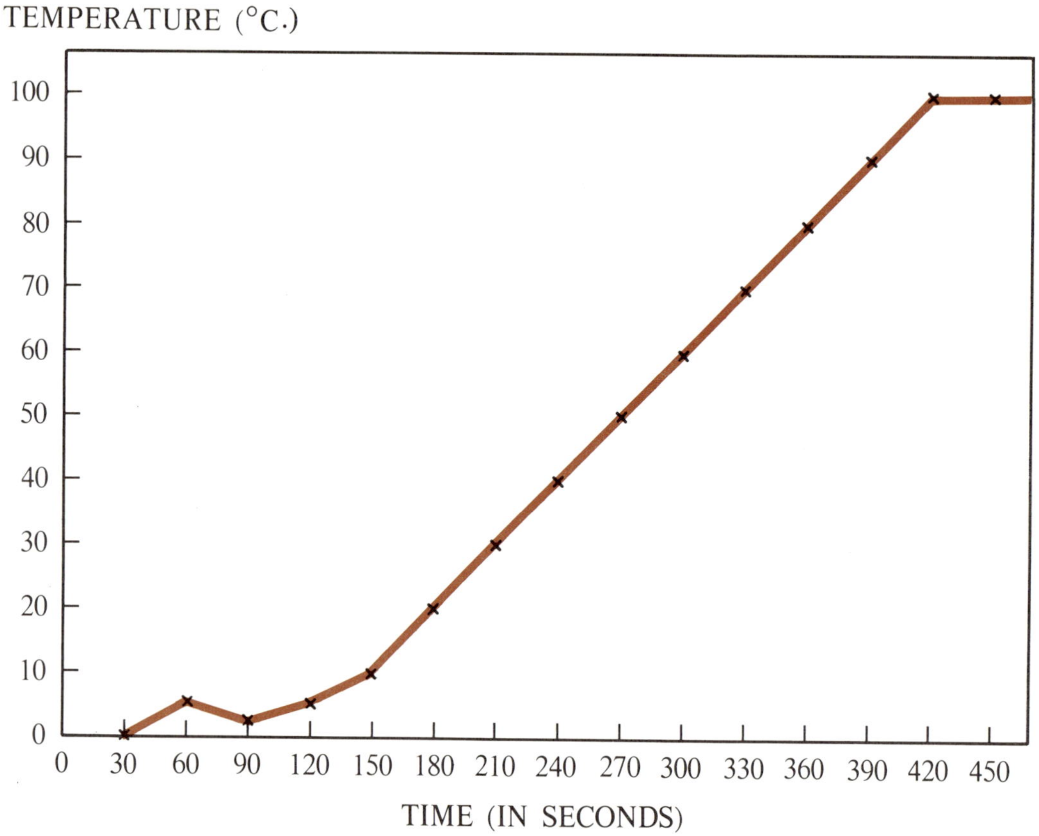

the temperature of the water. Record the readings of the thermometer every 30 seconds. After the water boils, continue taking readings for several minutes. Record your data on a graph like the one on page 120. Describe the temperature readings as you apply heat. When does the temperature begin to rise? When does it remain the same?

## The Theory of the "Caloric"

By the time of the American Revolution, scientists had collected a great number of observations about heat. They realized that heat could move from one object to another. All objects seemed to get larger when heated. Different substances absorbed heat at different rates. And, as matter changed from one state to another, no change in temperature could be observed.

To explain these observations, the **Theory of the Caloric** (kə lôr′ ik) was developed. This theory stated that heat was a fluid called **caloric,** which flowed from one substance to another. Particles of caloric were thought to **repel** each other, just as two magnets will push each other away if they are brought together in a certain way. This explained why, as a substance absorbed caloric, it seemed to get larger.

Specific heat was explained by the idea that some substances attracted caloric particles more strongly than did other substances. The various states of matter were caused, it was thought, by the ability of the caloric particles to combine with the substance to form a new substance—a gas or a liquid or a solid.

Scientific theories are constantly subjected to further experimentation by scientists, even those scientists who feel that the theories are probably correct. It was reasoned that if heat is a substance, it should have weight. Therefore, an object should weigh more when heated than when cool. Experiments were performed many times to test this idea, but no increase in weight was found.

The seeds of destruction of the Theory of the Caloric were sown long before the development of the theory. The earliest observers noticed that when one rubs one's hands together, they become warm. Plato, a Greek who lived about 2,400 years ago, wrote about heat produced by motion.

In the late 1700s no better theory had been developed, so most scientists had to assume that the mysterious substance, caloric, was weightless! However, a great doubt as to the truth of the theory of the caloric had been raised. As a result, more and more scientists began to try to find out the true nature of heat.

Later, convinced that the Theory of the Caloric was correct, scientists thought that friction produced heat by squeezing the substance and thereby forcing the caloric out of it. This idea was experimented on late in the eighteenth century by Benjamin Thompson, who was also known as Count von Rumford. He was a British-American scientist who, with the permission of the British Government, entered the civil and military service of Bavaria.

## Have You Learned?

Select the answer that best completes each statement. (Do not write in your book.)

1. The ability of a substance to absorb heat is called _____. (a) absolute heat; (b) specific heat; (c) heatability.
2. When a given amount of heat is applied to equal amounts of various substances, almost all of them will warm more rapidly than _____. (a) water; (b) iron; (c) sand.
3. The boiling point of water depends upon both temperature and _____. (a) density; (b) specific heat; (c) pressure.
4. When steam changes back into liquid water, we say that it has _____. (a) condensed; (b) evaporated; (c) expanded.
5. One of the first theories about the nature of heat held that heat was a fluid called _____. (a) water; (b) specific heat; (c) caloric.
6. The scientific study of the nature of heat could not begin until the _____ had been invented. (a) caloric; (b) barometer; (c) thermometer.
7. Understanding the idea of _____ helps explain why the temperature of a large body of water is usually cooler during the day than the surrounding land. (a) specific heat; (b) boiling temperature and pressure; (c) evaporation.
8. When water reaches its boiling temperature, the addition of more heat _____ the temperature of the water. (a) raises; (b) lowers; (c) does not change.
9. The substance caloric was thought to be _____. (a) a fluid; (b) a solid; (c) a magnet.

## 4. Heat = Molecules in Motion

**ARE YOU READY?**

Look up the following words if you are not sure of their meanings:

Conservation of Energy; friction; matter; mechanical energy; metric system; Theory of Caloric.

In the 1700s cannon barrels for the Bavarian army were made from solid pieces of brass that were hollowed out by boring. While supervising this process, Rumford (see page 121) noticed that a great amount of heat was produced by the friction of the drill against the brass barrel. He reasoned that if the heat produced by the boring was really due to the loss of caloric substance, the brass shavings from the cannon barrel should contain less caloric than similar pieces of brass that had had caloric added to them by being heated in a fire.

### Early Experiments with Heat

To test this theory, Rumford placed shavings from the cannon boring in a definite quantity of water and noted the rise in temperature of the water. He then took a quantity of brass shavings equal in weight to the cannon borings, heated them to the same temperature as the borings, and placed them in a second container of the same quantity of water as the first one. The rise in temperature in both cases was the same.

To investigate this discovery further, Rumford then fitted a chamber of water around a brass barrel. As the bit turned, heat was produced that caused the water to boil. Rumford reasoned that heat could not be matter, since the amount of heat produced by the friction seemed inexhaustible. He concluded, as Plato did, that heat was caused by motion.

Other experiments quickly followed. In 1799 Sir Humphry Davy, an English chemist, demonstrated that both wax and ice could be melted by friction even though their temperatures were below freezing. Another English scientist, James Joule (joul), carefully calculated the amount of mechanical energy necessary to raise the temperature of a pound of water by one degree Fahrenheit, and discovered that a given amount of mechanical energy always produced the same amount of heat. These experiments, and the work of many other scientists, opened the door for the discovery of the principle of the Conservation of Energy. This principle states that energy, like matter, can be converted from one form to another (for instance, mechanical energy can be converted to heat energy), but energy cannot be created or destroyed.

## The Modern Theory of Heat

The currently accepted idea of the nature of heat is based on the theory of the molecular structure of matter. According to the molecular theory, matter is composed of particles called molecules, which are in continuous motion. In the case of gases and liquids, the moving molecules rebound off each other like balls on a pool table. Even in solids this motion takes place, although the distance between the molecules is much shorter. The motion of the molecules of a solid has been described as being only **vibrations** (vī brā′ shən), with each molecule staying more or less in place while moving slightly toward its neighbor and then away again.

The modern theory explains heat as being the energy of motion of the molecules of matter. The hotter a substance is, the faster its molecules move. This in turn causes the average distance between them to become greater. This explains why objects increase in size when they are heated.

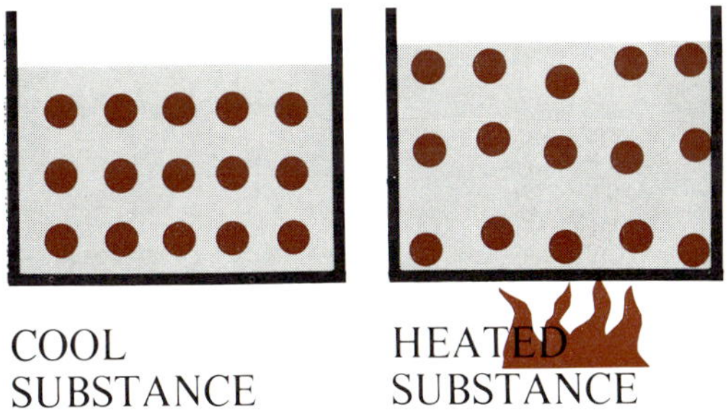

**4.10** What do the heated molecules do?

Since the molecules of every substance are in motion, heat energy is present in every bit of matter. Thus, what we call "cold" is not simply the absence of heat energy. To cool an object we slow down the motion of its molecules by transferring some of its energy to another bit of matter. An object is said to be "cool" if heat energy flows into it from its surroundings, and "warm" if heat energy flows away from it.

## Measuring Units Used

What would happen if we were to continue to remove heat energy until a substance had no more? Although this has not been accomplished in a laboratory yet,

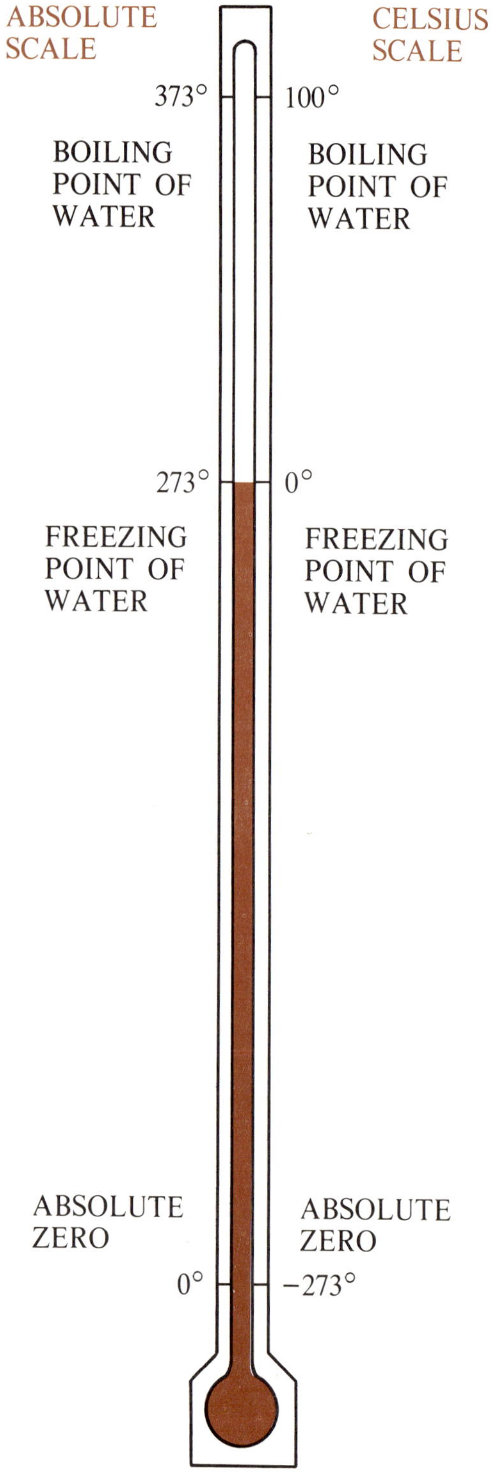


the lowest temperature possible has been calculated mathematically. This calculation indicates that the coldest temperature possible would be −273.16° C. This is known as **absolute zero,** and is used as the 0 degree point on a temperature scale known as the **absolute scale** or **Kelvin Scale.** In this system, the degree is equal in size to the Celsius degree, so that the melting point of ice is about 273° K, and the boiling point of water is about 373° K.

Scientists still use a word similar to "caloric," but it now means something entirely different from what it did during Rumford's time. The **calorie** (kal′ ə ri) is now used as a unit of heat. It is the amount of heat necessary to raise the temperature of one gram of water 1° C. As you might guess, this is a very small unit. When measuring the amount of energy in foods, biologists use the **kilocalorie** (kil′ ə kal′ ə ri), which equals 1,000 calories. You may see the kilocalorie referred to as the "Calorie," with a capital C.

The calorie, since it uses grams and degrees of Celsius, is part of the metric system of measurement. The unit of heat in the English system is the **British Thermal Unit,** or **BTU.** One BTU is the amount of heat necessary to raise the temperature of one pound of water 1° F.

**4.11** The absolute or Kelvin Scale as opposed to the Celsius. What does "absolute zero" mean?

## Have You Learned?

From the list at the right select the word that most accurately completes each of the following statements. (Do not write in your book.)

1. The coldest temperature possible is _____ zero.
2. The man who first melted ice by friction was _____.
3. The man who first wrote that heat was caused by motion was _____.
4. The modern theory explains heat as being the energy of motion of _____.
5. The BTU is a unit of heat in the _____ system of measurement.
6. The amount of heat necessary to raise the temperature of 1 gram of water 1° C is a _____.
7. The man who experimented with brass shavings heated by friction was _____.
8. The motion of molecules in solids is thought to be only _____.
9. The man who measured the amount of mechanical energy that is equal to one BTU was _____.
10. The amount of heat necessary to raise the temperature of 1,000 grams of water 1° C is a _____.

a. absolute
b. calorie
c. Davy
d. English
e. Galileo
f. Joule
g. kilocalorie
h. metric
i. molecules
j. Plato
k. Rumford
l. vibration

## 5. Transfer of Heat

**ARE YOU READY?**

Look up the following words if you are not sure of their meanings:

circulate; currents; distribute; expand; fluid; heat energy; transfer; universe.

The transfer of heat energy from one bit of matter to another can be done in several ways. One common method is through direct contact, called **conduction** (kən duk′ shən). If a cold piece of iron is put into warm water, the more rapidly moving molecules of the water strike against the molecules of the iron. The effect of this is to slow down the speed of the molecules of the water and to increase the motion of the iron molecules. Can you suggest what will happen to the temperature of the water and of the iron? Can you test your hypothesis?

Cooks use the conduction method of transferring heat every day: the rapidly moving molecules of burning fuel strike against the metal of the pan over the flame. In this way, the energy level of the molecules of the pan is increased and is, in turn, transferred to the food inside. An ice cube cools a drink partly through the conduction of heat energy out of the liquid and into the ice. Heat energy is conducted away from the food in a refrigerator and into the cold air around it.

A second method of heat transfer is called **convection** (kən vek′ shən). Here the heat is transferred from one place to another by the movement of matter itself.

## Observing Convection Currents

**MATERIALS:**

Two large glass jars of equal size and shape, hot water, cold water, a few drops of ink, a piece of thin cardboard large enough to cover the top of one jar

**PROCEDURE:**

Place a few drops of ink in one jar, and carefully add hot water until the jar is completely full. (CAUTION: If the water is too hot and is poured into the jar too quickly, the glass may break. Can you explain why this can happen?)

Pour the cold water into the second jar, filling it completely. Place the piece of cardboard over the mouth of the jar, like a lid. Turn the jar over quickly but carefully, holding the cardboard in place to prevent spilling the water. Put the jar of cold water upside down on top of the jar of hot water, so that their openings are opposite each other. Quickly remove the cardboard from between the two jars, being careful not to spill the water.

Observe the movement of the colored hot water and the colorless cold water.

**4.12** With a few drops of ink and some hot and cold water, you can see a liquid convention current.

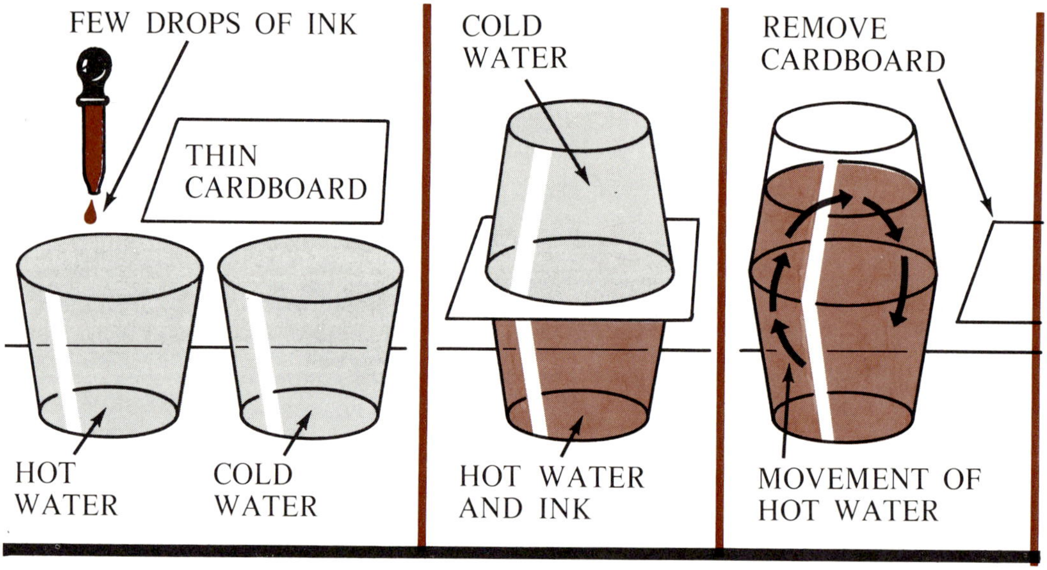


If you performed the above activity carefully enough, you should have observed currents in the water as the warm water moved upward and the cold water settled downward. These are **convection currents.**

Convection currents in air can be observed by using the instrument shown in the picture on page 127. A lighted candle is placed in the box directly under one of the lamp chimneys. By holding a lighted match above the other chimney and blowing it out to create smoke, you can easily see that the cooler air from outside is being pulled into the box as the air warmed by the candle rises.

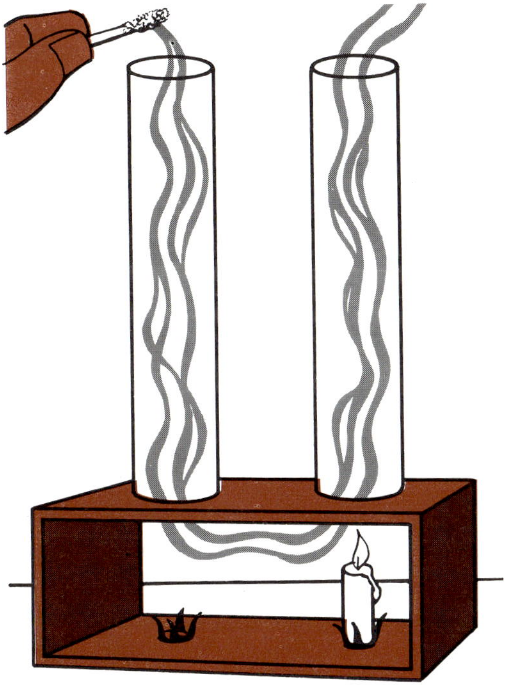

**4.13** A convection chamber in use

These currents occur in fluids (both gases and liquids) when they are heated unevenly. The molecules of the heated portion move farther apart as they receive energy is distributed through it. Try to describe the problems concerning heat in an indoor skating rink.
portion, and rises. The heavier, cooler fluid flows in to take the place of the rising fluid. As the fluid circulates, the heat energy is distributed through it. Try to describe the problems concerning heat in an indoor skating rink.

Both convection and conduction depend upon the presence of matter. But the most

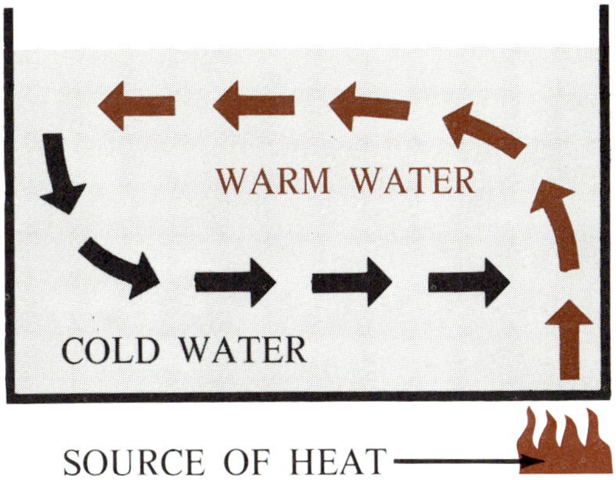


**4.14** Convection currents

important source of heat is the sun, which is separated from the earth by $149.6 \times 10^6$ kilometers of empty space. Thus it is not always necessary that matter be present

**4.15** When ice is made for an indoor skating rink, heat of the water must be removed (transferred) so that the water will freeze.

*Clif Garboden/Stock, Boston*

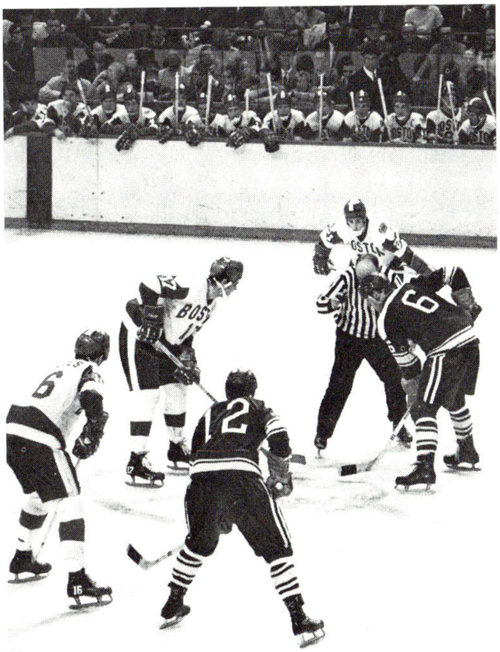

when heat is transferred from one place to another. A third method of heat transfer is called **radiation** (rā′ di ā′ shən). Energy in a form other than heat travels through space and is converted (kən vėrt′), or changed into heat when it strikes matter. This will be made more understandable when you study about light energy in Chapter 14.

Regardless of whether heat energy is being transferred by conduction, convection, or radiation, the heat energy moves from an area of high energy to an area of low energy. Like water, heat energy "flows only downhill."

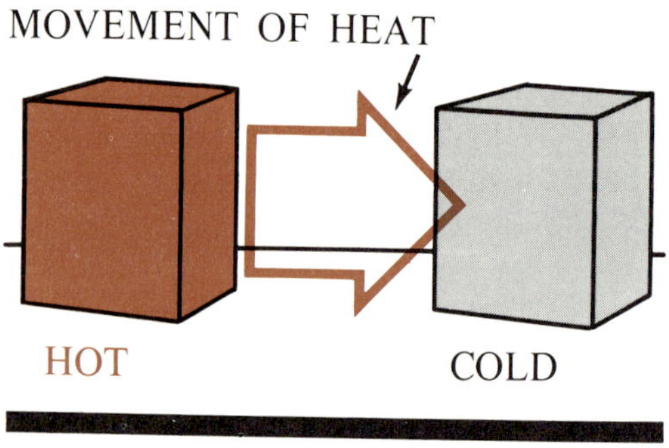


**4.16** Movement of energy

Imagine an iron bar that is completely insulated (in′ sə lāt′) in such a way that no heat energy is able to leave the bar, and none enters it from the outside. Suppose that the molecules at one end of the bar are moving very much faster than those at the other end. In other words, one end of the bar is very much hotter than the other.

The rapidly moving molecules at the hotter end of the bar collide with the molecules nearest to them and pass on some of their energy. But when they do so, their energy level becomes less. Thus, after a period of time, the heat energy will become *equally distributed* throughout the bar. No one spot will be cooler or warmer than any other spot.

Now imagine another such closed system. This time, a set of objects is surrounded by air, but the whole system is insulated from outside influences and from the loss of energy. If we place an object in the system that is hotter than the other objects, what will happen? The heat energy from the warm object will flow, primarily by convection currents, warming all of the other objects in the system. As this occurs, the warm object will become cooler. Eventually, just like the iron bar, all parts of the system will become the same temperature. (See Figure 4.18.)

Our earth is not a closed system, like those described here, since energy is constantly flowing to it from the sun. Because it is unevenly distributed over the earth, this energy constantly flows through the

**4.17** Movement of molecules in a bar heated at one end

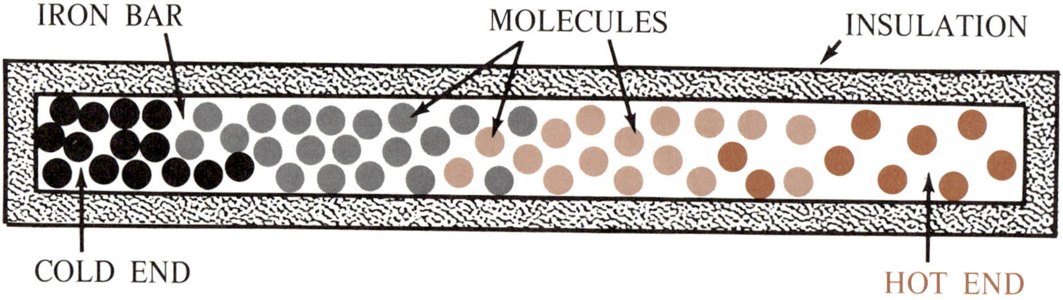

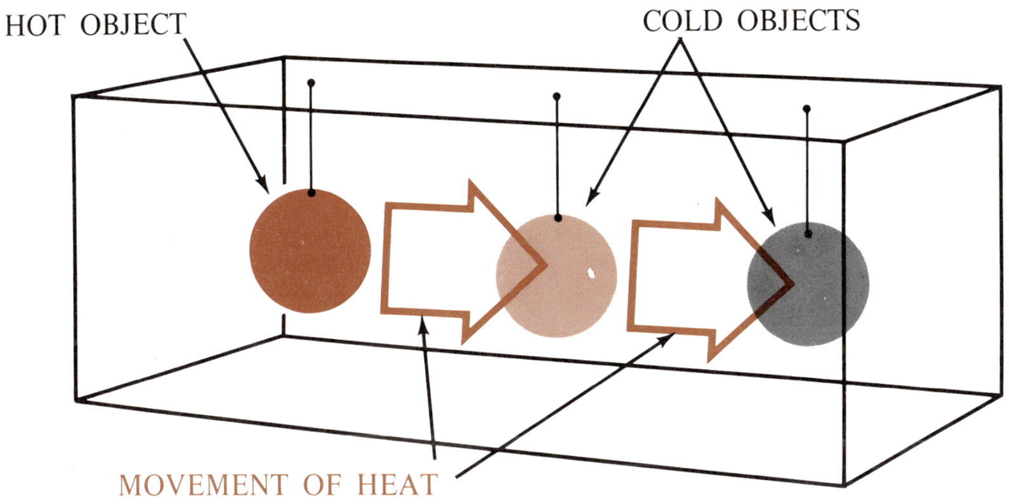


**4.18** Movement of heat in a closed system

atmosphere. One result of this transfer of heat energy from place to place is convection currents called *winds*.

The universe may be a closed system. If so, energy is in the process of being distributed evenly throughout all parts of the universe. When this even distribution is completed, energy will cease to flow from one place to another. If this occurs, what will happen to life on the earth?

## Have You Learned?

In each of the following situations heat is transferred from one place to another either by a. conduction, b. convection or c. radiation. Indicate which of these is the *primary* method of heat transfer in each case. Briefly explain your answer.

1. A silver spoon becomes heated when placed in a cup of hot liquid.
2. The handle of a frying pan becomes hot when the pan is put on a fire.
3. A campfire is built, and you warm your hands by holding them out toward the fire.
4. A fire is built in a fireplace, and the temperature of the air in the chimney increases.
5. The earth is heated by the sun.
6. An electric water-heating device is placed in one corner of a fish tank, and the temperature of all parts of the tank goes up.
7. You hold your hand over an electric toaster and feel the heat coming out.
8. You touch the outside of the electric toaster and it feels warm.
9. You walk down into the crater of an old volcano and find that the rocks are warm, even though the source of the heat is more than 50 kilometers below the surface.
10. A hot wind blows against you.

## 6. Change of State

> **ARE YOU READY?**
>
> Look up the following words if you are not sure of their meanings:
>
> average; calorie; contraction; expansion; state (of matter); vibration.

How does the modern theory of heat explain the fact that changing the amount of heat energy in a substance will sometimes change the state of the substance? How does slowing down the action of the molecules of a liquid cause it to become a solid? And how does an increase in the molecular action of a liquid produce a gas?

As you learned in Section 4, the molecules of a solid are held tightly in position. The only movement of molecules in a solid is thought to be vibration. As heat energy is added to the solid, this vibration increases, and the molecules move farther and farther apart. This continues until some of the molecules break away from their position in the solid. At this time, melting has begun.

When the substance is in the liquid form, its molecules are free to move around within the substance. In most substances, the average distance between molecules is much greater than when the substance was in the solid state. The molecules move in straight lines until they hit the walls of the container or other molecules.

If we could observe the molecules of a glass of water, we might notice that some are moving much faster than others. A thermometer that has been placed in the water is struck by many millions of molecules, some moving very rapidly and some moving more slowly. The expansion of the liquid in the thermometer measures the *average* speed of molecules that strike it.

The faster-moving molecules may have enough energy to break through the surface layer of the liquid and escape into the air. When this happens, we say that the water is **evaporating.** It is slowly changing from a liquid to a gas. Since the liquid is losing its most rapidly moving molecules, the average speed of the molecules of the liquid is reduced. What effect does this have on the temperature of the liquid? See Figure 4.19 on the next page.

### Feeling and Seeing the Effect of Evaporation

**MATERIALS:**

A small quantity of alcohol, water, medicine dropper, two identical saucers

**PROCEDURE:**

Using the medicine dropper, place 5 drops of water in one saucer and 5 drops of alcohol in the other. Observe the liquids every few minutes until one has completely evaporated. Which liquid evaporates more quickly?

Place a few drops of alcohol on the back of your hand, and fan them gently with your other hand. Can you feel a change in temperature? Why does fanning the surface of the alcohol speed up the evaporation? See Figure 4.19 on the next page.

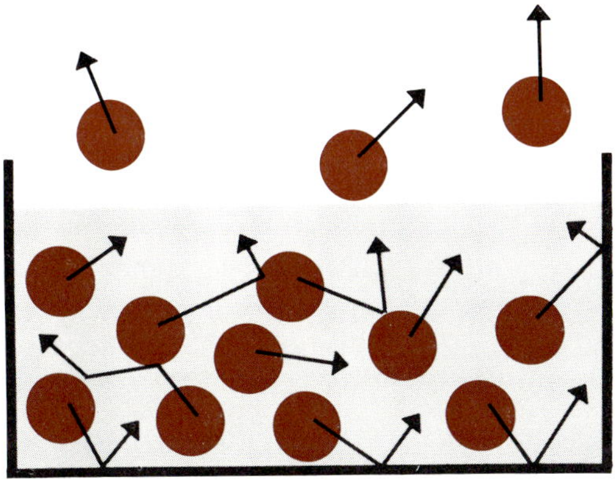

**4.19** Evaporation takes place when the most rapidly moving molecules escape from a liquid.

Since heating a liquid increases the speed of its molecular motion, heating increases evaporation. When we want damp clothing to dry, we hang it in the sun or put it in a dryer full of warm air.

Observe a container of water that is being heated. As the water becomes warm, small bubbles form along the sides of the container. This is air that has been dissolved in the water. As the temperature of the water rises, bubbles of steam form, and at about 100° C the liquid begins to boil rapidly. If we add more heat, the speed with which the water turns to a gas increases, but the temperature remains at 100° C.

This lack of change of temperature of a substance during a change of state is

**4.20** The heat of the sun would not evaporate the moisture on this tennis court fast enough. So surfacing material was spread on the court, and the fans were asked to walk on it to pack it down.

*Wide World Photos*

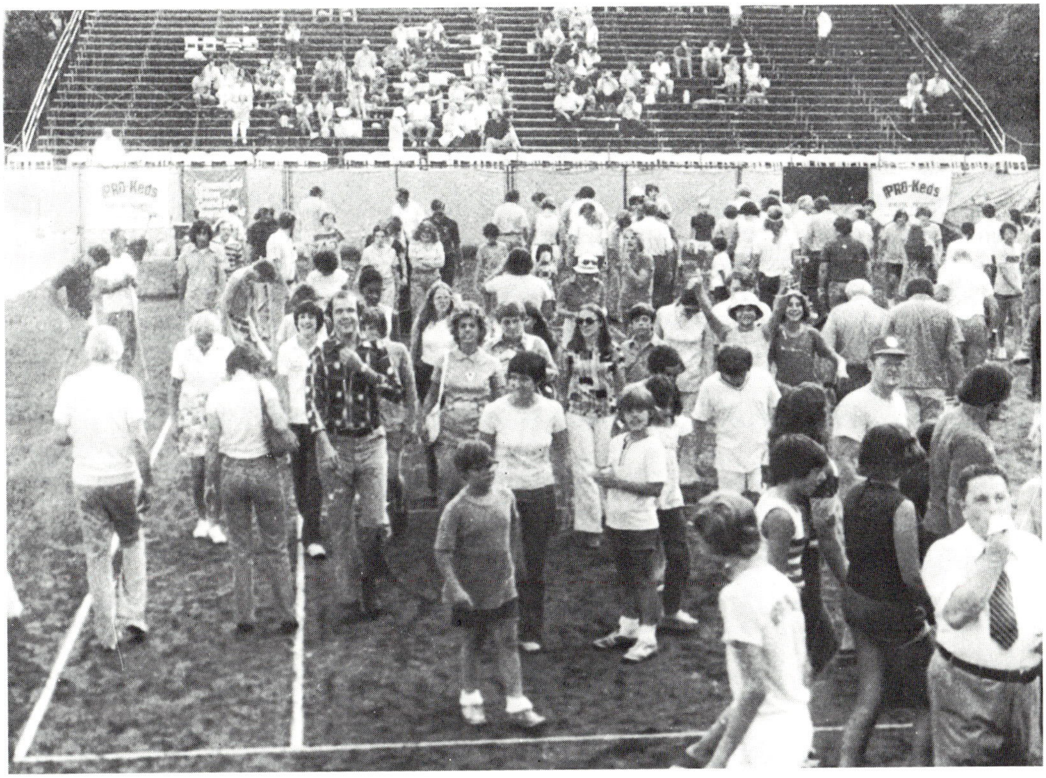

called **latent** (lā′ tənt) **heat.** The molecules of a solid or a liquid attract each other to some extent. The heat energy added to a boiling liquid or a melting solid is used to overcome these forces between molecules. Because it is used in this way, rather than in increasing the speed of the molecules, the temperature of the substance cannot increase.

The amount of latent heat for each substance is always the same. For example, to melt one gram of ice, 80 calories of heat are required. And it requires almost 540 calories to boil away one gram of water.

When a gas is being liquefied or a liquid is being solidified, the latent heat will be *released.* The amount of this heat energy is the same as that absorbed when the substance moves from the lower energy state to the higher one. In other words, when a quantity of gaseous water condenses into one gram of liquid water, 540 calories of heat will be given off. And when one gram of water freezes, 80 calories of heat are given off.

**4.21** Crystal structure of ice

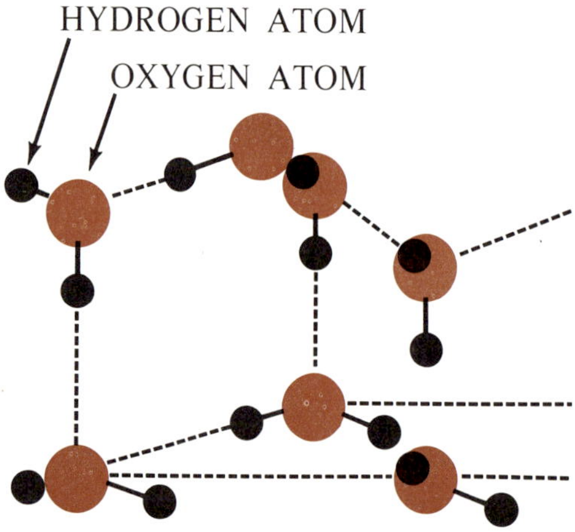


## Different Melting Points for Different Solids

Not all solids have a definite melting point. If a solid melts at a certain temperature, we know that its molecules are held in position by forces between them. These forces hold the molecules in certain positions, forming **crystals** (kris′ təl). Noncrystalline solids like wax are composed of molecules that are shaped like long strings. These long molecules are physically tangled together, and the attractive forces between them are very small. Because of this structure, noncrystalline solids soften slowly as heat is added to them.

Ice is a crystalline solid, as you can tell from its definite melting point. This crystalline structure is responsible for another important characteristic of ice. You have probably observed that as water freezes, it expands, rather than contracts as do most substances. Water pipes may burst as the water in them freezes and expands. Ice forming on the top of a lake may be pushed far up on the shore by this expansion (Figure 4.21).

As water cools, it contracts as almost all other substances do. At about 4° C, crystals begin to form, forcing the molecules farther apart. These crystal groups are small and do not attract each other, so at this stage the water is still fluid. As the temperature approaches 0° C, the number of crystals increases, and the volume of the liquid continues to increase. At the freezing temperature of 0° C, the liquid water is composed primarily of tiny ice crystals. With the removal of 80 calories of heat energy, solid ice is formed.

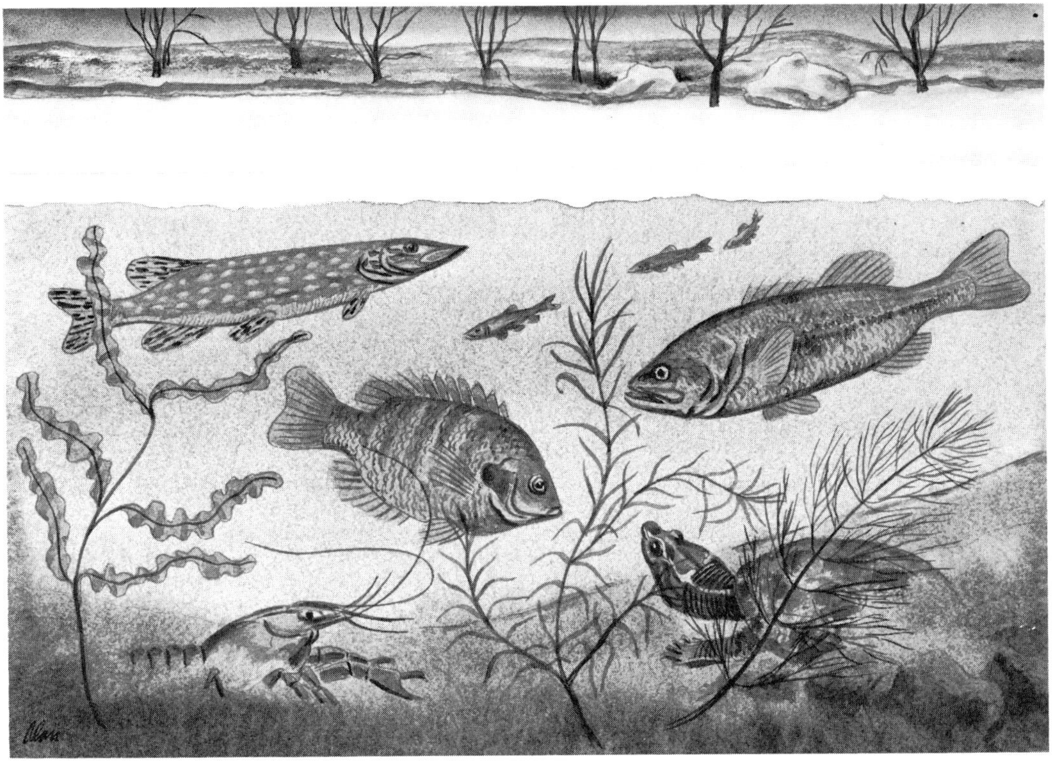

**4.22** Water expands as it freezes. Therefore, deep ponds rarely freeze to the bottom.

Since the volume of water is greater when its temperature is below 4° C, ice floats on water. Thus, when a lake freezes, the ice forms on the top of the water. Unless the lake is very shallow, water animals can live beneath the ice (Figure 4.22).

## Two Factors Affect Boiling

The temperature at which a liquid boils depends upon two factors. The first is the forces between the molecules making up the liquid. The second is the pressure of the air pushing down on the surface of the liquid. Enough energy must be added to the liquid to cause the molecules to overcome these forces before it will boil.

Changing the pressure on a liquid changes the boiling temperature. In Denver, Colorado, water boils at about 95° C because at 1,580 meters elevation the air pressure is much less than it is at sea level. Pressure cookers keep steam from escaping and build up pressure. Because of this increased pressure, the temperature of the water will go well above 100° C without boiling (Figure 4.23).

Changing a substance from a gas to a liquid and then to a solid is simply a matter of removing energy from it. As the molecular action decreases, the molecules move closer together. At a certain temperature and pressure the gas **condenses** into a liquid and at another temperature and pressure it **solidifies.**

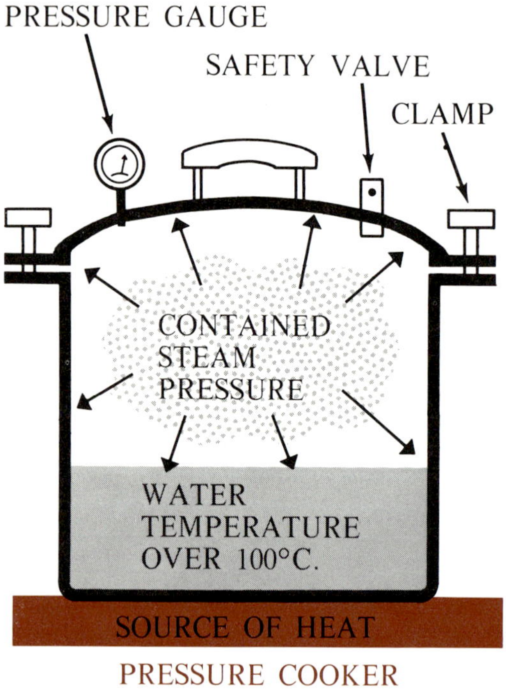


**4.23** By increasing the pressure, the boiling point of water is raised.

## Have You Learned?

Answer the following questions, using short complete sentences.

1. How does a thermometer measure temperature?
2. What happens to the molecules as ice melts into water and the water evaporates?
3. What is meant by the term "latent heat"?
4. How can plants and animals live in a deep lake when the air temperature is below freezing?
5. How is it possible for the water inside a pressure cooker to be above 100° C without boiling?

# 7. Putting Heat to Work

**ARE YOU READY?**

Look up the following words if you are not sure of their meanings:

calorie; combustion; compress; compressor; condense; convection; expand; liquefy; pressure (of the atmosphere); radiation; vaporize.

Long before the nature of heat was well understood, people learned to use heat energy. The control of fire was an early development, and most groups of very primitive peoples discovered that they could warm themselves by burning certain fuels. The use of fire to improve the taste of some foods and to preserve others was also discovered many thousands of years ago.

## The Invention of Several Kinds of Engines

But as the theory of heat energy became better developed, many more applications were possible. One of the most important of these was the practical steam engine, developed about 1765 by James Watt. By the use of a simple valve, Watt was able to use the pressure of steam to push a **piston.** Engines such as this were widely used during England's Industrial Revolution. (See Figure 4.24.)

The automobile engine is a modification of Watt's idea. In the automobile gasoline engine, gasoline and air are pulled into a **cylinder** (sil′ ən dər), where the mixture is burned. The heat necessary to start the

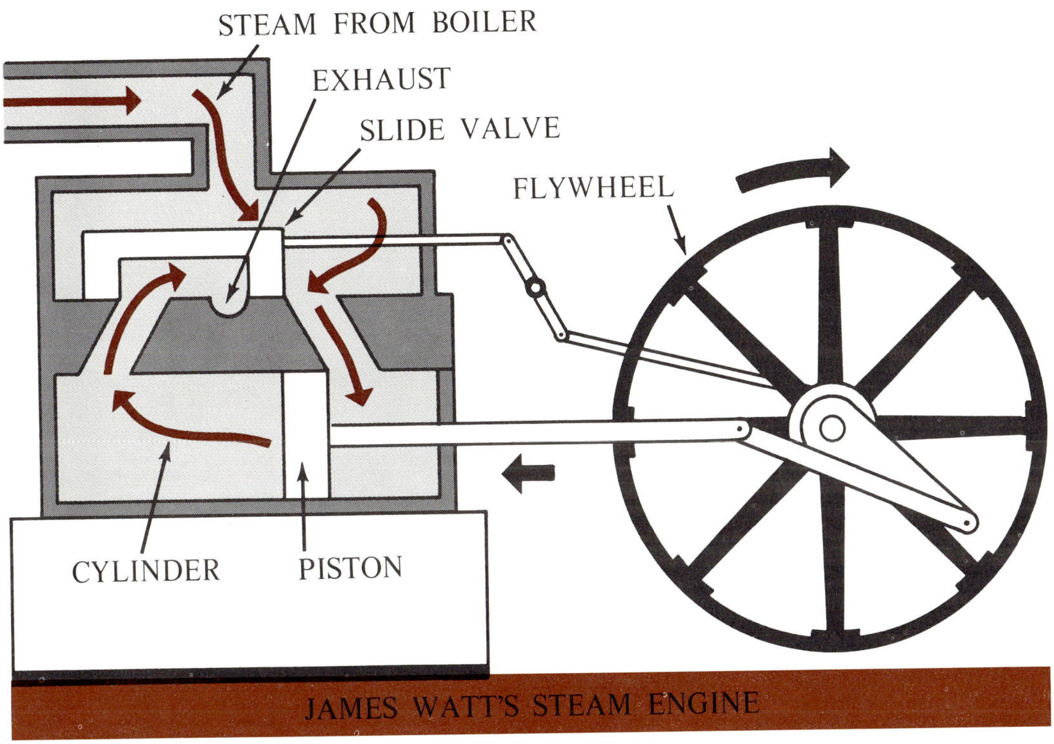


**4.24** James Watt's steam engine. Try to compare this engine with the one on the next page.

gasoline burning is supplied by an electric spark from the spark plug. As the gasoline burns, it expands rapidly. The pressure of the expanding gases pushes against the movable bottom of the cylinder, which is called the piston. As the piston moves down, its arm pushes against the **crankshaft,** which makes the wheels of the car turn. (See Figure 4.25 page 136.)

Another modification of the early steam engine is the turbine, shown in the diagram on page 137. Expanding steam rushes through sets of movable blades. This causes the central shaft to turn smoothly, unlike the jerky motion of a piston engine.

In a steam turbine, the steam enters the blades at a pressure more than 1,300 times the pressure of the atmosphere. As it cools, it condenses back into water, so that the pressure at the end of the turbine is actually lower than that of the atmosphere.

Some turbines are powered by gas from burning fuel. Air is compressed and combined with fuel that is then burned. This explosion further heats and expands the unused air that, along with the gases from the combustion, rushes through the turbine blades. Part of this energy is used to run the compressor and the remainder is used to do useful work.

Experiments are now being conducted that aim at adapting this type of turbine for use in an automobile. The useful work of the turbine shaft is in turning the wheels of the car. A turbine-powered car would have fewer moving parts and should be more efficient and less expensive.

In the **turbroprop** (tėr′ bō prop′) airplane

**4.25** Notice the position of the valves in each of the diagrams.

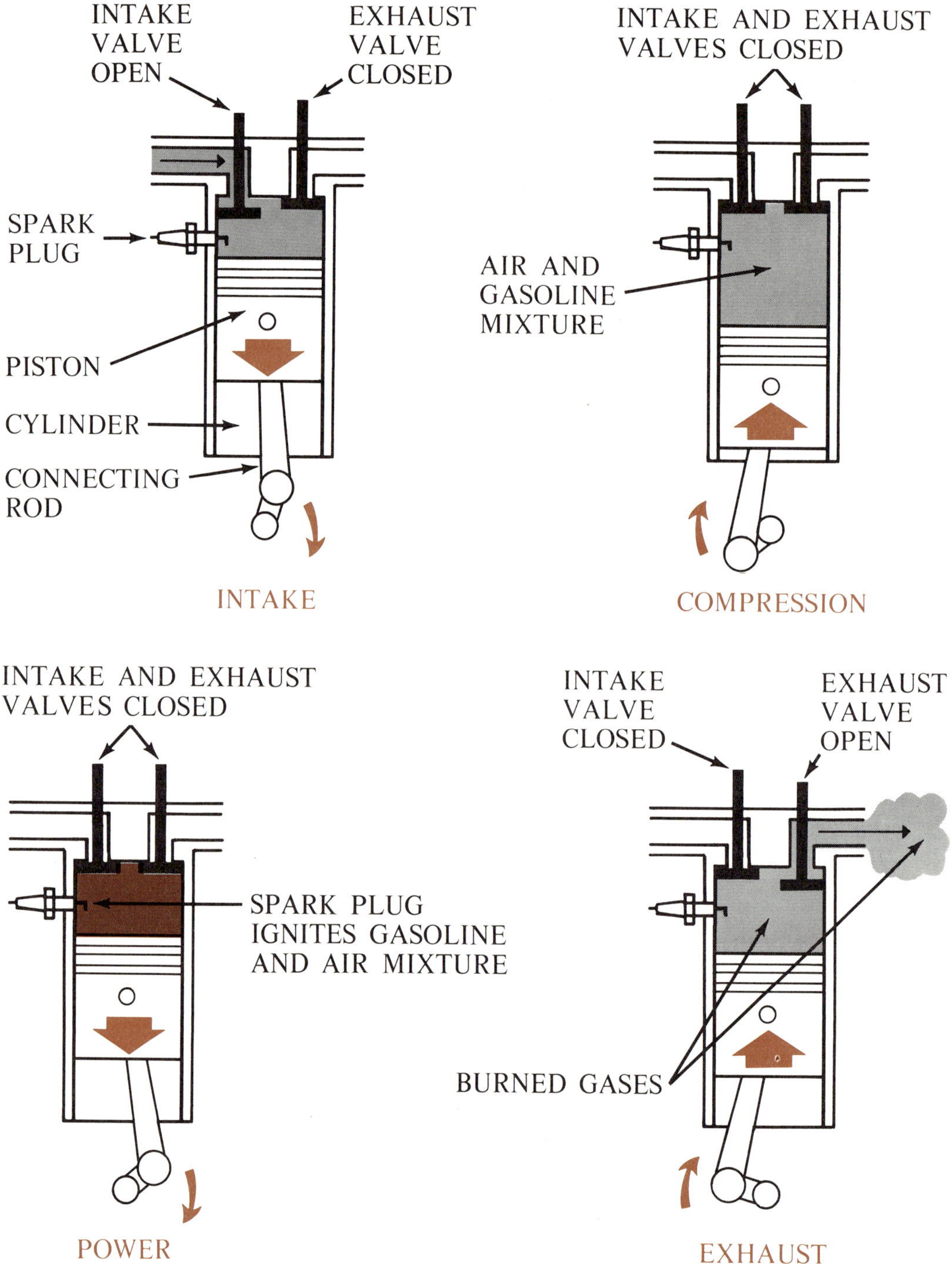


4-CYCLE GASOLINE ENGINE

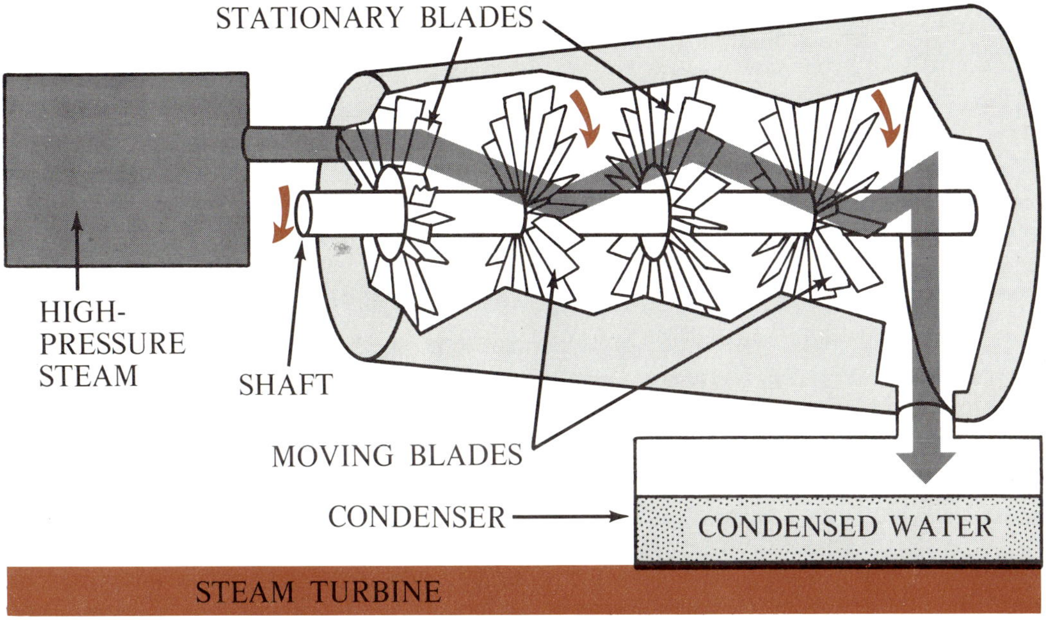


**4.26** Steam turbines are often used to turn generators that produce electricity.

engine, the turbine is used to turn the propeller. In the **turbojets** the turbine turns only the compressor, and the plane is pushed forward by the unequal pressure created when the gases and compressed air are discharged from the rear of the engine. The only difference between these airplane engines and the engine of a rocket is that the rocket carries its own supply of oxygen and is therefore not dependent upon the atmosphere. (See Figure 4.27 and Figure 4.28.)

**4.27** How is this engine different from the ramjet engine in Figure 4.28?

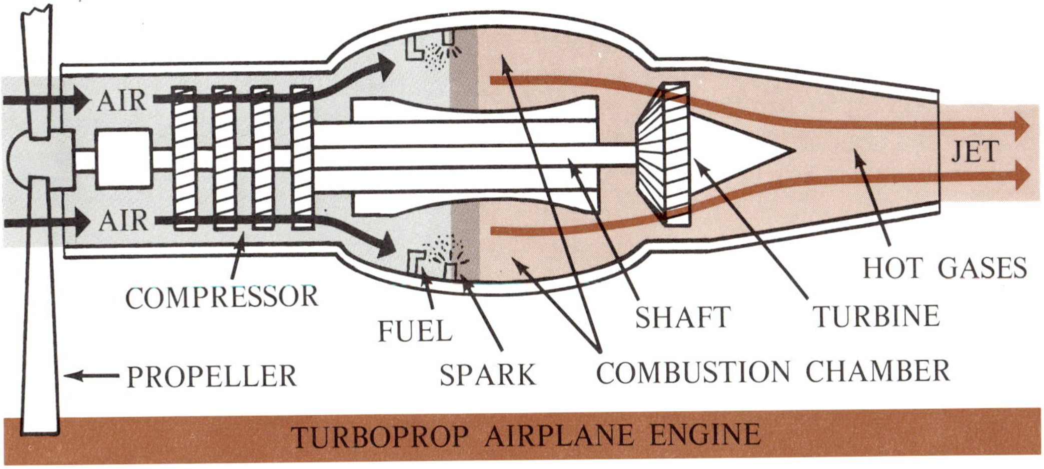

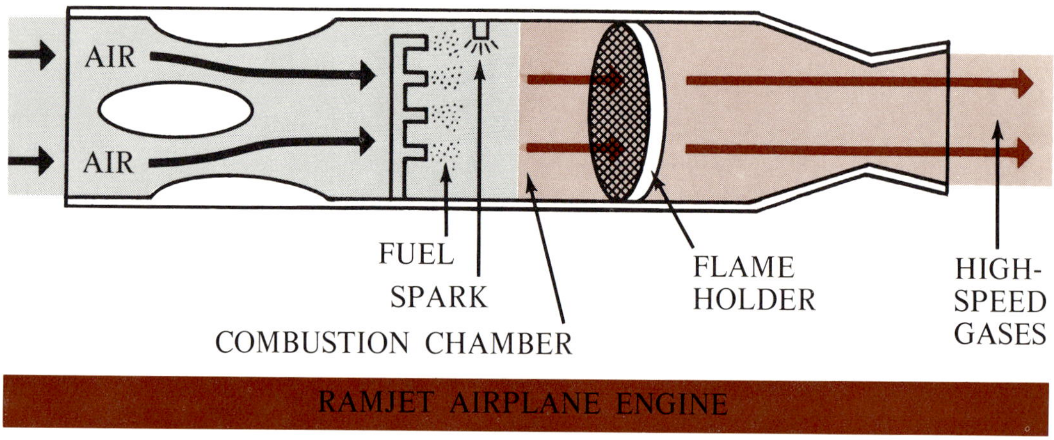


**4.28** Do you think that this type of engine could be used in outer space?

## Domestic Heating

In early times people had to spend a great deal of time simply collecting fuel in order to live through the winter. In the early days of this country's settlement, clearing the land of forest served the double purpose of making farmland available and providing a supply of fuel to last through the ensuing winter.

In prehistoric periods man warmed himself over fires in caves or in rough shelters, but it was long before he knew enough to cut a hole in the roof to permit the smoke to escape. Even in the fourteenth century, great manor houses in Europe had no chimneys. From about 1450 to the middle of the 1700s fireplaces remained much the same, but in the 1700s Benjamin Franklin invented the famous Franklin stove, the first real improvement in heating in centuries, and not long after that, Count von Rumford (page 121) developed a fireplace that threw out much more heat than was formerly available. Throughout the nineteenth century, stoves made of cast iron were generally used, the ancestors of our modern heating systems.

Today our homes may be heated in several ways. Most of these are easy to understand, since they use either convection currents of air or hot water to distribute the heat energy. Often radiation plays an important part also.

When a gram of water cools one degree Celsius, only one calorie of heat energy is released from it. But when steam condenses into a gram of water, 540 calories of heat energy are released. Because of this great difference, steam is often used in the heating systems of houses and large buildings. Inside the boilers water is changed to steam. The steam is forced by its own pressure through pipes until it condenses inside radiators placed in each room. The heat released by the condensation is distributed by both radiation and convection.

## Domestic Cooling

Modern refrigerators and air conditioners use a similar principle. Some gaseous substance, called the coolant or **refrigerant** (ri frij′ ər ənt), is put under a great deal of pressure by a piston inside

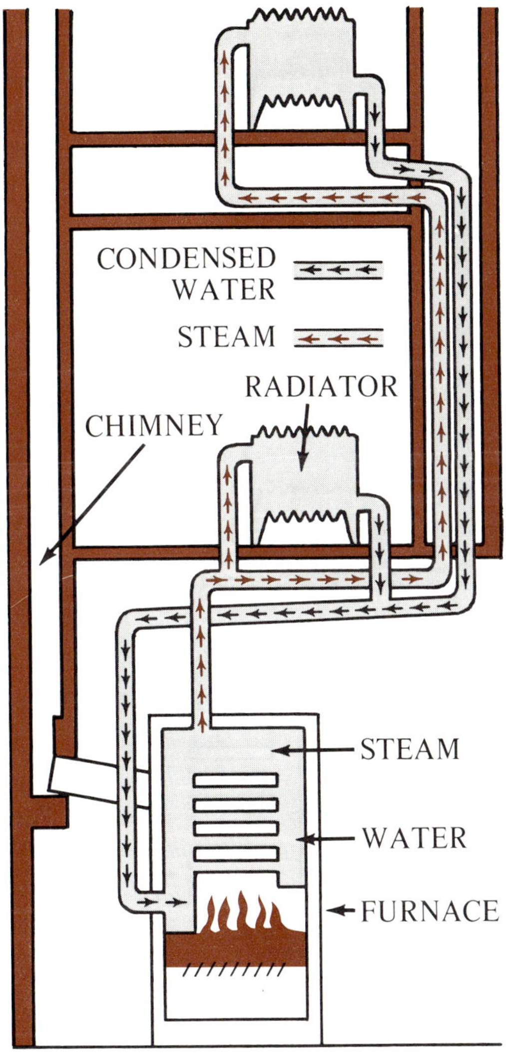


**4.29** Steam heating by radiation and convection

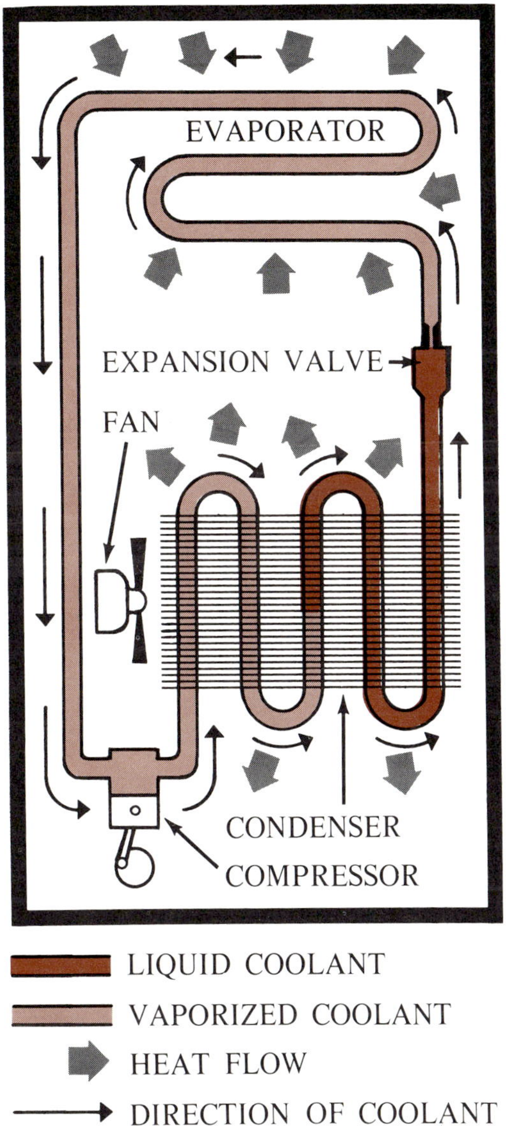


**4.30** The principle of refrigeration and air conditioning

the compressor and then cooled by blowing air across coils of tubes. Heat is given off and carried away by the flowing air. As a result, the coolant liquefies. The liquid coolant passes through a small opening and into a larger pipe. Because of the reduced pressure, the coolant again vaporizes. As it does, a large amount of heat is absorbed by it from the air.

The amount of heat taken from the air when the coolant vaporizes is equal to the amount of heat given off when the coolant liquefies. Can you explain why you cannot cool a room of a house by opening the door of a refrigerator? How can you warm a house in the winter by the use of a "heat pump" that removes heat from the cold air outside the house?

## Have You Learned?

From the list of words at the right, select those that will best complete the statements below. (Do not write in your book.)

In a gasoline engine, gasoline and air are pulled into a __(1)__ where the mixture is burned. The heat necessary to start the fuel burning is supplied by the __(2)__. As the fuel burns, it __(3)__. This pushes the __(4)__ down against the crankshaft, which makes the wheels of the car turn.

The __(5)__ engine has a set of blades that are moved by a gas that passes through them. This type of engine is used in a __(6)__ airplane, where it turns a propeller. The __(7)__ airplane engine does not turn a propeller but instead forces the airplane forward by the unequal pressure within the engine.

When a gram of water cools from 40° C to 39° C, only a single __(8)__ is released. When a gram of steam __(9)__, 540 times as much heat energy is released. In a refrigerator, a __(10)__ absorbs a great deal of heat as it vaporizes.

a. calorie
b. condenses
c. cylinder
d. expands
e. piston
f. refrigerant
g. spark plug
h. turbine
i. turbojet
j. turboprop

## 8. Behavior of Matter at High and at Low Temperatures

**ARE YOU READY?**

Look up the following words if you are not sure of their meanings:

absolute zero; atom; characteristic; conduction; electron; hypothesis; nuclear power; phenomena; solar system; viscosity.

One characteristic of life is that it cannot exist unless the temperature of its environment remains within a certain narrow range. What are the high and low temperatures that normally occur each year where you live? The highest officially recorded temperature is 58° C, observed in Azizia, Tripolitania, in northern Africa, on September 13, 1922. A record low temperature of −88.3° C was recorded in the Soviet Antarctica weather station Vostok on August 24, 1960. Consult the *World Almanac* or other reference books for the record high and low temperatures in your state.

Your understanding of the behavior of matter is based on observations made while the temperature of matter was within a narrow range of temperatures. At very high or very low temperatures, many of the characteristics of matter are very different.

### Matter at Low Temperatures

As heat energy is removed from a piece of matter, the molecules move more and more slowly. As this happens, gases become liquids, and liquids become solids. Some of the gases of the air and the temperatures at which they liquefy are below:

| | |
|---|---|
| Oxygen | −183.0°C |
| Argon | −185.7°C |
| Nitrogen | −195.8°C |
| Hydrogen | −252.7°C |
| Helium | −268.9°C |

Each of these different gases liquefies at a different temperature. Can you explain how this characteristic could be used to separate these gases?

The study of the behavior of matter at temperatures below −183° C (−297.4° F), where oxygen becomes a liquid, is known as **cryogenics** (krī′ ō jen′ iks). Many unexpected phenomena have been observed while working with matter at these temperatures.

For example, helium, an element having one of the smallest and least complex atoms, becomes a liquid at the lowest temperature of any gas—nearly 4° K (−268.9° C; −452 F). Below this temperature, liquid helium has no viscosity and is a good conductor of heat energy. It also tends to creep up the sides of its container.

As you may already know, electricity will pass through some substances easily and not through others. At temperatures very close to absolute zero (−273° C), all **resistance** (ri zis′ tens) to electrical current disappears in tin and lead. These materials are called **superconductors** (sü′ pər kən duk′ tər).

## Matter at High Temperatures

Increasing the heat energy of a substance drives the molecules farther apart, melting solids and evaporating liquids. Thus, at extremely high temperatures, we would expect all matter to exist as a gas.

The behavior of high-temperature gases is very much different from their behavior at lower temperatures. Because of this, physicists have given a special name to these gases—**plasma** (plaz′ mə). Thus, we can say that matter exists in *four* states —solid, liquid, gas, and plasma. Since the temperature of most of the universe is probably several hundred million degrees, most of the matter is in the plasma state.

When a gas is raised to temperatures of hundreds of millions of degrees, it no longer exists as molecules and atoms. At these temperatures, the molecules break up into single atoms, and then the electrons separate from the center part of the atoms. Therefore, a plasma is believed to consist of fragments of atoms with a shortage of electrons that are called **ions** (ī′ on), and of free electrons.

As you might guess from what you know about atoms, the free electrons are negatively charged, and the part of the atom that has lost electrons is positively charged. The entire mass of plasma is, of course, not charged, because for each positively charged particle there are negatively charged electrons that balance its charge. However, the free electrons make the plasma a good conductor of electricity. That is, an electric current will easily pass through it, because of the movement of the electrons of the plasma.

In the laboratory, matter does not remain in a plasma state very long. Any cooling of the plasma allows the electrons to recombine with the center part of the atoms, producing a whole atom again.

The science of the behavior of plasma is called **magnetohydrodynamics** (mag nē′ tō hī′ drō dī nam′ iks). Physicists use the principles of this science in many studies.

Experiments in the use of nuclear power require the use of plasmas. Electric generators have been built that produce electricity by passing plasma through magnetic fields. Arcs that produce high-velocity, high-temperature streams of plasma are now used to cut certain materials, and to study the effects of high temperature on space capsules that must reenter the earth's atmosphere.

The study of plasma has even produced a new theory of the origin of the solar system: that the sun was originally a cloud of plasma. As this cloud began to cool, atoms began to re-form. These atoms fell in toward the sun until they reached a plasma layer, where they again became plasma. In this state, the material was held away from the sun by its magnetic field, and eventually the planets formed as the plasma layers cooled. If this idea is correct, we can easily hypothesize that there are many solar systems, much like ours, formed in the same manner.

## Have You Learned?

On a sheet of paper list the numbers for the questions below. By each number write *T* if the statement is true and *F* if false.

1. At temperatures near absolute zero, the properties of some elements are very much different than at higher temperatures.
2. Materials that have almost no resistance to electrical currents are called plasmas.
3. Matter exists in four states.
4. The most common state of matter in the universe is gas.
5. Plasma consists of ions and free electrons.
6. The science of the study of plasma is called cryogenics.
7. A mass of plasma is always negatively charged.
8. Plasma is difficult to keep in the laboratory.
9. The study of magnetohydrodynamics is partly concerned with theories of the origin of the solar system.

### REVIEW QUESTIONS

*Select the answer that best completes each statement. (Do not write in your book.)*

1. The first thermometer was made about _____ years ago. (a) 100 (b) 250 (c) 350 (d) 500
2. The first attempt to build a thermometer was by _____. (a) Galileo (b) Fahrenheit (c) Newton (d) Rumford
3. The Centigrade thermometer is sometimes called the _____ thermometer. (a) Fahrenheit (b) Galileo (c) calibrated (d) Celsius
4. The coefficient of volume expansion of water is approximately _____. (a) 0.0002 (b) 0.2 (c) 2.0 (d) 20
5. A beam of steel is 20 meter long at 5°C. Its temperature is increased to 25° C. The coefficient of linear expansion of steel is 0.000013. How long is the steel beam at 25° C? (a) 0.0065 m (b) 20.0078 m (c) 20.0065 m (d) 20.0052 m
6. The gas nitrogen has approximately the same coefficient of volume expansion as which of the following? (a) oxygen (b) iron (c) water (d) none of these
7. The rate at which a substance absorbs

heat is called ____. (a) coefficient of expansion (b) specific heat (c) the refrigerant (d) BTU

8. As steam cools, it ____ back into water. (a) condenses (b) evaporates (c) conducts (d) freezes
9. At one time it was thought that heat was a fluid called the ____. (a) temperature (b) refrigerant (c) molecule (d) caloric
10. An eighteenth-century scientist named ____ performed experiments that helped destroy the Theory of the Caloric. (a) Plato (b) Galileo (c) Rumford (d) Einstein
11. If heat energy flows from an object into the air, we know that the temperature of the object is ____ that of the air. (a) higher than (b) lower than (c) the same as
12. Absolute zero is about ____ degrees Centigrade. (a) zero (b) −125 (c) −275 (d) − 1,000
13. The amount of heat necessary to raise the temperature of one pound of water one degree F. is one ____. (a) BTU (b) calorie (c) kilocalorie (d) specific heat
14. Heat transferred from one object to another through direct contact between the two bodies is ____. (a) convection (b) conduction (c) radiation (d) insulation
15. Heat transferred by the circulation of the matter itself is called ____. (a) convection (b) conduction (c) radiation (d) insulation
16. Heat reaches the earth from the sun through ____. (a) convection (b) conduction (c) radiation (d) insulation
17. If a solid melts at a definite temperature we know that it is ____. (a) crystalline (b) a wax (c) lacking latent heat (d) easily evaporated
18. As the temperature of water drops from 4° C to 0° C, its density will ____ (a) increase (b) decrease (c) remain the same
19. The movable bottom of a cylinder is called a ____. (a) crankshaft (b) turbine (c) spark plug (d) piston
20. A rocket can fly outside the atmosphere because it carries its own supply of ____. (a) coolant (b) refrigerant (c) oxygen (d) turbines
21. In a steam radiator, heat is given off when the steam ____. (a) vaporizes (b) evaporates (c) condenses (d) is compressed
22. In an air conditioner, the coolant absorbs heat when it ____. (a) vaporizes (b) is compressed (c) liquefies (d) condenses
23. One of the states of matter that consists of ions and free electrons is ____. (a) solid (b) liquid (c) gas (d) plasma
24. The study of the behavior of matter at temperatures below −183° C. is ____. (a) cryogenics (b) superconductors (c) magnetohydrodynamics (d) astronomy
25. One recent hypothesis of the origin of the solar system suggests that the sun was originally a ____. (a) solid (b) liquid (c) gas (d) plasma

## CAN YOU FIND OUT?

*It may be necessary to use an encyclopedia or other reference books in answering these questions.*

1. Galileo experimented with thermometers. What other types of experiments did he make?
2. What are deformation-type thermometers? How do they work? What are they used for?
3. What is the Réaumur scale for measuring temperature? How is it different from those scales you have learned about in this chapter?
4. When people are baking cakes, bread, etc. at high altitudes, what changes must they make in cookbook instructions that were written for lower altitudes?
5. What is meant by the term "standard atmosphere"?
6. Count von Rumford was born in America, and his real name was Benjamin Thompson. What else did he do besides experiment with the nature of heat? How did he become a count?

7. How many kilocalories (Calories) are there in some of the foods you normally eat? Why is it important to know about them? How many Calories should you take in each day?
8. What is liquid air? How is it made, and what are some of its properties?
9. What would be the advantages and disadvantages of using turbine engines in automobiles? Of using steam engines?
10. How do convection currents in the air cause winds?
11. Assuming that the universe is a closed system, explain what is happening to the distribution of heat energy. What will eventually happen to the heat of the universe? What will happen to the life of the universe?
12. How does a rocket engine work? How is it similar to a gasoline engine in a car? How is it different?
13. What are the current theories of the origin of the solar system?
14. How is a "heat pump" used to both heat and cool houses?

## REFERENCES FOR ADDITIONAL STUDY

CAREERS AND OPPORTUNITIES IN ENGINEERING by Phillip Pollack (Revised by John Alden). E. P. Dutton & Co., Inc.
Describes the many kinds of careers in engineering and the education needed for each

THE DEPTH OF COLD by A. R. Meetham. Barnes & Noble, Inc.
An introduction to the world of low temperatures, the uses of low temperatures, and the effects they have on various materials

ENGINES AND HOW THEY WORK by Geoffrey Boumphrey. Franklin Watts, Inc.
Contains descriptions of most of the different kinds of engines and the last chapter is on engines of the future

EXPERIMENTS WITH HEAT by Harry Sootin. W. W. Norton & Company, Inc.
Describes many experiments that can be done with simple equipment

GASES AND PLASMAS by Paul Thompson. J. B. Lippincott Company.
An excellent summary of the modern research on gases and plasmas

MODEL ROCKETRY: HOBBY OF TOMORROW by Peter Lowry and Field Griffin. Doubleday & Company, Inc.
The emphasis is on safety in discussing rocket construction, launching systems, and recovery methods

# *Workshop... Unit II*

**Experimenting with a Floating Object.** Fill a large test tube with water. Then fill a smaller test tube or vial about half full of water, invert it, and place it in the large test tube as shown in the first drawing of Figure W2.1. Adjust the amount of water in the smaller test tube so that the smaller tube just floats. Cover the mouth of the large test tube with a piece of rubber from a balloon.

Can you predict what will happen when you push down on the rubber covering the top of the large test tube? Try it to see if your prediction is correct. Can you explain what happened? *Hint:* Notice what happens to the level of the water inside the small test tube when you push downward on the rubber covering the top of the large test tube.

**W2.1** Apply your knowledge of floating.

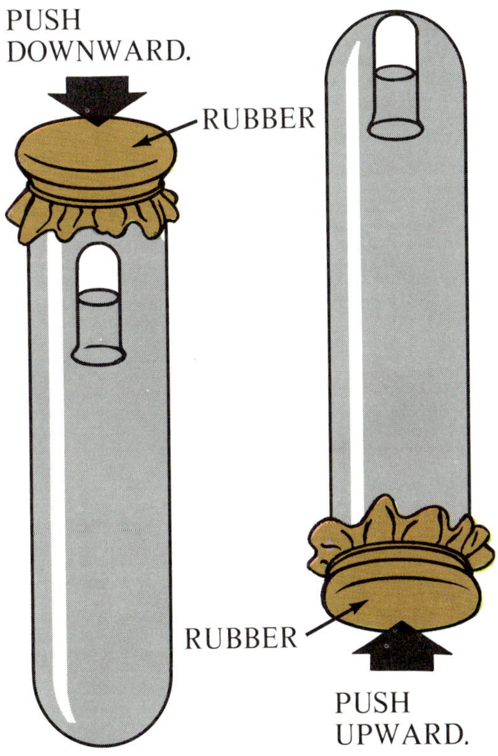


Change the apparatus so the small test tube is just floating in an inverted large test tube as shown in the second drawing of Figure W2.1. Predict what will happen when you push upward on the rubber covering the mouth of the large test tube. Test your prediction. Can you explain what happened?

If you would like to try this experiment at home and do not have any test tubes, try using a large glass jar and a small bottle.

**Building a Water Fountain.** Assemble the apparatus as shown in Figure W2.2 on page 146. Fill the flask about two-thirds full of water, stopper with a two-hole rubber stopper containing the glass tubes, and invert the flask. Be sure that the straight glass tubing is about an inch below the surface of the water in the upper dish. Explain what happens. Would the fountain work if the tube on the right side of the apparatus were made shorter?

**Does Water Flow Uphill?** Assemble the apparatus as shown in Figure W2.3 following on page 146. At the beginning of the experiment the bottom flask should be empty and the upper flask filled with water. Pour enough water into the funnel to get the flow of water started. If the water does not continue to flow, pour a little more water into the funnel. Can you explain

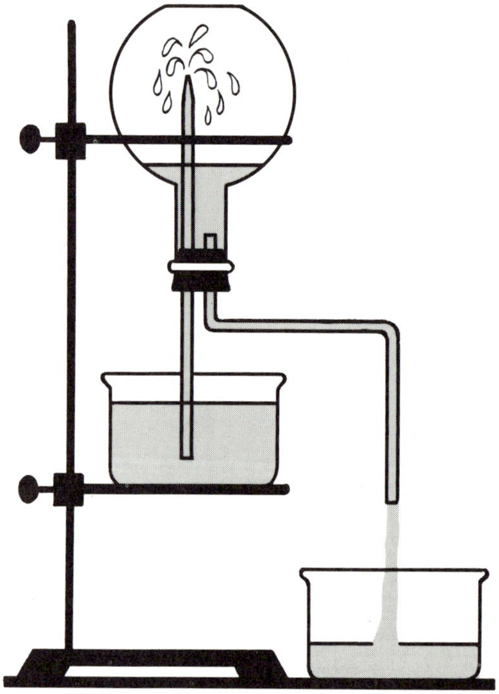

**W2.2** What makes the water fountain work?

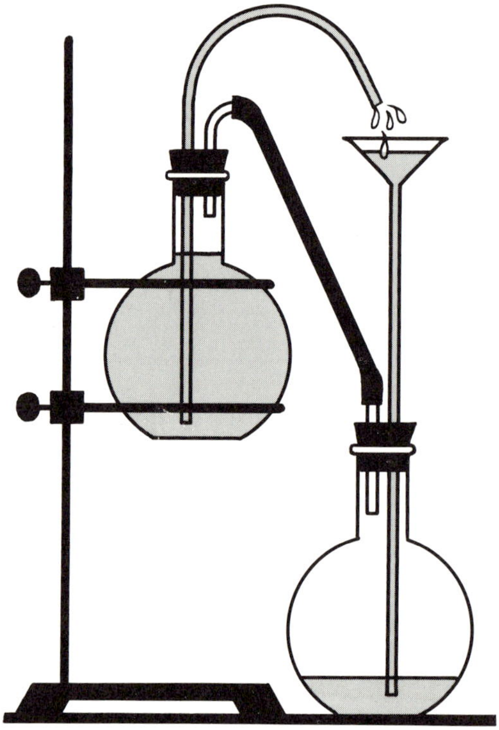

**W2.3** Does water flow uphill?

what makes the water appear to flow uphill?

Two gallon cans with screw tops can be used in place of the two glass flasks. Assemble the apparatus with two cans, and see if your friends can correctly figure out the arrangement of the glass tubes inside the cans. Do you think some "magic" tricks are based on scientific principles? (Figure W2.4 on page 147)

**Applying What You Know About Levers.** A wooden meterstick weighing 150 grams is placed on a table so that 40 centimeters of it extend beyond the edge of the table. How far out on the stick can a mouse weighing 50 grams walk before the stick tips off the table? *Hint:* The weight of the meterstick acts as if it all is concentrated at the center of the stick. (Figure W2.5)

You can check your prediction by using a meterstick and a weight to represent the mouse. Since metersticks vary in weight, it will be necessary to weigh the meterstick and use that weight in your calculations.

**Investigating Collisions.** A toy consisting of several steel spheres suspended in a frame can be used to investigate one kind of collision. (Figure W2.6)

Pull one sphere back and release it. Observe what happens. Now pull two spheres back, and release them at the same time. Experiment with other combinations, including pulling back more than half of the spheres and releasing them at the same time. When the collisions occur, is the number of spheres that bounce off always equal to the number of spheres that were released to cause the collision? Can you explain what you observe?

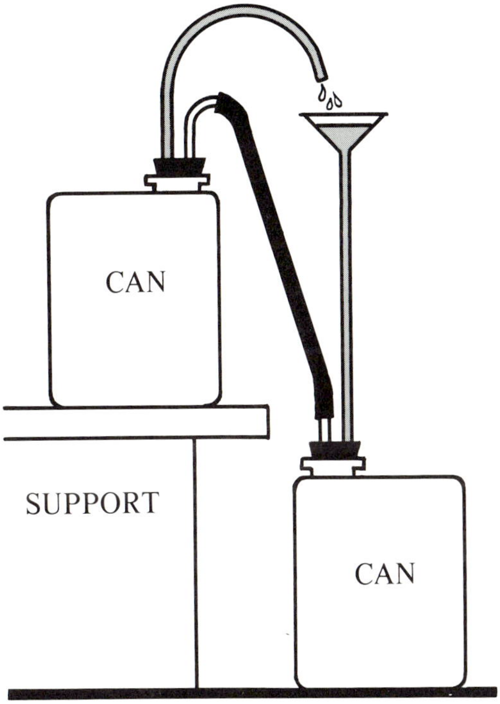


**W2.4** Compare this with Figure W2.3.

If you do not have a toy like the one in the diagram, you can experiment with collisions by rolling heavy marbles or steel spheres in a wooden trough. In this case there will be some friction between the spheres and the surface of the wood. You may also wish to try building a device like the one in Figure W2.6. String can be attached with glue or by drilling holes in the spheres.

**Studying the Expansion of Materials.** From a garage or service station obtain a discarded thermostat used in an automobile cooling system. Place the thermostat in a pan containing enough water to cover it. Heat the water on a burner until the thermostat opens. Use a thermometer to measure the temperature at which this occurs. Can you locate the part of the thermostat that expands when heated and that regulates the size of the opening?

**W2.5** Will the meterstick tip if the mouse moves all the way to the end?

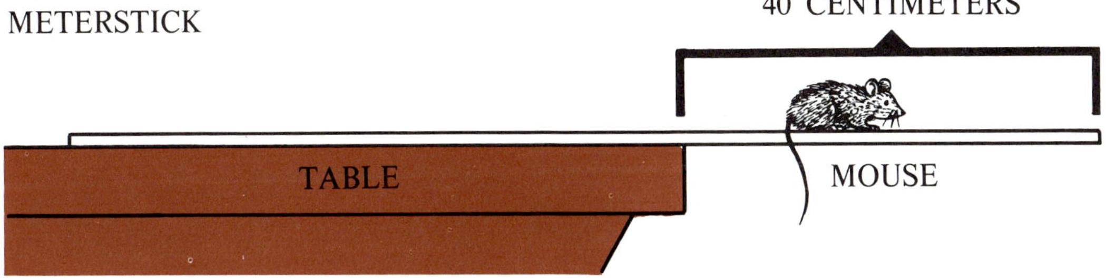


**W2.6** How many balls will move when one ball at the end is pulled back and released?

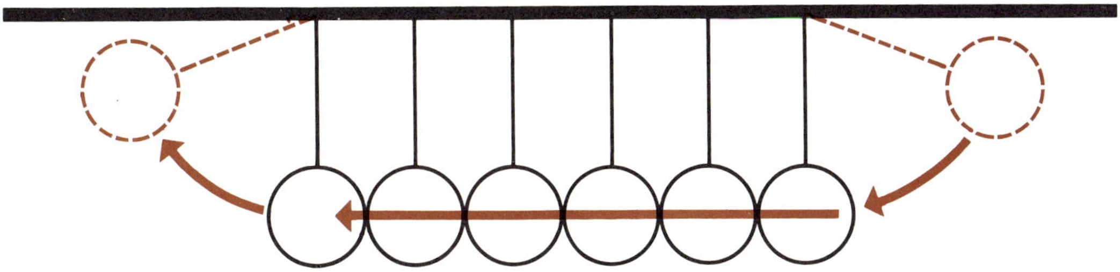

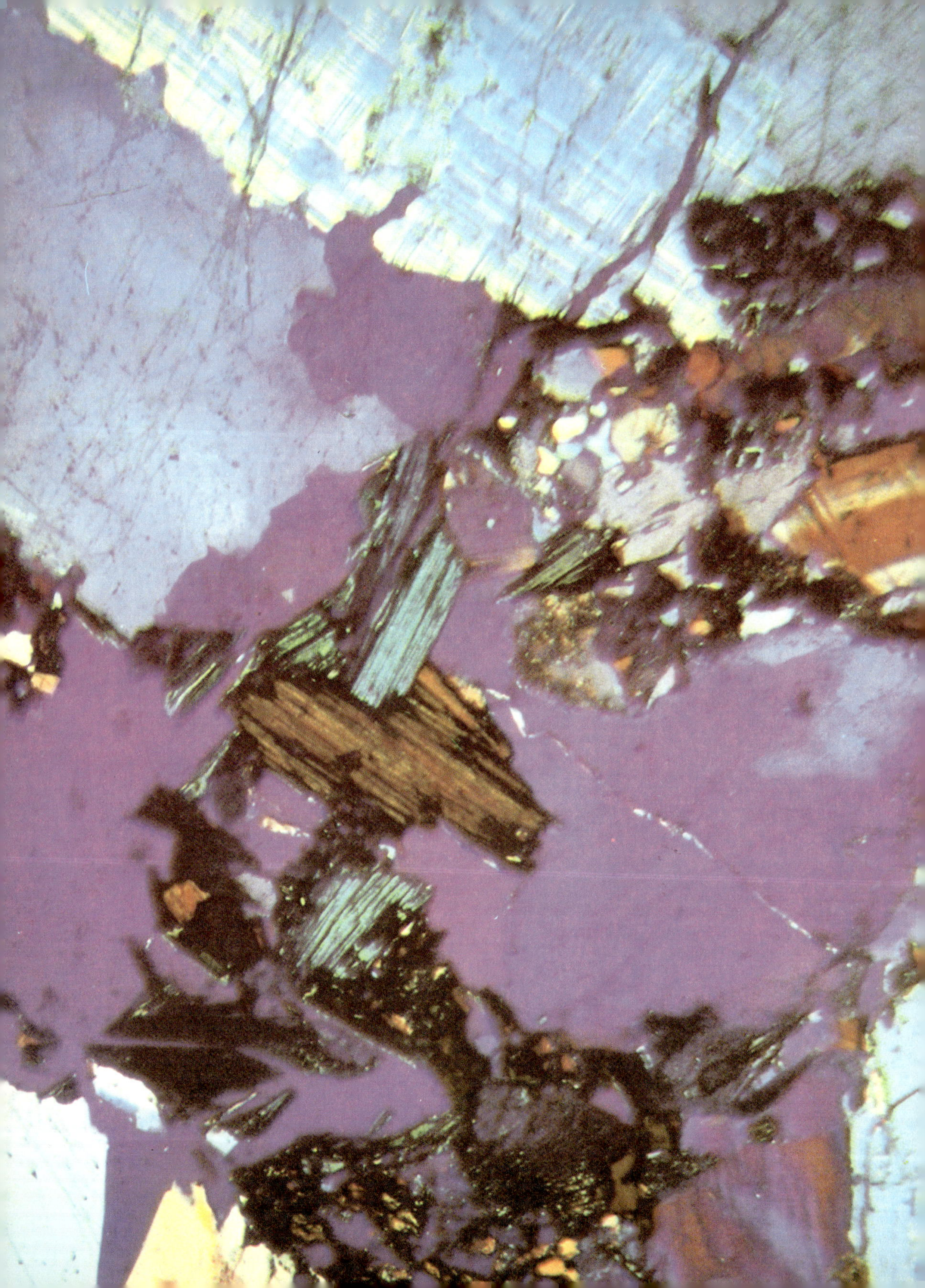

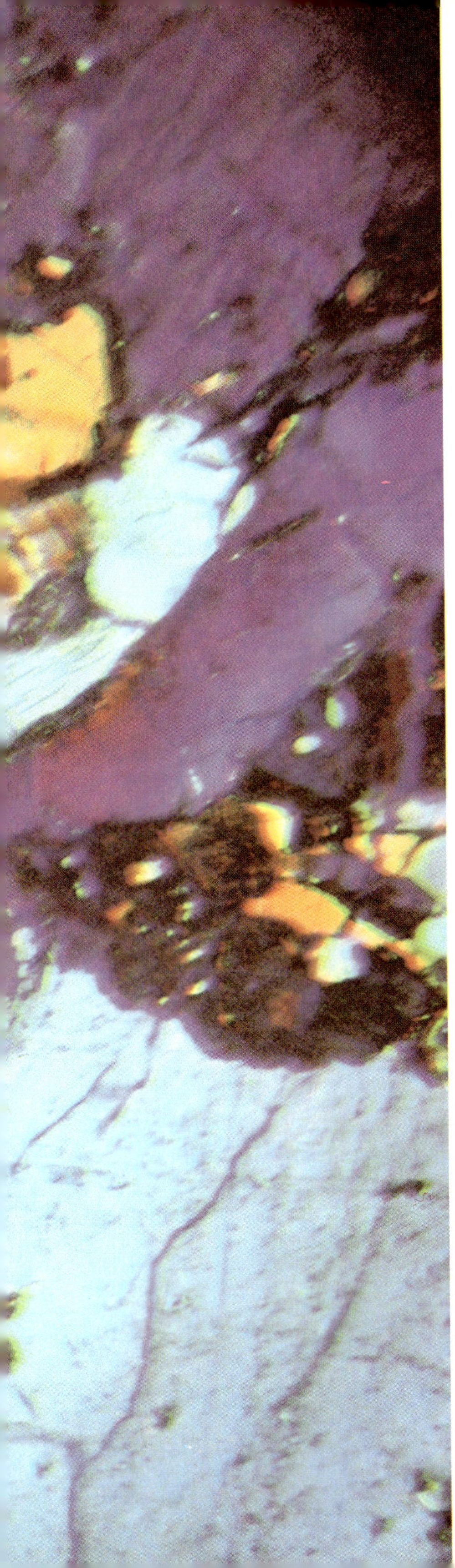

# unit III chemistry: a study of atoms

L. V. Bergman & Assoc., Inc.

CHAPTER **5**

# Building Blocks Called Atoms

TURN A DRINKING-GLASS UPSIDE DOWN, place it over a burning candle, and watch the candle go out. Pour some vinegar into a jar containing a small amount of baking soda, and observe what happens. Chew a soda cracker until it tastes sweet.

How can what happens in each case be explained? We must begin by investigating the building blocks of all matter—atoms.

## 1. Early Ideas in Chemistry

**ARE YOU READY?**

Look up the following words if you are not sure of their meanings:

atom; chemist; chemistry; element; mercury; oxygen.

Examine a few grains of sugar or sand and a drop of water. Think for a moment about what these substances are made of. Could it be that they all contain some of the same building blocks? The ancient Greeks thought so and suggested that everything on the earth was made of earth, air, water, and fire. Can you suggest observations that they might have made to lead them to believe that things on the earth were made of these four substances? For example, think what happens to a burning log.

Democritus (di mok′ rə təs), a Greek philosopher who lived about 420 B.C., taught his pupils that matter was made up of tiny particles called *atoms.* The name of these particles came from the Greek word *atoma,* which means something that cannot be divided into smaller parts. Aristotle (ar′ is tot′ əl) (384-322 B.C.), the most famous of the early Greek philosopher-scientists, supported the idea of the four elements rather than the atomic theory of Democritus. Because of his reputation, Aristotle's ideas about the makeup of matter were accepted for almost 2,000 years.

### Early Chemistry

**Alchemists** (al′ kə mists) worked in the period from about the time of the birth of Jesus to the 1700s. They searched for a way to change different metals to gold. They believed in a "philosopher's stone" that would change metals, such as mercury, into gold. They also tried to find the "elixir of life," a substance to make people live longer or forever. Much of their work involved the use of trial-and-error approaches and would not be classified as *science* by today's definition.

In spite of their strange beliefs, crude methods, and simple instruments, the alchemists made a number of important contributions. They discovered several elements such as **zinc** (zingk), **arsenic** (är′ sə nik) and **phosphorus** (fos′ fə rəs). They made chemicals, such as saltpeter, alcohol, and sulfuric and nitric acids, as well as chemicals used as drugs. They developed laboratory techniques, such as filtering and glass blowing, that were very useful in the new science of chemistry that began at about the time of the American Revolution.

## A Theory of Burning

In the last chapter, we learned how a *Theory of Caloric* was developed to explain heat energy and then later disproven. About 1700 a German scientist named Stahl (shtäl) suggested a theory of burning that, like the theory of Caloric, was also later disproven. According to Stahl, a substance called **phlogiston** (flō jis′ tən) escaped when wood burned or iron became rusty. The phlogiston theory was accepted by many famous chemists of the 1700s, and the story of this theory's rejection is the story of the birth of modern chemistry.

Joseph Priestley (prēst′ li), an English clergyman, experimented with chemistry as a hobby. He was especially interested in gases, and one of his experiments led to the discovery of oxygen. In 1774, with the aid of a lens, he heated a solid called "red ash" metal by focusing the sun's rays on it. He obtained silvery mercury and a colorless gas. When a candle was placed in a bottle of the gas, Priestley found that the candle burned brighter. Priestley tried other experiments with this strange gas, including putting a mouse in it as well as breathing some of it himself.

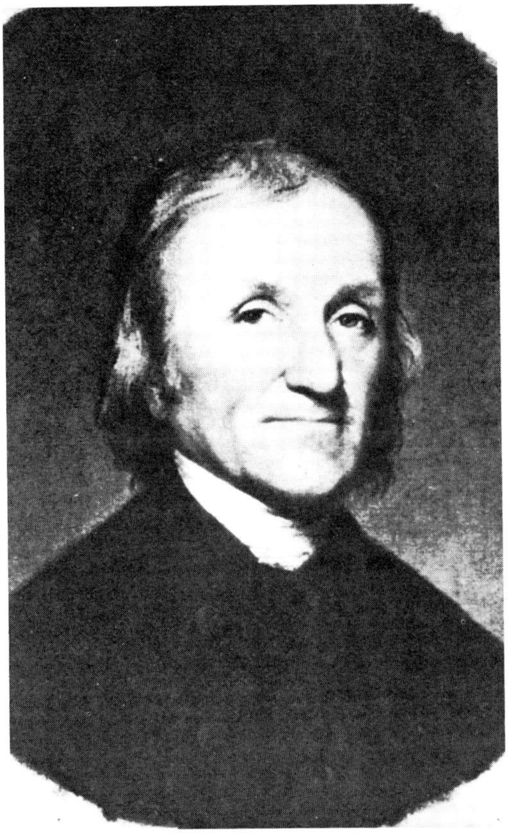

*Historical Pictures Service—Chicago*

**5.1** Joseph Priestly (1733-1804) was an English clergyman and an amateur chemist. He did experiments with air and separated oxygen from air.

Priestley told Lavoisier (lo vwo zyā′), a famous French chemist, about the results of his experiments. In 1775-77 Lavoisier repeated Priestley's experiments and reversed one by heating some mercury under a bell jar. He observed that about one-fifth of the air was used up, and part of the mercury was changed to "red ash." He found out also that a candle went out

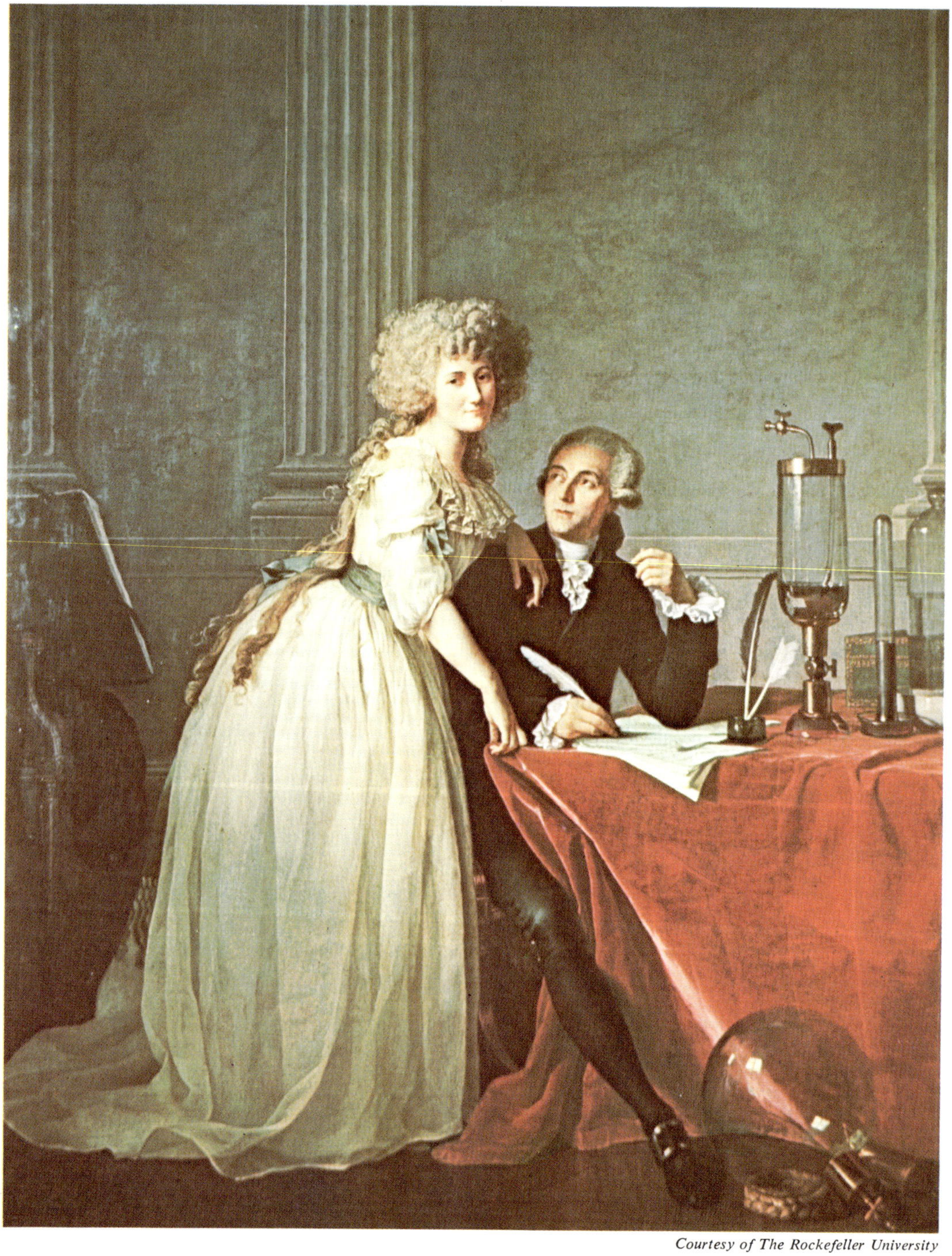

*Courtesy of The Rockefeller University*

**5.2** Antoine Lavoisier (1743-1793), with his wife and scientific equipment, discovered that about one-fifth of the air is oxygen—a life supporting element.

when it was placed in the air that remained in the bell jar.

Lavoisier concluded from this and other experiments that about one-fifth of the air is a gas that supports burning and helps to keep animals alive. He named this gas *oxygen*. He also found that when something burns, the weight of the substances formed is equal to the weight of the fuel plus the weight of the oxygen used in burning the fuel.

This illustrates an important principle of science. According to the *Law of Conservation of Matter*, matter cannot be created or destroyed. Do you see how this law is like the Law of the Conservation of Energy discussed in Chapter 2? The discovery of atomic energy made it necessary to combine these two laws.

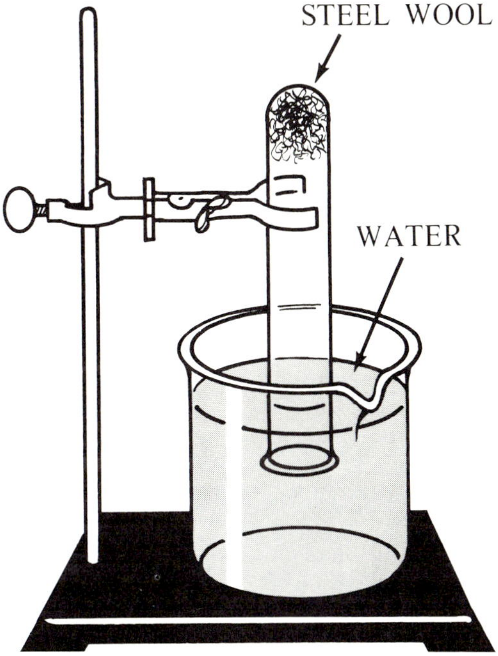


**5.3** What will happen to the air in the test tube?

## Determining the Amount of Oxygen in the Air

Place some wet steel wool in a bottle or jar, invert it, and place it in a pan of water. Use a ring stand and clamp as shown in Figure 5.3 to keep the jar from tipping and to keep the mouth of the jar off the bottom. Why is this necessary? Record the level of the water inside the jar each day for several days. Also observe what happens to the steel wool. Explain how what happens can be used as a crude measure of the amount of oxygen in air.

At the end of the experiment, remove the bottle from the pan, and quickly thrust a lighted candle into the bottle. Does the candle burn for a longer or shorter length of time than when the candle is placed in a bottle of air that has not had steel wool in it? Explain your results.

With the discovery of oxygen and new ideas about the nature of burning, the phlogiston theory was no longer accepted. At about this same time an Englishman, John Dalton (1766-1844), proposed an atomic theory similar to that suggested by Democritus 2,200 years earlier. Because of this new theory, the idea of the four elements of earth, air, fire, and water was discarded.

According to Dalton's theory, all matter is composed of tiny, invisible particles called *atoms*. Furthermore, the atom is the smallest particle of an element. For example, an *oxygen* atom is the smallest particle of the element *oxygen* and a *zinc* atom of the element *zinc*. Another way of saying it is that the elements represent different kinds of atoms—hydrogen atoms, copper atoms, carbon atoms, etc. How would you answer if you were asked what

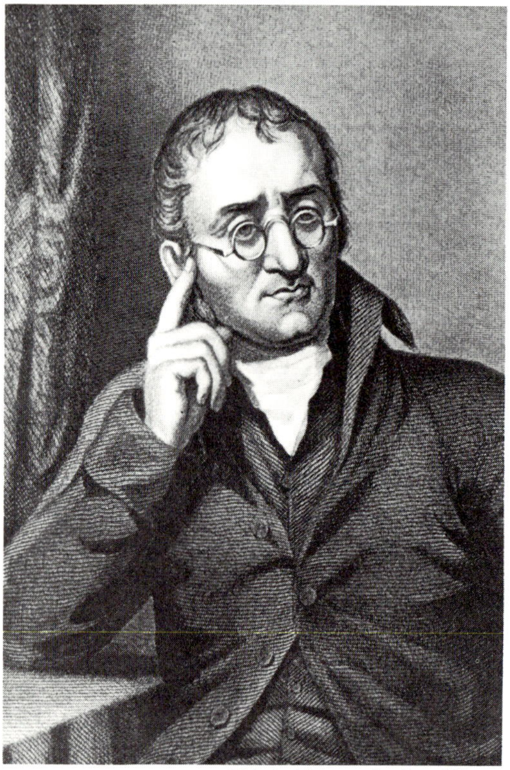

Historical Pictures Service—Chicago

**5.4** John Dalton said that matter is made of atoms.

is the smallest particle of oxygen that is possible?

Although chemists have modified and expanded Dalton's Atomic Theory since 1803, his basic ideas about atoms are still accepted. Since the beginning of the nineteenth century, chemists have also filled in many of the details. Elements unknown in Dalton's time have been discovered, and several elements have been produced artificially. We have discovered a great deal about the composition of atoms and how atoms of different elements are similar and how they differ. And, perhaps most importantly, we have discovered how atoms combine. This is the real story of chemistry.

### Have You Learned?

1. Name the four substances that the ancients believed everything was made of. Why did people continue to believe this idea for so long?
2. Describe what alchemists were trying to do and some of the things they managed to do.
3. What was the phlogiston theory? What did Priestley and Lavoisier do that caused this theory to be discarded?
4. What did Dalton propose about the nature of matter? Are his ideas still accepted?

## 2. Atoms and Molecules

**ARE YOU READY?**

Look up the following words if you are not sure of their meanings:

artificial; atom; element; Latin; molecule; respiration.

First, we talked about small particles called *molecules*, when we discussed heat energy. Now we talk about even smaller particles called *atoms*. Perhaps any confusion can be cleared up by considering the most common liquid on the earth—water.

As you may already know, water is made up of hydrogen and oxygen, and can be broken up into these two gases. However, this division is not done by dividing the molecules *physically*. The molecules are much too small for this. Instead, it is done by the use of electrical energy as shown in the following activity.

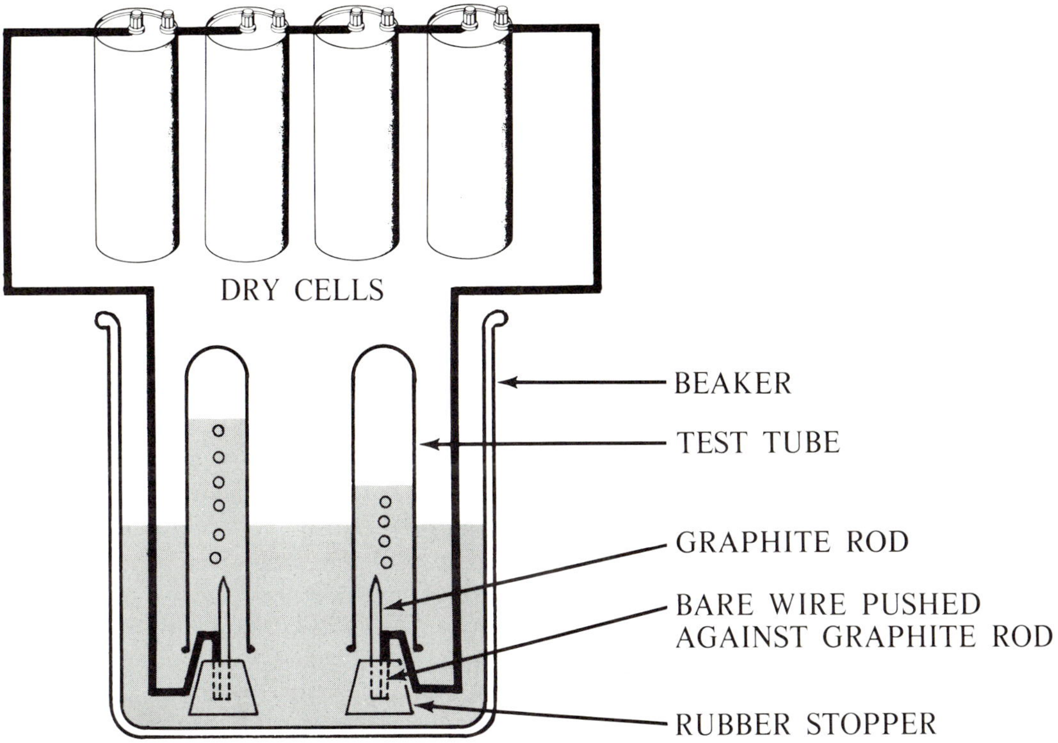


**5.5** Try to predict which test tube contains hydrogen and which contains oxygen.

## Splitting the Water Molecule

**MATERIALS:**

Water, beaker (or similar container), two large test tubes, two rubber corks to fit test tubes (each with a single hole), insulated bell wire, 6-volt dry cell, two dead flashlight batteries, metal-saw, file

**PROCEDURE:**

Cut the two flashlight batteries lengthwise, and remove the carbon rods that you find in their centers. File one end of each carbon rod until it is pointed. Cut the bell wire into two 50-centimeter lengths, and strip about 1 centimeter of insulation from each end.

Insert one end of one length of wire into the hole of one rubber cork, and wedge it into place with the *blunt* end of one of the carbon rods. Be sure that the bare wire is firmly touching the carbon rod. Repeat this process with the second cork, wire, and rod.

Place both corks in the bottom of the beaker in such a way that the pointed carbon rods point upward and the wire trails out of the beaker. Fill the beaker with water.

Fill each test tube completely full of water. Place your thumb over the mouth of the tube to hold in the water, turn the tube upside down, and place its mouth under the water in the beaker. Then remove your thumb. If done carefully, the test tube should remain completely full of water. If air leaks into the tube, try again.

Place the mouth of each test tube over the ends of the carbon rods, as shown in the diagram. Connect the wires to a dry cell. Gas bubbles should begin to appear on each carbon rod within a short time. If they do not, increase the size of the dry cell, or put a pinch of salt into the beaker to increase the flow of electricity.

You should have noticed in doing the above activity that one of the test tubes contained twice as much gas as the other. This indicates that water is composed of twice as much hydrogen as oxygen. From this experiment we conclude that *one molecule* of water is composed of *two atoms* of hydrogen and *one atom* of oxygen.

Earlier in this chapter you read about the work of Priestley and Lavoisier and investigated the rusting of steel wool. These experiments also show that molecules are made up of atoms. When mercury is heated, atoms of mercury combine with atoms of oxygen in the air to form molecules of the red powder. This red powder is called *mercuric oxide*. When the iron in steel wool rusts, atoms of iron combine with atoms of oxygen to produce molecules of *iron oxide*.

In the case of water, molecules of water were split apart to form atoms. The reverse process occurs when mercuric oxide is formed. Atoms of mercury combine with atoms of oxygen to form molecules of mercuric oxide. The same is true of iron atoms combining with oxygen atoms to form molecules of iron oxide.

You should note that when we talk about different kinds of atoms, we are talking about **elements** (el′ ə mənt). Hydrogen, oxygen, mercury, and iron are all elements. There are 92 natural elements, and at least 11 have been produced artificially.

## Using Chemical Shorthand

Rather than write out the names for *water*, *iron oxide*, and other chemicals, a shorthand method is used. A **symbol** (sim′ bəl), or abbreviation, for each of the elements is used to represent the different kinds of atoms. *H* is the symbol for hydrogen, *O* for oxygen, and *He* for helium. Other symbols are based on the Latin or latinized name for the elements—*Fe* for *ferrum* (iron), *Hg* for *hydragyrum* (mercury), and *Au* for *aurum* (gold).

A *formula* is used to represent a molecule. The formula for water, $H_2O$, shows that it is composed of the elements of hydrogen and oxygen. The $_2$, written below and after the symbol *H*, indicates that a molecule of water contains two atoms of hydrogen. If there is one atom of an element per molecule, as is the case of oxygen

5.6 How many atoms are there in a water molecule?

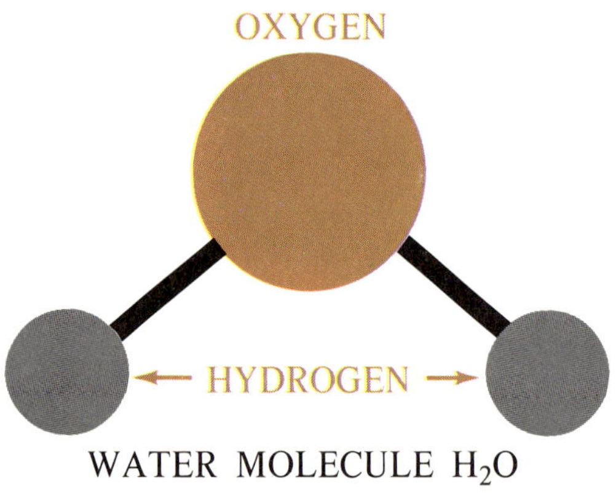

in water, we don't bother to write the 1 after the symbol.

Table salt, which is the chemical *sodium chloride*, has the formula of NaCl. Cane sugar is a combination of twelve atoms of carbon ($C_{12}$), twenty-two atoms of hydrogen ($H_{22}$), and eleven atoms of oxygen ($O_{11}$). The formula is written $C_{12}H_{22}O_{11}$. These formulas are read exactly as they are written—"H–two O" for water, "N–A C–L" for salt, and "C–twelve H–twenty-two O–eleven" for sugar.

The formulas for several substances frequently used by chemists are given in Table I. Although it is not necessary to memorize all the formulas, they will be useful in studying the later sections in this unit.

**TABLE I**

*Formulas for Some Common Chemicals*

| *Formula* | *Name* | *Common name or description* |
|---|---|---|
| $H_2SO_4$ | Sulfuric acid | Oil of vitriol; most widely used acid in industry |
| $HNO_3$ | Nitric acid | Used in the manufacture of fertilizers and explosives |
| HCl | Hydrochloric acid | Muriatic acid; found in the stomachs of human beings and animals |
| NaOH | Sodium hydroxide | Caustic soda or lye; used in making soap |
| $H_2O$ | Water | Most abundant liquid on the earth |
| NaCl | Sodium chloride | Table salt |
| $CO_2$ | Carbon dioxide | Gas produced by burning and in respiration |
| $CaCO_3$ | Calcium carbonate | Limestone or chalk |
| $CuSO_4$ | Copper sulfate | Blue when moist; used to kill fungi and algae |
| $C_{12}H_{22}O_{11}$ | Sucrose | Cane or beet sugar |

## Have You Learned?

Select the answer that best completes each statement. (Do not write in your book.)

1. NaCl is the (formula; symbol) for table salt.
2. Hydrogen, oxygen, and mercury are different kinds of (elements; molecules).
3. The formula for sugar, $C_{12}H_{22}O_{11}$, represents one (atom; molecule).
4. There are (92; 103) natural elements.
5. The symbol for iron is (Fe; I).
6. The formula for water, $H_2O$, shows that water is composed of (two; three) elements.
7. The red powder with which Priestley and Lavoisier experimented was (iron oxide; mercuric oxide).
8. (Formulas; Symbols) are used to represent the different kinds of atoms.

## 3. How Atoms Differ

> **ARE YOU READY?**
>
> Look up the following words if you are not sure of their meanings:
>
> atom; average; decompose; element; particle.

An atom is defined as the smallest particle of an element. Thus the smallest particle of gold is a gold atom, and the smallest particle of oxygen is an oxygen atom. However, atoms are apparently composed of several kinds of yet smaller particles, since some atoms decompose or can be broken up in certain kinds of high-energy machines. No one knows how many different kinds of particles there are within an atom, but there are three that are important in explaining differences among atoms and how atoms combine to form molecules.

### Three Kinds of Particles

Near the center of each atom is a **nucleus** (nü′ kli əs) that, with the exception of the hydrogen atom, is composed of two types of particles. Each of these is about the same size and about equal in weight. One, the **proton** (prō′ ton), has an electrical charge. The other does not appear to have any type of electrical charge. In other words, it is neutral, and the name given to this particle is **neutron** (nü′ tron).

Around this nucleus revolve the **electrons** (i lek′ tron). The speed of these electrons is very great, and the result is to surround the nucleus with a "cloud of energy." The weight and size of the electron is very small when compared to that of the proton and neutron. Each electron has an electrical charge that is opposite to that of the proton. In order to identify these opposite electrical charges, the proton is said to have a positive (+) charge, and the electron to have a negative (−) charge. (Figure 5.7 below)

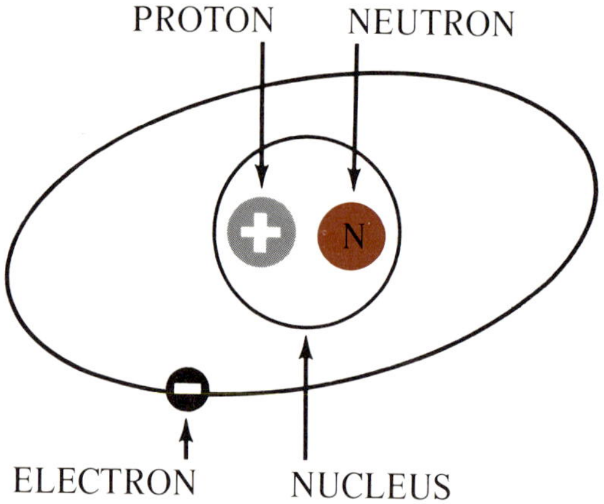

5.7 A model of a hydrogen atom of atomic weight 2.

We can picture an atom as consisting of a certain number of protons in the nucleus with an *equal number* of electrons revolving around the nucleus. In addition to the protons, the nucleus will also contain neutrons. Since the neutrons are electrically neutral, they will have no effect on the chemical action of the atom except to give it weight.

Each element has two important numbers associated with it, as shown in the Table on page 160. The number in the upper left-hand corner of each box is known as the **atomic number.** From it we can tell how many protons each atom of the element has. Carbon (C), for example, has 6 protons, and sodium (Na) has 11. The atomic number also tells us how many electrons an atom has. An atom has the same number of electrons as protons, and thus carbon has six electrons and sodium has 11. As we shall see a little later, the number of electrons has a lot to do with how an atom behaves chemically.

The number in the upper right corner of the box in Figure 5.8 is called the **atomic weight.** The unit of atomic weight is the weight of one proton or neutron. Remember that the weight of the electron is so small that we can ignore it. The weight of an atom, then, is the weight of its protons *plus* the weight of its neutrons.

The atomic weight of carbon, as shown in Figure 5.8, is approximately 12. Since we know from the atomic number that a carbon atom has 6 protons, we know, too, that it must also have 6 neutrons (12 − 6 = 6). Sodium has an atomic weight of approximately 23. With an atomic number of 11, we know that sodium has 11 protons. Therefore, 12 neutrons would be present in the nucleus of the sodium atom (23 − 11 = 12).

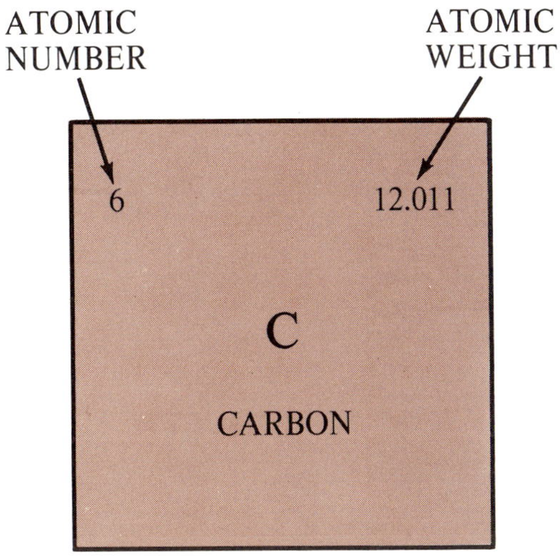


**5.8** Check this in the table on page 160.

## Determining the Number of Particles

Complete the following chart by determining the number of protons, neutrons, and electrons each atom would have.

| *Element* | *Atomic Number* | *Atomic Weight* | *Number of Protons* | *Number of Neutrons* | *Number of Electrons* |
|---|---|---|---|---|---|
| Carbon | 6 | 12 | 6 | 6 | 6 |
| Nitrogen | 7 | 14 | | | |
| Sodium | 11 | 23 | | | |
| Iron | 26 | 56 | | | |
| Copper | 29 | 64 | | | |
| Zinc | 30 | 65 | | | |
| Gold | 79 | 197 | | | |
| Lead | 82 | 207 | | | |
| Uranium | 92 | 238 | | | |

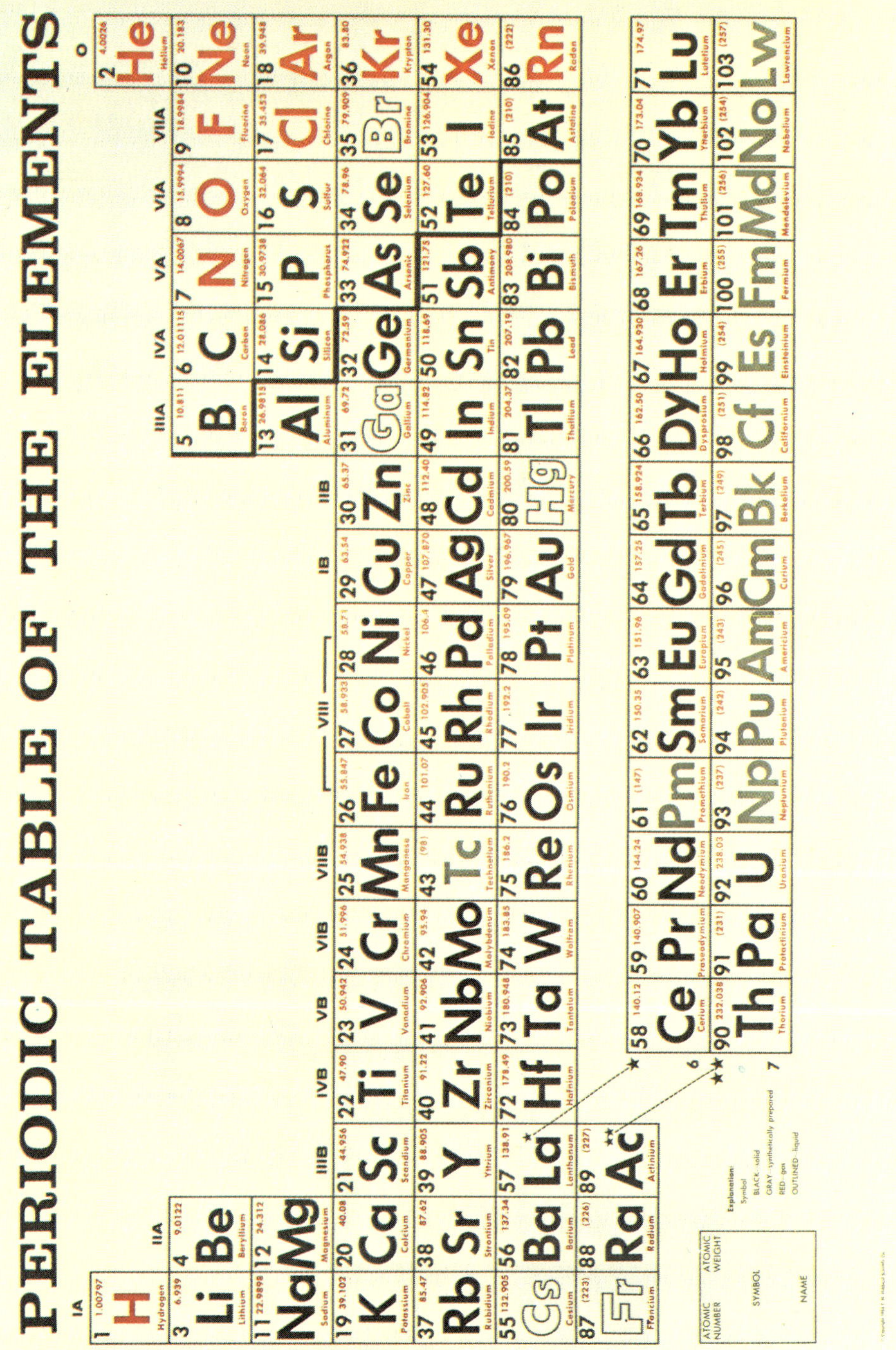


5:9 Periodic Table of the Elements (Courtesy of the Hubbard Scientific Company)

## Explaining Why Atomic Weights Are Not Whole Numbers

You have noticed perhaps that only a few of the atomic weights listed in the Table are whole numbers. Carbon has a weight of 12.011, and chlorine (Cl) has a weight of 35.453. Since the weight of an atom is determined by the number of protons and neutrons in the nucleus, it would seem logical that these weights should all be whole numbers.

The fractional weights listed on page 160 are accounted for by the fact that not all atoms of an element have the same number of neutrons in their **nuclei** (nü′ cli ī) (plural of nucleus). For example, some atoms of carbon have an atomic weight of 12 (6 protons plus 6 neutrons). Other carbon atoms have an atomic weight of 13 (6 protons plus 7 neutrons), and 14 (6 protons plus 8 neutrons). Any piece of carbon, as it appears in nature, will contain atoms of all three weights. These will normally occur in such a combination that the *average* weight of the atoms will equal 12.011. Would you expect the carbon in nature to contain more carbon-12 atoms or more carbon-14 atoms?

These atoms of the same element that have different weights are called **isotopes** (ī′ sə tōp) of the element. Carbon has three: carbon-12, carbon-13, and carbon-14. Carbon-12 is the atom used as a standard in determining the weight of all isotopes of all the elements (Figure 5.10).

Earlier it was stated that atoms of all of the elements except hydrogen had two particles in their nuclei—protons and neutrons. This statement is true for the most common isotope of hydrogen. It has an atomic number of 1 and contains one

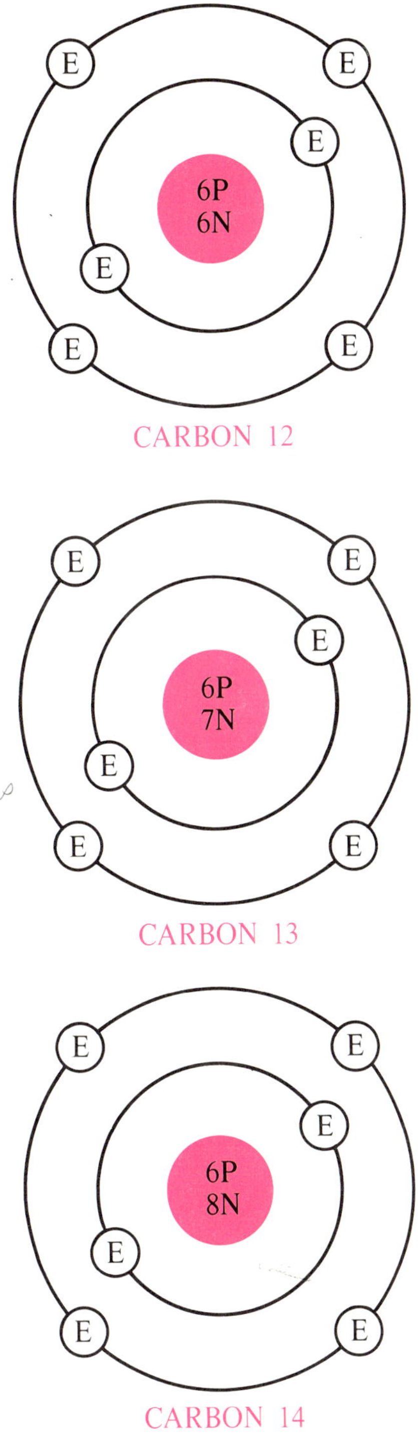


**5.10** The isotopes of carbon

proton and no neutrons. However, hydrogen has two other isotopes, one with an atomic weight of 2 (1 proton and 1 neutron) and) the other 3 (1 proton and 2 neutrons. Therefore the statement should be: "The nucleus of every atom contains protons and neutrons except the one isotope of hydrogen."

You will recall that it was stated earlier that the neutron had no effect on the action of the atom, other than to add weight to it. For this reason, all of the isotopes of an element act the same way chemically, and are therefore considered to be the same element. That is, the $C^{12}$ isotope and the $C^{14}$ isotope both react the same way. The only difference is their weights.

If the number of protons were to be changed, the nature of the atom would change, and a new element would be created. Scientists have been able to make several new elements, and this is described in Chapter 12.

### Have You Learned?

Select the word from Column B that best corresponds with each definition in Column A. (Do not write in your book.)

| *Column A* | *Column B* |
|---|---|
| 1. Tells how many electrons an atom has | a. atomic number |
| 2. Center part of the atom | b. atomic weight |
| 3. Has no charge and is found in the nucleus | c. electron |
| 4. Equals the number of protons plus the number of neutrons | d. isotopes |
| 5. Has positive charge and is found in the nucleus | e. neutron |
| 6. Atoms of the same element that have different weights | f. nucleus |
| 7. Has negative charge and revolves around the nucleus | g. proton |

## How, Then, Are Atoms Different?

In summary, atoms differ in two important ways. First, an atom of one element has a different number of protons and electrons than an atom of another element. The number of protons and electrons is indicated by the atomic number, and each element has its own atomic number.

Second, atoms of the same element differ in their atomic weights and are called isotopes. The heavier isotopes contain more neutrons than do the lighter ones.

## 4. Building a Model of the Atom

**ARE YOU READY?**

Look up the following words if you are not sure of their meanings:

electron; model; neutron; nucleus; orbit; proton.

In the last section, the atom was pictured as a particle having protons and neutrons in the nucleus, with electrons revolving around the nucleus. This mental picture is called a *model*. Of course we can also construct a physical model of an atom, using different colored spheres to represent the protons, neutrons, and electrons. A model of the argon atom is shown in Figure 5.11.

Models are useful because they help us explain things we observe, and, of course, this is the principal aim of science. With the model described in the last section, we were able to explain how atoms of the different elements differ. For example, how do atoms of sodium differ from atoms of calcium? We also were able to explain how atoms of the same element differ in weight. Can you explain the difference between $Uranium^{235}$ and $Uranium^{238}$?

There are many things that cannot be explained by using our model of the atom. Why does hydrogen combine with oxygen to form water? Why does it take *two* atoms of hydrogen and only *one* atom of oxygen to form a molecule of water? Why do atoms of calcium combine with atoms of chlorine and not with atoms of hydrogen?

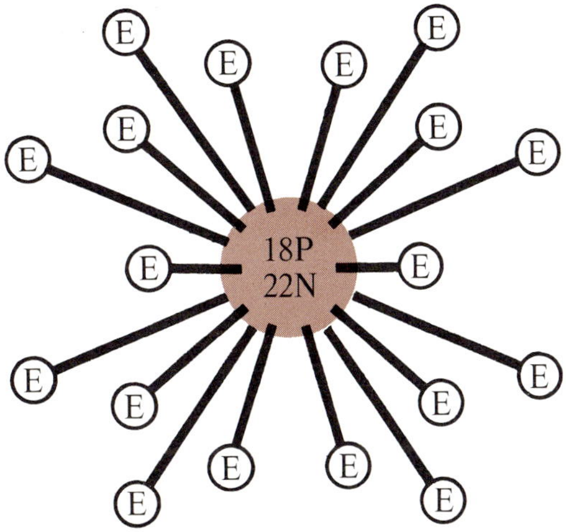


MODEL OF ARGON ATOM

**5.11** A model of argon—a gas. How is it like the model of the carbon atom on page 161?

## Placing Electrons in Shells

The chemist is interested in questions like these, and to answer them it is necessary to add something to our model of the atom. Instead of just picturing electrons revolving around the nucleus, we will now think of them as revolving in definite orbits, or **shells** as the chemist calls them. Unlike each of the planets revolving around the sun in its own orbit, each shell of an atom may contain more than one electron.

The chemist has worked out a model to show how the electrons of atoms of each element are arranged. The first eighteen elements in *The Periodic Table of the Elements* on page 160 can be used to show how this works. As you look at the table, remember that the number in the upper left corner of the box is the atomic number. It tells how many protons there are in the nucleus and the number of electrons revolving around the nucleus. Hydrogen has one, helium has two, lithium has three, and so on.

The shells of an atom fill up in a definite way. The first shell can contain up to two electrons, the second shell up to eight electrons, and the third shell up to eighteen electrons. It is also important to note that the first shell always fills up first, then the second shell, and then the third shell.

You can think of this being like a hotel that has room for two guests on the ground floor, for eight guests on the second floor, and eighteen guests on the third floor. In order to save money, the hotel fills up the ground floor first, then the second floor, and then the third floor. In the case of atoms, the electrons in the inner shells do not have as much energy as electrons in outer shells.

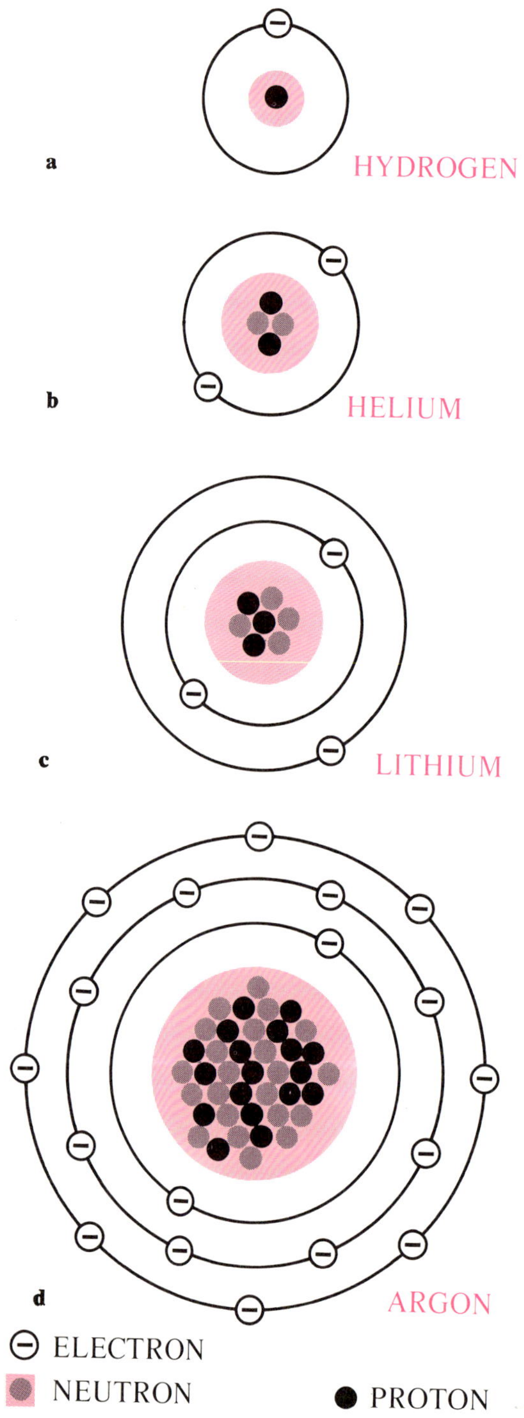


**5.12** Models of hydrogen, helium, lithium, and argon

Knowing how the shells fill up, we can now draw a picture of our new model of the atom. Starting with *hydrogen* that has an atomic number of one and an atomic weight of one, we would have the atom shown in Figure 5.12a. Next is *helium*, shown in Figure 5.12b, with an atomic number of two and atomic weight of four. Figure 5.12c shows *lithium*, with atomic number three and an atomic weight of seven. The eighteenth element on the chart is *argon*, the model of which is shown in Figure 5.12d. Notice that helium (Figure 5.12b) and argon (Figure 5.12d) have outer shells that are filled up. As you will see a little later, this has important effects on the properties of these two elements.

## Drawing Atomic Models

Draw models like those in Figure 5.12 for the elements having atomic numbers four through seventeen (beryllium through chlorine). You can obtain the atomic number of each element from the Table on page 160. Be sure to label each model with its correct name. With the models you draw and those in Figure 5.12, you will have models for the first eighteen elements.

You may be wondering how the electrons arrange themselves for elements having atomic numbers greater than eighteen. As you already know, the first shell can have up to two, the second shell up to eight, and the third shell up to eighteen. The fourth and fifth shells can contain up to thirty-two electrons each.

As you can see, this would total up to 92 (2+8+18+32+32). Uranium, the natural element with the highest atomic number, has ninety-two electrons. However, the electrons of uranium are not arranged in shells of 2-8-18-32-32. Instead, the arrangement is 2-8-18-32-21-9-2.

This can be explained by going back to the element having atomic number nineteen on the periodic chart, *potassium*. From the models you drew and those in Figure 5.12, you might expect the electrons of potassium to be in a pattern of 2-8-9. Instead, the electron distribution is 2-8-8-1. In other words, the fourth shell starts filling up before the third shell is full. Using our hotel example, guests start occupying the fourth floor before all the beds are occupied on the third floor.

You can look in a chemistry textbook or encyclopedia if you are interested in how the electrons are arranged in atoms of elements having atomic numbers larger than eighteen. These references also will explain how the chemist's model of the atom has shells that are broken into subshells and yet still smaller divisions. However, for the things we want to explain, our model of the atom with the electrons in shells will work very well.

This illustrates an important point about a scientific model or theory. We try to build a model or theory that will help us to explain our observations. When things occur that we cannot explain, we must do one of two things. We can modify our model or theory as we have done in the way we arrange electrons in their orbits around the nucleus; the other possibility is to discard the theory, as was done in the case of the phlogiston theory and of the earlier idea that everything was composed of air, earth, fire, and water.

It is also important to recognize that a scientific model does *not* represent an object in the same way a model airplane resembles a real airplane. Atoms do not look like the drawings you have made, nor do atoms resemble the balls of wood or plastic that are sometimes used to represent them. Atoms can be represented by many models, and some phenomena are explained using a mathematical model. But regardless of the model being used, it is important to remember that we are talking about a *model* and not the real thing.

### Have You Learned?

1. Explain how models, or mental pictures, are used. What kinds of things do chemists explain, using a model of the atom?
2. Describe how electrons are arranged around the nucleus of the atom. How many electrons can each of the first three shells contain?
3. Draw a picture showing how the electrons are arranged in hydrogen, oxygen, and carbon.

## 5. How Atoms Combine

**ARE YOU READY?**

Look up the following words if you are not sure of their meanings:

conduct; distilled water; electron; inert; minus; model (scientific); negative; plus; positive; shell (electron); stable.

Early chemists were puzzled about how atoms combined and why they combine the way they do. For example, why does *one* atom of oxygen combine with *two* atoms of hydrogen? Why not *one* atom of hydrogen and *one* atom of oxygen? Why do metals like iron and mercury combine with oxygen but not with each other? Why do some elements like argon and helium, which are called **inert** (in ėrt′) elements, combine with other elements only under very special conditions?

One suggested model for explaining how atoms combine showed atoms as if they were tiny spheres with hooks attached.

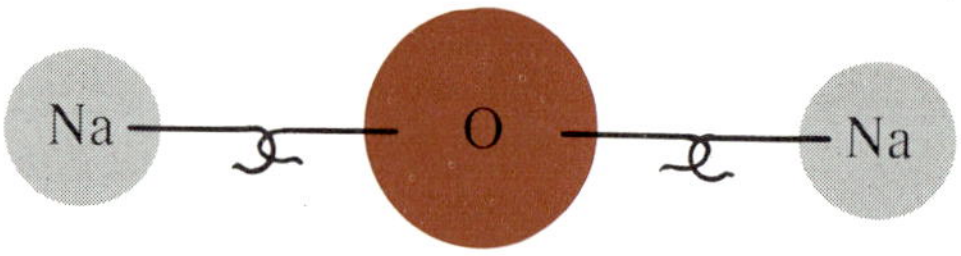


**5.13** A model of an old idea of how atoms of sodium combine with an atom of oxygen

The formation of water could be explained by having two hooks on each oxygen atom and one hook on each hydrogen atom. To explain why the metals iron and mercury do not combine, it was reasoned that something about the hooks prevented their joining together. The behavior of argon and neon could be explained by their not having any hooks.

As scientists learned more about the electrical nature of the atom, their ideas changed about how atoms combine. To understand how we now believe they combine, let's reexamine the electron arrangement of several atoms.

Study carefully how the electrons are arranged in the four atoms diagramed in Figure 5.12. Notice that the outer shells of the two inert elements are filled, whereas the shells of the other two are not. For instance, lithium has one electron in its outer shell, and oxygen has six. Chemists have found that atoms are most stable when their outer shells are filled. In other words, they are most stable when their electrons are arranged like those of an inert gas.

It has also been found that atoms tend to change from a form that has an incomplete outer shell to a form that has the outer shell filled. How is this accomplished? One way is for atoms to gain or lose electrons through a process similar to borrowing and lending. Another way is for atoms to combine in such a way that electrons are shared.

## Electron Gainers and Losers

Look at the electron arrangement of sodium and chlorine in Figure 5.14.

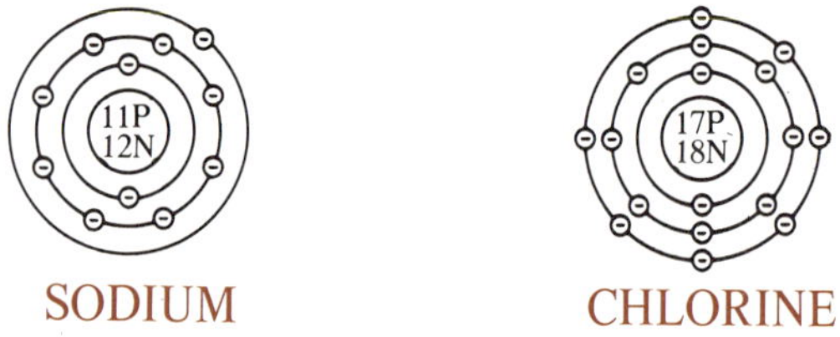


**5.14** The outer ring is important.

Note that sodium has one electron in its outer shell and chlorine has seven. This should give you a clue as to how sodium and chlorine combine to form sodium chloride, or table salt.

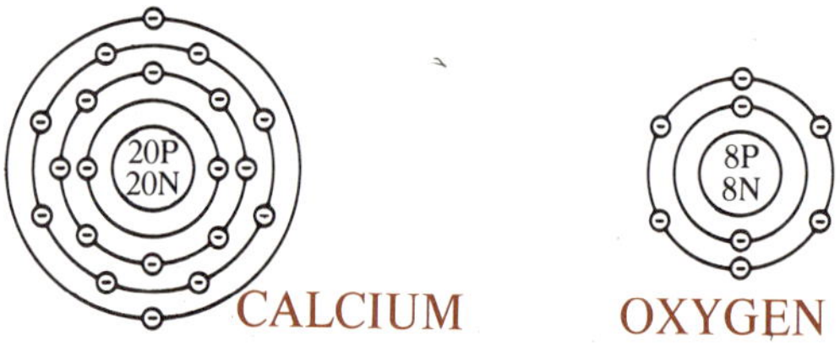


**5.15** Can you predict how calcium and oxygen combine?

An experiment on how well certain solutions conduct electricity should provide additional information.

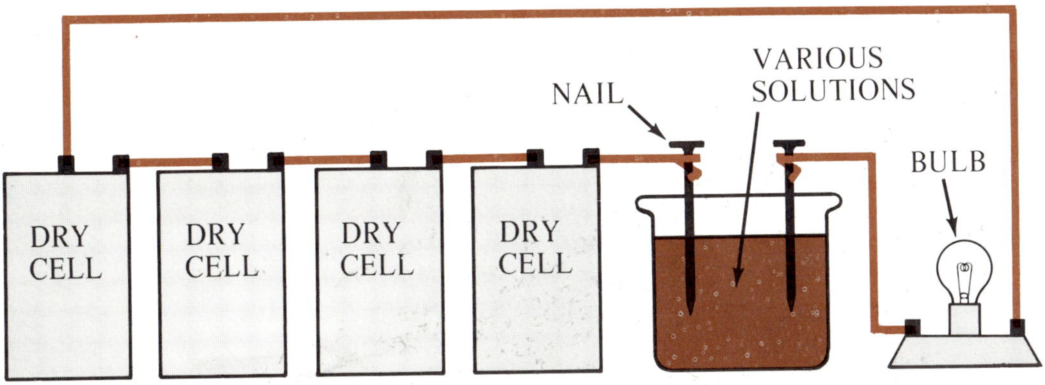


**5.16** How does the brightness of the bulb vary when the nails are placed in the various substances?

## Observing Solutions Conduct Electricity

**MATERIALS:**

Four dry cells or other source of low-voltage electricity, light bulb and socket, beakers, wire, nails, distilled water, table salt, calcium chloride, sugar

**PROCEDURE:**

Connect the dry cells and lamp as shown in Figure 5.16. Touch the nails together. The lamp should light up. If it doesn't, check the connections, the dry cells, and the bulb.

(1) Place the two nails in a beaker of distilled water, keeping them on opposite sides of the beaker. Does the lamp light up?

(2) Repeat the experiment, placing the nails first into a solution of table salt, then in the calcium chloride and sugar. Be sure to rinse off the nails with distilled water before putting them into each of the solutions. Why is this necessary?

(3) You may wish to test how well solutions of other chemicals, such as vinegar, ammonia, and rubbing alcohol conduct electricity. Also try sticking the nails about an inch apart in a lemon, orange, or tomato.

When sodium chloride is placed in water, *ions* are formed. The sodium atom gives up the single electron in its outer shell to the chlorine atom. As a result, the sodium atom has the stable arrangement of a filled shell. But it also has 11 protons and only 10 electrons. As a result of having one more proton than it has electrons, it has a positive charge of one. *An ion is any atom, or group of atoms, that is electrically charged because of a loss or gain of electrons.*

The chlorine atom gains an electron that completes its outer shell. Because it now has 18 electrons and only 17 protons, it has a negative charge of one. The chlorine atom has become a negative ion.

One way that compounds are formed is by the combining of oppositely charged ions. These ions are held together because bodies with opposite electrical charges attract each other. This attractive force is called a *bond.*

Let's go back to our investigation of how well certain solutions conduct electricity. You should have found that the lamp burned brightly when the nails were placed in the solutions of table salt and calcium chloride. This is because both of these compounds are composed of ions. When placed in solution, these ions are very good conductors of electricity.

## The Combining Power of Certain Elements

The combining power of an element that forms ions is called its **valence** (vā′ ləns). A sodium atom loses one electron to form a sodium ion with a positive charge of one. We say that it has *a positive valence of one.*

The combining power, or valence, of several common elements is given in Table II. First, compare the valences of calcium and oxygen with their electron arrangements, shown in Figure 5.15 on page 166. Do you see why calcium has a valence of a positive, or plus, 2, and oxygen has a valence of a negative, or minus, 2? Do you think you would be able to predict the valences of the elements in Table II by drawing pictures of their electron arrangements?

**TABLE II**

*Combining Power of Some Common Elements*

| *Metals* | *Valence* | *Nonmetals* | *Valence* |
|---|---|---|---|
| Aluminum (Al) | +3 | Bromine (Br) | −1 |
| Calcium (Ca) | +2 | Chlorine (Cl) | −1 |
| Hydrogen (H) | +1 | Iodine (I) | −1 |
| Lead (Pb) | +2 | Nitrogen (N) | −3 |
| Magnesium (Mg) | +2 | Oxygen (O) | −2 |
| Mercury (Hg) | +2 | Phosphorus (P) | −3 |
| Potassium (K) | +1 | Sulfur (S) | −2 |
| Silver (Ag) | +1 | | |
| Sodium (Na) | +1 | | |
| Zinc (Zn) | +2 | | |

The information in Table II can be used in writing the formulas for many compounds that are formed by the combination of ions. For example, if we want to write the formula for calcium oxide, we first look up the valence of calcium and oxygen. For calcium it is plus two (+2), and for oxygen it is minus two (−2). Since calcium and oxygen have exactly opposite charges that will offset each other, the formula for calcium oxide is CaO. Be sure to note that the name or symbol of the metal, or the element with the positive valence, is written *before* that of the nonmetal.

What is the formula for calcium chloride

that we used in the investigation on how well solutions conduct electricity? The valence of calcium is +2, and that of chlorine is −1. In order for the charges of the ions to be balanced, there must be two chlorine ions for each calcium ion. Thus, the formula is $CaCl_2$.

As a final example, let's try writing the formula for aluminum sulfide. The valence of aluminum is +3, and that of sulfur is −2. One possibility would be $Al_{2/3}S$, and another would be $AlS_{1\frac{1}{2}}$. But these formulas will not work because it is impossible to have two-thirds of an aluminum atom or one-and-a-half sulfur atoms.

What we do instead is something like using a common denominator in adding fractions. How can we group aluminum ions and sulfide ions so that the charges will balance? The formula $Al_2S_3$ should solve the problem. The two aluminum ions have a total charge of +6, and the three sulfide ions have a total charge of −6.

### Practice Writing Formulas

Write the formulas for the following compounds. Remember that the total positive charge, or valence, must be equal to the total negative charge.

Potassium chloride
Zinc oxide
Sodium iodide
Magnesium oxide
Aluminum iodide
Lead sulfide
Silver chloride
Calcium bromide

### Have You Learned?

Complete the following summary of this section by writing on a sheet of paper or in your notebook the word or words that best completes each statement.

Chemists have found that atoms of the __(1)__ elements, that have their outer shells filled, do not usually combine with other atoms. They have learned also that some elements borrow or lend __(2)__, thus resulting in their outer shells' being filled. When an atom gains or loses electrons, __(3)__, or electrically charged particles, are formed. The attractive force between two oppositely charged particles is called a __(4)__. The combining power of an element is called its __(5)__. Using this, correct __(6)__ can be written for compounds such as *calcium chloride* and *aluminium oxide*.

## 6. More About How Atoms Combine

**ARE YOU READY?**

Look up the following words if you are not sure of their meanings:

compound; formula; ion; solution; valence.

Thus far we have seen how ions, such as those of sodium and chloride, combine to form compounds. When you look at the formula *NaCl*, you might think that a sodium ion and a chlorine ion combine to form a particle called a molecule. In Section 2, it was stated that a formula is used to represent a molecule, and that $H_2O$ represents a molecule of water. This is not exactly correct, however, in cases like sodium chloride. Ions of sodium and chloride do not combine in the same way as atoms of hydrogen and oxygen combine to form water. Instead, they form clusters of sodium and chloride ions called *crystals*. A single tiny crystal contains billions of sodium and chloride ions. (See Figures 5.17 and 5.18.)

Because of the way ions combine to form crystals, we do not speak of "sodium chloride molecules" or "calcium chloride molecules." Instead, we say that sodium ions and chloride ions combine to form a **compound.** A compound is a substance that contains two or more elements that are united chemically. Most compounds held together by forces between ions are solids composed of crystals, and they melt at high temperatures.

## Groups of Atoms That Stay Together

Not all ions are single atoms that have gained or lost electrons. Frequently we find groups of atoms that stay together during chemical reactions and that form ions when they are in solution. We call these groups of atoms **radicals** (rad′ ə kəl).

The formulas and valences of several common radicals are given in Table III. These radicals combine with elements or other radicals to form compounds. To see how this works, let's write the formula for two such compounds.

What is the formula for sodium bicarbonate? The valence of sodium is +1 and that of bicarbonate is −1. The positive charge of one sodium ion would be counterbalanced by the negative charge of one bicarbonate ion. Thus the formula for sodium bicarbonate is $NaHCO_3$.

**TABLE III**

*Common Radicals*

| *Radical* | *Formula* | *Valence* | *Compounds containing radical* |
|---|---|---|---|
| Ammonium | $NH_4$ | +1 | Ammonium hydroxide ($NH_4OH$); used as a household cleaner |
| Bicarbonate | $HCO_3$ | −1 | Sodium bicarbonate ($NaHCO_3$); common name for baking soda |
| Carbonate | $CO_3$ | −2 | Calcium carbonate ($CaCO_3$); makes up limestone and chalk |
| Chlorate | $ClO_3$ | −1 | Potassium chlorate ($KClO_3$); used to make oxygen |
| Hydroxide | OH | −1 | Calcium hydroxide ($Ca(OH)_2$); common name is limewater |
| Nitrate | $NO_3$ | −1 | Nitric acid ($HNO_3$); a strong acid |
| Phosphate | $PO_4$ | −3 | Calcium phosphate ($Ca_3(PO_4)_2$); found in bones and teeth |
| Sulfate | $SO_4$ | −2 | Calcium sulfate ($CaSO_4$); common name is gypsum, used in making plaster |

What is the formula for aluminum sulfate? Aluminum has a valence of +3, and sulfate has a valence of −2. This means two aluminum ions ($+3 \times 2 = +6$) will combine with three sulfate ions ($-2 \times 3 = -6$). The formula is written $Al_2(SO_4)_3$. Parentheses are placed around the sulfate radical to show that there are three sulfate groups. The formula is read "A-L taken twice, parentheses S-O-four taken three times." The formula for ammonium sulfate, $(NH_4)_2SO_4$, is read "parentheses N-H-four taken twice, S-O-four."

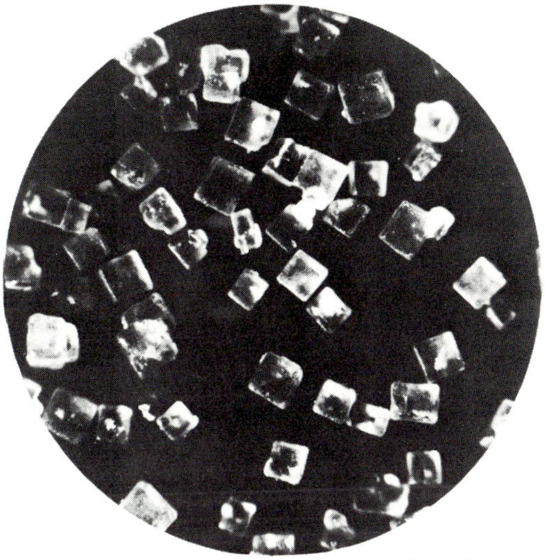

*Morton International, Inc.*

**5.17** Sodium chloride crystals (table salt)

### Practice Writing Formulas with Radicals

Write formulas for the following compounds and decide how to read them.

calcium carbonate
magnesium sulfate
sodium hydroxide
potassium phosphate
lead nitrate
ammonium hydroxide

**5.18** Crystal lattice of sodium chloride

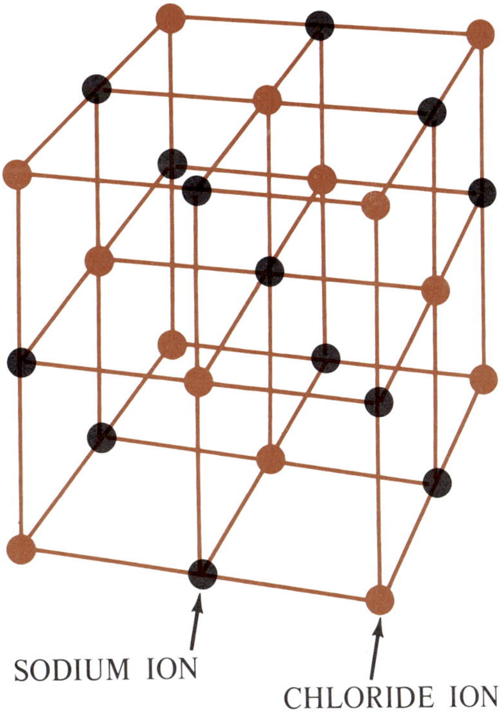


## Sharers of Electrons

Earlier, when you placed the nails in a beaker of distilled water and in a solution of sugar water, the lamp burned very dimly or not at all. This is because the atoms in water and sugar are not held together in the same way as in compounds composed of ions. Instead of being held together because of gains and losses of electrons, molecules of water and sugar are held together by atoms sharing electrons.

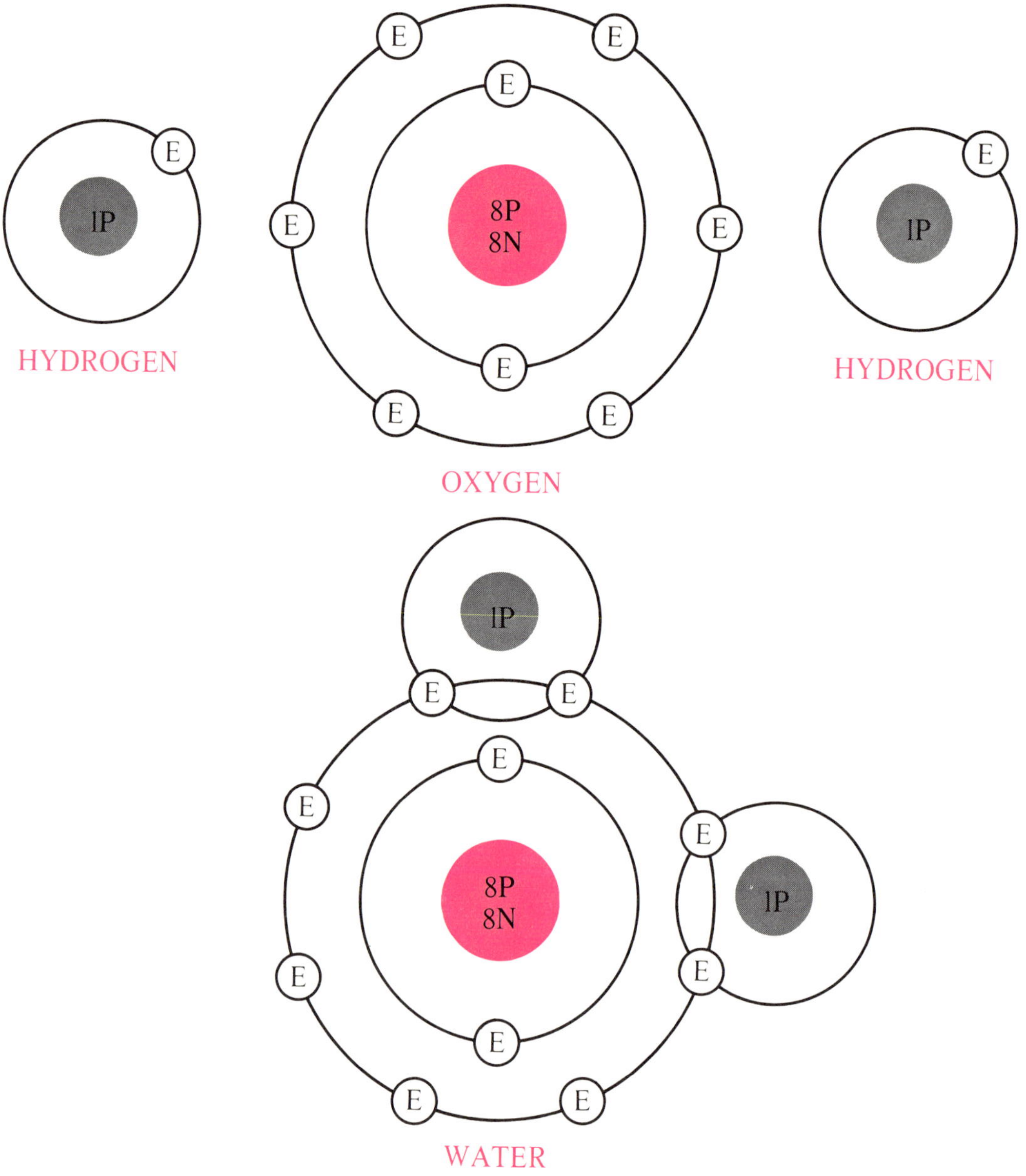


**5.19** When oxygen and hydrogen atoms combine, each of the two hydrogen atoms shares a pair of electrons with the oxygen atom (not at right angles as shown).

Look at Figure 5.19 above. Shown at the top are two atoms of hydrogen and one atom of oxygen. Each hydrogen atom has one electron in its shell and the oxygen has six electrons in its outer shell. As shown in the lower part of Figure 5.19, in a water molecule a pair of electrons is shared by the oxygen atom with each of the two hydrogen atoms.

Each of these pairs of shared electrons

is called a *bond*. Because of the cooperative arrangement, the sharing power of these atoms is called **covalence** (kō vā′ ləns). Bonds formed by the sharing of electrons are called **covalent bonds.**

The sharing power or covalence of some common elements is given in Table IV. Since electrons are shared rather than gained or lost, covalences do not have + and − signs.

TABLE IV

*Sharing Power of Common Elements*

| *Element* | *Covalence (Pairs of Electrons Shared)* |
|---|---|
| Hydrogen | 1 |
| Chlorine | 1 |
| Carbon | 4 |
| Nitrogen | 3 |
| Oxygen | 2 |

Carbon is one of the most important elements that forms covalent compounds. How would you expect an atom of carbon to combine with hydrogen? Since carbon has a covalence of four, it should combine with four atoms of hydrogen, each with a covalence of one.

There is a compound with the formula $CH_4$. It is **methane** (meth′ ān), a very light-weight gas used in gas stoves and furnaces. You will learn more about this compound and other carbon compounds in Chapter 7.

## Writing Formulas Using Covalence

Write formulas for the following compounds using the covalences given in Table IV. Check to see if you can find out if such compounds actually exist and what they are called.

carbon and chlorine
nitrogen and hydrogen
carbon and oxygen

## Summary

By studying the electron arrangement in the outer shell of most atoms, we can predict if the element will combine with other elements and, if so, how. Most of the forces holding atoms together are due either to electron borrowing and lending or to electron sharing. The combining power of an element, because of electron gains and losses, is *valence*, and that resulting from electron sharing is *covalence.*

## Have You Learned?

On a sheet of paper list the numbers for the questions below. By each number write *T* if the statement is true and *F* if false.

1. A compound is a substance that contains two or more elements that are united chemically.
2. A crystal of sodium chloride never contains more than one sodium ion and one chloride ion.
3. Groups of atoms that stay together during chemical reactions and form ions in solution are called *radicals.*
4. The formula for ammonium sulfate is $(NH_4)_3(SO_4)_2$.
5. Molecules of water and molecules of sugar are held together by atoms borrowing and lending electrons.
6. Bonds formed by the sharing of electrons are called *covalent bonds.*
7. Carbon has a covalence of +4.
8. The formula for methane is $CH_4$.

## 7. Classifying the Elements

**ARE YOU READY?**

Look up the following words if you are not sure of their meanings:

atomic number; atomic weight; chemically active; classify; density; predict; row; solubility; valence.

In working with a large number of objects or a lot of information, it is helpful to have a system for classifying them. For example, in a library, books are grouped together, magazines placed in another group, and so on. Books in turn are divided into smaller groups according to their subject. This makes the books easier to catalog and find.

In a like manner, plants and animals are classified. All animals with backbones are placed in one group. The birds are a subgroup and have several characteristics in common. As soon as it is determined that an unknown animal is a bird, it can be predicted that it has feathers, lays eggs, has two feet, and has a body temperature that does not change with the temperature of its surroundings.

In addition to the predictive value of a classification system, scientists have other reasons to classify things. They believe that there is order in the universe and they always try to get information to fit into a pattern. They are also interested in how things are related. How are birds alike and different from other groups of animals having backbones? How are the elements alike, and how do they differ?

Soon after Dalton's proposed atomic theory of 1803, scientists attempted to

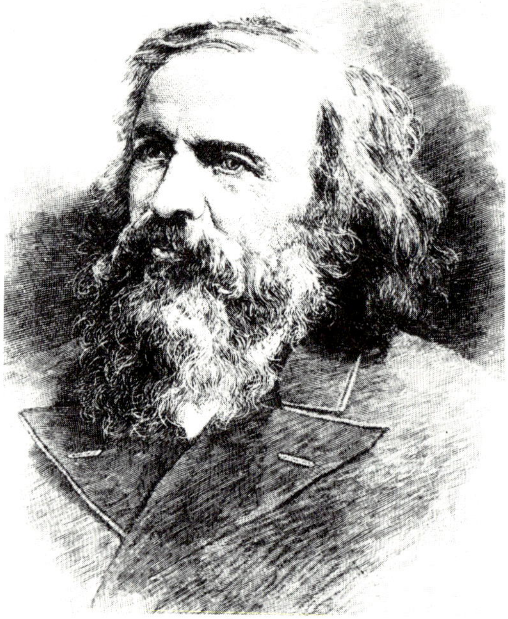

*Historical Pictures Service—Chicago*

**5.20** Mendeleev classified the elements.

classify the elements on the basis of their characteristics or properties. In 1869 Mendeleev (men′ də lā′ əf), a Russian chemist, proposed a chart of the elements arranged on the basis of their atomic weights.

Mendeleev's chart had eight vertical rows and seven horizontal rows, making a total of 56 boxes. He arranged the 59 elements known at that time so that elements with similar properties were lined up under each other. For example, lithium, sodium, and potassium were lined up, one under the other, because they are chemically alike in many ways. In some boxes he had to place two or three elements, and, in a few cases, he placed no elements in a box. He reasoned that the blank spots represented elements that had not yet been discovered. By studying the properties of the elements above, below, and to either side of the blank spots, he was able to predict the properties and atomic weights of some unknown elements.

One of the elements predicted by Mendeleev was **Germanium** (jėr mā′ ni əm), discovered later in 1886. Compare Mendeleev's prediction of characteristics with the actual properties of the element.

**Germanium (Ge)**

| | *Predicted Properties* | *Actual Properties* |
|---|---|---|
| 1. Atomic Weight | 72 | 72.60 |
| 2. Melting Point | High | 958° C. |
| 3. Density | 5.5 g/cc | 5.36 g/cc |
| 4. Color | Dark gray | Gray |
| 5. Solubility | Will dissolve in HCl | Does dissolve in HCl |
| 6. Combination with oxygen | Will form $GeO_2$ | Forms $GeO_2$ |

Since Mendeleev's time, an additional thirty-three natural elements have been discovered, bringing the total number of natural elements to ninety-two. In addition, at least eleven elements have been made in the laboratory, and thus most periodic tables show at least 103 elements.

Since Mendeleev's work many new techniques and instruments for studying the atom have been developed. As a result of work which involved making X rays of the elements, the chart of the atoms was revised. In the revised chart, the elements were arranged on the basis of their atomic number. Our present system of classifying the elements still has them arranged in order of increasing atomic number.

## The Periodic Table of the Elements

The chart on page 160 is one version of the Periodic Table of the Elements used by chemists and other scientists. For each element the atomic number is in the upper left-hand corner, and the atomic weight is in the upper right-hand corner. The large letters are the symbols for the elements. What other information does the chart contain?

By studying the arrangement of the elements, it is possible to make predictions about an element on the basis of the properties of its neighbors. Look at the elements on the left-hand side of the chart. They are all **metals,** and many have names ending in *ium.* They are usually electron lenders and thus have plus valences. Compare the elements in Table II (on page 168) that have positive valencies, with their positions on the chart on page 160. Elements to the right side of the dark stair-step-shaped line are **nonmetals.** They are electron gainers and have minus valences.

The elements in a vertical row are called a **family** or group. The elements in Row VIIA—fluorine, chlorine, bromine, and iodine—are called the **halogen** (hal′ ə jən) family. Just as you would expect of a family of humans, members of a family of elements have many similar characteristics. For example, members of the halogen family all combine with sodium to form the compounds NaF, NaCl, NaBr, and NaI.

However, there are also differences within a family. In families on the right side of the chart, elements near the top of the chart (fluorine) are chemically more active than elements near the bottom (iodine). In the case of the metals on the left side of the chart, just the opposite is true. Elements near the bottom are more active than those higher in the row. Cesium is more active than potassium, which in turn is more active than either sodium or lithium.

The elements in Row 0 on the right side of the chart are called the **inert gases.** They were so named because it was believed that they would not combine with any other elements. This is understandable when one draws a picture of their electron arrangement and in each case finds the outer shell filled. In 1962, **xenon** (zē′ non) was made to combine chemically with **fluorine** (flü′ ə rēn). As is so often true in science, we had to revise our ideas. We now use *inert* to describe the elements in Row 0, which *usually* do not combine with other elements.

You may be wondering about the two horizontal rows at the bottom of the chart. They are called the **lanthanum** (lan′ thə nəm) **series** and the **actinium** (ak tin′ i əm) **series,** and each includes the element after which it is named. Horizontal rows on the chart are called **series.**

The elements in the lanthanum and actinium series are commonly called the **rare earths.** However, this name is misleading because they are neither rare nor earths. They are metals that are widely used in the manufacture of many products Elements in the lanthanum series are used to add to or take away color from glass, and to make many heat-resistant parts such as those in jet engines and rockets. Elements in the actinium series are the "heavyweights" of the elements, and all of them are **radioactive** (rā′ di ō ak′ tiv). This means that they break up by a natural process into two or more simpler parts. Can you name ways that elements such as uranium and plutonium are used?

### Have You Learned?

Write on a sheet of paper the word that best completes the statement. (Do not write in your book.)

1. _____, a Russian chemist, developed a chart of the elements arranged on the basis of their atomic weights.
2. In the Periodic Table of the Elements that we now use, the elements are arranged on the basis of their atomic _____.
3. The _____, which are electron lenders, are found on the left side of the chart, and the _____, which are electron borrowers, are on the right side of the chart.
4. Fluorine, chlorine, bromine, and iodine are members of the _____ family.
5. The elements in the lanthanum and actinium series are commonly called the _____ _____.
6. Elements that break up by a natural process into two or more simpler parts are _____.
7. A _____ system has several advantages, including making it easier to work with a large number of objects and to make predictions.

## 8. Acids and Bases

> **ARE YOU READY?**
>
> Look up the following words if you are not sure of their meanings:
>
> chemical reaction; compound; formula; indicate; ion; radical; symbol.

*Acids* and *bases* are two important groups of chemical compounds. These two groups of compounds include thousands of important chemicals, many of which are found in nature. Taking acids as an example, one of the first many people think of is *citric acid*, found in lemons, oranges, and grapefruit. Sour milk contains *lactic acid*, and rancid butter has *butyric acid* in it. The *acetic acid* in vinegar is another acid found in foods.

### Acids

The most common way of defining an **acid** is to say that it is a compound that releases hydrogen ions when placed in a water solution. We can show how this works for hydrochloric acid by the use of an **equation** (i kwā′ zhən). Just as *symbols* and *formulas* are shorthand ways of representing elements and compounds, an equation shows what happens when a compound forms ions. As we shall see in the next chapter, equations also are used to show what happens during a chemical reaction.

The formula for hydrochloric acid is HCl and this is the equation that shows how it yields ions. The arrow in an equation points toward the products.

$$HCl \xrightarrow{\text{(in water)}} H^+ + Cl^-$$

It has been found that there is a strong attractive force between water molecules and hydrogen ions. They combine to form **hydronium** (hī drō′ nē əm) ions, $H_3O^+$. The equation for the **ionization** (ī′ ən ə zā′ shən) of hydrochloric acid is modified to show this.

$$HCl + H_2O \longrightarrow H_3O^+ + Cl^-$$

Because acids in water result in the formation of hydronium ions, our definition of an acid should be changed. Accordingly: *An acid is a compound that, when placed in water, yields hydronium ions.*

Look back to the list of common compounds on page 157. The first three in the list are acids that are frequently used in

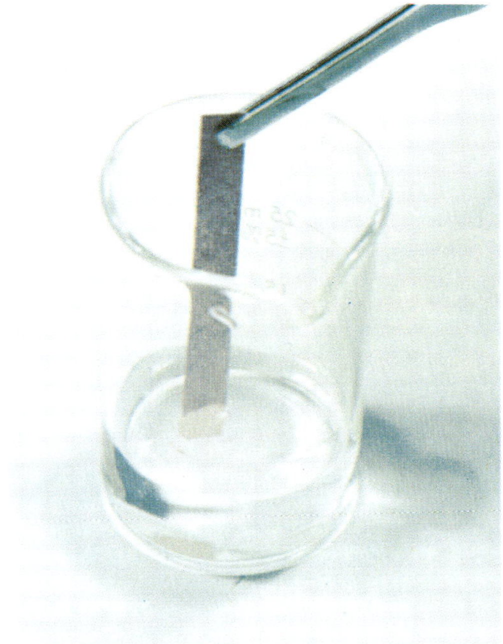

J. W. McDonald

**5.21** What has caused this blue litmus paper to become this color? (See the following page.)

chemistry laboratories and in industry. Chapter 6 describes several ways that these acids react with other compounds.

## Bases

A compound that yields hydroxide ions in water solutions is described as being a **base.** It is said to be **basic,** or **alkaline** (al′ kə līn). For example, when sodium oxide reacts with water, sodium hydroxide is formed. This compound ionizes to form sodium ions and hydroxide ions.

$$Na_2O - H_2O \longrightarrow 2\ NaOH \longrightarrow 2\ Na^+ - 2\ (OH)^-$$

We classify sodium hydroxide as a base. It has a flat bitter taste as do all bases.

## Determining How Acidic or How Basic

Suppose you have a water solution of an unknown compound, and you want to know if it is an acid or base. There are several methods you can use to find out. You can test the solution with **litmus** (lit′ məs) **paper.** Acids turn blue litmus red, and bases turn red litmus blue. Although litmus paper can be used to find out if the unknown solution is an acid, we still will not know if it is a strong acid or a weak acid. (See Figure 5.21 on the preceding page.) In addition to litmus, there are other chemicals called **indicators** that change color when placed in acids or bases. Some of these indicators are one color in strong acids and a different color in weak acids. Strips of paper are now manufactured that contain indicators that show several shades of color, depending on how acidic or basic a solution is.

Figure 5.22 shows a scale used by scientists to describe how acidic or how basic a solution is. The numbers go from a pH of 0 to a pH of 14. Solutions with a pH less than 7 are acidic, and those with pH's greater than 7 are basic. Strong acids have pH's near 0, and strong bases have a pH near 14. The pH scale finds common usage in describing such things as the acid condition of soil or drinking water.

A pH meter is an electrical instrument used to measure the pH of a solution. Remember the experiment in which nails connected to a dry cell and lamp were placed in several solutions, and the brightness of the lamp was observed? Can you suggest the scientific principle on which a pH meter works?

---

## Investigating Acids and Bases

**MATERIALS:**

Red and blue litmus paper, pH or universal indicator paper if available, indicators such as **phenolphthalein** (fē′ nōl thal′ ēn), **bromothymol** (brō′ mō thī′ məl) **blue,** and **methyl** (meth′ əl) **orange,** solutions to be tested (such as vinegar, various kinds of fruit juice, ammonia water, and laboratory chemicals, such as HCl, $H_2SO_4$, and NaOH), distilled water, a few leaves of purple cabbage, test tubes, beakers, forceps, medicine dropper, hot plate or Bunsen burner

**PROCEDURE:**

*Testing with litmus paper.* Place a small amount (10-25 cc) of each solution to be tested in a test tube or beaker. Be sure to label each container so you can keep a

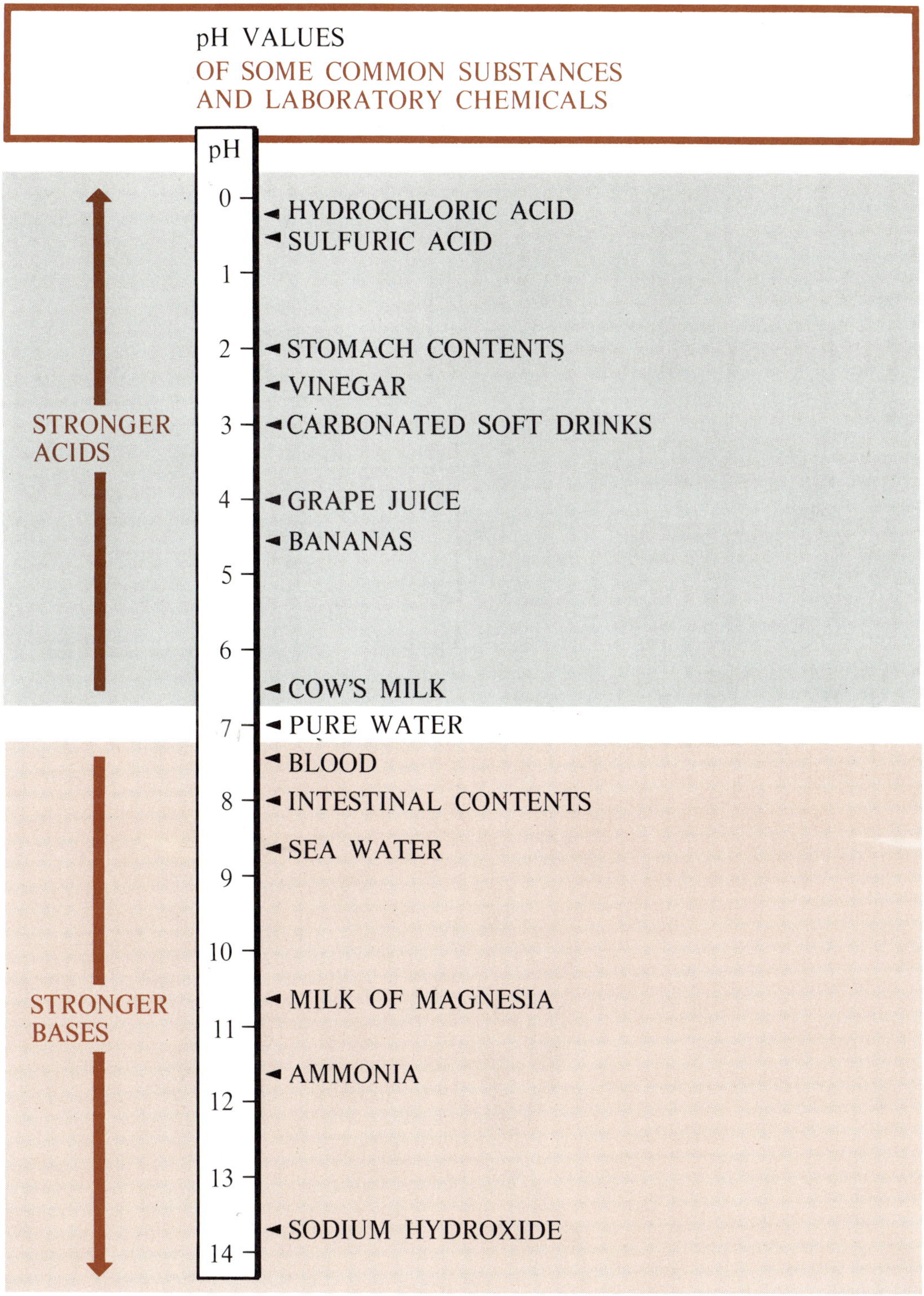


**5.22** What are the two strongest acids and the two strongest bases in this diagram?

record of your results. Dip a piece of red litmus paper in each of the solutions, and record any color changes you observe. **(Caution: In order to avoid getting strong acids or bases on your skin, use a pair of forceps to hold the litmus paper.)** Repeat testing each solution with blue litmus paper.

Which of the solutions were acids? bases? neutral? If you have some pH or universal indicator paper, repeat the tests to see if you can determine the approximate pH of each solution.

*Testing with other indicators.* If indicators such as phenolphthalein or bromothymol blue are available, place about 10 cc of an indicator solution in a test tube, and add, drop by drop, the solution you wish to test. Record any color changes that occur. By comparing these results with those obtained using litmus paper, explain how these color changes can be used to tell if a solution is acidic or basic.

*Making your own indicator.* Cut up a few leaves of purple cabbage, place in a beaker of water, and bring to a boil. Allow the leaves to simmer for about 15 minutes, remove the leaves, and filter the remaining juice into a clean beaker.

Fill several test tubes about half full of the cabbage juice. Add a few drops of the solution you wish to test. You may wish to start with a known acid such as vinegar and a base such as ammonia water. Observe any changes in the color of the cabbage juice. Explain how cabbage juice can be used to determine if a solution is an acid or a base. Can you tell from your results if it is a strong acid or a strong base?

**5.23** (*From left to right*) Acid and phenolphthaein; base and phenolphthalein; acid and bromothymol blue; and base and bromothymol blue.

*Norman D. Anderson*

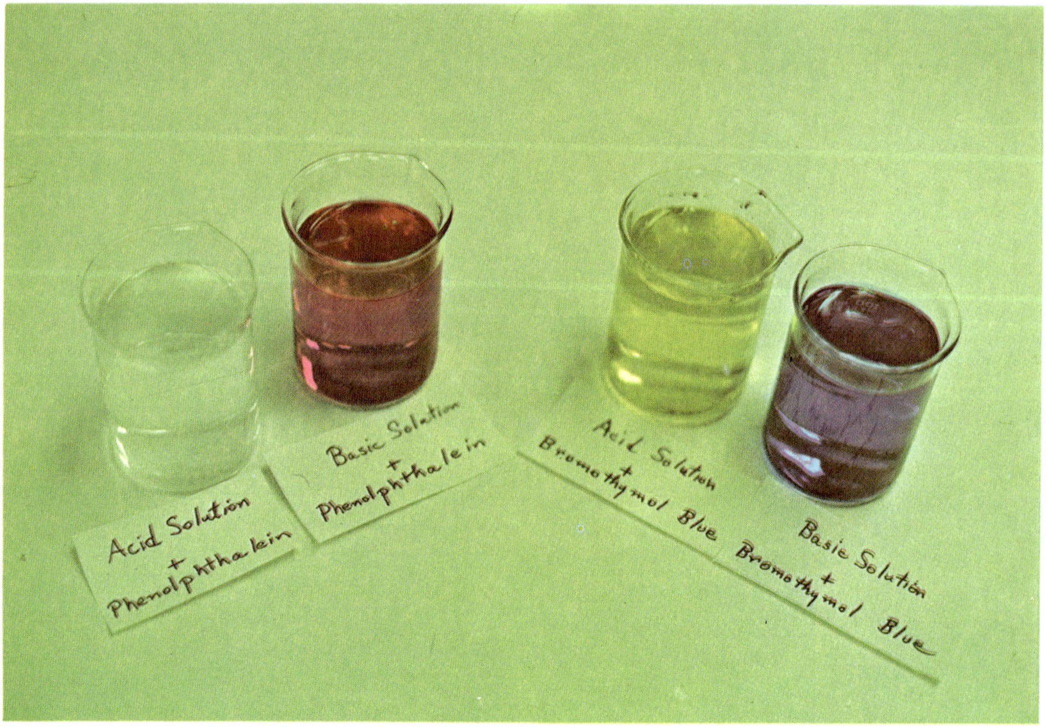

## Have You Learned?

Select the answer that best completes each statement. (Do not write in your book.)

1. A shorthand way for showing how a compound forms ions is a(n)
   a. equation.
   b. formula.
   c. ionization.
   d. symbol.
2. An acid is a substance that
   a. produces hydroxide ions in solution.
   b. produces hydronium ions in solution.
   c. turns red litmus paper blue.
   d. has a pH greater than seven.
3. A base is a substance that
   a. produces hydrogen ions in solution.
   b. produces hydronium ions in solution.
   c. turns red litmus paper blue.
   d. has a pH of less than seven.
4. Which of the following is an acid?
   a. NaCl
   b. $Na_2O$
   c. $H_2SO_4$
   d. NaOH
5. Which of the following is not an indicator?
   a. bromothymol blue
   b. methyl orange
   c. phenolphthalein
   d. vinegar

## REVIEW QUESTIONS

1. Briefly describe the early ideas that people had about chemistry. Include the following names and terms in your answer: ether; Democritus; Aristotle; alchemists; phlogiston; Priestley; Lavoisier.
2. Write the formulas for five common substances such as table salt and sugar. Tell what elements each of these substances contain.
3. Draw a picture of an atom that has an atomic number of 6 and an atomic weight of 12. How many electrons are there in the outer shell? How many neutrons does it have? Which element is it?
4. Explain how atoms combine and the difference between valence and covalence. What is a radical?
5. List as many things as you can about an element that can be learned from the Periodic Table of the Elements.
6. Define *acid* and *base*, and describe several properties of each.

## CAN YOU FIND OUT?

*You may find it necessary to use an encyclopedia or other reference books in answering these questions.*

1. Can you find out what particles in atoms have been identified in addition to electrons, protons, and neutrons?
2. How are the elements with atomic numbers larger than 92 made? What is the largest atomic number believed to be possible?
3. How are the electrons arranged within the shells of atoms?
4. Experiments show that the two hydrogen atoms in a molecule of water are not on opposite sides of the oxygen atom, but are at approximately right angles to each other. How can this be explained?
5. Are atoms all the same size? Does this affect the way that they combine with other atoms?
6. Examine a Periodic Table of the Elements such as a wall chart or one found in a chemistry textbook or encyclopedia. How many things can you tell about each element using the chart?

## REFERENCES FOR ADDITIONAL STUDY

ANTOINE LAVOISIER, SCIENTIST, ECONOMIST, SOCIAL REFORMER by Douglas McKie. Abelard-Schuman Limited.
A biography of one of the pioneers of modern chemistry

BUILDING BLOCKS OF THE UNIVERSE (Revised Edition) by Isaac Asimov. Abelard-Schuman Limited.
The story of the 102 elements known at the time the book was written

CAREERS AND OPPORTUNITIES IN CHEMISTRY by Phillip Pollack, E. P. Dutton & Co., Inc.
Describes careers in chemistry and chemical engineering, including duties and college preparation required

CRYSTALS AND CRYSTAL GROWING by Alan Holden and Phylis Singer. Doubleday & Company, Inc.
The story of the world of crystals, with ideas for growing crystals

ELEMENTS OF THE UNIVERSE by Glen Seaborg and Evans Valens. E. P. Dutton & Co., Inc.
Compares early beliefs and later ideas with recent discoveries in chemistry, including element 102

MENDELEYEV: PROPHET OF CHEMICAL ORDER by Peter Kelman and A. Harris Stone. Prentice-Hall, Inc.
A biography of the chemist who contributed so much to the development of the periodic table

METALS by Raymond Wohlrabe. J. B. Lippincott Company.
Treats all phases of metallurgy—history of metals, alloys, processes for extracting ores, and prospecting for metals

THE NOBLE GASES by Isaac Asimov. Basic Books, Inc., Publishers.
A complete treatment of the noble gases, from the early work in the seventeenth century to the new chemistry of the gases formerly believed to be inert

THE SEARCH FOR THE ELEMENTS by Isaac Asimov. Basic Books, Inc., Publishers.
Describes the history of chemistry and the recent work involving the production of the new elements

TEST TUBES AND BEAKERS: CHEMISTRY FOR YOUNG EXPERIMENTERS by E. H. Coulson, A. E. J. Trinder, and Aaron E. Klein. Doubleday & Company, Inc.
Contains directions for doing many chemical experiments, some of which require only little equipment

MR. TOMPKINS EXPLORES THE ATOM by George Gamow. Cambridge University Press.
Describes how Mr. Tompkins, a fictional character, discovers molecular motion, the electron, and atom-smashers

CHAPTER 6

# Chemical Reactions: Atoms in Action

WITH OUR KNOWLEDGE FROM CHAPTER 5 of how atoms combine, we are ready to investigate **chemical reactions.** A chemical reaction is a process by which one or more new substances are formed. We shall see that this may involve combining atoms or breaking up of combinations of atoms. Atoms also sometimes change partners during chemical reactions. We shall also see that there are several things that can be done to change the rates of reactions.

## 1. Combining the Elements

> **ARE YOU READY?**
>
> Look up the following words if you are not sure of their meanings:
>
> chemical properties; compound; crystalline; element; equation; formula; luster; molecule; physical properties.

Weigh out 4 grams of sulfur on a piece of filter paper. Next weigh out 2 grams of iron filings or iron powder on a second piece of filter paper. Examine each of these elements, noting their color, luster, whether or not they are crystalline, and any other visible characteristics. In Chapter 2 we learned that these characteristics are called *physical properties.* How many physical properties of iron and sulfur can you name?

If the iron filings are heated to a high enough temperature, they will become a liquid. If the liquid iron is cooled, a solid will form. Instead of thousands of tiny particles of iron, however, you will have a single piece of iron. A change of this kind is called a **physical change.** Dissolving a substance or grinding up crystals are other examples of a physical change. The atoms of a substance are not altered during a physical change. Atoms uncombined remain uncombined and those in combination with other atoms remain in combination.

Mix the 4 grams of sulfur with the 2 grams of iron. Pass a magnet over the pile of iron and sulfur. Can a magnet be used to separate the iron from the sulfur? Since the iron and sulfur apparently are not combined, or held together in any way, we call this a **mixture.** A mixture is two or more substances that can be separated by physical means.

## Separating Mixtures

Suggest as many ways as you can for separating these mixtures.

| *Mixture* | *Suggestions for separating* |
|---|---|
| Pocketful of pennies, nickels, and dimes can be separated by . . . | |
| Solution of salt and water can be separated by . . . | |
| Sack of iron and aluminum nails can be separated by . . . | |
| Cow's milk that has not been processed (cream has not been separated from milk) can be separated by . . . | |
| White sand and sugar can be separated by . . . | |

In some cases the materials in a mixture can be combined to form a compound.

## Making a Compound from a Mixture

Place some of the iron-sulfur mixture in a Pyrex test tube, and heat it over a Bunsen burner (Figure 6.1). Be careful not to point the test tube toward anyone while you are heating the mixture. After the mixture has been thoroughly heated, remove the test tube from the flame, and allow it to cool. Wrap the test tube in a paper or cloth towel, and break it by tapping it with a hammer.

Examine the material inside the test tube. The iron and sulfur have combined to form a compound, iron sulfide. Does it have the same properties as iron and sulfur? Is it attracted by a magnet?

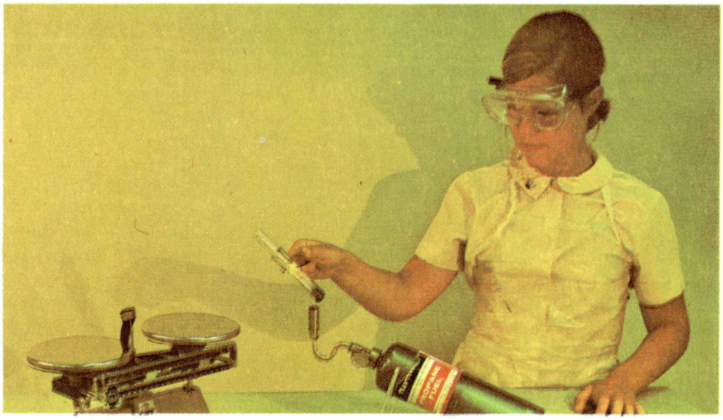

**6.1** Name the safety precautions this student is taking as she heats a mixture of iron and sulfur.

*Norman D. Anderson*

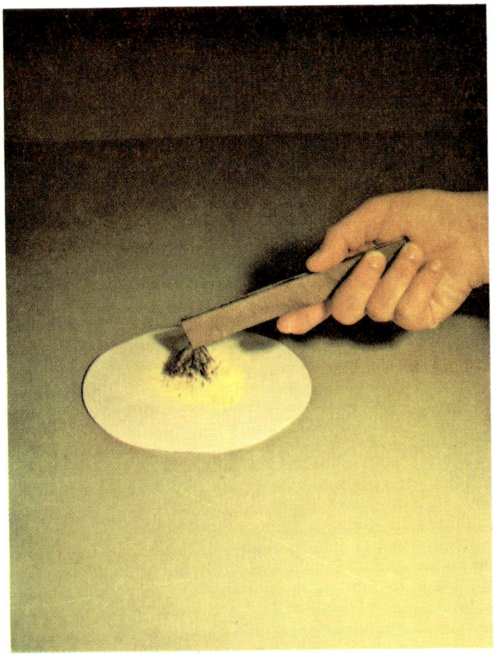

*Norman D. Anderson*

**6.2** Magnet separating iron and sulfur

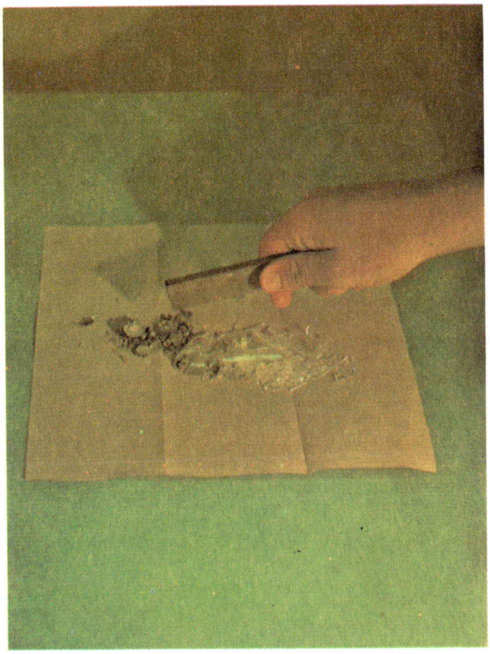

*Norman D. Anderson*

**6.3** The iron sulfide, formed when iron and sulfur are heated, is not attracted by a magnet.

The combining of iron and sulfur is an example of a **chemical change.** Chemical changes occur when new substances are formed during a chemical reaction. Unlike physical changes, chemical changes involve combinations of atoms being formed or broken up.

Whether or not an element or compound will react with another substance is called a **chemical property.** As you have seen, one chemical property of iron is that when heated it combines with sulfur. Remember when, in Chapter 5, you placed some steel wool (iron) in a jar and inverted it over a beaker of water? Another chemical property of iron is that it combines with oxygen to form iron oxide, or rust.

Why did iron and sulfur combine? If we draw a picture of the electron arrangement of an iron atom and a sulfur atom, we have the answer (Figure 6.4 page 186). The iron atom gives up two electrons, leaving its outer shell filled. The sulfur atom accepts the two electrons to fill its outer shell. Because of the positive charge on the iron atom and the negative charge on the sulfur atom, they are held together.

## Writing Equations for Combination-Type Reactions

Iron and sulfur are not the only elements that combine to form compounds. Iron combines with oxygen to form rust. Liquid mercury combines with oxygen to form the red powder, mercuric oxide. This is

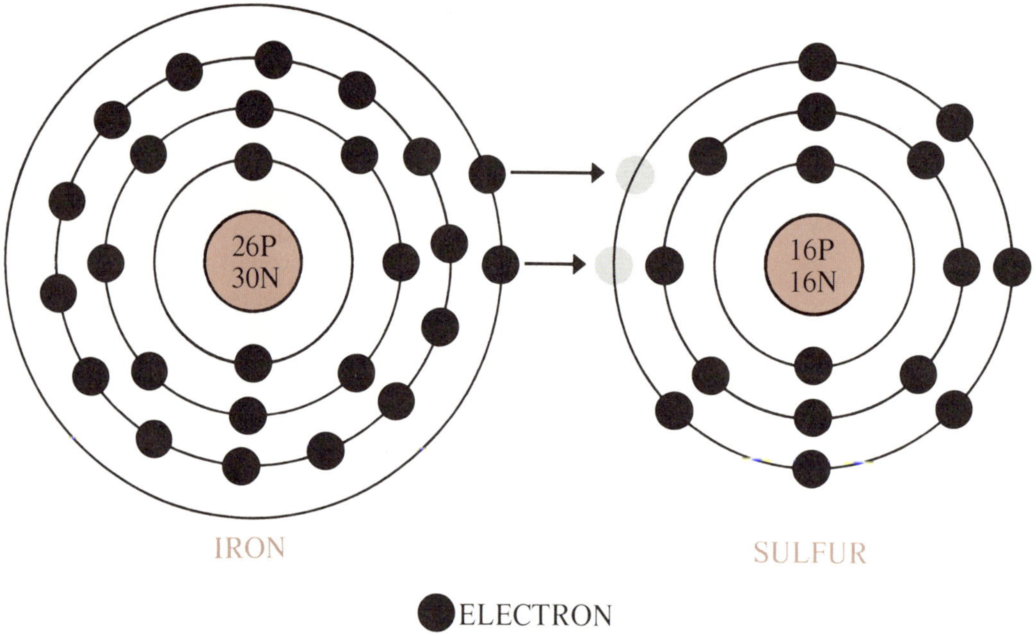


**6.4** An atomic model that shows where iron and sulfur atoms share electrons.

the reaction that Lavoisier and Priestley worked with. When a mixture of hydrogen and oxygen come in contact with a flame or spark, they combine with an explosive force, forming water.

Some compounds combine with other compounds. Calcium oxide combines with water to form calcium hydroxide. Ammonia gas combines with water to form ammonium hydroxide.

All of these reactions can be represented by an *equation*. The first step in writing an equation is to write the correct formulas for all the elements and compounds involved in the reaction. To show how this works, write the equations for the reactions just mentioned. For the combination of iron and sulfur, the equation is:

$$Fe + S \longrightarrow FeS$$

From this equation, you might predict the equation for the reaction of iron and oxygen to be:

$$Fe + O \longrightarrow FeO$$

This is not the correct equation, however, since the formula we have written for oxygen is not correct. Two oxygen atoms in the air combine to form a molecule, so the correct formula for oxygen is $O_2$. This is also true of several of the other gaseous elements: hydrogen ($H_2$), nitrogen ($N_2$), fluorine ($F_2$), chlorine ($Cl_2$), and bromine ($Br_2$).

We can rewrite the equation:

$$Fe + O_2 \longrightarrow FeO$$

The first step of writing an equation has now been done correctly since we have the correct formulas for oxygen, iron, and iron oxide. The second step in writing an equation is to *balance the equation*. In using equations in mathematics, the total value of the numbers and other symbols on the left side of the equal sign is always equal to what appears on the right side. In writing chemical equations, we do something very similar. We must have the same number of atoms of an element on the left side as on the right side of the equation.

The equation for the reaction of iron and oxygen has two oxygen atoms on the left side and only one oxygen atom on the right side. The equation does not balance. To balance the equation, the number of molecules must be juggled. We know that each atom of iron combines with an atom of oxygen. It follows that it will take two iron atoms to combine with the two oxygen atoms. Two pairs of iron-oxygen atoms, or iron oxide molecules, will be formed.

The equation is rewritten to show this.

$$2\ Fe + O_2 \longrightarrow 2\ FeO$$

The number to the left of the formula stands for the number of molecules. If there is only one molecule, we don't bother to write the number 1. The equation is now balanced because the number of iron atoms on the left side equals the number of iron atoms on the right side. There is also the same number of oxygen atoms on each side of the equation.

The first step in writing the equation for the formation of water is to write the correct formulas for all the elements and compounds involved in the reaction.

$$H_2 + O_2 \longrightarrow H_2O$$

The equation does not balance because we have two oxygen atoms on the left side and only one on the right side. So we change it to

$$H_2 + O_2 \longrightarrow 2\ H_2O$$

Now we have more hydrogen atoms on the right side than on the left side. To get the hydrogen atoms to balance, we change it to

$$2\ H_2 + O_2 \longrightarrow 2\ H_2O$$

Does it balance now?

The first step in writing the equations for the three following reactions has been done for you. In other words, the formulas are correct. Examine each equation to see if it is balanced. If not, change the number of molecules so that it does balance.

(1) $Hg + O_2 \longrightarrow HgO$
(2) $CaO + H_2O \longrightarrow Ca(OH)_2$
(3) $NH_3 + H_2O \longrightarrow NH_4OH$

### Have You Learned?

1. Describe the difference between a physical property and a chemical property. Give as many examples as possible of each.
2. Describe the difference between a physical change and a chemical change. Give examples of each.
3. Write the equation for three examples of elements combining to form compounds. Be sure that the equations are balanced.

## 2. Investigating an Important Gas of the Atmosphere

**ARE YOU READY?**

Look up the following words if you are not sure of their meanings:

decompose; dense; displacement; filter paper; oxygen; soluble.

For man and other animals, oxygen is the most important gas in the atmosphere. Without a supply of oxygen, man can survive for only a couple of minutes. Oxygen also plays an important role in burning or **combustion** (kəm bus′ chən) and in many other chemical reactions.

## Investigating Oxygen

**MATERIALS:**

Large Pyrex test tube, one-hole rubber stopper, two lengths of glass tubing (each about 15 centimeters long), rubber hose about two feet long, ring stand and test tube clamp, Bunsen burner or propane torch, water trough or large cake pan, five collecting bottles or large test tubes, glass plates large enough to cover mouth of collecting bottles or test tubes, balance, glass dish or crucible, tongs, potassium chlorate ($KClO_3$), manganese dioxide ($MnO_2$), wooden splints, steel wool

**PROCEDURE:**

*Part I—Preparing Oxygen.* Set up the equipment as shown in Figure 6.5. Weigh out 14 grams of potassium chlorate and 7 grams of manganese dioxide. **(Caution: Potassium chlorate should not be mixed with any material except manganese dioxide. It is a very good supplier of oxygen and may cause an explosion if mixed with powdered metals or substances that burn.)** *Gently* mix the potassium chlorate and manganese dioxide together in a glass dish or crucible. Remember—do not grind the mixture or mix it on a filter paper. The filter paper is combustible.

**6.5** A method of preparing and collecting oxygen

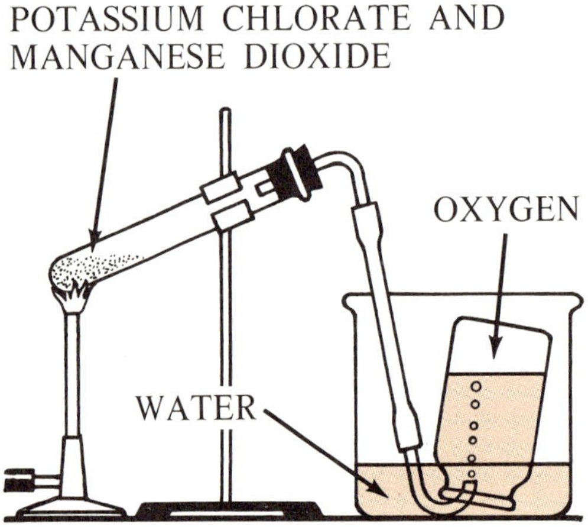


Place enough of the mixture in the test tube to fill it to a depth of about an inch and a half. Mount the test tube with the mouth pointing slightly upward (see Figure 6.5). Place the rubber stopper, glass tubing, and rubber hose as shown in the diagram. Fill several bottles or large test tubes with water, invert, and place in the water trough.

Gently start heating the potassium chlorate-manganese dioxide mixture. Place the end of the hose under the mouth of a bottle, and keep it there until bubbles of gas have pushed all of the water out of the bottle. Discard the first bottle of gas you collect because it will contain mainly the air that was in the test tube and rubber hose.

Continue to heat the potassium chlorate until all of the bottles have been filled. When each bottle is full, raise it enough to slip a glass plate over the mouth, and store *mouth upward.* Would you be able to use this water displacement method of collecting a gas if the gas were soluble in water? Why not?

When you stop heating the potassium chlorate, the rubber hose should be removed from the water at once. As the contents of the test tube cool, the pressure will be reduced. As a result, the outside atmospheric pressure will be greater, and the water in the trough will be pushed up the rubber tube into the hot test tube. Do you see why this could be dangerous?

After the test tube has cooled, examine its contents. Was the manganese dioxide used up in the experiment? The potassium chlorate?

*Part II—Investigating the Properties of Oxygen.* (Figure 6.6) Bottle 1: What do you see when you look at the bottle of gas you have collected? You are pretty sure that a gas pushed the water out of the bottle. Since the gas is colorless, you will have to test for its presence.

The test for oxygen is to light a wooden

6.6 A method of testing for oxygen

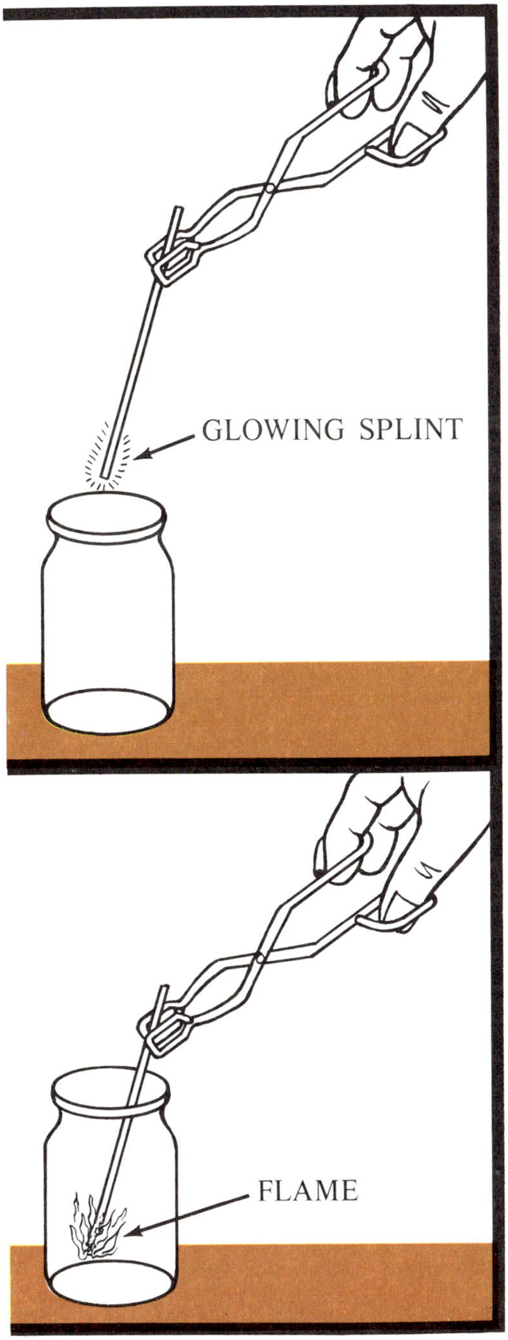


splint, blow it out, and thrust the glowing splint into the gas. It is a good idea to hold the glowing splint in a pair of tongs when you do this. If the glowing splint bursts into flame, the unknown gas is oxygen.

Thrust a glowing splint into one of the bottles of gas you have collected. Does the splint burst into flame? Repeat this several times. Do you have to place the splint a little lower in the bottle each time? Try pouring some of the gas over a burning splint. On the basis of your results, would you predict that oxygen is more dense or less dense than air? Explain.

Bottle 2: With a pair of tongs, hold a small wad of steel wool in a flame until it glows. Thrust it into a bottle of oxygen. Explain what happens. Can you see how welders can cut a piece of hot steel with a stream of pure oxygen?

Bottle 3: To find out if iron rusts faster in pure oxygen than in air, place equal amounts of steel wool in a bottle of oxygen and in a bottle of air (Figure 6.7). Stop each bottle with a one-hole rubber stopper that has a piece of glass tubing inserted. Invert the bottles and place them over beakers of water.

6.7 In which tube will water rise more rapidly?

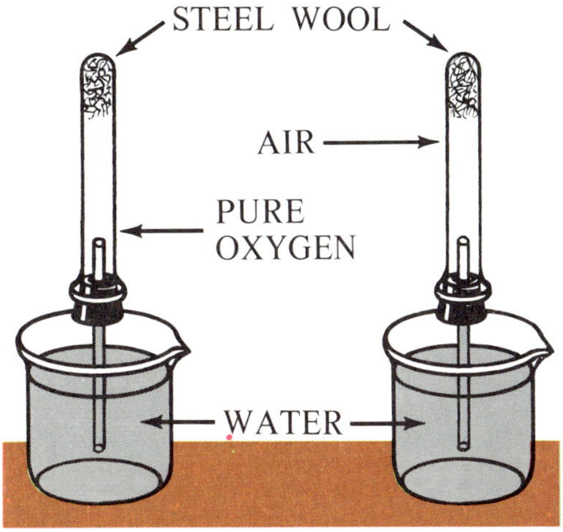

Bottle 4: Devise an experiment that you can do with the fourth bottle of oxygen. For example, compare the brightness of a candle flame in pure oxygen with one burning in air. **Caution: Have your teacher approve your experiment before you perform it!**

---

When potassium chlorate is heated, it is decomposed and oxygen is one of the products formed.

$$2\ KClO_3 \longrightarrow 2\ KCl + 3\ O_2\uparrow$$

The equation for the reaction shows that potassium chloride is the other product. The arrow pointing upward indicates that the oxygen produced is a gas.

Why was the manganese dioxide used? And why wasn't it included in the equation? If potassium chlorate is heated, you will find that oxygen is given off, but not as fast as when manganese dioxide is present. The manganese dioxide acts as a **catalyst** (kat′ ə list). A catalyst is a substance that either speeds up or slows down a reaction but is not itself changed by the reaction. Many important chemical reactions, including some that occur in your body, involve one or more catalysts.

The breakdown of $KClO_3$ to produce KCl and $O_2$ is classified as a decomposition reaction. In this type of reaction, a molecule decomposes to form two or more new substances. You have already read about two other decomposition reactions that can be used to produce oxygen, and a third one is easy to do in the laboratory.

1. *Heating of mercuric oxide.* If about 3 grams of mercuric oxide are placed in a Pyrex test tube and heated, a thin coating of mercury should form on the upper inside wall of the test tube. Test to see if oxygen is given off by thrusting a glowing splint into the mouth of the test tube.

Note that the equation for this reaction is just the reverse of the combination-type reaction of mercury and oxygen described in the last section.

$$2\ HgO \longrightarrow 2\ Hg + O_2\uparrow$$

2. **Electrolysis** (i lek′ trol′ ə sis) *of water.* In Chapter 5, an electric current was used to decompose water. This reaction is one method of producing the gases hydrogen and oxygen, as shown in the equation for the electrolysis of water.

$$2\ H_2O \longrightarrow 2\ H_2\uparrow + O_2\uparrow$$

3. *Decomposition of hydrogen peroxide.* "Peroxide blondes" have made hydrogen peroxide a well-known compound. In addition to its use as a bleaching agent, it can be used to generate oxygen in the laboratory. If a small amount of manganese dioxide is added to about two-thirds of a test tube of hydrogen peroxide, bubbles of gas are given off. Placing the test tube in a beaker of warm water should speed the reaction. A glowing splint reveals that the gas given off is oxygen.

$$2\ H_2O_2 \longrightarrow 2\ H_2O + O_2\uparrow$$

As in the case of the decomposition of potassium chlorate, the manganese dioxide acts as a catalyst in this reaction. In this case, it is a simple matter to see if any of the catalyst is used up. Weigh the amount of manganese dioxide placed in the hydrogen peroxide at the beginning of the experiment. After the reaction has been completed, filter out the $MnO_2$, dry it, and reweigh it. It should then weigh the same.

## Have You Learned?

1. Define each of the following terms, and give an example of each.
   a. Combustion
   b. Catalyst
   c. Electrolysis
   d. Decomposition reaction
2. How is a gas tested to see if it is oxygen?
3. Name four ways that can be used to prepare oxygen.

## 3. One Element for Another

**ARE YOU READY?**

Look up the following words if you are not sure of their meanings:

acid; active (chemically); mass; replace.

Certain elements have a stronger tendency to form compounds than some other elements. If some zinc metal is placed in hydrochloric acid, some of the zinc replaces the hydrogen in the acid. As a result, hydrogen gas is given off.

$$Zn + 2\ HCl \longrightarrow ZnCl_2 + H_2\uparrow$$

This type of reaction is called **simple replacement.** As you can see in the equation, the hydrogen was *replaced* by the more active zinc.

### Making a Silver Star

Dissolve about one gram of silver nitrate in 250-300 cc of distilled water, and place the solution in a medium-sized beaker or drinking glass. Cut a star or other figure about the size of a half dollar from a piece of aluminum foil. Hang the aluminum figure in the silver nitrate solution by a string. In a few minutes it should be covered with tiny crystals of pure silver!

On the basis of your results, is aluminum or silver the more active? Can you write a balanced equation for the reaction of aluminum and silver nitrate solution? Try the experiment again, this time using a piece of steel wool shaped like a Christmas tree. Explain what happens (Figure 6.8).

You are probably already familiar with the action of most acids on many metals. It is easy to set up an experiment to see which metals react with acid.

### Observing an Acid Reacting with Various Metals

**MATERIALS:**

Test tubes, test tube rack, dilute hydrochloric acid or vinegar, pieces of metal (such as magnesium, aluminum, zinc, iron, lead, and copper)

**PROCEDURE:**

Place equal amounts of acid in several test tubes. Place a piece of each kind of metal to be tested in a test tube of acid, and mark the name of the metal on the outside of the test tube. The pieces of metal should be approximately the same size.

Keep a record of the time it takes for the metal to disappear and whether or not the solution changes color. Also note if bubbles are formed in any of the test tubes, and if so, the approximate rate.

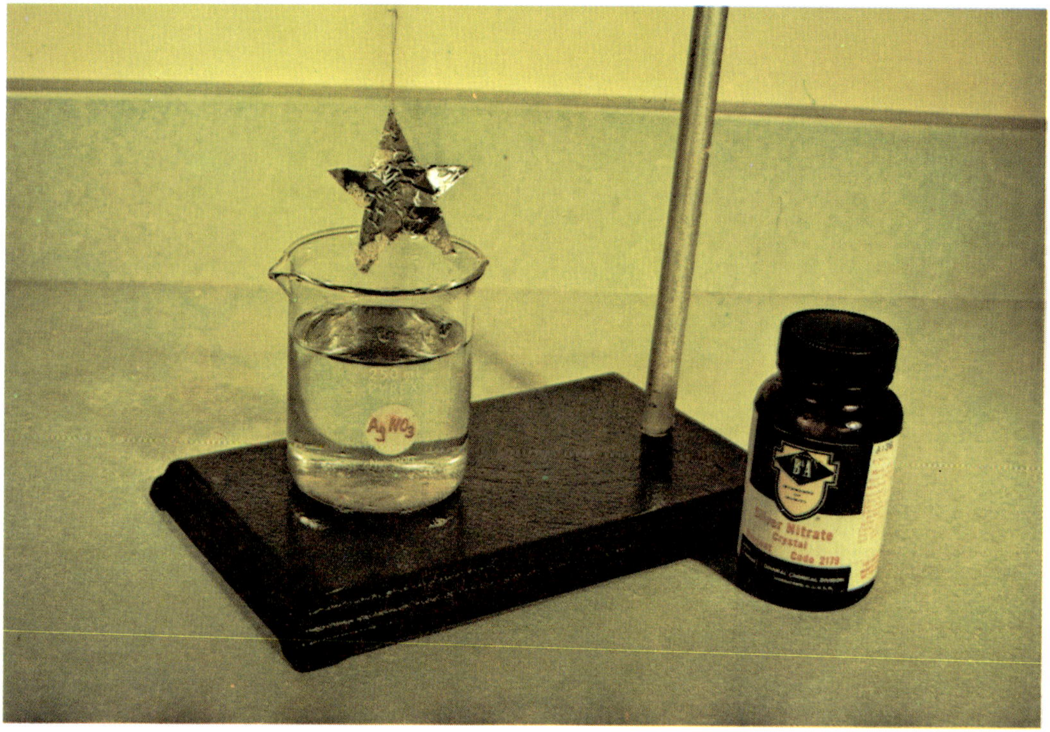


Norman D. Anderson

**6.8** Making a silver star (page 191)

From the results of this experiment, we can conclude that some metals replace the metallike hydrogen in an acid. As a result hydrogen is released as a gas. In the case of iron, the equation shows how this works.

$$Fe + 2\,HCl \longrightarrow FeCl_2 + H_2\uparrow$$

If you used vinegar, the reaction was probably slower since vinegar is a weaker acid, but the results would be similar.

$$Fe + 2\,HC_2H_3O_2 \longrightarrow Fe(C_2H_3O_2)_2 + H_2\uparrow$$

Thus far you have seen that iron replaces copper, aluminum replaces silver, and several metals replace hydrogen from an acid. From these and similar experiments, chemists have figured out an activity series of the metals (Table I). This is a list of metals with the most active metal at the top and the least active of the group at the bottom. Notice that hydrogen, which is a gas, is included in the list of metals. This is because hydrogen acts like a metal in many reactions.

Using the list, one can predict that iron will replace copper. Since it is higher on the list, iron is more active than copper. Using this same reasoning, one would expect aluminum to replace silver as it did in the experiment with the silver star. Do the results you obtained when various kinds of metals were placed in acid agree with the results you would predict using the activity series?

Would you expect to find the elements at the top of the list free in nature or in the form of compounds? Why?

**TABLE I**
*Activity Series of Metals*
(Most active at top and least active at bottom)

Potassium
Calcium
Sodium
Magnesium
Aluminum
Zinc
Iron
Nickel
Lead
*Hydrogen*
Bismuth
Copper
Mercury
Silver
Platinum
Gold

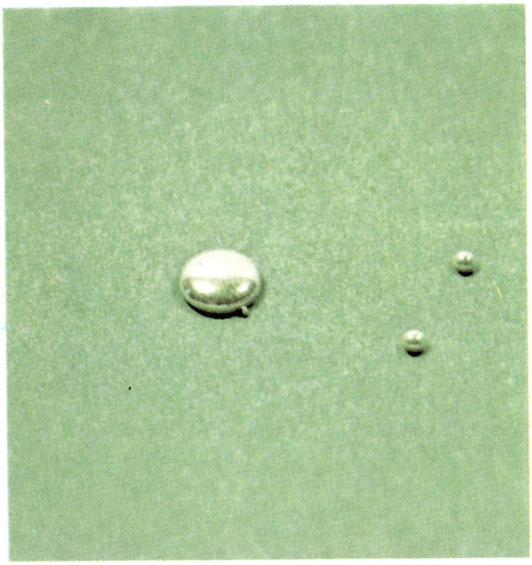

*J. W. McDonald*

**6.9** Mercury (page 83) resting on cloth

**6.10** Explain why the three metals at the bottom of Table I are used in jewelry.

*Museum of the American Indian*

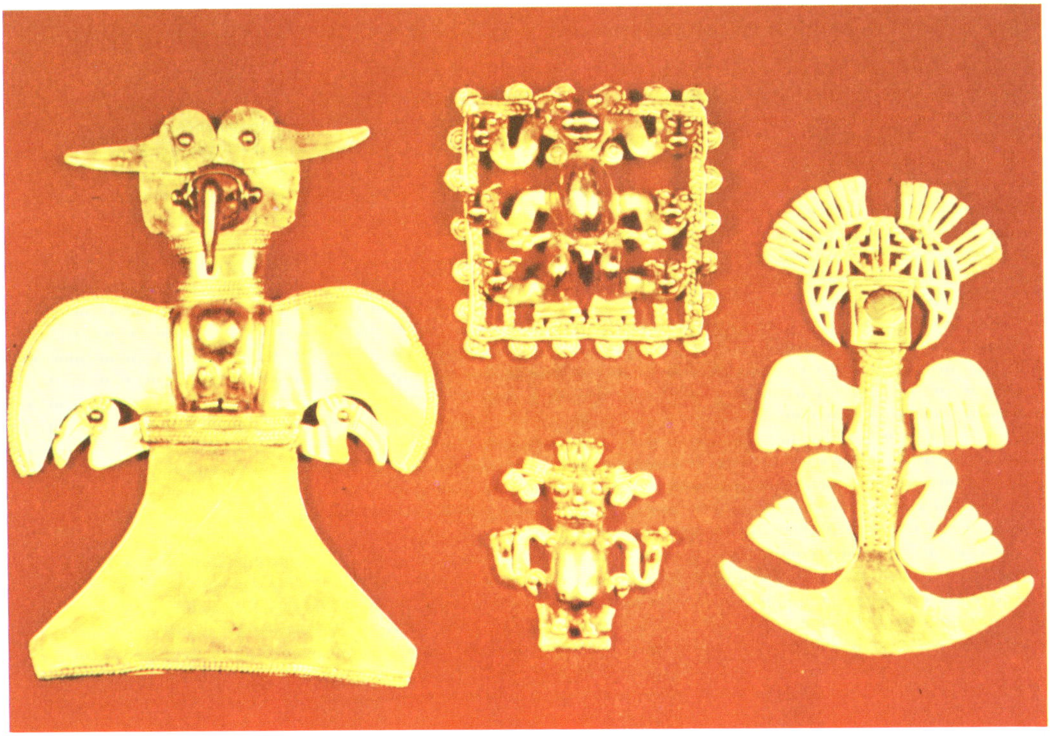

## Generating the Most Abundant Element in the Universe

Scientists estimate that over 90 percent of the universe is composed of hydrogen atoms and hydrogen ions. Furthermore, it is thought that over 70 percent of the *mass* of the universe is hydrogen, although it is the lightest of the elements.

Here on the earth practically all of the hydrogen is found combined with other elements. Water, the most abundant liquid on our planet, is a combination of hydrogen and oxygen. Hydrogen, of course, is the identifying element of compounds called acids. Many of the carbon compounds, such as those that make up plants and animals, contain hydrogen.

However, here on the earth, oxygen is king. By weight, about one half of the earth's crust, oceans, and atmosphere is oxygen. Only about one percent of the earth is estimated to be hydrogen. But in space it is a different story. Stars contain great amounts of hydrogen, and it is believed that about 75 percent of our sun is hydrogen.

In the laboratory, a common method of making hydrogen involves the reaction of a metal, such as zinc, with an acid, such as dilute sulfuric acid. The equation for the reaction is $Zn + H_2SO_4 \longrightarrow ZnSO_4 + H_2\uparrow$. As with oxygen, the gas is collected by water displacement (Figure 6.11).

Since a mixture of hydrogen and oxygen is very explosive, this experiment should not be performed unless proper safety precautions are taken and adequate supervision is available. The flask should be wrapped in a cloth towel and the experiment carried out away from flames. The test for hydrogen is to bring a test tube of gas, mouth downward, near a flame. Pure hydrogen burns quietly with a pale blue flame. Often the test tube also contains some oxygen mixed with the hydrogen. When it is brought near a flame, the result is a *loud pop*! To appreciate fully the explosive nature of hydrogen, read the story of the dirigible *Hindenburg*.

**6.11** Making hydrogen in the laboratory

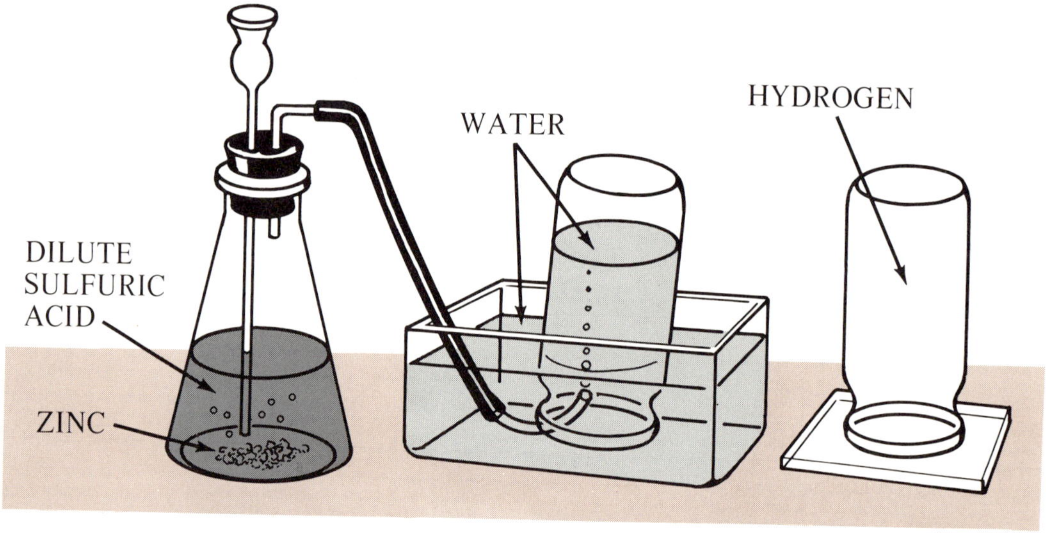

If you wish to test some hydrogen, reassemble the apparatus you used in Chapter 5 to split water molecules. Run it long enough to fill a test tube with hydrogen. Hold the test tube, mouth downward, with a test-tube holder, and bring it near the flame. How can you test the gas in the other tube to see if it is oxygen? (See Figure 6.12.)

**6.12** A method of testing for hydrogen

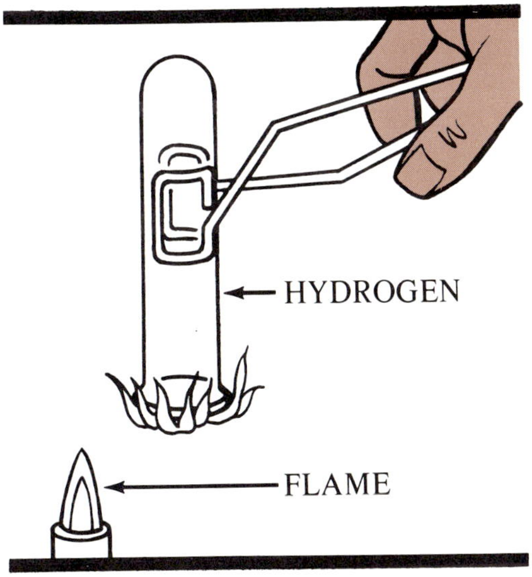


> ### Have You Learned?
> 1. Explain how a simple replacement reaction differs from combination and decomposition types of reactions.
> 2. Which of the metals in the following pairs is more active: potassium and silver? copper and silver? platinum and gold?
> 3. What is the most abundant element in the universe? What is the test for this element? How is it prepared in the laboratory?

## 4. Exchanging Partners

> **ARE YOU READY?**
>
> Look up the following words if you are not sure of their meanings:
>
> base; crystal; decompose;
> litmus paper; pH; replacement;
> respiration; salt; starch; sugar.

If about 10 cc of dilute sodium hydroxide is poured into a dish containing a piece of red litmus paper, the litmus paper turns blue. This indicates that the solution is basic or alkaline. If dilute hydrochloric acid is *slowly* added while the solution is stirred, the litmus paper will change from blue to pink. The pink color means that the solution is now a little on the acid side. Sodium hydroxide is then added, drop by drop, until the color of the litmus paper is between pink and blue. This indicates that the solution is about neutral or has a pH of 7. If pH paper is available, the solution can be checked to see if more acid or more base is needed to make the solution as close to a pH of 7 as possible.

When the solution is heated gently over a water bath, the liquid evaporates leaving behind tiny white crystals. It is not a good idea to taste chemicals in a laboratory. However, in this case it is all right to taste a very small amount. The white crystals taste salty.

The equation for the reaction shows why the white crystals taste salty.

$$NaOH + HCl \longrightarrow \underset{\text{(table salt)}}{NaCl} + H_2O$$

Notice how the sodium changes place with the hydrogen and two new compounds are formed. This type of reaction is called a **double replacement** reaction. In some ways a double replacement reaction is like what happens when two couples exchange partners on the dance floor.

The reaction of an acid and base is a special kind of double replacement reaction called **neutralization** (nü′ trə li zā′ shən). In a neutralization reaction, an acid and base react to form a salt and water. When we add an acid to a base, it is said that we **neutralize** (nü′ trə līz′) it. The same is true when a base is added to an acid. Have you heard advertisements for tablets that *neutralize* the excess acid of the stomach?

## Making a Smoke Ring

Remove the stopper from a bottle of ammonium hydroxide, and hold near the mouth of the bottle a stopper from a bottle of hydrochloric acid. This will give you an idea of what happens when $NH_4OH$ and HCl react.

Clamp a glass tube about 2-3 cm in diameter and 1 meter long in a horizontal position. Stuff a piece of cotton into each end of the glass tubing. Use a medicine dropper to wet the cotton at one end with HCl and at the other end with $NH_4OH$. Place a stopper or cork in each end of the tubing. Record the time the acid and base were placed on the cotton. (See Figure 6.13 below.)

Watch for a white smoke ring to appear near the center of the tube. Can you suggest reasons why the ring is not exactly in the center? How long does it take for the ring to appear? Why didn't it appear as soon as the acid and base were placed on the cotton? Suggest as many ways as you can to reduce the time it takes for the ring to appear.

The reaction of HCl and $NH_4OH$ is a neutralization reaction, and the products are a salt and water. The salt in this case is $NH_4Cl$. It is a solid and gives the appearance of white smoke when it forms. Can you write the equation for this reaction?

**6.13** What causes the smoke ring to form in the tube? What is it made of?

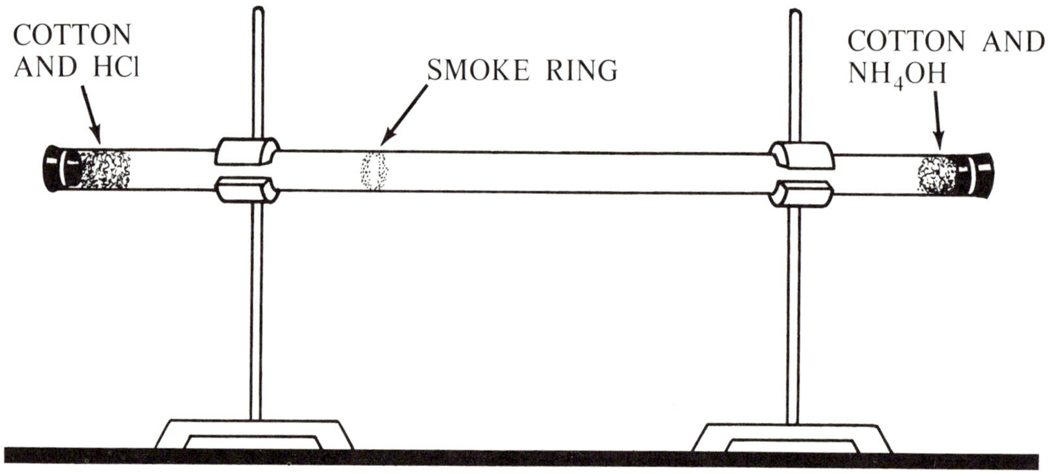

## Making an Important Oxide of Carbon

Carbon combines with oxygen to form carbon dioxide, or $CO_2$. Carbon dioxide is formed during the burning of fuels containing carbon, such as charcoal and coal, and during respiration in living things. Carbon dioxide is used up during photosynthesis in green plants. Carbon dioxide is one of the basic building blocks of the sugars, starches, and other compounds produced in green plants. Although only about 0.03 percent of the air is $CO_2$, the gas is very important because of its link between the living and the nonliving world.

A double displacement reaction can be used to make the gas in the science laboratory.

### Investigating Carbon Dioxide

**MATERIALS:**

Flask, thistle tube or funnel with long stem, glass tubing, rubber hose about 60 cm long, water trough or cake pan, bottles or large test tubes, stoppers or glass plates, marble chips ($CaCO_3$), dilute hydrochloric acid (HCl), limewater, candles, cardboard about 15 cm × 45 cm, pins

**PROCEDURE:**

Set up a gas generator as shown in Figure 6.14. The thistle tube should be adjusted so that the bottom of the tube is below the surface of the acid. Why is this necessary? Place about 10 grams of marble chips in the flask. Before adding the HCl, run the test for carbon dioxide.

*Test for $CO_2$.* Place a clean glass tube or soda straw in a test tube about half full of clear limewater. Blow through the straw until the limewater turns to a milky white. This is the test for $CO_2$. The equation shows what happens. The arrow pointing down-

**6.14** A method of preparing and collecting carbon dioxide. Now pour it as shown on page 198.

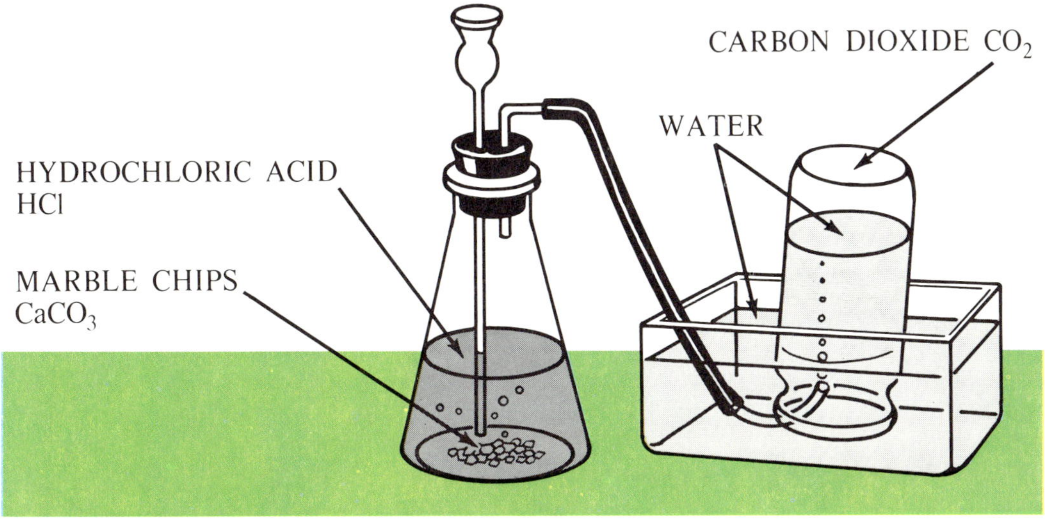

ward is used to show that the product is not soluble in water.

$$CO_2 + Ca(OH)_2 \longrightarrow CaCO_3\downarrow + H_2O$$

*Generate $CO_2$.* Add about 25 cc of dilute hydrochloric acid to the flask of marble chips by pouring it down the thistle tube. Gas bubbles should start to form at once around the marble chips. Place the end of the rubber tube in a test tube half full of limewater. How long does it take for the limewater to turn milky?

Collect several bottles or large test tubes of carbon dioxide by water displacement. As each container is filled, remove it from the water trough and cover it with a glass plate or rubber stopper. When you have finished, be sure to remove the end of the rubber hose from the pan of water. Why is this necessary?

Bottle 1: Lower a burning candle into a bottle of $CO_2$. Does the result suggest why $CO_2$ is used to put out fires?

Bottle 2: Fold a piece of cardboard, about 15 cm × 45 cm, to form a V-shaped trough. Place five or six short birthday candles upright in the trough by pushing pins through the bottom of the trough into the candles. Prop the trough so that one end is about 25 cm off the table. Light the candles. Pour some carbon dioxide on the top candle. What happens? Continue to pour the $CO_2$ on the top candle. Even though carbon dioxide is colorless and therefore invisible, you should be able to observe its effects. Is it more dense or less dense than air? Explain. (Figure 6.15)

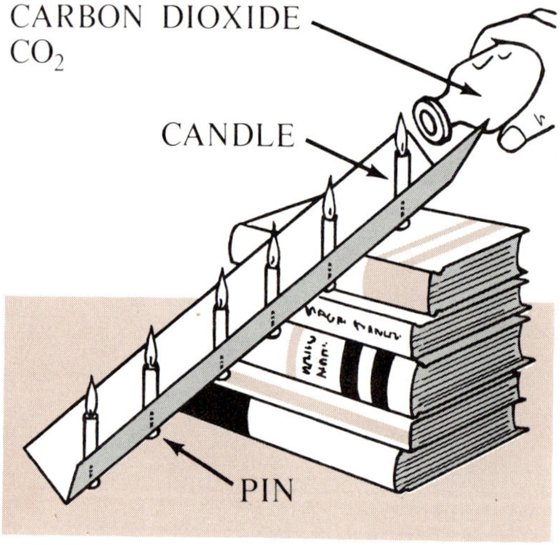


**6.15** What will happen to the candles?

Bottle 3: Devise your own experiments for using the remaining bottles of carbon dioxide. For example, can you find out if it will combine with steel wool? Will some of it dissolve in water, and if so, is the water still neutral? **CAUTION: Be sure to have your teacher approve your experiments before you perform them.**

The equation for the reaction of calcium carbonate and hydrochloric acid shows why the reaction can be classified as a double displacement reaction.

$$CaCO_3 + 2\ HCl \longrightarrow H_2CO_3 + CaCl_2$$

But something is wrong. When calcium carbonate and hydrochloric acid react, carbon dioxide is formed. The explanation is that carbonic acid, $H_2CO_3$, decomposes to form water and carbon dioxide.

$$H_2CO_3 \longrightarrow CO_2\uparrow + H_2O$$

The formation of a product that decomposes or reacts with another substance is not at all uncommon. As we will see in Chapter 7, many of the chemical reactions in living things involve long chains of reactions. A product is formed, that product reacts, then another product is formed, and so this reaction continues at length.

### Have You Learned?

1. Which of the following reactions are double displacement reactions? Which are neutralization reactions?
   a. $H_2SO_4 + 2\ NaOH \longrightarrow Na_2SO_4 + 2\ H_2O$
   b. $CaCl_2 + Na_2CO_3 \longrightarrow 2\ NaCl + CaCO_3$
   c. $H_2CO_3 \longrightarrow CO_2\uparrow + H_2O$
   d. $Zn + 2\ HCl \longrightarrow ZnCl_2 + H_2\uparrow$
2. What products are usually formed in a neutralization reaction?
3. Describe how carbon dioxide can be prepared in the laboratory. What is the test for this gas? What are some of the physical properties of carbon dioxide?

## 5. Rates of Reaction

**ARE YOU READY?**

Look up the following words if you are not sure of their meanings:

catalyst; cold-blooded (animals); concentration; dilute; ion.

By now you probably have noticed that some reactions appear to take place faster than others. There are several factors that affect the *rate of a reaction.* In the experiment in which various metals were placed in an acid solution, gas bubbles formed faster in some test tubes than in others. The rate at which the bubbles of hydrogen formed is a good indicator of how fast the substances reacted.

From the results of the reaction of metals with acid, it was concluded that some elements are more active than others. If a very small piece of sodium is placed in a dish of water, the sodium darts around on the surface of the water like a speedboat. Hydrogen gas is released, and the reaction also gives off heat. CAUTION: Because of the explosive nature of hydrogen, this reaction is very dangerous.

If other metals below sodium in the activity series are placed in water, they either react more slowly or not at all. One of the factors that affects the rate of reactions is the nature of the substances themselves. This is why it is never a good idea to add two substances together without having first checked in a reference book to see what would happen. *Explosions* are the result of reactions that occur very rapidly.

A factor that can control the rate of a reaction was involved in the preparation of oxygen by heating $KClO_3$. The catalyst, $MnO_2$, made the reaction go much faster. Catalysts, or **enzymes** (en′ zīm) as they are called in the case of living things, can also slow a reaction.

Three other factors that commonly affect the rate of chemical reactions can be illustrated by some easily performed experiments.

### Investigating the Effect of Heat on Rate of Reaction

Place test tubes containing equal amounts of dilute acid in a beaker of ice water (0° C.), in a beaker of warm water (about 40° C.), and in a beaker of hot water (about 60-70° C.), and keep a fourth test tube at room temperature (20-25° C.). Place an equal-sized strip of aluminum or magnesium in each test tube. Judge the

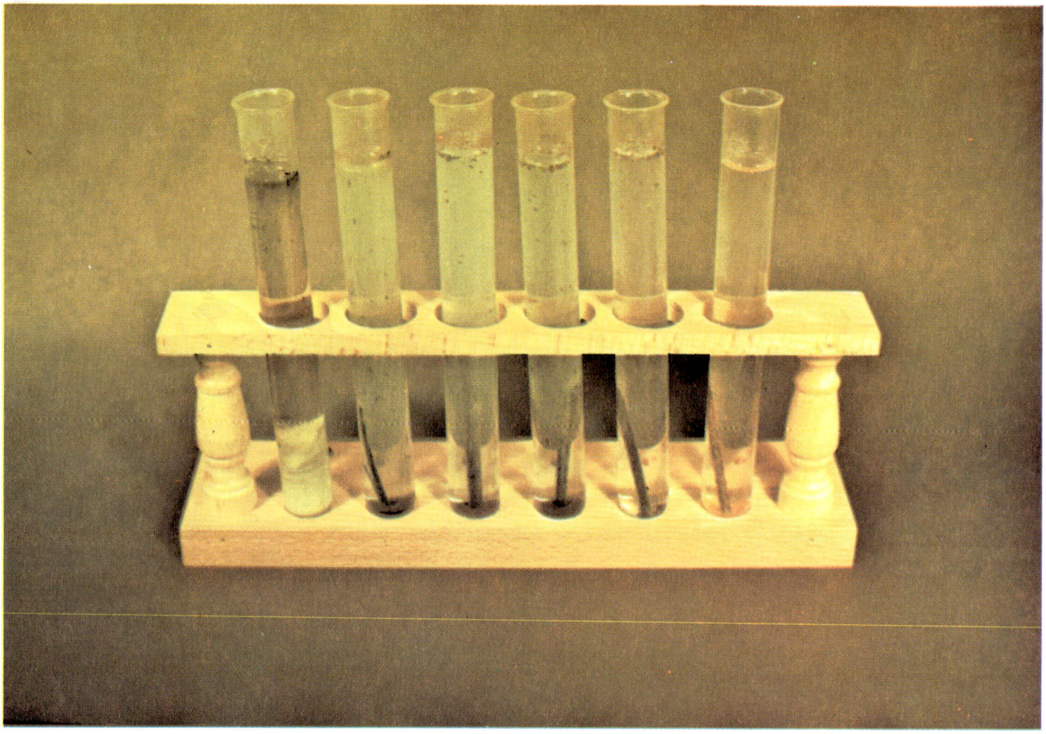

*Norman D. Anderson*

**6.16** Why do you think the metal strip that was in the far-left test tube has disappeared?

rate of reaction in each test tube by the number of hydrogen bubbles or by the length of time it takes for the metal strips to disappear.

An increase in temperature generally increases the rate of a reaction. Do you remember the reason why warm water evaporates more rapidly than cold water? As a substance is heated, the molecules and atoms move more rapidly and thus possess more energy. In many cases, reactions occur only between these energy-rich atoms.

In many reactions, there is a very definite relationship between temperature and rate of reaction. The rate of reaction is doubled for every increase in temperature of 10° C. Can you devise an experiment to test this? Can you write a formula or draw a graph to show this relationship?

The effect of temperature on the rate of chemical reaction can be easily observed in a frog. The frog is a cold-blooded animal. The body temperature of a frog and of other cold-blooded animals varies with the temperature of their surroundings. If a frog is placed in a beaker of ice water, the chemical activity in its body slows down and so does the rate of breathing.

Verify this by observing the rate of breathing of a frog in cold water compared to the rate when it is in water that is 10° C. warmer.

## Investigating the Effect of Concentration on Rate of Reaction

Place some acid in a test tube. Place some acid that has been diluted with equal parts of water in a second test tube. (CAUTION: **Acid should be slowly added to the water and stirred as it is being diluted.**) In a third test tube, put some acid that has been diluted one part acid to five parts water. The fourth test tube should contain acid diluted one part acid to ten parts water. Each test tube should contain the same amount of solution, the only difference being the **concentration** (kon′ sən trā′ shən) of the acid.

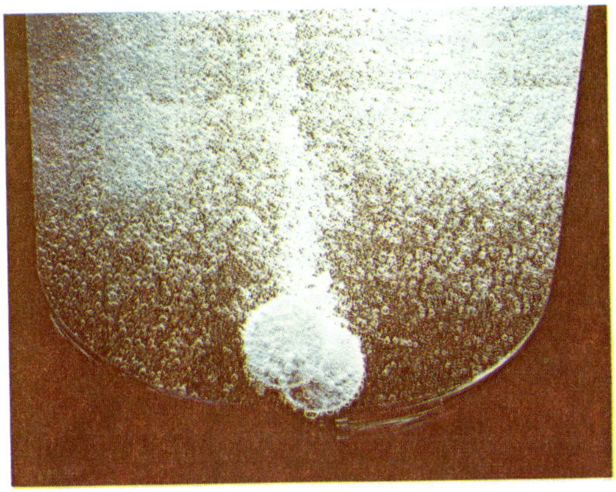

*Miles Laboratories, Inc.*

**6.17** How is the rate of reaction changed by grinding up the tablets?

Place strips of aluminum or magnesium of equal size in each test tube. As before, judge the rate of reaction by the number

**6.18** Cobalt chloride paper is used to test for the presence of water. (See page 207, right column.)

*J. W. McDonald*

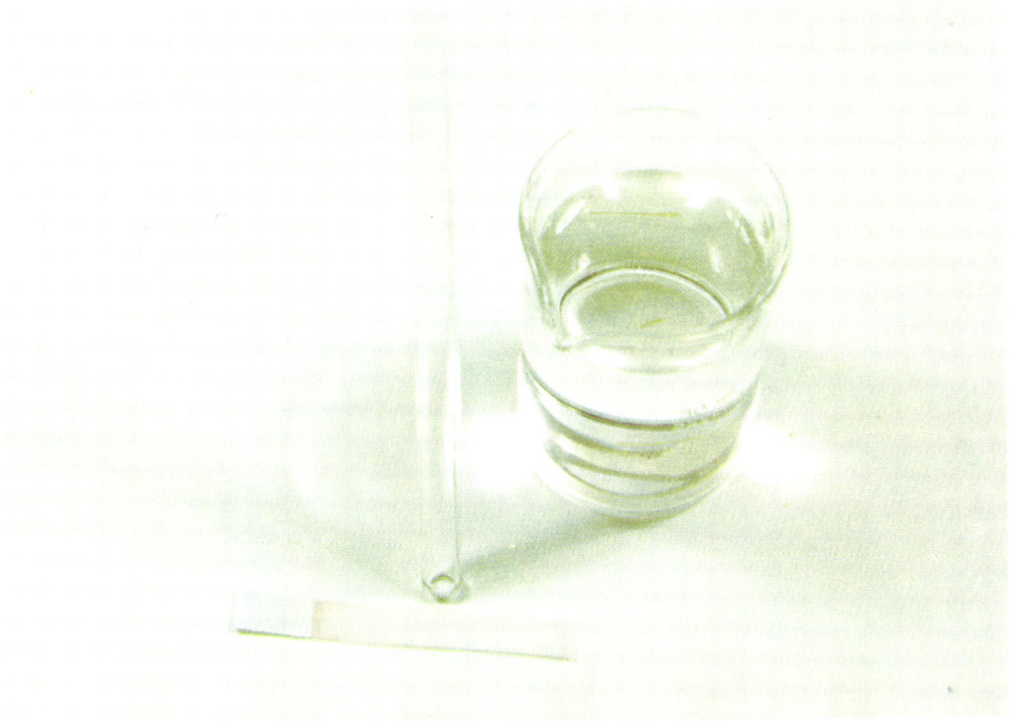

of hydrogen bubbles or by the length of time it takes for the metal strips to disappear. (See Figure 6.16.)

Since the pieces of metal were about the same size, the number of metal atoms in each case was about the same. However, the number of ions formed by the acid would be much greater in the concentrated acid than in the more dilute solution. Therefore, the chances of a reaction's occurring are greater in the concentrated solution.

If you are wandering around in a crowd, the chances of your bumping into a friend are increased if the number of friends in the crowd is increased. Likewise the chances of atoms' reacting are increased when their numbers, or concentration, is increased.

The surface area of the reacting substances is closely related to concentration. Do you think the rate of reaction would be increased if powdered metal were placed in the acid?

### Investigating the Effect of Increasing Surface Area on Rate of Reaction

Drop an antacid tablet, such as Alka-Seltzer, into a large test tube of water. In a second test tube of water, place a tablet that has been broken into several pieces. Grind a tablet in a mortar, and place the powder in a third test tube of water. In which case did the reaction appear to occur at the most rapid rate? At the slowest rate? How do you explain the results? (Figure 6.17 page 201)

Special precautions have to be taken in flour mills and coal mines because the amount of surface area affects the rate of reaction. Finely divided flour or coal mixed with air is an explosive mixture. The apparatus in Figure 6.19 is used to demonstrate this.

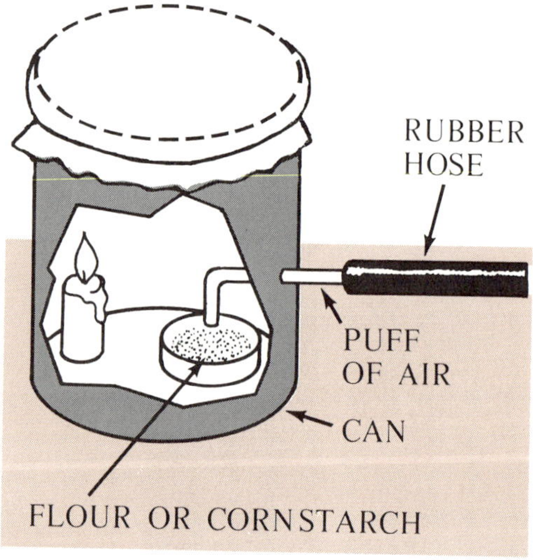


**6.19** How to make a dust explosion

A few grams of flour or cornstarch are placed in the small dish. The candle is lit, and the can covered with a *loose* lid such as a piece of cardboard. When a small puff of air strikes the fine powder in the dish, it is blown out into the can. The mixture is ignited by the candle flame.

All of this takes place in a fraction of a second. Do you see now why places like flour mills and coal mines must be very careful to prevent dust explosions?

## Have You Learned?

Listed in Column A are examples of chemical reactions being slowed down or speeded up. In your notebook or on a piece of paper, write the letter corresponding to the factor in Column B that best explains the examples listed in Column A. (Do not write in your book.)

*Column A*

1. Wood is cut into small pieces to start a fire.
2. Benzoate of soda is added to catsup to slow down spoilage.
3. Steel wool burns brightly in pure oxygen.
4. Zinc is plated with copper at a faster rate when placed in $CuSO_4$ than is lead.
5. Copper, which oxidizes slowly at room temperature, is heated to speed up the reaction.

*Column B*

a. catalyst
b. concentration
c. nature or activity of substances reacting
d. surface area
e. temperature

## 6. The Chemist as a Detective

**ARE YOU READY?**

Look up the following words if you are not sure of their meanings:

absorption; botanist; characteristic; classify; distilled water; litmus paper; pigment; radiation; X ray.

Chemists and other scientists frequently have the job of identifying an unknown substance. They work much like detectives, using their knowledge of chemistry to look for clues that they can use in solving the mystery.

Imagine that you have been given a beaker of a clear colorless liquid. You are told that the beaker contains either one substance or two substances. You are asked to find out what the liquid is. From what you have already learned about chemistry and the physical properties of matter, there are several things you can do in the search for clues. In addition, some methods described later in this section can be used.

As we have said before, it is important to organize or classify information in trying to figure something out. For this reason, some of the things that can be done in trying to identify the unknown liquid have been organized in the form of the chart on page 206.

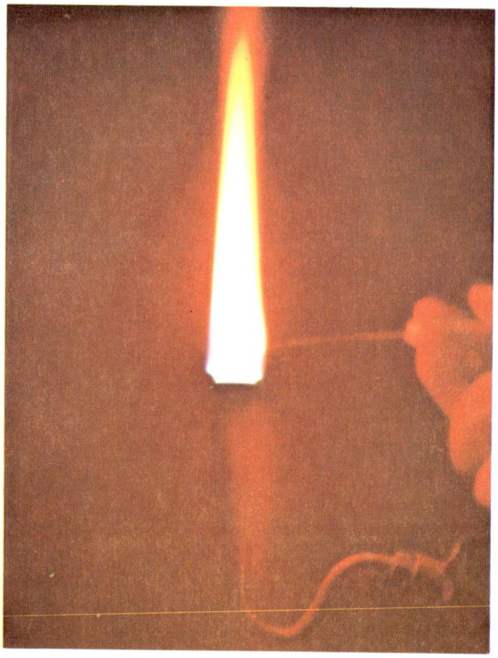

6.20a

6.20b

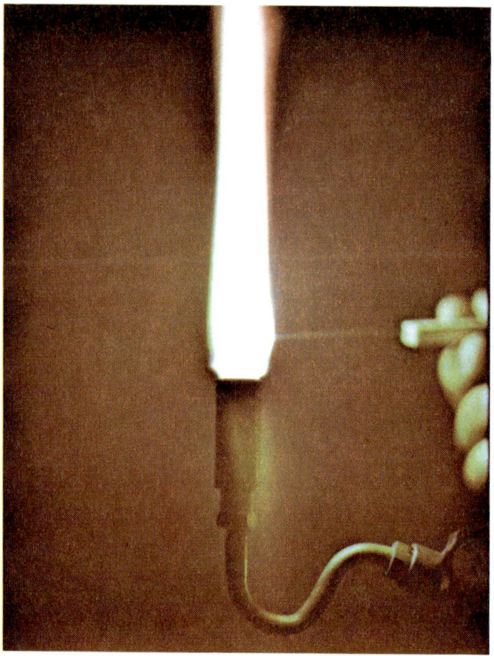

6.20c

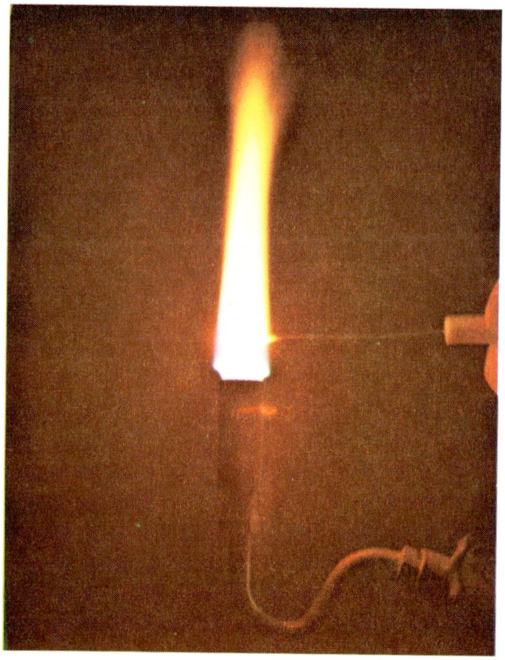

6.20d

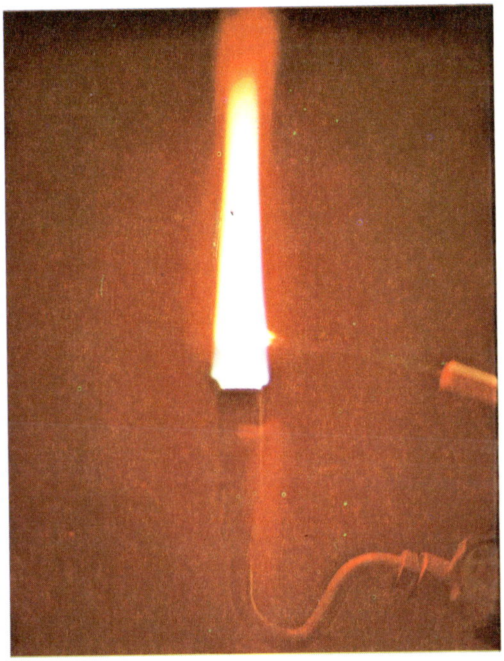

6.20e

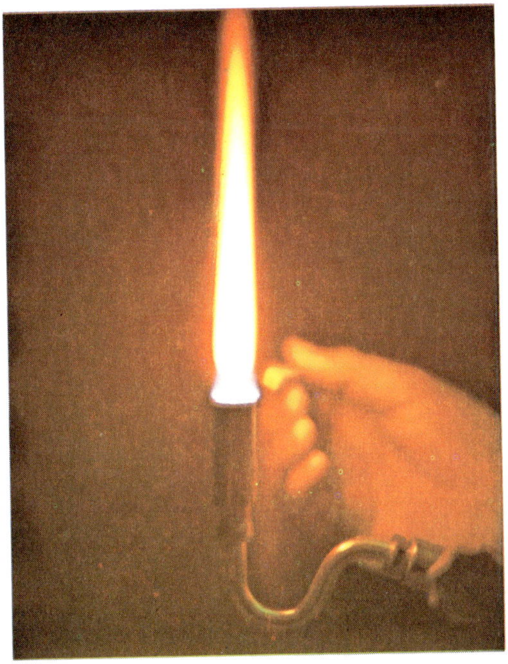

6.20f

FLAME TESTS

**6.20a** Strontium Compound

**6.20b** Potassium Compound

**6.20c** Copper Compound

**6.20d** Calcium Compound

**6.20e** Lithium Compound

**6.20f** Sodium Compound

*Norman D. Anderson*

## Identifying the Colorless Liquid

| *Steps Taken* | *Results* | *What Results Indicate* |
|---|---|---|
| 1. Liquid is cautiously smelled. | No odor | Some substances, such as $NH_4OH$, have a characteristic odor. This rules out these substances. |
| 2. Test with litmus paper. | Does not change color of litmus paper | This is not an acid or a base. |
| 3. Weigh 25 cc of liquid. | 25 cc weighs 27.4 g | Since 25 cc of water would weigh about 25 gm, this suggests the liquid is not water or is water with something dissolved in it. |
| 4. A drop of the unknown liquid is placed on a strip of dry cobalt chloride paper. | Paper turns from blue to pinkish-red. | This indicates the presence of water. (Now the problem is to find what is dissolved in the water.) |
| 5. A few drops of the unknown liquid are placed in a watch glass and heated over a beaker of boiling water. | Liquid disappears leaving behind a white solid. | This confirms that there is something dissolved in the water. The white solid has no visible characteristics, other than color, that can be used to identify it. |
| 6. A platinum needle is dipped into the unknown solution and placed in the flame of the Bunsen burner. | Flame turns yellow. | The yellow color indicates the presence of sodium. Now suspect a sodium compound dissolved in water. Which sodium compound? |
| 7. Check table in chemistry book to see which sodium compounds are soluble in water. | All sodium compounds listed are soluble in water. | We cannot eliminate any possibilities this way. |

Although we have only been able to identify the unknown liquid as a sodium compound dissolved in water, this should give you the general idea how chemists go about identifying a substance. We would have to do additional tests to find out which sodium compound it is. Do you understand why each step was taken? Explain how each step helped rule out certain possibilities and build a case for a sodium compound dissolved in water. Were any steps taken that were not necessary? Can you suggest other things that could have been done to gain information useful in identifying the unknown?

The use of cobalt chloride paper in step 4 illustrates an interesting property of certain compounds. Some crystals, such as cobalt chloride and copper sulfate, contain water. If they are dissolved in water and the water is evaporated away, some of the water remains locked up in the crystals. If these crystals are heated, the water is driven off, and the powder that remains is a different color. This difference in color of the crystals containing water and of the dry powdered form can be used as a test for water. In the case of copper sulfate, the dry form is a whitish color. When water is added, it turns to a dark blue. (See Figure 6.18 on page 207.)

### Flame Tests

In step 6, the sodium was identified by means of a flame test. A piece of platinum or nichrome wire is welded into the end of a piece of glass tubing which serves as a handle. (Nichrome wire is used in toasters and other electrical appliances.) The wire is cleaned in distilled water and held in the flame of a Bunsen burner until it no longer colors the flame. The wire is dipped into the solution to be tested, and then placed in the flame. In the case of solids, moisten the wire with distilled water, and touch it to the crystals or powder to be tested.

Several of the metals, as shown in Table II, give the flame a color. When elements are heated to high temperatures, each gives off a specific pattern of colors. In a sense, each element has its own set of fingerprints. This idea is described in greater detail in Chapter 15.

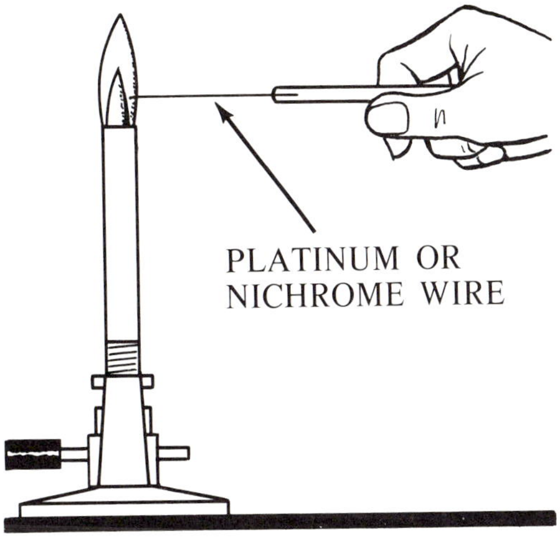


**6.21** How to do a flame test

On pages 204-205 you will find color photographs of six elements being used in flame tests, Figures 6.20a-f.

**TABLE II**
*Flame Test*

| *Element* | *Color* |
|---|---|
| Sodium | Yellow |
| Potassium | Violet |
| Calcium | Yellow-red |
| Strontium | Deep red |
| Lithium | Crimson |
| Barium | Green-yellow |
| Copper | Blue-green |

Try your hand at using flame tests by placing the salt of each of these elements in a flame. For example, salts of potassium such as potassium chloride, potassium sulfate, or potassium carbonate can be used.

### Identifying Unknowns

Listed below are five pairs of substances. Name as many things as you can that could be done to determine which of the substances an unknown is. In each case, the unknown will be one of the two substances. Explain how the results of your suggestions could be used in identifying the unknown. You may wish to organize your answers in the form of a chart.

Pair 1: Dilute hydrochloric acid and dilute sodium hydroxide

Pair 2: Crystals of table salt and crystals of table sugar

Pair 3: Test tube of oxygen and test tube of carbon dioxide

Pair 4: Water solution of $CuSO_4$ and water solution of $FeSO_4$

Pair 5: Beaker of water and beaker of white syrup

You may wish to test your ideas in the laboratory. If so, have your teacher give you one of the substances, and see if you can correctly identify it. (Your teacher will probably wish to check your suggested method of attack before you begin.)

**6.22** A method for doing chromatography

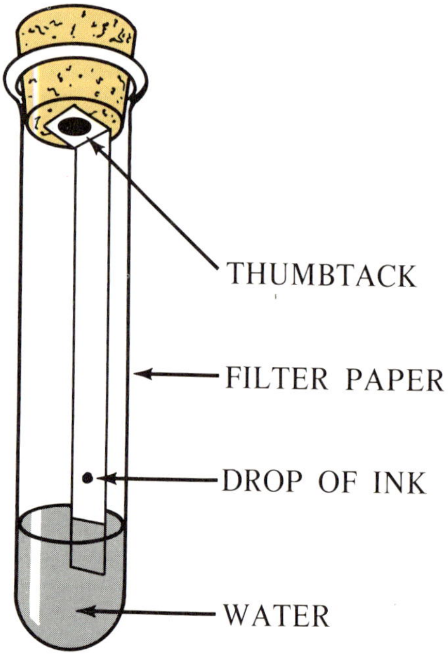


## Using Strips of Paper to Analyze

Cut a strip of filter paper so that it will fit freely inside a large test tube. Attach the strip to the bottom of a cork with a thumbtack. Place enough water in the test tube so that when the cork is inserted, the bottom of the paper strip will be about 2 cm in the water. Put a drop or two of water soluble ink on the filter paper about 3 cm from the bottom. Insert the paper strip into the test tube and observe what happens (see Figure 6.22).

As the water moves up the filter paper by absorption, the substances in the ink are carried along. But notice that they do not all move at the same rate. In one kind of black ink, the black moves faster than the violet and yellow. This method of separating substances is called **chromatography** (krō′ mə tog′ rə fi). *Chromato* means *color* and *graphy* means *writing* or *record*. As you can see, chromatography provides us with a record in color.

Chromatography was first used by a Russian botanist in the early 1900s to separate the compounds found in leaves. It is still one of the easiest ways to separate the pigments in leaves, and directions for doing so are found in most biology or life science textbooks. Chromatography is also used in laboratories to separate many other compounds, including many that are colorless. In the case of those that can't be seen, techniques have been developed for finding where the substances are on the paper strip.

In scientific laboratories much of the identification of unknown substances is done with the aid of specially designed instruments. In many cases, only a drop or few specks of the material are needed in order for it to be identified. One instrument operates on the same principle as flame tests. Other instruments measure what happens when a substance is struck by X rays, a special kind of red light, and other kinds of radiation. But regardless of how complicated these instruments may seem, the principles involved are ones you have been learning about in this book.

### Have You Learned?

On a sheet of paper list the numbers for the questions below. By each number write *T* if the statement is true and *F* if false.

1. Cobalt chloride paper is used to test for the presence of a salt.
2. Sodium chloride gives a yellow color when placed in a flame.
3. The deep red color produced when strontium chloride is placed in a flame is due to the strontium.
4. Substances dissolved in water are removed from the water by filtering the solution through filter paper.
5. Chromatography can be used to separate substances because different substances are absorbed at different rates.

## 7. Finding Out How Much

**ARE YOU READY?**

Look up the following words if you are not sure of their meanings:

atomic weight; crucible; mineral; ratio.

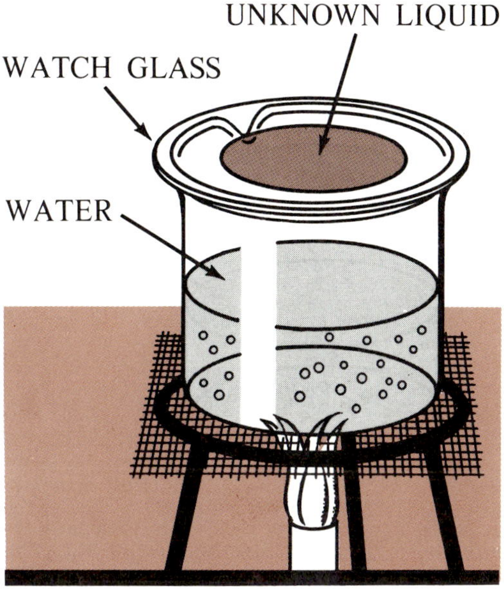


**6.23** Removing water from an unknown liquid

In the last section were described ways that chemists use to find out *what* a substance contains. Often chemists also want to know *how much* of each element or compound a substance contains. Take, for example, the unknown liquid that we found to be a water solution of a sodium compound. It would be a simple matter to find out what fraction of the liquid was water and what fraction the sodium compound.

Place 10 grams of the liquid in a watch glass, and let the water evaporate. The weight of the sodium compound remaining could be easily found by reweighing the watch glass. To make the problem easy, let's say that we find that the sodium compound weighs 1 gram. Of course this means that the water which evaporated weighed 9 grams. Do you see why? (See Figure 6.23 above.)

From these results it can be reported that the unknown liquid is 90% water and

10% sodium compound. In the case of water, the percentage was calculated by comparing the weight of water to the total weight of the liquid $\left(\frac{9 \text{ grams}}{10 \text{ grams}} = {}^{9}/_{10}\right.$ or $0.9 = 90\%\left.\right)$. Can you suggest two ways to show that the sodium compound makes up the remaining 10% of the solution?

## Determining the Chemical Composition of a Raw Potato

Cut a white potato into small pieces. Place exactly 50 grams of the potato pieces in a pan. Heat the pan of potato pieces in an oven at 90°-120° C until they no longer lose any weight. The weight lost is the weight of the water that was in the potatoes.

Place the pieces of dry potato in a crucible and heat them with a Bunsen burner. The food or fuel part of the potato will combine with oxygen to form mainly carbon dioxide and water. The material remaining in the crucible is the mineral content of the potato (Figure 6.24).

Record your data in a chart in your notebook:

| | |
|---|---|
| Raw potato (water + food part + minerals) | = 50 grams |
| Dry potato (food part + minerals) | = __ grams |
| Ashes remaining after heating (minerals) | = __ grams |

Calculate what percentage of the raw potato was water, what percentage was the food part, and what percentage was mineral. Compare your answers with those of your classmates. Your teacher may wish to divide the class into groups and have each group use a different vegetable or fruit. Which ones do you think will contain the highest percentage of water? The lowest percentage of water?

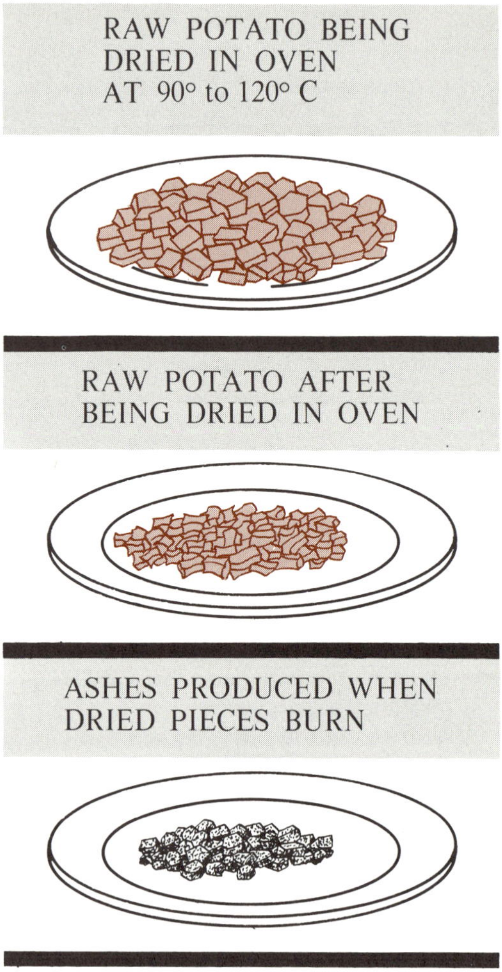


**6.24** Is water the largest part of the raw potato?

## Finding How Much of Each Element

What if we want to go one step further and find out what the percentage is of each element in the unknown solution? What percent is hydrogen, what percent is oxygen, and so on? In order to show how we find these percentages, let's assume that the sodium compound is our old friend sodium chloride. We know that out of 10 grams of solution, 9 grams are water. The remaining 1 gram would be NaCl.

One way to find the percentages of hydrogen and oxygen would be to use an electric current to split the water apart as was done in the experiment in Chapter 5. The hydrogen and oxygen could then be weighed and the percentages calculated. There is an easier way, however, and the formula for water, $H_2O$, provides the clue.

On the Periodic Table of the Elements (page 160) we see that the atomic weight of hydrogen is about 1 and that of oxygen is about 16. This tells us that an atom of oxygen is 16 times heavier than an atom of hydrogen. Look at sodium and chlorine on the chart. Sodium has an atomic weight of about 23 and chlorine of about 35½. The sodium atom is only about ⅔ as heavy as a chlorine atom.

Just as we can talk about atomic weights, we also can refer to **molecular** (mə lek′ ū lər) **weights.** The molecular weight of a compound is found by adding up the atomic weights of all the atoms that it contains. The molecular weight of water is 18.

| | | |
|---|---|---|
| 2 Hydrogen Atoms (2 × 1) | = | 2 |
| 1 Oxygen Atom (1 × 16) | = | 16 |
| Total | | 18 |

The molecular weight of NaCl is 58.5 (23 + 35.5) and of HCl is 36.5 (1 + 35.5). What is the molecular weight of FeO? $FeSO_4$? Table sugar, $C_{12}H_{22}O_{11}$? Hemoglobin in the blood, $C_{3032}H_{4816}Fe_4N_{780}O_{872}S_8$?

In order to help you understand ratios better, let's imagine that you have three times as much money as a friend has. If you combine your money with his, you will have contributed 75% and the friend 25%. This will be true regardless of the *amount* of money involved. If you contribute 3¢ and the friend 1¢, it will be true. If you contribute $3.00 and the friend $1.00, it also will be true. Will it also be true if you give $3.12 and the friend $1.04? $12.36 and $4.12?

Now back to the problem of finding what percent of the water is hydrogen and what percent is oxygen. As in the case of money, we can find the percentages if we know the ratio of the weights in a compound. In $H_2O$, the weight of hydrogen accounts for $^2/_{18}$, or $^1/_9$, of the total weight of the molecule. (Two atoms of hydrogen weigh 2 and the molecular weight of water is 18.) Oxygen accounts for $^{16}/_{18}$, or $^8/_9$. Converted to percentages, water is 11.1% hydrogen and 88.9% oxygen.

The sodium atom in sodium chloride represents $^{23}/_{58.5}$ of the molecular weight of NaCl and the chlorine atoms, $^{35.5}/_{58.5}$. Expressed as percentages, sodium chloride is 39.7% sodium and 60.3% chlorine. Can you find the percentages of iron and oxygen in iron oxide? Of carbon, hydrogen, and oxygen in table sugar?

We now know what percentage of water is hydrogen and what percentage is oxygen. We also know what percentage of sodium chloride is sodium and what percentage is chlorine. The percentage of each of these elements in this solution is 90% water and 10% sodium chloride. This means that out of each 100 grams of solution, 90 grams is $H_2O$, and 10 grams is sodium chloride.

We can find out how much of the solution is hydrogen by multiplying the amount of water (90 grams) times 11.1% (percent of hydrogen in water). By doing this, we find that 90 grams of water contains about 10 grams of hydrogen (90 × .111). The 90 grams of water also contain about 80 grams of oxygen (90 × .889). Check these answers by adding the weight of the hydrogen and the weight of the oxygen. The total should equal the weight of the water. Does it?

The 10 grams of NaCl are 39.7% sodium and 60.3% chlorine. Multiplying, we find that the 10 grams of NaCl contains about 4 grams of sodium and 6 grams of chlorine.

We can represent our findings in the form of a bar graph (Figure 6.25). It can be seen that of each 100 grams of the 10% NaCl solution, 80 grams are oxygen, 10 grams are hydrogen, 6 grams are chlorine, and 4 grams are sodium. It is an easy matter to convert to percentage.

| Element | Percentage of Unknown Solution |
|---|---|
| Oxygen | 80% |
| Hydrogen | 10% |
| Chlorine | 6% |
| Sodium | 4% |

Thus we know not only what the unknown solution contained, but how much of each compound and how much of each element.

**6.25** This diagram shows the weight of each element and compound in the solution.

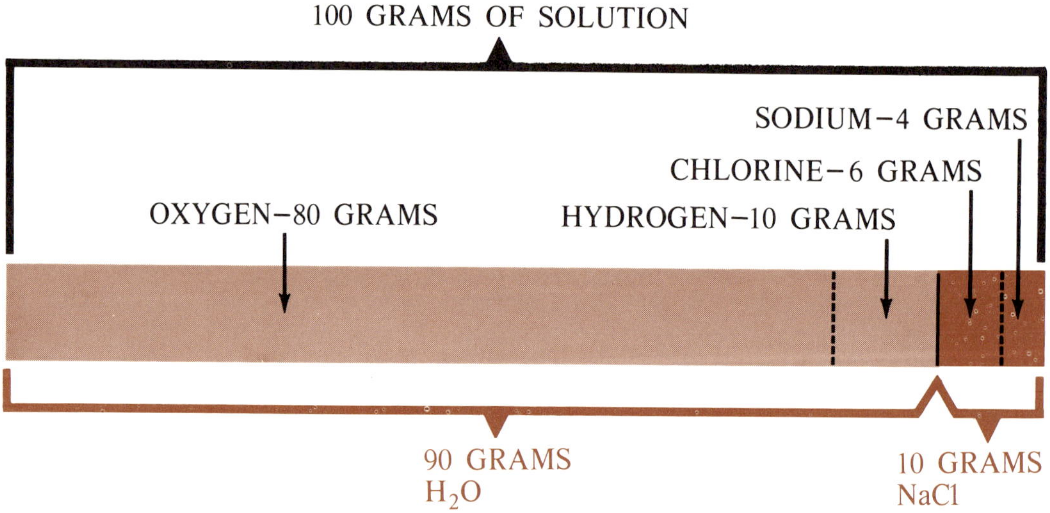


## Have You Learned?

1. If an apple that weighs 100 grams weighs only 14 grams after it has been dried in an oven, what percentage of the raw apple was water?
2. Explain how you would go about finding out how much of an apple is made up of minerals.
3. What percent of $CaCO_3$ is calcium? Carbon? Oxygen?

## 8. Using Equations to Write Recipes

> **ARE YOU READY?**
>
> Look up the following words if you are not sure of their meanings:
>
> molecular weight; ratio; react; reaction; recipe.

Chemists use molecular weights to figure out how much of a substance to add during a reaction or how much product will be formed. In Section 4, HCl was added to NaOH, and the products were NaCl and $H_2O$. In doing this, chemists would want to know how much acid to add to a certain amount of NaOH. If too much acid is added, the salt will contain acid. If not enough acid is added, the salt will contain some basic sodium hydroxide. Do you see why this is so? What was done in the experiment so that just the right amount of acid and base were added and only salt and water remained in the dish?

What the chemist often really needs is a recipe. Recipes in cookbooks tell how much of each ingredient to use and often also tell how much this will make. If more is wanted, the amount of each ingredient in the recipe can be increased.

### Using Molecular Weights in Writing Recipes

Molecular weights can be used to work out a recipe for chemical reactions. The first step is to write a balanced equation. The molecular weight of each element and compound is determined and written under it. The equation for the reaction of NaOH and HCl shows how this is done. As a check, the total of the molecular weights on the left side of the equation is equal to the total of the molecular weights on the right side of the equation.

$$\underset{40}{NaOH} + \underset{36.5}{HCl} \longrightarrow \underset{58.5}{NaCl} + \underset{18}{H_2O}$$

$$40 + 36.5 = 58.5 + 18$$

(Molecular weights)

Think a moment again about the situation of you and your friend pooling your money. The ratio between the amount you gave and the amount he gave remains the same regardless of whether it was 3¢ to 1¢ or \$3.00 to \$1.00. The ratio between molecular weights works the same way.

Imagine that you have a very sensitive balance that can weigh one molecule! If you weighed one molecule of the NaOH and it weighed 40, then one molecule of hydrochloric acid would weigh 36.5. Using the same balance and system of weights, one molecule of sodium chloride would weigh 58.5, and one water 18.

### Using Ratios in Writing Recipes

Unfortunately we do not have a balance that can weigh one molecule. However, we can use our knowledge of ratios to solve the problem. If we weigh 40 grams of NaOH, we will have a very large number of molecules. Because of the ratio between the weight of NaOH and HCl (40 to 36.5), we know that 36.5 grams of HCl will contain about the same number of molecules as 40 grams of NaOH. In like manner, 40 kilograms of NaOH would contain about the same number of molecules as 36.5 kilograms of HCl. The important thing to remember is that if the weight of one of the compounds is in grams, then the weights of all the other compounds must also be expressed in grams.

The equation for the reaction of NaOH and HCl indicates that 40 grams of NaOH would react with 36.5 grams of HCl to form 58.5 grams of NaCl and 18 grams of water. If 80 grams, or twice as much NaOH is used, 73 grams of HCl would be required, and 117 grams of NaCl and 36 grams of water would be produced. If we wish to make 9 grams of water, 20 grams of NaOH is added to 18.25 grams of HCl. Can you explain why this is so?

Can you figure out how much sulfuric acid would be required to react with 65.4 grams of zinc? How many grams of $ZnSO_4$ would be produced? How many grams of hydrogen? To get you started, the equations for the reaction and the molecular weights are as follows:

$$Zn + H_2SO_4 \longrightarrow ZnSO_4 + H_2\uparrow$$

$$65.4 + 98.1 = 161.5 + 2.0$$

(Molecular weights)

## Writing Recipes When One Molecule Reacts with Two Molecules of Another Compound

The two previous equations have involved one molecule reacting with another molecule in a 1 to 1 ratio. One NaOH molecule reacts with one HCl molecule, and one zinc atom reacts with one sulfuric acid molecule. In a reaction like the following one, the compounds do not react in a 1 to 1 ratio.

$$2\ H_2 + O_2 \longrightarrow 2\ H_2O$$

$$4.0 + 32 = 36$$

(Molecular weights)

The equation indicates that two molecules of hydrogen react with one molecule of oxygen to form two molecules of water. In order to have twice as many hydrogen molecules as oxygen, the molecular weight of hydrogen is multiplied by 2 ($2 \times 2.0$). Two water molecules will be formed for each oxygen molecule used up in the reaction, so its molecular weight has to be multiplied by two also ($2 \times 18$). Thus the recipe for the reaction with the ingredients measured in grams is:

4 grams of $H_2$ plus 32 grams of $O_2 \longrightarrow$ 36 grams of $H_2O$

The total weight of the gases on the left equals the weight of the water on the right side.

To make sure you have the idea, let's write the recipe for one more reaction.

$$CaCO_3 + 2\ HCl \longrightarrow CaCl_2 + H_2O + CO_2\uparrow$$

| $CaCO_3$ | $2\ HCl$ | $CaCl_2$ | $H_2O$ | $CO_2$ |
|---|---|---|---|---|
| 100.1 | 36.5 | 111.1 | 18 | 44 |

(Molecular weights)

$$100.1\ g + 73\ g = 111.1\ g + 18\ g + 44\ g$$

(Recipe in grams)

In writing the recipe, the molecular weight of HCl was doubled because two molecules of HCl are required for every one molecule of $CaCO_3$. Does the total weight of the compounds on the left side of the equation equal the total weight on the right side?

Mathematics, as you have seen in the last two sections, is a very useful tool to the chemist. It can be used in figuring out how much of an element or compound a substance contains. It also is useful in working out the recipe for a chemical reaction. Look again at the last equation.

A chemist also uses mathematics to figure out how many milliliters of hydrochloric acid solution would contain 73 grams of HCl. He could also predict the volume of the 44 grams of $CO_2$ gas at a certain pressure and temperature.

### Have You Learned?

The following equation is for the reaction of hydrochloric acid and ammonium hydroxide. The molecular weight of each compound appears below the formula.

$$\underset{36.5}{HCl} + \underset{35}{NH_4OH} \longrightarrow \underset{53.5}{NH_4Cl} + \underset{18}{H_2O}$$

1. How many grams of ammonium hydroxide are needed to react with 36.5 grams of hydrochloric acid?
2. How many grams of $NH_4Cl$ will be produced?
3. How many grams of $H_2O$ will be produced?
4. How much HCl and how much $NH_4OH$ would be needed to produce 9 grams of water?

## 9. Putting Chemistry to Work

**ARE YOU READY?**

Look up the following words if you are not sure of their meanings:

catalyst; enzyme; epidemic; fabric; fertilizer; fiber; microorganism; neutralize; soluble.

Chemistry affects our lives in many ways. The food we eat, the water we drink, the clothes we wear, and many of the things in our homes are at least in part products of chemistry. A few of the new products that have been made during the last 30 to 40 years with chemistry are listed in the chart on page 217.

The future undoubtedly holds an even larger role for chemistry. As the population of the world increases, new sources must be found for food, new fibers for clothing, new materials for shelter, and new sources for fuel. Nor are we content to continue to live the same way we have lived in the past. We expect improvements. Therefore, chemistry is involved in developing faster and safer means of transportation and new and improved methods of communication.

In this section, several of the ways in which chemistry is involved in our daily lives are discussed.

### Drinking Water

Most of us take for granted that we shall have an adequate supply of water that is safe to drink. This is not always the case in this country, nor is it true in many parts of the world. Wells still provide many people in small towns and rural areas with a safe supply of water. However, the water used in large cities generally comes from surface sources such as lakes and streams. Impurities must be removed and living organisms killed before it is safe to use.

Chemicals play an important role in water treatment plants. They are used to speed the water purification process and to kill harmful microorganisms.

### Treating Muddy Water

Make two beakers of muddy water by

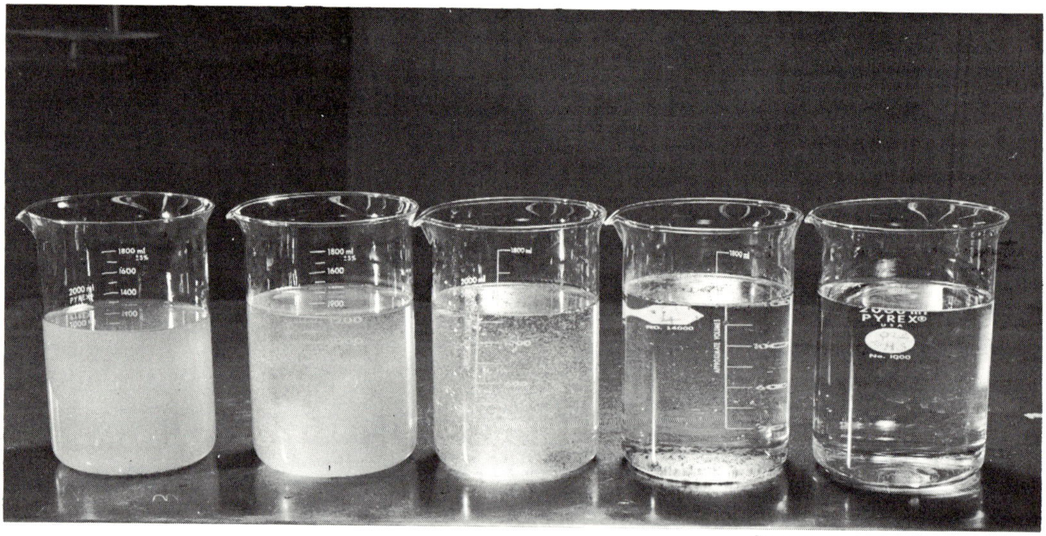


*City of Philadelphia Water Department*

**6.26** Water treatment. The beaker at the extreme left contains only murky river water without the addition of chemicals. In the next beaker (second from left), alum and lime have been added. The other three beakers show the settling process in sequence, with clarified water in the beaker at the extreme right.

stirring some dirt and water together. To one beaker add some alum and enough ammonium hydroxide or lime to make the solution basic. Stir the solution.

Observe what happens in the two containers. In which container do the dirt particles settle to the bottom sooner? How do you explain this?

The alum reacts with the $NH_4OH$, or lime, to form aluminum hydroxide, which is not soluble in water. It is a sticky substance called "floc" and as it settles to the bottom, it drags the fine dirt particles down with it. The equation for the reaction of the alum and lime used in water treatment plants is as follows:

$$\underset{\text{Filter alum}}{Al_2(SO_4)_3} + \underset{\text{Lime}}{3\,Ca(OH)_2} \longrightarrow \underset{\text{Aluminum hydroxide floc}}{2\,Al(OH)_3} + 3\,CaSO_4$$

Chlorine is added to water to kill the microorganisms in it. Extra chlorine is added to the water in swimming pools. This makes the water slightly acid. To neutralize this acid condition, lime is usually also added to the water in swimming pools.

Most water contains very small amounts of fluorine. Scientists have found that water containing about 1 part of fluorine to each 1,000,000 parts of water reduces tooth decay. Some communities add a fluorine compound to the water supply. Some individuals and groups have objected to this practice on religious grounds or because they have no choice in deciding whether or not to consume the fluorine compounds. Others say that in addition to reducing tooth decay, fluorine may affect the body in undesirable ways. Can you name other things to which fluorine compounds have been added to reduce tooth decay?

**Some Recent Products of Chemistry That Affect Our Lives**

| *Food and Agriculture* | *Clothing* | *Health* | *Shelter* | *Transportation and Communication* |
|---|---|---|---|---|
| Artificial flavors<br>Improved fertilizers<br>Selective weed killers<br>Insecticides<br>Fungicides<br>Foods such as oleomargarine and "instant" coffee | Fabrics such as nylon and Orlon<br>Water repellents<br>Shrink-proofing chemicals<br>Permanent "starch"<br>Dyes<br>Flame-retardant finishes | Sulfa drugs<br>Synthetic detergents<br>Synthetic vitamins<br>Antibiotics<br>Synthetic hormones<br>Radioisotopes<br>Antihistamines<br>Plastic replacement parts for blood vessels, etc. | Plastic building parts<br>Resin-adhesive for plywood<br>Insulation material<br>Latex-based paints<br>Simulated wood finishes | Plastic parts<br>Heat-resistant metals<br>Fuels<br>Synthetic rubber<br>Improved lubricating compounds<br>Transistors<br>Materials for television receivers |

## Chemistry in the Kitchen

All of the cooking ingredients in a kitchen are chemicals. Some, such as sugar and salt, are single compounds, but most are mixtures of tens or even hundreds of different compounds. Making a cake or a loaf of bread involves chemical reactions, and cooking is nothing more than applied chemistry. We heat things to speed up reactions. We add ingredients in certain definite amounts just as we do in performing a chemical experiment. Scientists who develop new foods or cooking techniques rely on chemistry to solve their problems.

Let's take the baking of bread and pastries as an example. In making bread or cake, it is important that it "rise." We start out with dough or batter. During a chemical reaction, bubbles of carbon dioxide are given off and trapped in the dough or batter. When the food is baked, the carbon dioxide expands, leaving the bread or cake full of holes (Figure 6.27).

Cooks use two methods of producing the desired carbon dioxide. Yeast may be added to the dough of foods such as bread and rolls. The yeast produces an enzyme, or catalyst, that converts sugar to carbon dioxide and alcohol. The alcohol is driven off during the baking process.

$$\underset{\text{(sugar)}}{\underset{\text{Glucose}}{C_6H_{12}O_6}} \longrightarrow 2\ \underset{\text{Alcohol}}{C_2H_5OH} + 2\ CO_2\uparrow$$

Baking powder also is used to produce carbon dioxide. It contains baking soda, which is a source of carbon dioxide, and an acidlike substance such as cream of tartar. Baking powder also contains cornstarch to keep the mixture dry. When water is added, the baking soda reacts with the acid in the cream of tartar to produce carbon dioxide.

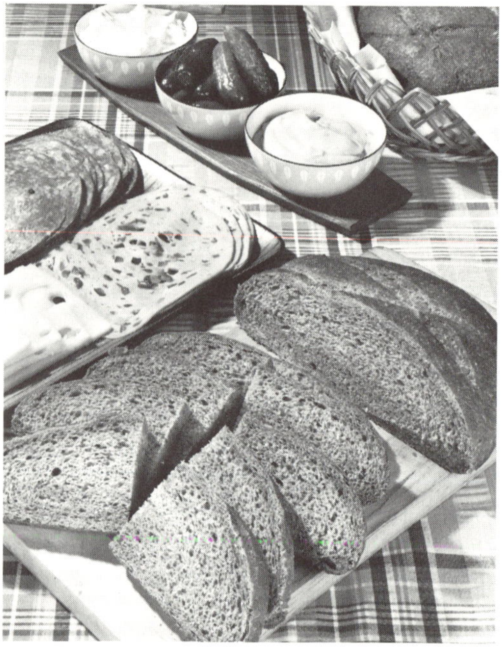

*Wheat Flour Institute*

**6.27** Carbon dioxide made the holes in the bread.

## Using Baking Soda and Powder

Add some water to a few grams of baking soda. What happens? Now add some vinegar, an acid, to some baking soda. Observe what happens. Test the gas that is given off by bubbling it through limewater. Do you think baking soda and an acid such as vinegar could be used to make foods "rise"?

Add some water to a few grams of baking powder. How do your results differ from those obtained when water is added to baking soda? Add some water to a small amount of an "instant" cake mix. Do you think it contains baking powder? Explain.

Experiment making biscuits using baking powder as the recipe calls for. Make a second batch in which baking soda is substituted for the baking powder, and a third batch leaving out both baking soda and baking powder. Which biscuits do you prefer? Explain your results.

## Chemistry in the Garden

Both farmers and amateur gardeners make use of many of the products of chemistry.

1. *Fertilizers.* Fertilizers supply plants with the minerals necessary for proper plant growth. The minerals contain the elements calcium, nitrogen, phosphorus, and potassium. They also contain smaller amounts of the **trace elements,** which include sulfur, magnesium, iron, manganese, boron, zinc, copper, molybdenum, and chlorine. In most parts of the country, the soil contains enough of the trace elements for most plants.

Fertilizers are made which contain the proper amounts of the elements needed by certain kinds of plants. For example, special fertilizers are made for grass, for roses, for flowering shrubs, and so on. These are sold under various brand names and often with the misleading name of "plant foods." Plants make their own food and the minerals they get from the soil are not considered by scientists to be a food.

Farmers frequently buy fertilizer that is labeled "4-6-8," "8-8-8," or with some other series of three numbers. These numbers indicate the amount of nitrogen, phosphorus, and potassium in the fertilizer. It is easy to remember which number is which since the numbers refer to the three elements in alphabetical order. Thus 4-6-8 means four percent nitrogen, six percent phosphorus (in the form of $P_2O_5$), and eight percent potassium (in the form of $K_2O$). The production of low-cost fertilizer custom designed for a variety of plants is a major accomplishment of modern chemistry.

2. *Insect Killers.* Each year insects do millions of dollars worth of damage. It is estimated that in the United States alone insects cause over $1,600,000,000 worth of damage to crops and livestock each year. Chemicals called **insecticides** (in sek′ tə sīd) have been made to fight these enemies. Perhaps the most famous insecticide, DDT, became well known during World War II when it was used in Italy to stop an epidemic of typhus fever. DDT kills body lice that carry the microorganisms causing typhus fever.

Since that time DDT has been widely used to control insects. In the last few years some people have waged a battle against the use of DDT. They claim that the insecticide accumulates in some animals and is harmful to them. Watch for stories in the newspaper and magazines on this controversy. Where do you stand on this issue? Collect as much information as you can before you answer.

3. *Weed Killers.* **Herbicides** (hėr′ bi sīdz) are chemicals used to kill weeds and other plants. Two commonly used herbicides, 2,4-D and 2,4,5-T, were developed at about the same time as DDT. The 2,4-D is what we call a selective weed killer. When properly applied, it kills most broad-leaved plants but not the narrow-leaved grasses. Since the appearance of 2,4-D and 2,4,5-T, chemists have developed dozens of other herbicides to perform certain specialized jobs.

Some people have the same objection

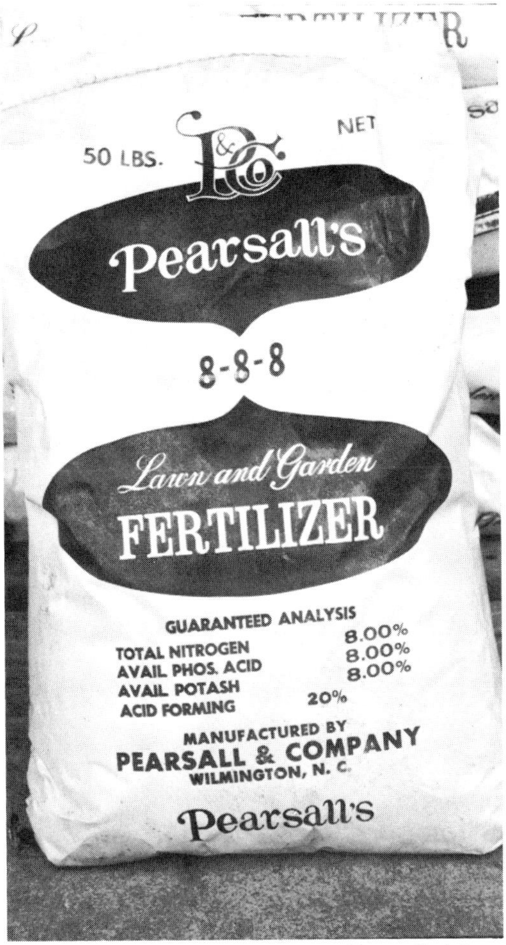


Norman D. Anderson

**6.28** What is the significance of "8-8-8"?

to the use of herbicides as they do to the use of insecticides. This controversy illustrates what often happens in the case of scientific contributions. Science can make possible insecticides, herbicides, the release of atomic energy, and space travel. It is another matter to decide how they should be used. These decisions are eventually made by elected public officials and by voters at the polls. It is important that all of our citizens know something about science so that they can make intelligent decisions on issues involving scientific knowledge.

## Have You Learned?

Write on a sheet of paper the word that best completes the statement. (Do not write in your book.)

1. _____ is added to water to kill microorganisms in the water.
2. Some communities add _____ to the drinking water to reduce tooth decay.
3. The gas that makes bread rise is _____.
4. A fertilizer marked "4-6-8" contains four percent _____, six percent _____, and eight percent _____.
5. Chemicals used to kill insects are called _____.
6. 2,4-D and 2,4,5-T are examples of _____.

## REVIEW QUESTIONS

1. Define the terms *physical property, chemical property, physical change*, and *chemical change*. Give an example of each.
2. Name the four types of chemical reactions, and illustrate each with an example.
3. Write balanced equations for the following reactions:
   a. Combination of hydrogen and oxygen to form water
   b. Decomposition of mercuric oxide into mercury and oxygen
   c. Reaction of magnesium with $H_2SO_4$
   d. Reaction of $H_2SO_4$ and $Al(OH)_3$
4. Tell at least one way that hydrogen, oxygen, and carbon dioxide can be prepared in the laboratory. What is the test for each gas?
5. Explain how the activity series can be used to predict if a chemical reaction will occur.
6. What factors affect the rate of a reaction? Give an example of how each factor is used to change the rate of a chemical reaction.
7. Name as many ways as you can that are used in identifying an unknown substance and the elements it contains.
8. Explain how molecular weights are used in writing recipes for chemical reactions.
9. List examples of how we use chemistry in our daily lives.

## CAN YOU FIND OUT?

*You may need to use an encyclopedia or other reference book in order to answer the following questions:*

1. Can you find out about important chemical reactions used in industry, such as the contact process for making sulfuric acid, the Haber process for making ammonia, and the Ostwald process for making nitric acid?
2. Investigate the chemistry involved in photography. Can you learn how to develop a negative and make a contact print?
3. Find out how chemistry is used in extracting metals from ores, such as iron from iron ore. Also investigate how chemistry is involved in making steel from iron and in making mixtures of metals called alloys.
4. What evidence made scientists first suspect that oxygen and hydrogen molecules contained two atoms each?
5. How is hydrogen peroxide used to bleach cloth and yarn? What is the formula for hydrogen peroxide? How does it bleach the color from various substances?
6. Helium is not so light as hydrogen, yet it is used for blimps by the U.S. Navy. Can you find out why?
7. How does a $CO_2$ fire extinguisher work? What other uses are made of carbon dioxide?
8. How do catalysts act to speed or slow a reaction?
9. What are some of the instruments used by the chemist to identify chemicals? How do they work?

## REFERENCES FOR ADDITIONAL STUDY


EXPLORATIONS IN CHEMISTRY by Charles Gray. E. P. Dutton & Co., Inc.
Describes a set of experiments designed to teach the major ideas of chemistry, with one section devoted to setting up a home laboratory and another on research

EXPERIMENTAL CHEMISTRY (Revised Edition) by Nathan Feifer.
Sentinel Books Publishers, Inc.
Directions for doing 200 chemistry experiments, accompanied by explanations

YOUR CAREER IN CHEMISTRY by Arnulf Esterer. Jullian Messner.
Describes careers in chemistry and chemical engineering, including academic requirements

EXPERIMENTS IN CHEMISTRY by Nelson Beeler and Franklin Branley. Thomas Y. Crowell Company.
A popular book containing many experiments that can be done in a home or school laboratory

SCEINCE EXPERIMENTS YOU CAN EAT by Vicki Cobb. J. B. Lippincott Company.
Describes chemistry experiments that involve cooking—most of the experiments can be eaten when you have finished!

# CHAPTER 7

# The Story of Carbon

HOLD A BEAKER over the tip of a candle flame. Do you notice the black stuff that forms on the bottom of the beaker? Rub a piece of graphite or some graphite powder between your fingers. Does it feel greasy? Then, the next time you pass a jeweler's window, look at a diamond. Would you have ever guessed that the soot on the beaker, the graphite, and the diamond are all different forms of one element—carbon?

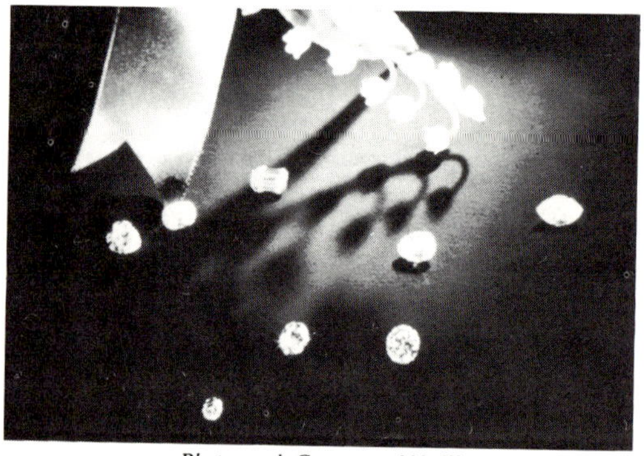

*Photograph Courtesy of N. W. Ayer & Son, Inc.*

**7.1** This is one form of carbon.

## 1. Introduction to the Element Carbon

> **ARE YOU READY?**
>
> Look up the following words if you are not sure of their meanings:
>
> abrasive; bond (chemical); diamond; graphite; petroleum; soot; synthetic.

Chemistry is divided into two major divisions called **organic** (ôr gan′ ik) **chemistry** and **inorganic** (in′ ôr gan′ ik) **chemistry.** There was a time when organic chemistry was defined as the chemistry of living things. *Organic* means "alive," and *inorganic* is used to describe nonliving materials such as water, minerals, and air.

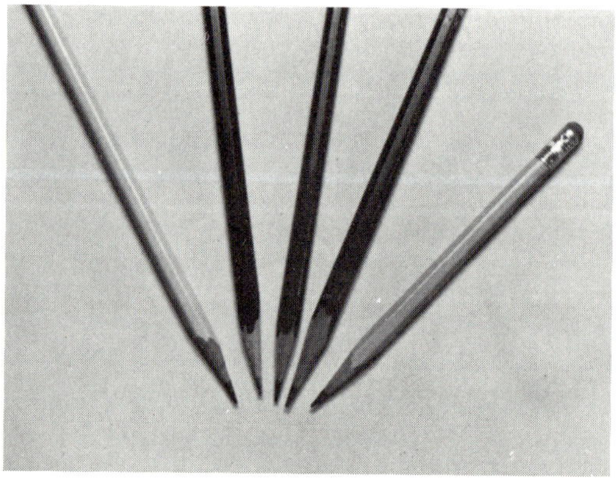

*Norman D. Anderson*

**7.2** Graphite in "lead" pencils is also carbon.

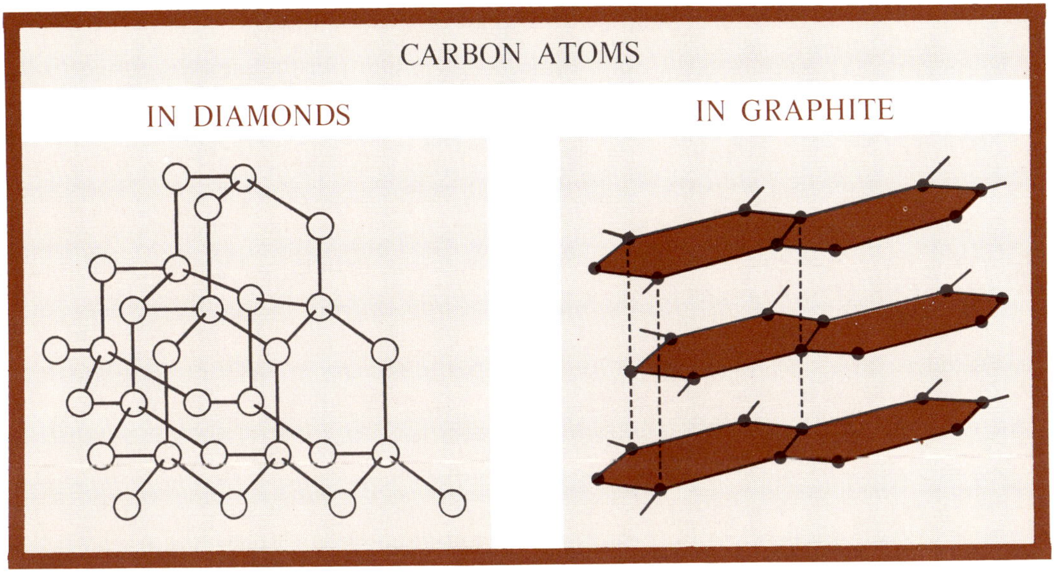


**7.3** Notice that the carbon atoms are arranged differently in diamond than in graphite.

Chemists have found that carbon atoms are the backbone of most of the compounds found in living things. They have found also that many of these carbon compounds can be made in the laboratory, and thus organic chemistry is no longer limited to living things. Organic chemistry is now defined as the chemistry of carbon compounds.

The key to understanding organic chemistry is learning how carbon atoms are bonded to each other and to atoms of other elements. Let us start by finding out how carbon can be something as beautiful as a diamond and can also form soot.

Diamonds are found mainly in South Africa, the East Indies, and Brazil. When they are taken from the ground, they are not the sparkling stones we see in the jeweler's showcase. They must be "cut" so that light reflects from them the way that it does. Diamond is one of the hardest known substances, and it is used as an *abrasive*. Perhaps you have heard of cutting stones with a diamond saw. Diamonds are crystals of carbon atoms arranged in a pattern that looks a little like a Junglegym on a playground or an interlocking pattern of Tinker Toy sticks. Study the arrangement of carbon atoms in the diagram in Figure 7.3. Notice that the atoms of carbon are arranged in the form of **hexagons** (hek′ sə gon), or six-sided figures. Close inspection will reveal that each of the carbon atoms except those on the edges is attached to four other carbon atoms.

The diagram of the arrangement of carbon atoms in graphite reveals why its physical properties differ from those of diamond. The carbon atoms in crystals of graphite are arranged in *layers* of hexagons. The layers are so far apart that they are not held together very firmly. When a force is applied, the layers slide over each other like sheets of paper.

Graphite is mined in Ceylon, Siberia, some parts of the United States, Canada, and Mexico. It is used as a lubricating agent and in powdered form is sprayed in locks. A gray mark is made when a piece of graphite is rubbed across paper. Powdered graphite is mixed with clay and baked to make the "lead" in lead pencils.

Scientists have made both synthetic graphite and diamonds in the laboratory. To make diamonds, carbon is placed under pressures of 100,000 kilograms per square centimeter and temperatures of 2,800° C. It is estimated that these are the conditions that exist about 400 kilometers beneath the surface of the earth. A process of making graphite, which is much simpler than that for making diamonds, was patented in 1896. Much of the graphite now used by industry is synthetic graphite.

Carbon also exists in a noncrystalline form. Soot, or *carbon black*, is a very fine powder used in the manufacture of printer's inks, phonograph records, and shoe polish. *Bone black*, made from bones, and *lampblack*, made by burning oil or coal gas, are other forms of powdered carbon.

## Carbon and Fuels

Coal and petroleum are the two most important fuels, and both contain carbon. They are used to heat our homes, generate electricity, and supply energy for cars, trains, and airplanes. These fuels are important as sources of heat and as the raw material for thousands of products.

Coal dates back millions of years to a time when the earth was very different from the way it is today. In one stage of the earth's history, much of its surface was covered with very thick vegetation. As the vegetation died, a layer of decaying material collected much as it does on the floor of a forest today. As conditions on the earth changed, parts of the earth's surface sank. The decaying vegetation was covered by mud and sand, and the pressure caused by these materials changed the decaying vegetation to coal. If you look carefully at a piece of coal, you may be able to see a fernlike leafprint or some other sign of plant remains.

## Making Coke and Charcoal

**MATERIALS:**

Pyrex test tube, ring stand and test tube clamp, Bunsen burner, one-hole and two-hole rubber stoppers, glass tubing, beaker, several pieces of wood and soft coal

**PROCEDURE:**

*Coke.* Set up the apparatus as shown in Figure 7.4 on page 225. Place a few pieces of the soft coal in the test tube, and heat it. Test to see if the *coal gas* will burn by bringing a match near the nozzle. Continue heating until all of the gas is given off.

After the test tube has cooled, examine the coke in the test tube. How does it differ from coal? Burn a piece of coke and a piece of coal. Which one burns better? Coke is widely used in the steel industry to remove the oxygen from iron oxide ores.

Examine the liquid in the vertical test tube. It is called *coal tar*. Coal tar is used in industry to make hundreds of compounds ranging from coal-tar dyes to aspirin, nylon, and mothballs.

*Charcoal.* Repeat the experiment using pieces of wood instead of coal. Heat the wood, and check to see if a gas that burns is given off. After the tube has cooled, examine the remains of the wood. Charcoal, which is mainly carbon, is the product of heating wood in the absence of air. How does a piece of charcoal burn compared with a piece of wood?

Grind up a few pieces of charcoal into a fine powder. Place some of the charcoal powder in a test tube containing some water and a few drops of ink. Cover the test tube with a stopper and shake it thoroughly. Filter the liquid through a filter paper. The color should have been absorbed by the charcoal. How do you know that the color wasn't removed by the filter paper? Devise an experiment to test your answer. Because of its ability to absorb substances, charcoal is used in gas masks and in some kinds of smoke filters.

Also examine the liquid that remains in the vertical test tube. Test with cobalt chloride paper to see if it contains water and with litmus to see if it is an acid or base. At one time this liquid was an important source of wood alcohol, acetic acid, and several other important chemicals. As more and more of our wood supply is used to make paper and other products, other methods have been developed for making these chemicals.

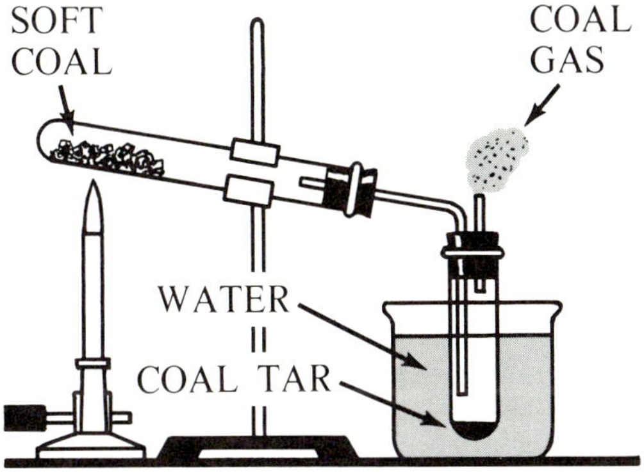


**7.4** Making coke and charcoal

Scientists do not know for sure how petroleum was formed. Most believe that it was formed from the plants and animals that lived in the oceans and shallow seas that covered much of the earth millions of years ago. Whereas coal was formed from the remains of land plants and animals, it is thought that the remains of marine plants and animals are the source of petroleum. Some of the chemistry of petroleum is described in the following sections.

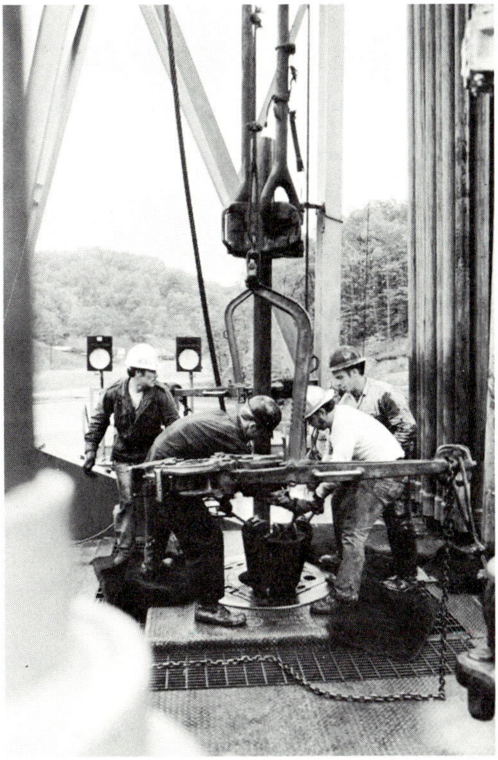

*An Exxon photo*

**7.5** Petroleum, like diamonds, coal, and graphite, contains carbon, and is important in industry.

### Two Gaseous Oxides of Carbon

Several methods of preparing carbon dioxide were described in Chapter 6. This important gas is produced when an acid reacts with limestone or marble ($CaCO_3$) or baking soda ($NaHCO_3$), when enzymes of yeast act upon sugars, and when any one of the thousands of carbon compounds is burned. Burning carbon compounds without an adequate supply of oxygen also produces another gas, *carbon monoxide*. Carbon monoxide, CO, is an odorless, tasteless, and colorless gas. It combines with the hemoglobin or red part of the blood. As a result, not enough oxygen can be carried to the cells of the body, and the victim suffocates. Hundreds of people are killed by carbon monoxide each year. To reduce the number of deaths, stoves and furnaces should be properly vented, and gasoline engines should not be operated inside a building unless the doors and windows are open.

**7.6** Electron arrangement of the carbon atom

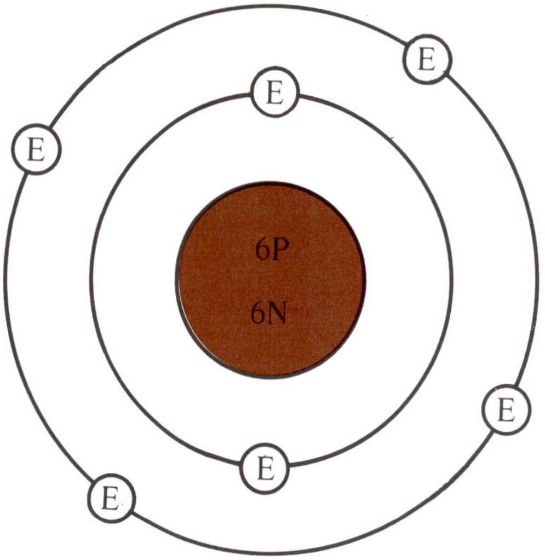

CARBON

### Have You Learned?

Select the word from Column B that best corresponds with each definition in Column A. (Do not write in your book.)

| Column A | Column B |
|---|---|
| 1. Produced by heating coal | a. boneblack |
| | b. carbon dioxide |
| 2. Produced when sugar is acted on by yeast | c. carbon monoxide |
| | d. charcoal |
| | e. coal |
| | f. coke |
| 3. Made by burning oil or coal gas | g. diamond |
| | h. graphite |
| | i. lampblack |
| 4. Is dangerous to humans because it causes suffocation | j. petroleum |

5. Thought to have been formed from the remains of marine plants and animals
6. Produced by heating wood
7. One of the hardest known substances
8. A form of carbon made from bones
9. Used in lead pencils
10. Formed from decaying vegetation

## 2. Chains and Rings

**ARE YOU READY?**

Look up the following words if you are not sure of their meanings:

boiling point; covalence;
organic chemistry; styrofoam; valence.

In the last section it was stated that the secret of understanding organic chemistry is learning how carbon atoms are bonded to each other and to atoms of other elements. To see how this works, we start by drawing the electron arrangement of the carbon atom (Figure 7.6). Carbon has four electrons in its outer shell and four unfilled spaces. A carbon atom forms compounds by *sharing* electrons with other atoms. The covalence, or sharing power, of carbon is four since it can share four pairs of electrons with other atoms. The covalence of several other common elements is given in Table IV, page 173.

The covalence, or electron-sharing power, of hydrogen is one. In other words, a hydrogen atom has one electron it can share. From what we know about valence, we would expect one carbon atom to combine with four hydrogen atoms, and this combination does exist. $CH_4$ is a compound called *methane*. A diagram of this combination can be shown by using dots to represent the electrons in the outer shell of carbon and crosses to represent the electrons of hydrogen.

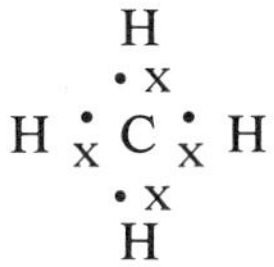

An easier way to write this formula is to use dashes to represent each pair of electrons. A dash then represents a covalent bond between two atoms. Using dashes, the formula for methane looks like this.

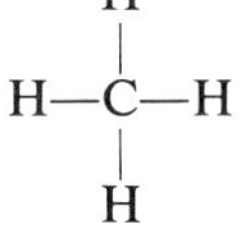

Note that hydrogen has one dash because it has a covalence of one, and carbon has four dashes because it has a covalence of four. How many dashes would you expect oxygen to have? chlorine?

A carbon atom can share electrons with another carbon atom. Using dots and crosses or using dashes, the following shows how two carbon atoms combine with six hydrogen atoms to form **ethane** (eth′ ān).

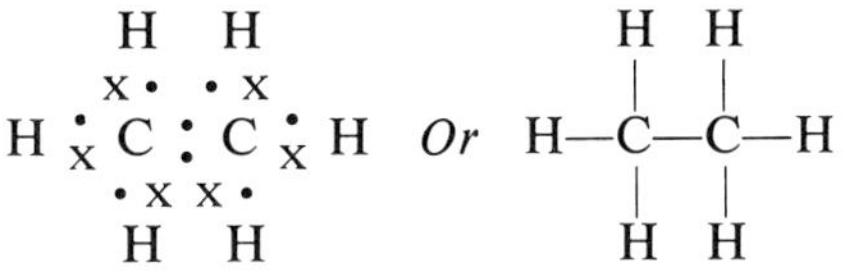

The formula showing how the carbon and other atoms are arranged is called a **structural formula.** Organic chemists often use structural formulas in describing a molecule. To see how structure can be important, let us write the structural formula for the **hydrocarbon** (hī′ drō kär′ bən) that contains 4 atoms of carbon and ten atoms of hydrogen. Hydrocarbons are compounds made up of carbon and hydrogen atoms.

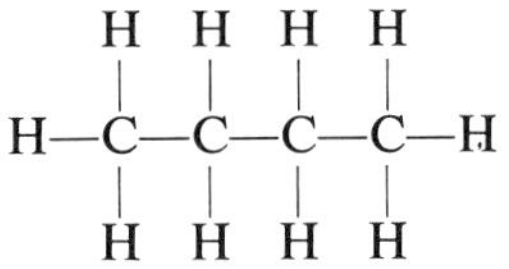

This structural formula represents a molecule of **butane** (bū′ tān). The chain is four carbon atoms long. There is another possibility for arranging four carbon atoms and ten hydrogen atoms. In this case, the chain is only three carbon atoms long with a side chain of one carbon atom.

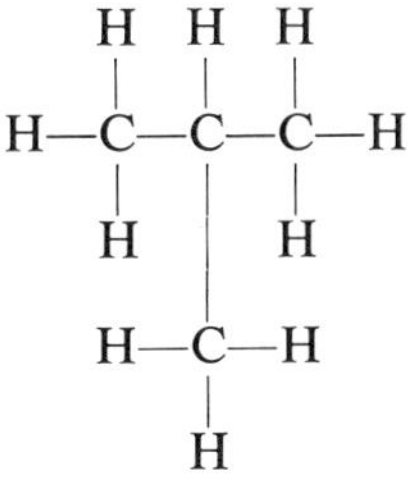

This compound is called **isobutane** (ī sə bū′ tān). Although butane and isobutane have the same formula, $C_4H_{10}$, they have different structural formulas and, therefore, different properties (Figure 7.7). Although both are gases at room temperature, the boiling point of butane is −0.5° C. and that of isobutane is −11.7° C.

Compounds that have the same formulas but different structural formulas are called **isomers** (ī′ sə mər). As you can see in Table I below, as the number of carbon atoms in a hydrocarbon increases, so does the number of possible isomers. Can you write the structural formulas for the three isomers of **pentane** (pen′ tān)? *Hint:* one chain is five carbons long, in the second the longest chain is four carbons long, and in the third, the longest chain is three carbons long.

**TABLE I**

*Some Simple Hydrocarbons*

| *Name* | *Formula* | *Physical State at Room Temperature* | *Number of Isomers* | *Source or Common Name* |
|---|---|---|---|---|
| Methane | $CH_4$ | Gas | 1 | Natural Gas |
| Ethane | $C_2H_6$ | Gas | 1 | |
| Propane | $C_3H_8$ | Gas | 1 | |
| Butane | $C_4H_{10}$ | Gas | 2 | |
| Pentane | $C_5H_{12}$ | Liquid | 3 | Naphtha |
| Hexane | $C_6H_{14}$ | Liquid | 5 | |
| Heptane | $C_7H_{16}$ | Liquid | 9 | Gasoline |
| Octane | $C_8H_{18}$ | Liquid | 18 | |

Can you suggest a way to help remember how many carbon atoms there are in each of these compounds? Does **hexane** (heks′ ān) suggest six? How many carbon atoms would you predict in **octane** (ok′ tān)? Some hydrocarbons have extremely long chains. For example, paraffin is a mixture of hydrocarbons with 20 to 30 carbon atoms per molecule.

## Building Models of Hydrocarbons

Kits are sold that contain wooden balls painted various colors to represent different kinds of atoms. Black is frequently used for carbon, red for oxygen, and yellow for hydrogen. The balls representing carbon have four holes corresponding to its covalence of four, oxygen has two, and hydrogen has one. Short sticks are used to connect the atoms, and these sticks represent the bonds, or the electrical attraction, between atoms.

Small styrofoam balls, such as those sold to make Christmas decorations, or gumdrops of various colors can be used if a kit is not available. If you are using styrofoam balls, several should be painted black to represent carbon, others painted red for oxygen, and still others painted yellow for hydrogen, and so on. Use toothpicks to represent the bonds. Study the model of methane, and notice how the bonds are at the greatest possible angle to each other. Compare the angle between them to the angle between the bonds of a carbon atom and its neighbors in a crystal of diamond (Figure 7.3 page 223). You should place the toothpicks in the styrofoam balls or gumdrops representing carbon so that they stick out in the same way as shown in the methane diagram on page 227.

Using either a kit or objects such as styrofoam balls or gumdrops, assemble the model for each of the hydrocarbons listed in Table I. By rearranging the molecule so it has one or more side chains, see how many isomers you can make for each hydrocarbon. Compare your results with the number of isomers possible (see Table I on the opposite page).

## Double and Triple Bonds

Carbon atoms can share two pairs of electrons to form a double bond and three pairs of electrons to form a triple bond. The structural formulas for **ethylene** (eth′ ə lēn) and **acetylene** (ə set′ ə lēn) illustrate how this is shown in a structural formula.

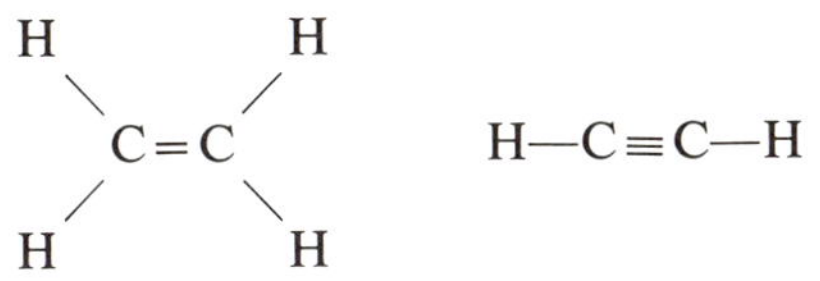

*ethylene* *acetylene*

Perhaps you have heard of **polyethylene** (pol′ i eth′ ə lēn), which is a plastic used to wrap foods. As you will see a bit later, it is a close relative of ethylene. Acetylene

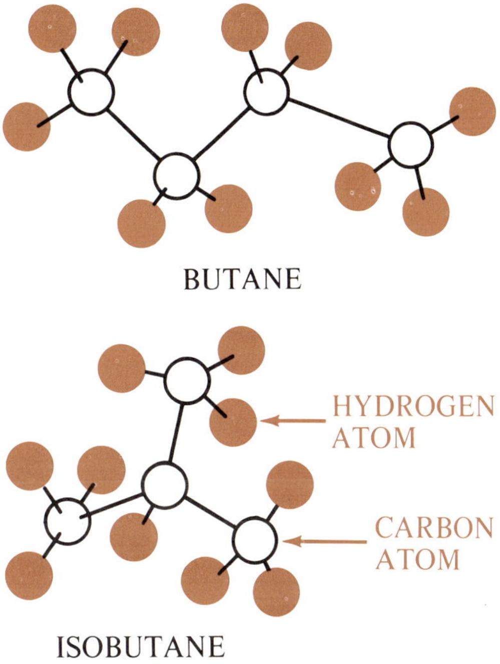


**7.7** Models of two isomers of butane

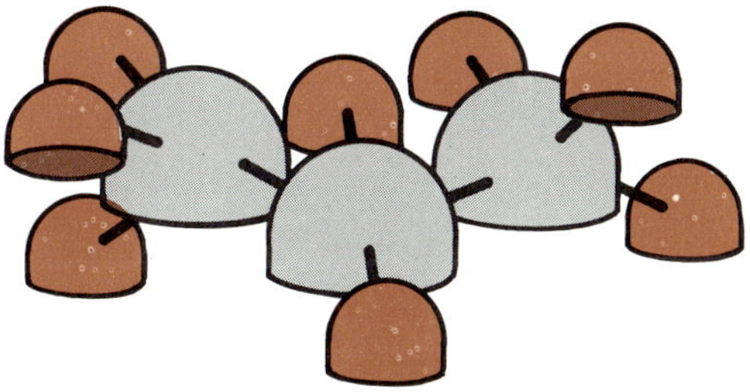

**7.8** Gumdrop model of propane molecule

is a gas that is used in welding metals. It combines with oxygen to produce a very hot flame.

You will have difficulty building models of ethylene and acetylene using wooden balls with four holes in them for carbon atoms. The sticks are usually replaced with small springs that can be bent so that the atoms can be joined. Since the springs tend to slip out of the holes, this is not a very stable arrangement. In a way, compounds

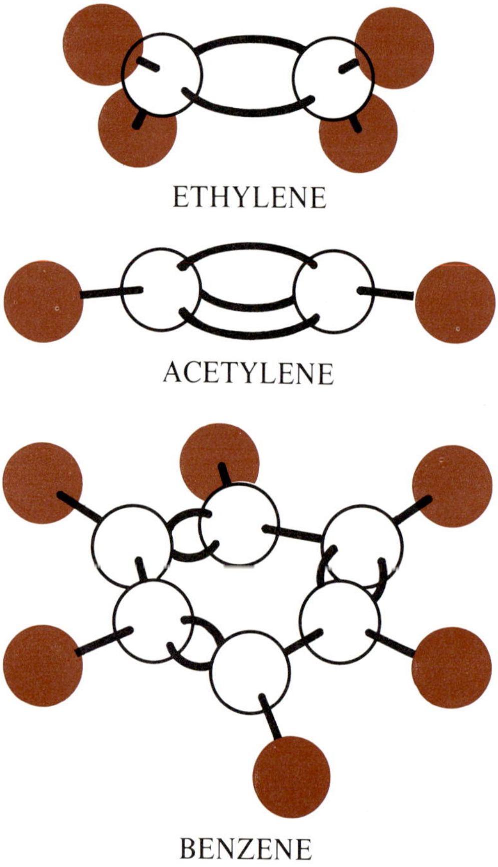


**7.9** Models of ethylene, acetylene, and benzene

with double and triple bonds are much like this. These compounds are not so stable as hydrocarbons with single bonds. The double and triple bonds open to form new compounds during many chemical reactions. For example, both acetylene and ethylene react with chlorine to form a more stable compound.

## Carbon Atoms in Rings

One of the compounds in coal tar is **benzene** (ben′ zēn), which has the formula $C_6H_6$. This compound does not act the same way that most of the other hydrocarbons do, and chemists were puzzled about its behavior. Nor were they able to write a structural formula to show how six carbon atoms could combine with six hydrogen atoms. Finally Kekule (kā′ kü lā), the German chemist who had invented structural formulas, suggested that the carbon atoms were arranged in a ring in which every other bond was a double bond.

The structural formula for a molecule of benzene shows how six carbon atoms and six hydrogen atoms can combine.

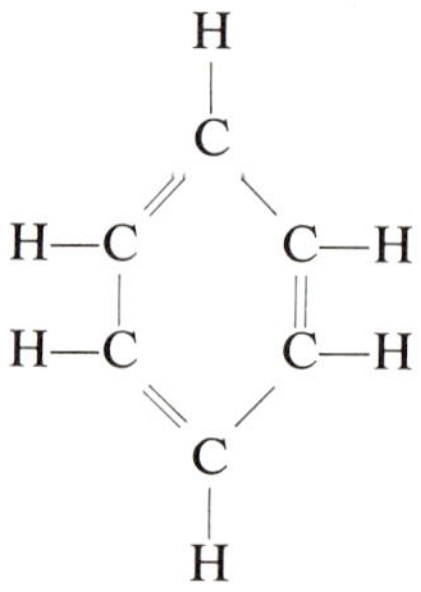

*benzene*

When you look at the structural formulas for many carbon compounds, you will see one or more benzene rings. Many organic compounds are combinations of chains of carbon atoms and one or more rings.

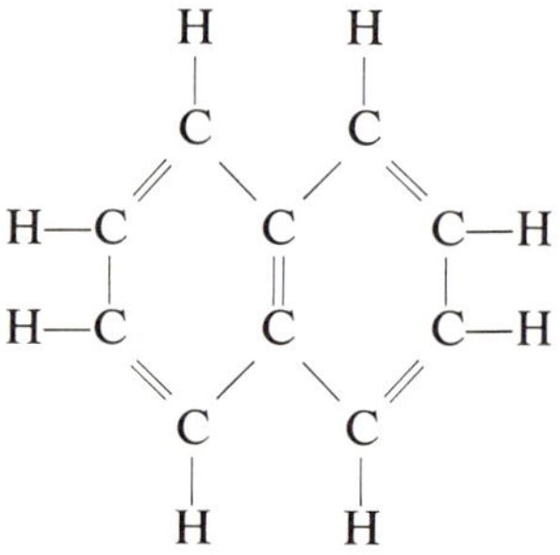

*naphthalene*

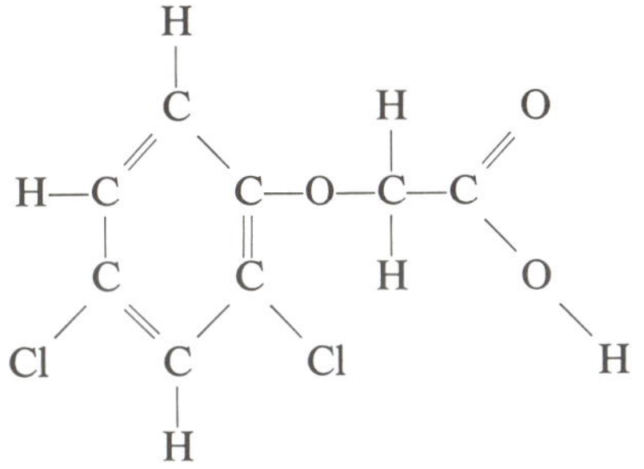

*2,4-D (weed killer)*

## Have You Learned?

1. Define or explain the following:
   a. hydrocarbon
   b. covalence
   c. isomer
   d. structural formula
2. Draw structural formulas for the following:
   a. $C_3H_8$
   b. ethylene
   c. acetylene
   d. benzene

## 3. How Are Carbon Compounds Classified?

**ARE YOU READY?**

Look up the following words if you are not sure of their meanings:

anesthetic; dissolve; hydrocarbon; isomer; organic; system of classification.

There are more compounds of carbon than of any other element. Over 30,000 carbon compounds have been found in nature, and more than 500,000 compounds have been made by chemists in the laboratory. A system of classification is needed because it would be impossible to learn about each of these half-million or more compounds. It is much easier to learn about the properties of a group of compounds that are chemically alike. The way that chemists classify carbon compounds is related to an explanation of how it is possible for carbon to make so many different compounds.

To explain how it is possible to make so many different compounds, let us start with the simplest hydrocarbon, $CH_4$. If one or more hydrogen atoms are replaced with chlorine atoms, new compounds are formed.

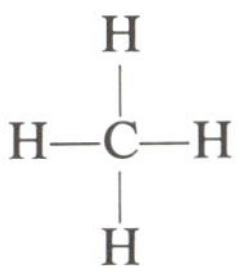

*methane*

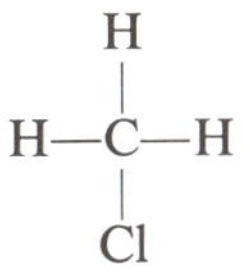

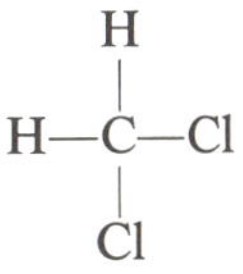

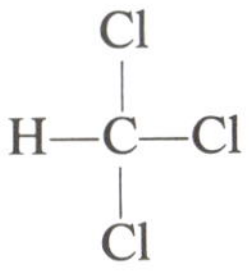

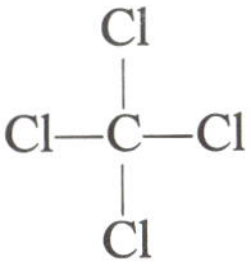

You can see by examining the formulas that four new compounds have been formed. The second compound in the second row that contains four chlorine atoms is called **carbon tetrachloride** (kär′ bən tet′ rə klô′ rīd). It is used in dry cleaning clothes because it dissolves fats and greases well. **Chloroform** (klô′ rə fôrm), or $CHCl_3$, is used as an **anesthetic** (an′ is thet′ ik). Can you find its structural formula in the group?

But wait, there is more to the story. Other atoms besides chlorine can replace hydrogen atoms in methane. For example, two atoms of chlorine and two atoms of fluorine can replace the hydrogen atoms to form $CCl_2F_2$, which has the long name of **dichlorodifluoromethane** (dī klô′ rō dī flü′ ə rō meth′ ān). The common name for this gas is Freon, and it is the gas used in refrigerators and air conditioners.

If you look carefully at the scientific name for Freon, you will see that it is not so complicated as it first appears. *Di* means "two," and thus the name indicates a methane molecule with two hydrogen atoms replaced with chlorine ("dichloro-") and two replaced with fluorine ("difluoro-"). Because of the large number of carbon compounds, it is easier to use a system of scientific names than it is to use common names. Can you name other examples of things that have both a scientific name and a common name?

To explore further the idea of how hydrogen atoms are replaced in carbon compounds, let us build some more models.

## Building Models of Modified Hydrocarbons

Use the materials you used earlier to build models of hydrocarbons. The objects used to represent hydrogen should be a different color from those used for chlorine. Start by building models of the two isomers of butane ($CH_3$—$CH_2$—$CH_2$—$CH_3$ and $CH_3$—$CH$—$CH_3$). These are the

|

$CH_3$

shortened forms of structural formulas for the two isomers of butane. They are often used in books to save space. Can you draw the regular structural formula for each of these two isomers?

Once you have built the isomers of butane, see how many ways you can replace hydrogen atoms with chlorine atoms. In addition to the two isomers, there is another thing to complicate the problem. This is illustrated by an example showing three of the ways that three chlorine atoms can replace three hydrogen atoms. As in the case of isomers, each of these three molecules has its own physical and chemical properties and thus is considered a separate compound.

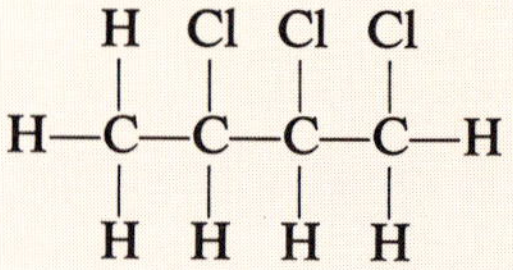

*Or*

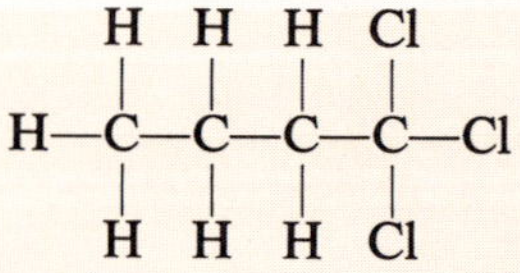

*Or*

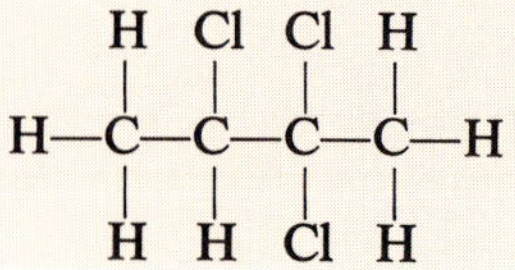

See how many ways you can replace one or more chlorine atoms on the two isomers of butane. Chemists use mathematics to figure out the number of different possibilities. Using balls and sticks, how many can you make?

Do you see now why it is possible for chemists to have made hundreds of thousands of different carbon compounds? The organic chemist works much as an architect does. He designs new compounds by putting together combinations of chains and rings with atoms of other elements also attached. The number of possibilities is unlimited. And who knows? One of the future compounds may be a cure for cancer or one of the many other diseases not yet conquered. Or it may be a new food, or a plastic for building homes or making clothes, or a key to explaining one of the mysteries of life!

You have seen that atoms of other elements can replace hydrogen in hydrocarbon molecules. There are groups of atoms, or radicals, that also can replace hydrogen. Compounds containing one of these radicals have similar properties and thus can be grouped together. Several of the common groups of carbon compounds are discussed in the next section.

### Have You Learned?

1. Explain why it is possible to have many different carbon compounds.
2. Write the formulas for methane, carbon tetrachloride, chloroform, and Freon. How is each used?

## 4. A Catalog of Carbon Compounds: Part 1

**ARE YOU READY?**

Look up the following words if you are not sure of their meanings:

enzyme; hydroxyl; nitroglycerin; solvent; synthetic.

Thousands of different carbon compounds can be made by replacing the hydrogen atoms on hydrocarbon chains with other groups of atoms. These groups of atoms give the compounds certain properties that can be used in classifying them.

### Alcohols

**Alcohols** are one of the most important groups of carbon compounds. They contain a hydroxyl group (—OH) in place of the hydrogen atoms. The structural formula for three common alcohols shows how the hydroxyl group is attached to the carbon atoms.

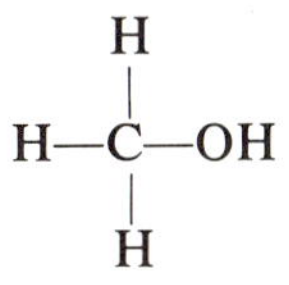

*methyl alcohol*

$CH_3OH$

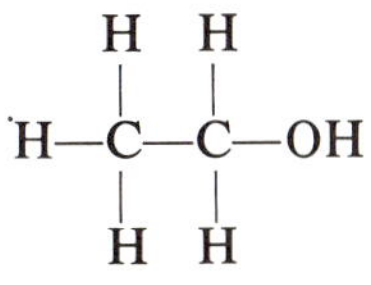

*ethyl alcohol*

$CH_3CH_2OH$

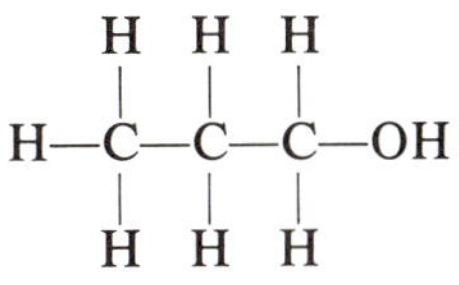

*propyl alcohol*

$CH_3CH_2CH_2OH$

**Methyl** (meth′ əl) alcohol is sometimes called *wood alcohol* because it can be made by heating wood. It was one of the compounds in the liquid you collected when you made charcoal earlier in this chapter. Methyl alcohol is used in making shellac, and since methyl alcohol is very poisonous, vapors from shellac should not be inhaled. Because it has a low freezing point, it is used as an antifreeze in automobile cooling systems.

The common name for ethyl alcohol is *grain alcohol* since it can be made by the **fermentation** (fėr′ men tā′ shən) of grain such as corn and barley. Fermentation is a chemical reaction in which enzymes produced by yeast aid in changing sugars to alcohol. Ethyl alcohol is used as a solvent and in the manufacture of many materials such as synthetic rubber and plastics. Alcoholic beverages contain ethyl alcohol.

## Preparing Ethyl Alcohol

Add 25 ml of molasses to 175 ml of water in a flask. If molasses is not available, use a 10 percent solution of table sugar. Mix ⅛ of a package of yeast with 20 ml of water. Add the yeast mixture to the molasses and water, and stir. You may wish to stopper the flask with a one-hole rubber stopper and test with limewater the gas that is given off. What will this show? Do not leave the mixture of molasses and yeast stoppered. Why would this not be a good idea?

After the mixture of molasses and yeast has set for several hours, smell the contents of the flask. Can you detect the odor of alcohol? Check in reference books to see if you can find out how to separate the alcohol from the rest of the mixture.

There are two kinds of **propyl** (prō′ pəl) alcohol. The one that has the hydroxyl group attached to carbon on the end of the chain is called normal propyl alcohol. This is the kind that is pictured on page 233. If the hydroxyl group is attached to the middle carbon atom in the chain, we have a different compound. It is called **isopropyl** (ī′ sə prō′ pəl) alcohol and is used as rubbing alcohol.

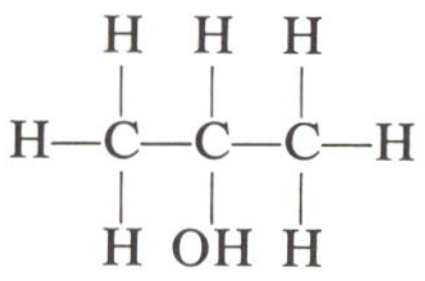

*isopropyl alcohol*

$CH_3CHOHCH_3$

As the number of carbon atoms in the chain increases, the number of different possible alcohols increases almost beyond imagination. The number of possible alcohols is also increased because some alcohols contain more than one hydroxyl group.

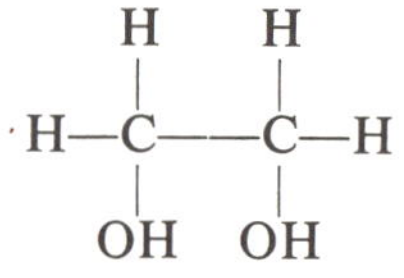

*ethylene glycol*

$CH_2OHCH_2OH$

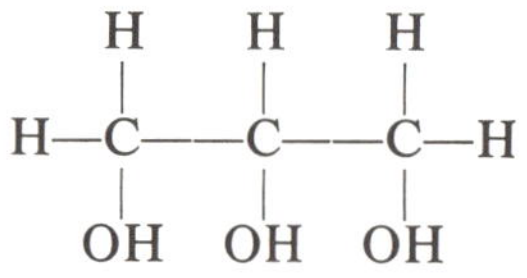

*glycerol*

$CH_2OHCHOHCH_2OH$

**Ethylene glycol** (glī′ kōl) is used as an antifreeze for automobile radiators. It has a higher boiling point than methyl alcohol, and thus there is less danger of its boiling away when the engine gets hot. **Glycerol** (glis′ ər ōl) is used in the manufacture of plastics and **nitroglycerin** (nī′ trə glis′ ər in). Nitroglycerin, which is a liquid explosive, is very dangerous to handle. Dynamite, which is made by soaking sawdust in nitroglycerin, is much safer.

## Aldehydes

Perhaps you have smelled **formaldehyde** (fôr mal′ də hīd), a compound used in biological laboratories to preserve animals. It is the simplest of the **aldehydes** (al′ də hīd′) and has the formula H—CHO. The formula is written this way to show the group 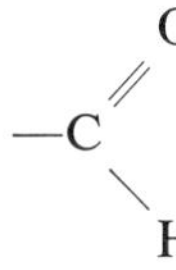 that distinguishes aldehydes from other compounds. This group may be added to a hydrogen atom as is the case of formaldehyde, or to a carbon atom in a carbon chain.

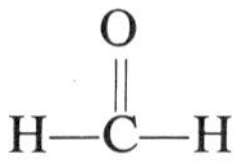

*formaldehyde*

HCHO

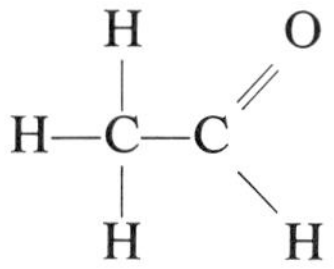

*acetaldehyde*

(*used to make acetic acid*)

$CH_3CHO$

## Ketones

The **ketones** (kē′ tōn) are compounds closely related to the aldehydes. The group that distinguishes ketones from other compounds is 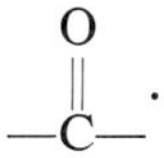. A ketone has a carbon atom or carbon chain attached to each of the bonds. The simplest ketone has a methyl group attached to each side. What would you have if a methyl group were attached to one bond of the ketone group and a hydrogen atom to the other bond? Look at the formula for acetaldehyde for a clue.

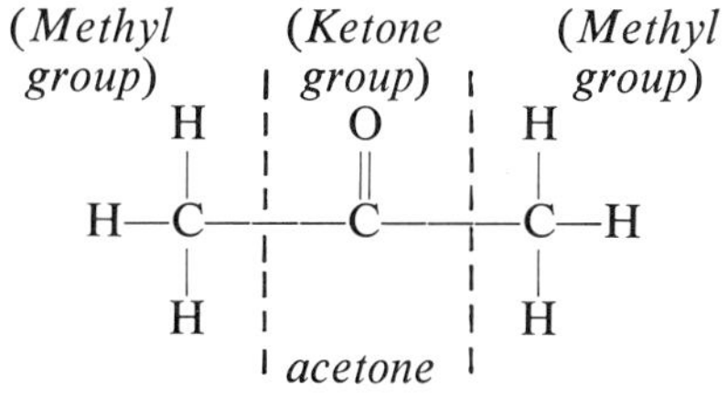


$CH_3COCH_3$

Acetone is used as a solvent for lacquers and in fingernail polish.

### Have You Learned?

Summarize what you have learned about alcohols, aldehydes, and ketones by completing the following chart. The boxes for alcohol have been filled in for you.

| | *Distinguishing Group* | *Formula for a Member (Example)* | *Name of Example* | *How Example Is Used* |
|---|---|---|---|---|
| Alcohol | –OH | $CH_3CH_2OH$ | Ethyl Alcohol | Solvent |
| Aldehyde | | | | |
| Ketone | | | | |

## 5. A Catalog of Carbon Compounds: Part 2

> **ARE YOU READY?**
>
> Look up the following words if you are not sure of their meanings:
>
> aldehyde; anesthetic; bacteria; enzyme; fermentation; ketone; organic.

In addition to alcohols, aldehydes, and ketones, there are several more groups of compounds composed of hydrocarbon chains and a distinguishing group. Among these are acids, esters, and ethers.

### Acids

Acetic acid, which is found in vinegar, is an important organic acid. The formula

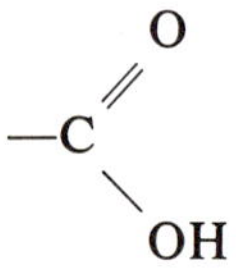

illustrates the group that distinguishes acids from the very similar aldehydes and ketones.

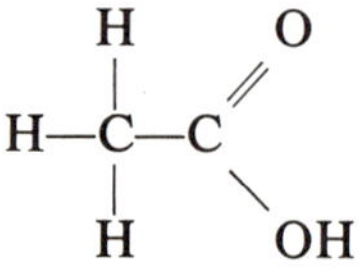

*acetic acid*

$CH_3COOH$

One way that vinegar is made illustrates the relationship between alcohols, aldehydes, and acids. If fruit juices such as apple juice or cider are allowed to ferment, sugars in the juices are the raw materials for a chain of reactions.

$$C_6H_{12}O_6 \xrightarrow{(enzymes)} 2\ CH_3CH_2OH + 2\ CO_2\uparrow$$

(*Sweet cider contains sugar.*) (*ethyl alcohol*)

The ethyl alcohol through the action of bacteria in the cider is combined with oxygen to form an aldehyde. The aldehyde in turn combines with more oxygen to form an acid.

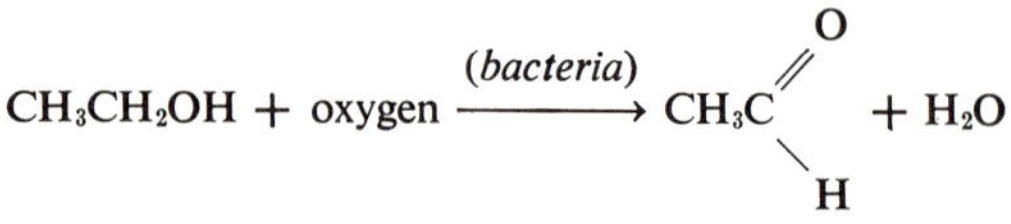

(*acetaldehyde*)

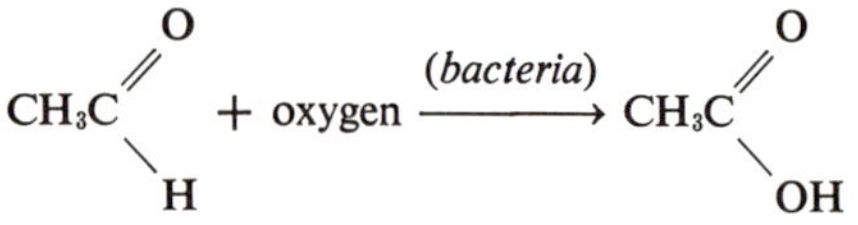

(*acetic acid*)

Foods contain many acids including the following:

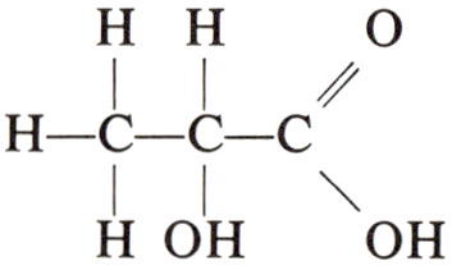

*lactic acid*

Forms when the sugar in milk ferments

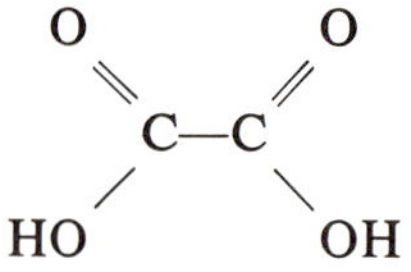

*oxalic* (oks al′ ik) *acid*

Found in foods such as spinach and rhubarb

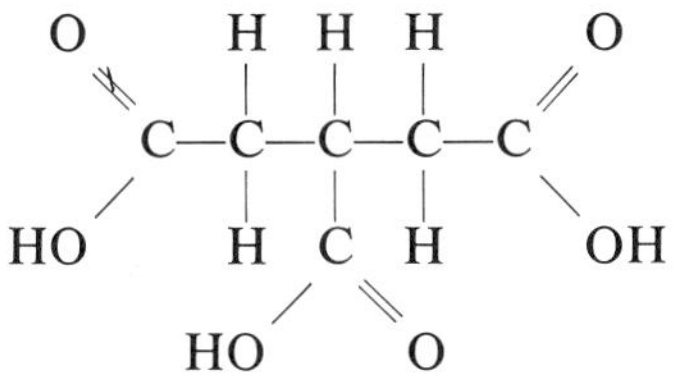

*citric acid*

Found in foods such as oranges, lemons, and grapefruit

An examination of the structural formulas for these acids reveals that some acids contain more than one acid group:

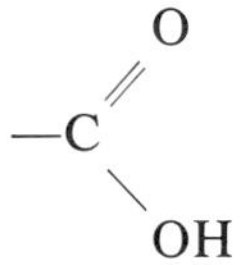

## Esters

**Esters** (es′ tər) are a group of compounds of which many of the members have the odor of ripe fruit. An ester is the product of a reaction between an acid and an alcohol. The equation below (Figure 7.10) shows how this reaction takes place. The dotted line shows the part that splits off from each molecule. Note how similar this reaction and the products are to the reaction of an acid and base.

The group that distinguishes esters from other compounds is 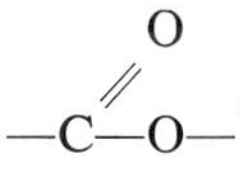. This group is written in the shorter form as —COO—. A methyl group or hydrocarbon chain can be attached to each of these bonds, as you can see in the structural formula for methyl acetate, Figure 7.11.

Formulas for several other esters show how the —COO— group is always conducted to a methyl group or hydrocarbon chain.

**7.10** Notice what is split off each molecule forming water and methyl acetate.

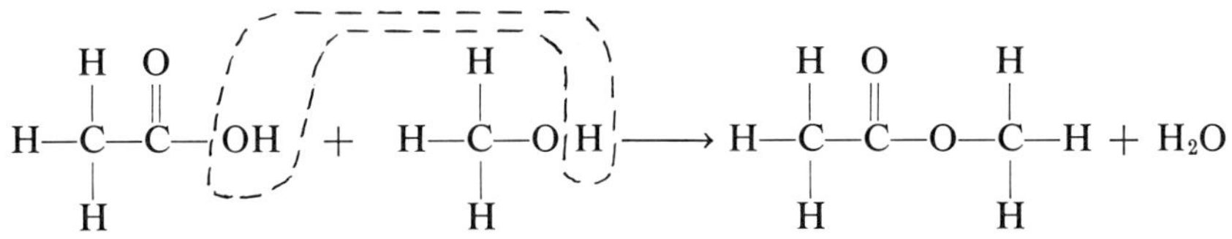


**7.11** These are formulas for esters with their odors.

| *Formula* | *Odor* |
|---|---|
| $CH_3COOCH_2CH_2CHCH_3$ (with $CH_3$ branch on the CH) | banana |
| $CH_3COOCH_2CH_2CH_2CH_2CH_2CH_2CH_2CH_3$ | orange |
| $CH_3CH_2CH_2COOCH_3$ | pineapple |
| $CH_3CH_2CH_2COOCH_2CH_3$ | apricot and peach |

### Making an Ester

Add 6 ml of acetic acid to 4 ml of ethyl alcohol in a large test tube. Carefully add 4 or 5 drops of concentrated sulfuric acid. Heat the test tube by placing it in a beaker of hot water. (**CAUTION: Avoid getting any of the sulfuric acid on you!**)

Carefully sniff the vapors by waving your hand over the top of the test tube. **Do not place your face over the test tube.** Note the odor of the product, ethyl acetate.

Other esters can be made using the same procedure. **Always handle sulfuric acid with care, and never point the test tube toward anyone.**

| *Odor* | *Materials and Procedure* |
|---|---|
| Wintergreen | Add 1 ml of methyl alcohol to 1 gram of salicylic acid, and then 3 drops of sulfuric acid. Heat in water bath. |
| Banana | Add 3 ml of amyl alcohol to 5 ml of acetic acid, and then 1 ml of sulfuric acid. Heat in water bath. |
| Pineapple | Add 2 ml of ethyl alcohol to 2 ml of butyric acid, and then 1 ml of sulfuric acid. Heat in water bath. |

## Ethers

Have you ever smelled **ether** (ē′ thər)? It has a very characteristic odor that you are not likely to forget. Ethers are good solvents, but they should be handled with care. They are very *flammable*, and their vapors can cause an explosion.

The formula for *diethyl ether*, the compound used as an anesthetic, shows that ethers are made up of two hydrocarbon groups connected by an oxygen atom (—O—).

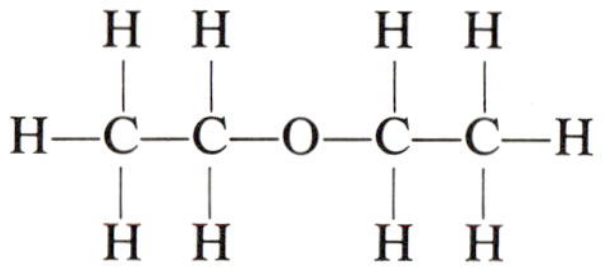

*diethyl ether*

$CH_3CH_2OCH_2CH_3$

## Fats

Fats can also be classified with the groups that have been described in the last two sections of this chapter. However, since many fats are eaten, they are described in the next section that deals with the chemistry of groups of compounds found in foods.

### Have You Learned?

Summarize what you learned about acids, esters, and ethers by completing a chart like the one in the last section. You may wish to include your answers from this section on the same chart you made in the last section. In this way, you will be able to describe the different groups of carbon compounds by glancing at your chart.

## 6. Chemistry of Foods

**ARE YOU READY?**

Look up the following words if you are not sure of their meanings:

alcohol; aldehyde; carbohydrate; digestion; energy; ester; ketone; structural formula.

When you sit down to a big breakfast of pancakes covered with syrup and butter, bacon cooked just the way you like it, and a glass of fruit juice or milk, you probably think about how good it tastes. There is also a lot of science in that big breakfast. Why do we need food? What do various kinds of foods contain? What happens to food in our bodies?

The **biochemist** (bī′ ō kem′ ist) specializes in the chemistry of living things, and food is one of the things he investigates. He and other scientists have found that we need food for two reasons. First, food supplies us with the energy we need to remain alive, play basketball, mow the yard, and clean the house. Second, we need food to grow and to replace worn-out parts of the body. As you shall see in Chapter 11, the atoms and molecules of the human body are continually replaced by new atoms and molecules from the food we eat.

## Carbohydrates

Carbohydrates contain the elements carbon, hydrogen, and oxygen and are the chief source of the body's energy. They are sometimes called "energy foods." If you ate the breakfast described above, you would have taken into your body some *sugar* that was in the syrup and fruit juice. You would also have consumed some *starch* that was in the flour used to make the pancakes. Sugars and starches are two important kinds of carbohydrates.

The sugar in the syrup and the fruit juice is what chemists call **monosaccharide** (mon′ ə sak′ ə rīd). *Mono* means "one," or "single," and *saccharide* means "sugar." Many monosaccharides, which are also called single sugars, have the formula $C_6H_{12}O_6$. There are several different six-carbon monosaccharides, each having the same formula but different properties. You are correct if you guessed that they have different structural formulas. The structural formulas for two common single sugars show how they differ. Notice that **glucose** (glü′ kōs) contains an aldehyde group and five alcohol groups. **Fructose** (fruk′ tōs) also contains five alcohol groups, but a *ketone* instead of an aldehyde group.

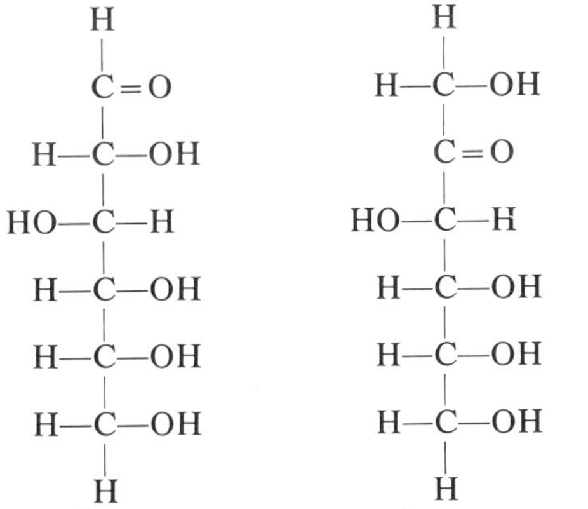

*glucose* (found in fruits and corn syrup) *fructose* (found in ripe fruit and honey)

**Sucrose** (sü′ krōs), or table sugar, has the formula $C_{12}H_{22}O_{11}$. It is called a **disaccharide** (dī sak′ ə rīd), or double sugar. By comparing its formula with that of glucose or fructose, you can see that it contains twice as many carbon atoms. During digestion and in cooking certain foods, sucrose splits apart to form two monosaccharides.

$$\underset{sucrose}{C_{12}H_{22}O_{11}} + H_2O \longrightarrow \underset{glucose}{C_6H_{12}O_6} + \underset{fructose}{C_6H_{12}O_6}$$

When two or more saccharides like glucose and fructose combine, the compound is called a **polysaccharide** (pol′ i sak′ ə rīd). *Poly* means "many." Starch is a polysaccharide that contains 20 to 400 saccharide groups. During digestion the large starch molecules are split into smaller sugar molecules. You can experience this by slowly chewing a soda cracker until it tastes sweet. An enzyme in the saliva in your mouth aids in the breakdown of starch into sugar.

**Cellulose** (sel′ ū lōs), like starch, is a polysaccharide. Molecules of cellulose are generally even larger than starch molecules, being made up of 50 to 5,000 saccharide groups. Cellulose for the most part does not break down during digestion in humans, but serves to provide the needed *roughage* in the diet. Your breakfast of pancakes and bacon contained little cellulose. Foods like celery, cabbage, and lettuce contain a great deal of cellulose.

## Proteins

**Proteins** (prō′ tēn) contain nitrogen in addition to carbon, hydrogen, and oxygen. Some proteins also contain sulfur, phosphorus, and iron. The lean part of the bacon in your imaginary breakfast contained protein, as do eggs, nuts, and meats. Proteins are the source of much of the materials used in body growth and repair.

Proteins are giant molecules composed of simpler substances called **amino** (ə mē′ nō) **acids.** The structural formulas for two amino acids, **glycine** (glī′ sēn) and **tyrosine** (tī′ rə sēn), show that they contain an acid

group 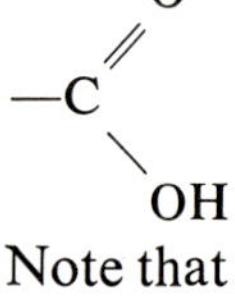 and at least one nitrogen

atom. Note that tyrosine is a glycine group attached to a benzene ring. All amino acids, and thus all proteins, contain one or more glycine groups per molecule.

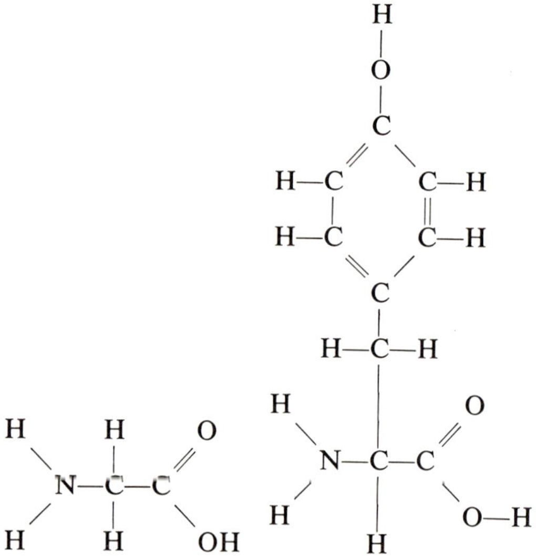

*glycine* *tyrosine*

During digestion in the body, the proteins are broken down into amino acids. The amino acids are transported by the blood to the cells, where they are reassembled to form protein. Since amino acids play such a vital role in living things, they are one of the groups of compounds scientists look for in exploring outer space. The presence of amino acids could indicate the possible presence of life!

## Fats

Bacon and the shortening or cooking oil, used to make the pancakes, contain compounds classified as fats. Fats are *esters* that form when *glycerol*, an alcohol, combines with an acid that has a long carbon chain. The equation (Figure 7.12) shows how glycerol combines with stearic acid to form a fat found in beef and lamb as well as in bacon and other pork.

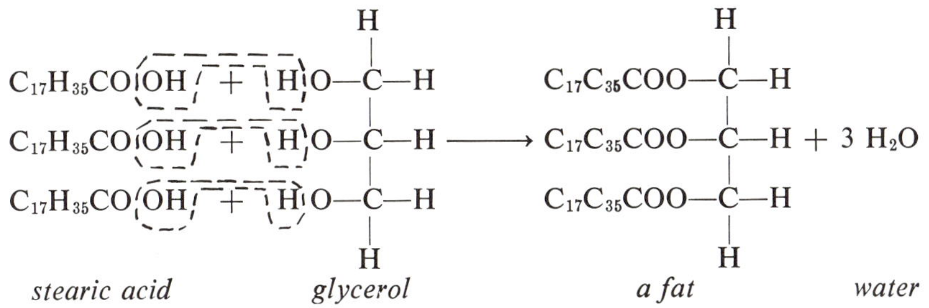

**7.12** Three molecules of stearic acid combine with one of glycerol forming fat and water.

The body uses fats as a source of energy. When more food is eaten than the body uses, some of this surplus is stored in the body as fat.

## Vitamins

**Vitamins** (vī′ tə min), chemical compounds that are necessary for good health, are also found in food. They act as catalysts, and without them many of the chemical reactions in the human body cannot take place. A well-balanced diet usually supplies us with an adequate amount of each vitamin. The vitamins vary in complexity, as shown by the formulas for four of them.

| | |
|---|---|
| Vitamin A | $C_{20}H_{29}OH$ |
| Vitamin $B_1$ | $C_{12}H_{17}ON_4SClHCl$ |
| Vitamin C | $C_6H_8O_6$ |
| Vitamin D | $C_{28}H_{44}O$ |

## Testing Foods

*Testing for Starch*

Add a few drops of iodine solution to a slice of white potato. A bluish-black color indicates the presence of starch. Does the potato contain starch? Test other foods for starch.

*Testing for Sugar*

Place 10 cc of Benedict's solution in a test tube and gently heat over a Bunsen burner. When it begins to boil, add a few pieces of apple. What is the color of the Benedict's solution now? Test foods such as oranges, corn syrup, and table sugar. Do all sugars make Benedict's solution change color?

*Testing for Fat*

Rub a piece of bacon over some unglazed paper such as wrapping paper or paper toweling. A clear spot on the paper is a test for fat. Does butter contain fat? Cooking oil? What other foods?

*Testing for Proteins*

Place some egg white in a test tube. Using an eyedropper, add concentrated nitric acid to the sample. **CAUTION: Be careful not to get acid on your skin.**

Gently heat the sample until it boils. This can be done by passing the tube in and out of the flame. Be careful not to point the top of the test tube toward anyone. A yellowish color indicates the presence of protein.

Pour off the acid, and let the test tube cool. Add a few drops of ammonium

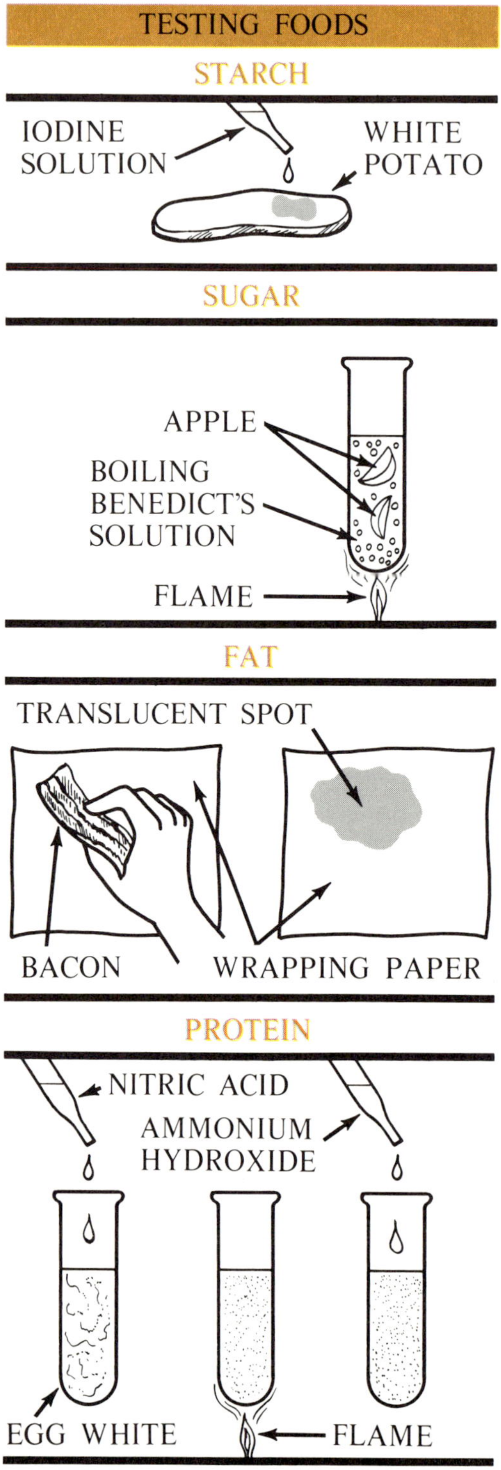


hydroxide. The protein should turn to an orange color. Try testing other foods to see if they contain proteins.

---

### Have You Learned?

Select the word from Column B that best corresponds with each definition in Column A. (Do not write in your book.)

| *Column A* | *Column B* |
|---|---|
| 1. Starch | a. carbohydrate |
| 2. Food stored in the body | b. fats |
| 3. Cellulose | c. proteins |
| 4. An ester of an alcohol and acid | d. vitamins |
| 5. Disaccharide | |
| 6. Act as catalysts | |
| 7. Contain amino acids | |
| 8. Sugars | |
| 9. Known as "energy foods" | |
| 10. Used in growth and body repair | |

## 7. Two Important Life Processes

**ARE YOU READY?**

Look up the following words if you are not sure of their meanings:

carbohydrate; cellulose; digestion; glucose; protein; sucrose.

An entire breakfast—pancakes, syrup, butter, bacon, fruit juice, and milk—once was part of a green plant. The flour in the pancake was made from the grain of wheat. The bacon represents a new form of the corn eaten by a hog. Can you explain how the rest of the breakfast was once part of a green plant?

## Food Factories

Green plants make food by a process called **photosynthesis** (fō′ tō sin′ thə sis). *Photo* means "light" and *synthesis* means "built up" or "put together." The following equation shows how during photosynthesis carbon dioxide and water combine to form glucose and oxygen. Since this process occurs only in the presence of **chlorophyll** (klô′ rə fil), the green pigment in plants, and sunlight, they are included in the equation.

$$6\ CO_2 + 6\ H_2O \xrightarrow[\text{sunlight}]{\text{chlorophyll}} C_6H_{12}O_6 + 6\ O_2$$

If you think about the equation for a moment, you'll probably begin to suspect that it doesn't tell the whole story. The equation shows that glucose and oxygen are produced. From your study of foods, you know that many molecules making up food are really much more complex than glucose.

The manufacture of glucose is just the first step in a series of reactions. The glucose molecules are building blocks for making double sugars, such as sucrose, and the giant molecules of starch and cellulose. Of course, the plant also takes in nitrogen and other mineral elements through its roots. These are combined with carbohydrates and thus they form proteins.

**7.13** Green plants make food by photosynthesis.

*David Telfair*

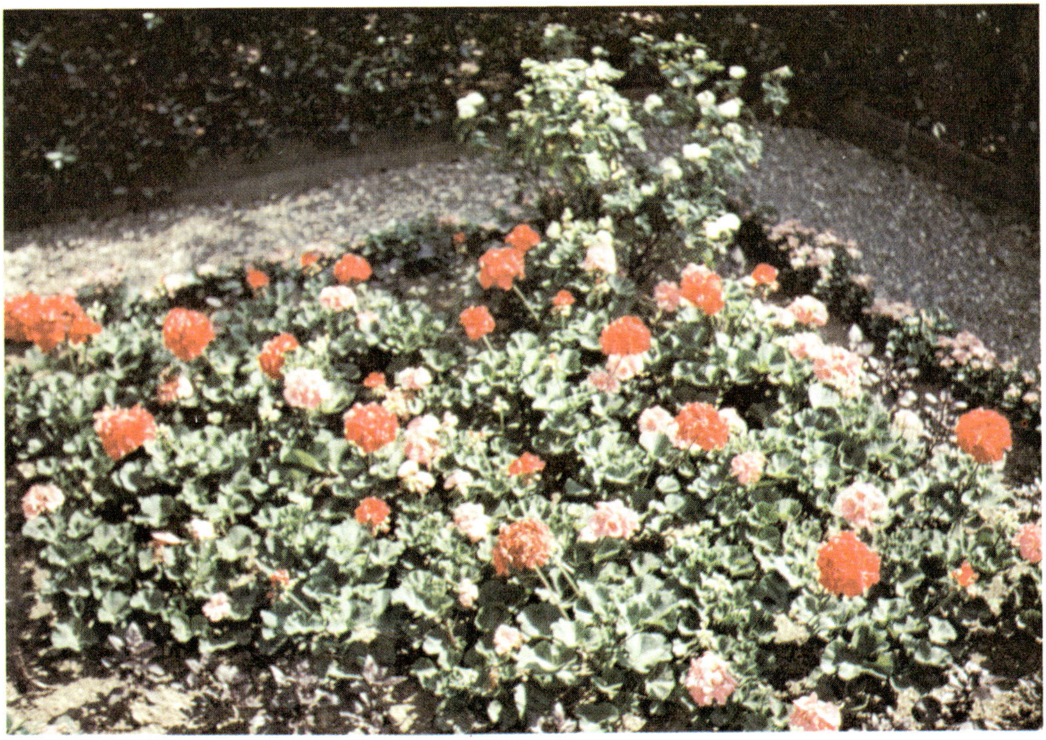

## Using Food

When the food manufactured by green plants is eaten by animals, the large molecules are broken down by the process of digestion. The smaller molecules pass through the walls of the stomach and intestines and into the blood. The blood carries the food to the cells of the body.

It is in the cells that the food combines with oxygen, or is "burned," and energy is released. This energy-producing process is called **respiration** (res′ pə rā′ shən). The term *respiration* is also used to mean breathing, the process by which cells receive oxygen and get rid of carbon dioxide.

The following equation shows how oxygen and carbon dioxide are involved in one type of respiration.

$$C_6H_{12}O_6 + 6\,O_2 \xrightarrow{enzymes} 6\,CO_2 + 6\,H_2O + \text{energy}$$

Notice how this reaction for respiration is just the opposite of the simplified reaction for photosynthesis shown earlier. The energy released is the energy that was stored in the food and that originally came from the sun. As in the case of photosynthesis, there is much more to the story than this equation for respiration actually shows.

Although the combination of glucose and oxygen in cells actually involves dozens of steps, the reaction can be shown in four main steps. This is done to give you some idea of the nature of the chemistry that goes on in living things. The equations have been written using structural formulas for some of the compounds to help you see what happens. They have not been balanced because they are rather complicated.

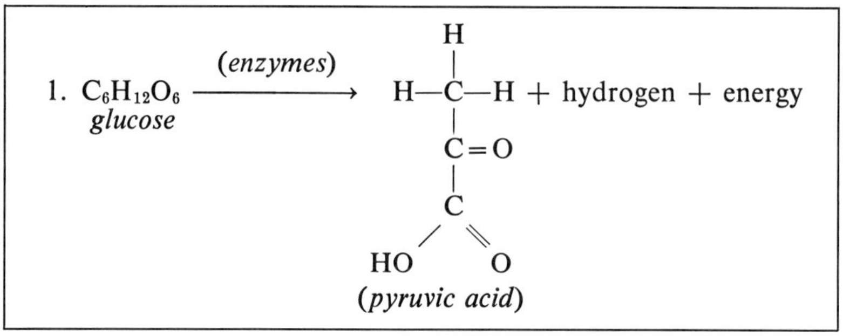


The glucose molecule is split in half to form two molecules of **pyruvic** (pī rü′ vik) acid, four atoms of hydrogen, and a relatively small amount of energy.

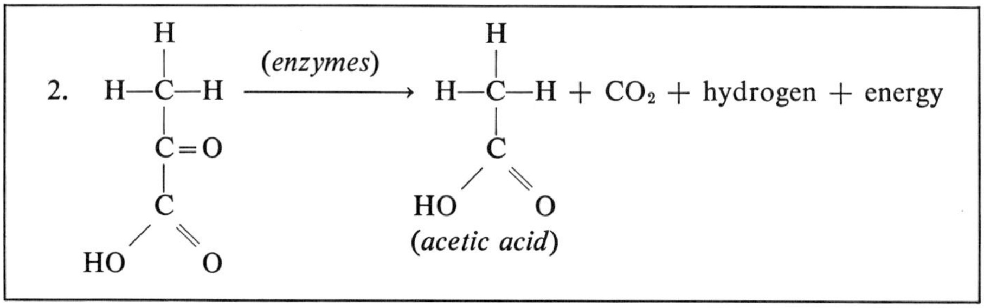

The pyruvic acid is broken down into acetic acid, carbon dioxide, and hydrogen atoms. More energy is released than in step one.

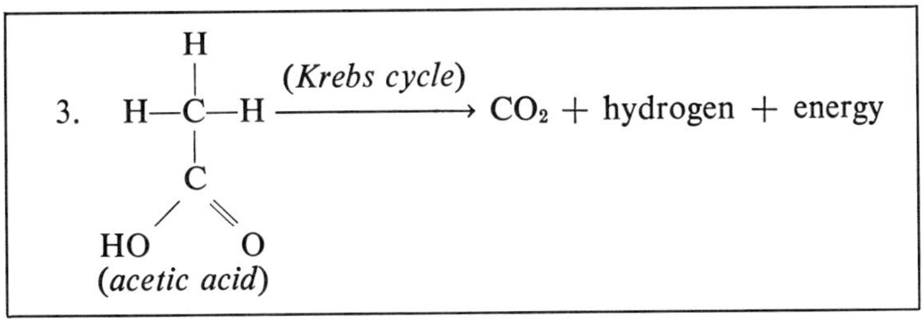


Through a series of reactions known as the **Krebs** (krebz) **Cycle,** the acetic acid is broken down into carbon dioxide and hydrogen, and much energy is produced.

$$4.\ \text{hydrogen} + O_2 \xrightarrow{(enzymes)} H_2O$$

In this, oxygen combines with the hydrogen produced in the preceding reactions.

If oxygen is not available during respiration, as in the case of fermentation, pyruvic acid is changed to ethyl alcohol and carbon dioxide. Do you understand how apple juice can be used to make both acetic acid (vinegar) and alcohol?

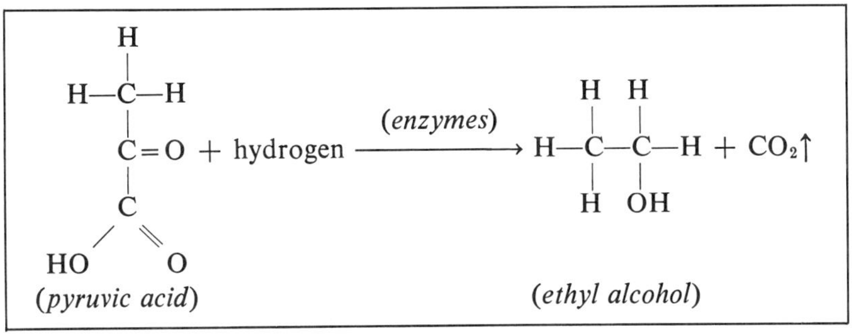


During exercise, the blood in the body cannot carry enough oxygen to the cells. When this happens, the pyruvic acid in the cells is changed to lactic acid.

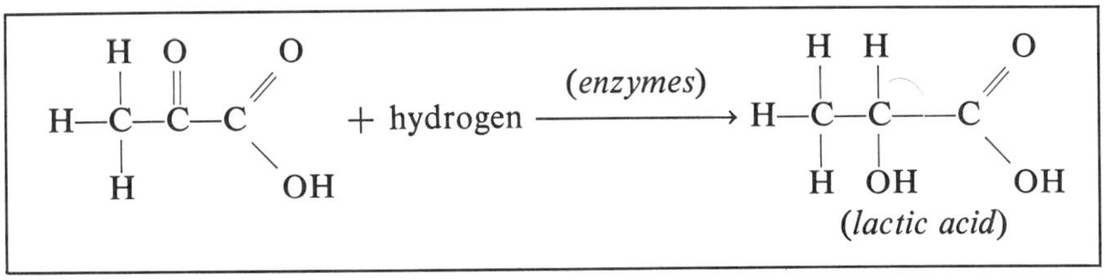

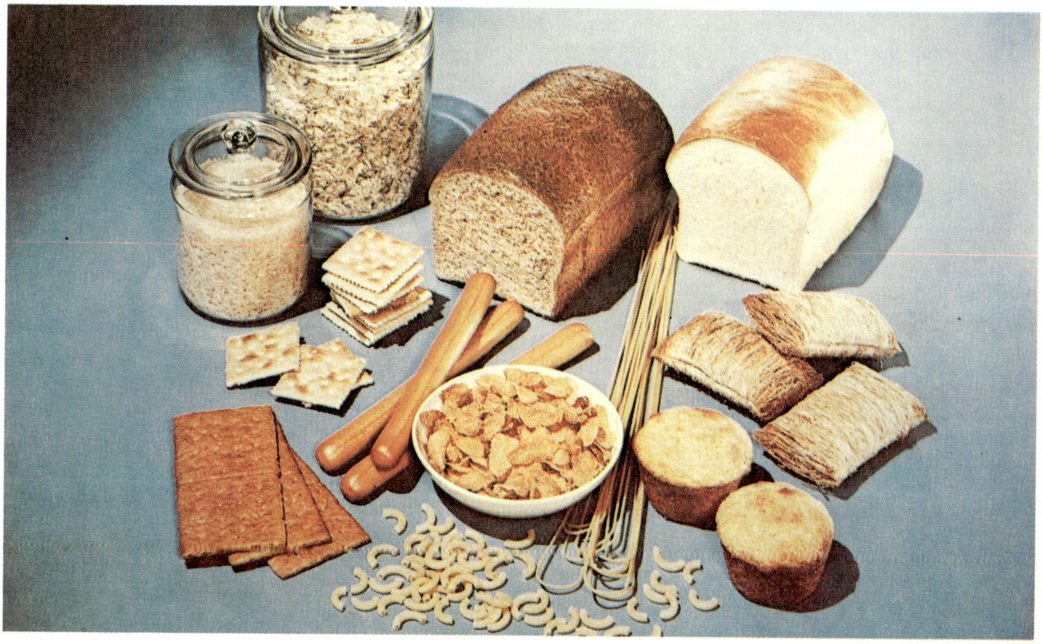

National Dairy Council

**7.14** Cereal group

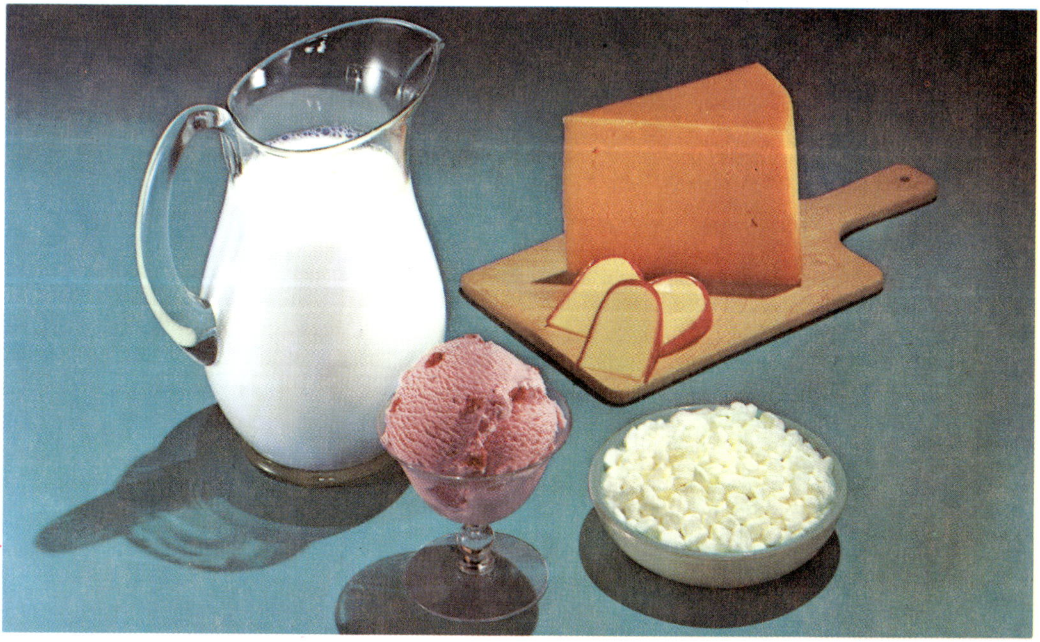

National Dairy Council

**7.15** Dairy group

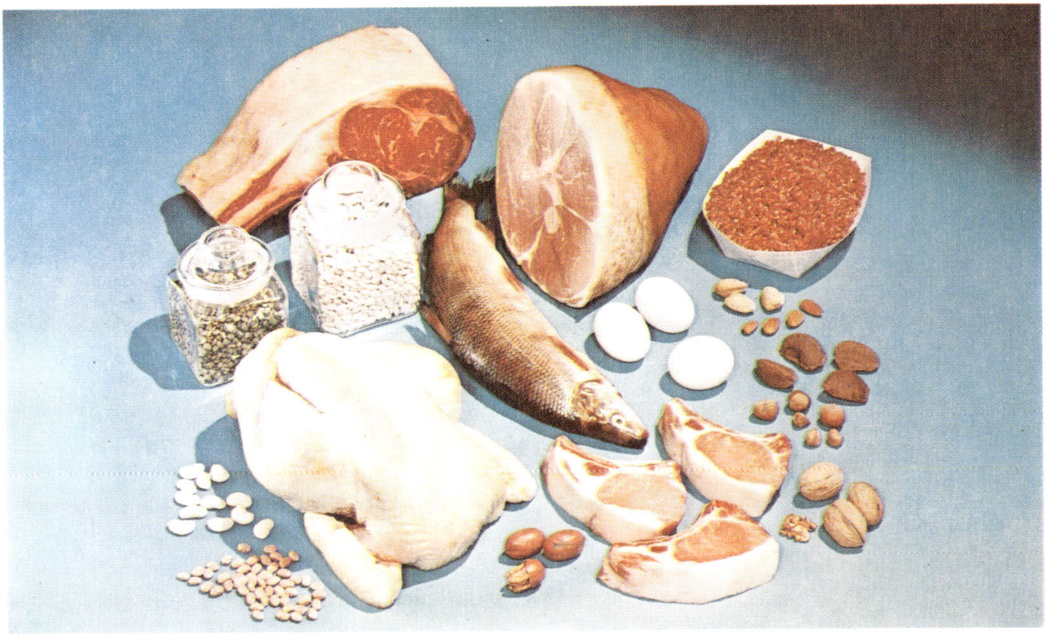

National Dairy Council

**7.16** Meat and protein group

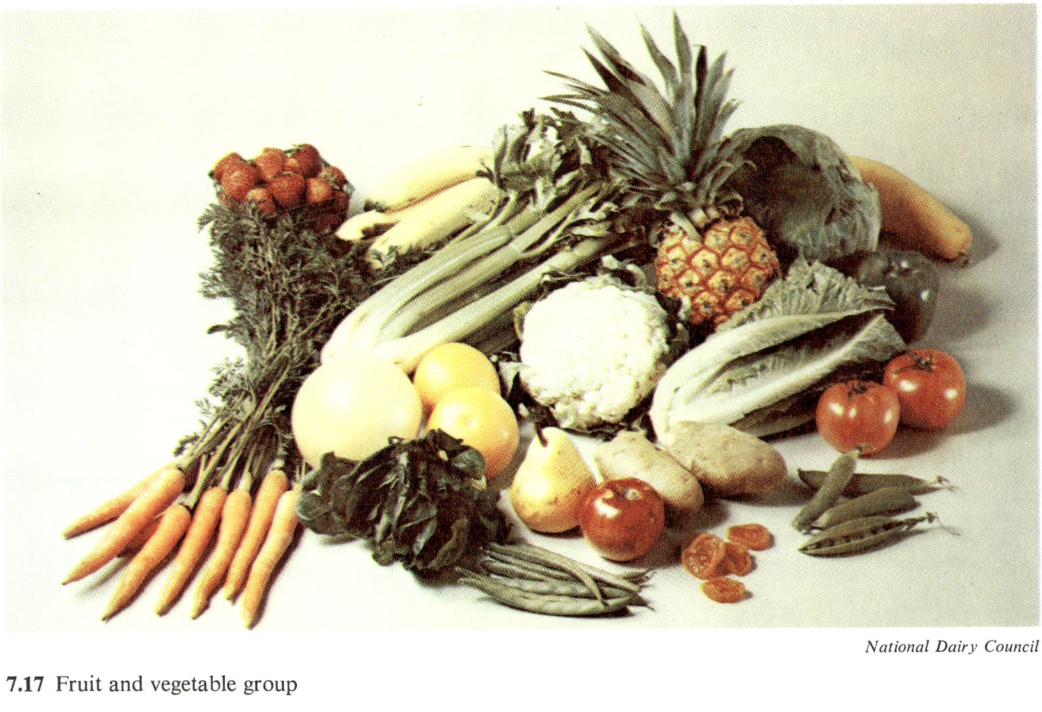

National Dairy Council

**7.17** Fruit and vegetable group

It is this lactic acid in the muscles that makes you feel tired. When you stop your exercises, the oxygen supply catches up with the demand, and the lactic acid is changed to carbon dioxide and water.

These reactions should show you that the basic life processes, such as photosynthesis and respiration, are a series of chemical reactions.

### Have You Learned?

In your notebook indicate which of the following definitions are best described by *photosynthesis* and which by *respiration.*

1. Carbon dioxide used and oxygen produced
2. Occurs only in green plants
3. Glucose produced
4. Occurs in both plants and animals
5. Pyruvic acid changed to lactic acid
6. Oxygen used and carbon dioxide produced
7. A type of reaction that occurs without oxygen and called fermentation
8. Occurs only in the presence of chlorophyll and sunlight

## 8. Putting Organic Chemistry to Work

**ARE YOU READY?**

Look up the following words if you are not sure of their meanings:

cellulose; fabric; fiber; glycerol; stearic acid; synthetic.

People have used chemistry for a long time to make useful products. Pliny (pli′ ni) (A.D. 23–79), a Roman writer, described how soap was made by cooking together fats and *potash* obtained from the ashes of wood. Later the Spanish used olive oil to make Castile (kas tēl′) soap, and the English used whale oil. Pioneer housewives in this country saved all the fats from cooking and combined these with wood ashes to make soap.

A few people still make soap this way, and you can also. It is suggested, however, that you use sodium hydroxide and fat first. Later you may wish to try making soap with wood ashes.

### Making Soap

MATERIALS:

Beaker, ring stand, Bunsen burner, funnel, flask, glass stirring rod, filter paper or screen wire, fat such as lard or bacon grease, sodium hydroxide (approximately 10% solution), table salt

PROCEDURE:

Warm about 50 milliliters of fat in a beaker, and then slowly add enough 10 percent solution of NaOH solution to cover the fat with about 2 cm of solution. (**CAUTION: You should be wearing goggles and an apron. The mixture may splatter. If any gets on you, wash it off with water at once.**) Gently boil the mixture for about 10 minutes, stirring it with a glass rod as it cooks.

After the mixture has cooled for about 10 minutes, "salt" the mixture by adding two tablespoons of salt (NaCl). The soap floats in the salt water and can be skimmed off with a plastic spoon. The soap should be washed by placing it in a filter and running cold water through it several times. This should get rid of most of the excess sodium hydroxide. A piece of screen wire in place of the filter paper can be used to speed the process.

Check with your teacher before you use a little of the soap to wash your hands. It probably still contains some sodium hydroxide and should not be used as a face soap.

You may wish to experiment making soap using other fats. Cottonseed oil, olive oil, coconut oil, and linseed oil can be used. In some cases, the soap will be a liquid. Can you devise a way to separate the liquid soap from the excess sodium hydroxide solution?

---

The equation in Section 6 (page 241) for the formation of a fat found in bacon and other pork shows how stearic acid combines with glycerol.

The following equation (in the ruled box) shows how NaOH reacts with this fat to form a soap, with glycerol as a *by-product*.

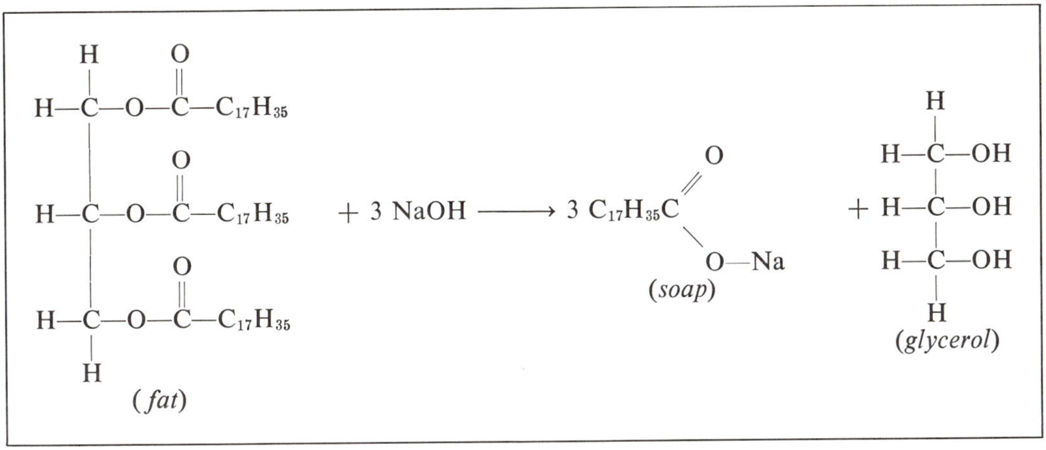


Soaps have the disadvantage of forming a scum when used with "hard" water. Hard water contains calcium and magnesium ions, and the soap molecules combine with these ions to form compounds that do not dissolve in water. This is what causes the ring to form around the inside of the bathtub.

Chemists have developed **synthetic detergents** (sin thet′ ik di tėr′ jənt) that do not form scums in hard water. "Synthetic" comes from the word "synthesis" and is used to describe things made or put together by man. Synthetic soaps and other substances used in cleaning are called *detergents*. Most of the soap powders used in washing machines and dishwashers are synthetic detergents. Some have been developed for use in cold water, and some clean without suds. Unlike soap, some synthetic detergents cannot be broken down into simpler compounds by bacteria. Because of this they have become a serious pollution problem in streams and lakes.

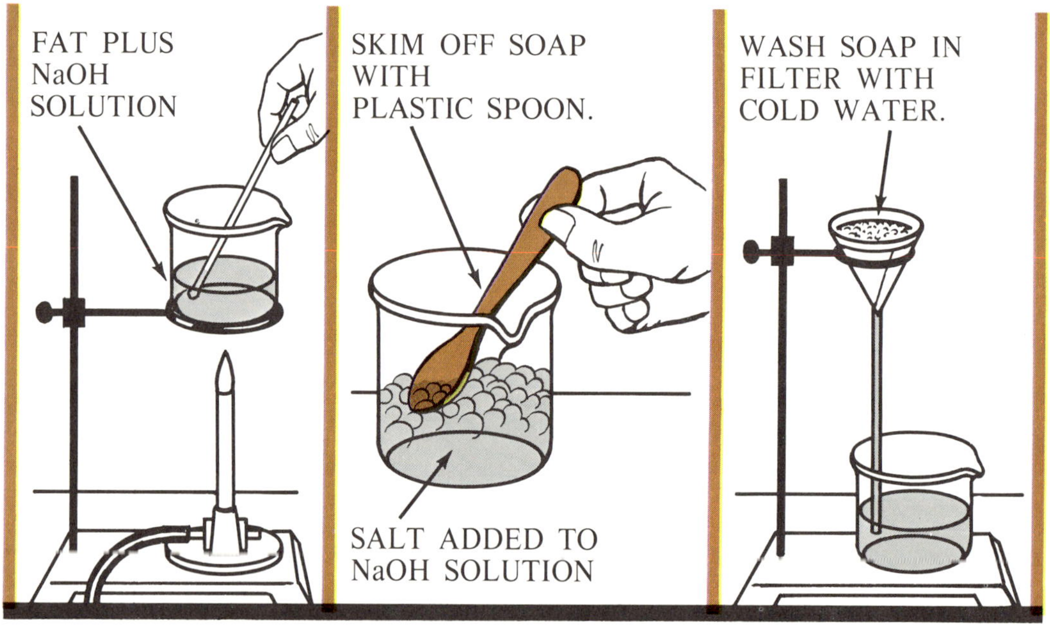


**7.18** Get some fat from home and use it to make soap at school.

## New Fibers for Our Clothing

Chemists have not only developed synthetic detergents to wash our clothes, but they have also developed synthetic fibers for making them. **Rayon** (rā′ on), the first synthetic fiber, was made as a substitute for silk. It is made by dissolving cellulose in a solution and forcing the solution through very small holes into a solution of acid. The acid changes the dissolved cellulose back to a solid in the form of long fibers. Many of our clothes contain rayon. It also has many other uses, such as making the cords used in automobile tires. A method of making rayon in the laboratory is described in the Workshop on page 256.

**Nylon** is a synthetic material made by a

**7.19** This equation shows only part of the formula for a molecule of nylon.

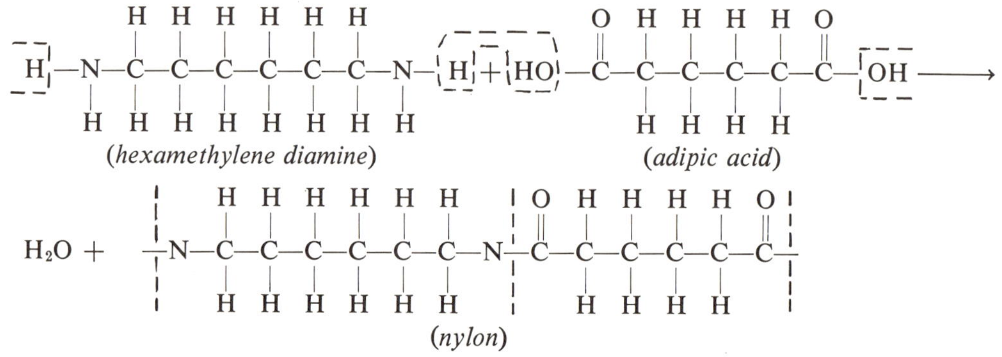

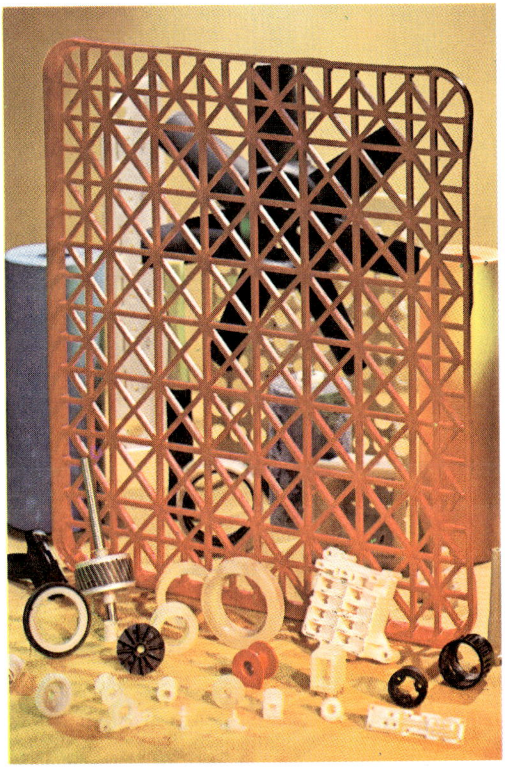

E. I. du Pont de Nemours & Company

**7.20** Various mechanical components of plastic

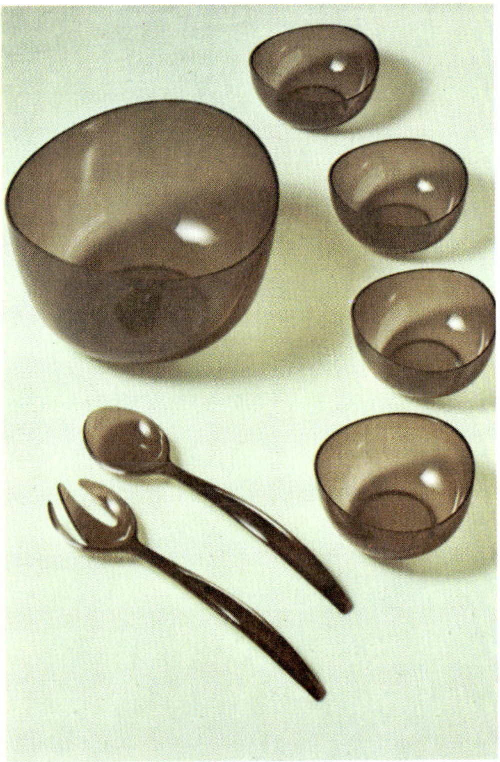

E. I. du Pont de Nemours & Company

**7.21** Salad bowls and utensils of plastic

process called **polymerization** (pə lim′ ər i zā′ shən). In this process, large molecules or **polymers** (pol′ ə mər), are made out of smaller molecules. You have already read about starch and cellulose, which are two polymers found in nature.

In the case of nylon, two compounds with the long names of **hexamethylene diamine** (hek′ sə meth′ ə lēn dī′ ə mēn′) and **adipic** (ə dip′ ik) **acid** combine to form long chains that make up nylon. Figure 7.19 shows how these compounds combine. Be sure to note that only a small part of the nylon molecule is shown. How many ways can you name that nylon is used? Don't overlook its many uses in addition to clothing.

**Dacron** (dā′ kron) and **Orlon** (ôr′ lon) also are produced by the process of polymerization. Fabrics made using these two polymers are resistant to creasing and wrinkling. Dacron also has the advantage of having a high resistance to sunlight.

## Plastics

Look around your classroom or one room in your home such as the kitchen. How many ways can you see plastics being used? The synthetic fibers, such as nylon and Orlon, are just two examples. Chemists have developed hundreds of other synthetic materials, which are called plastics.

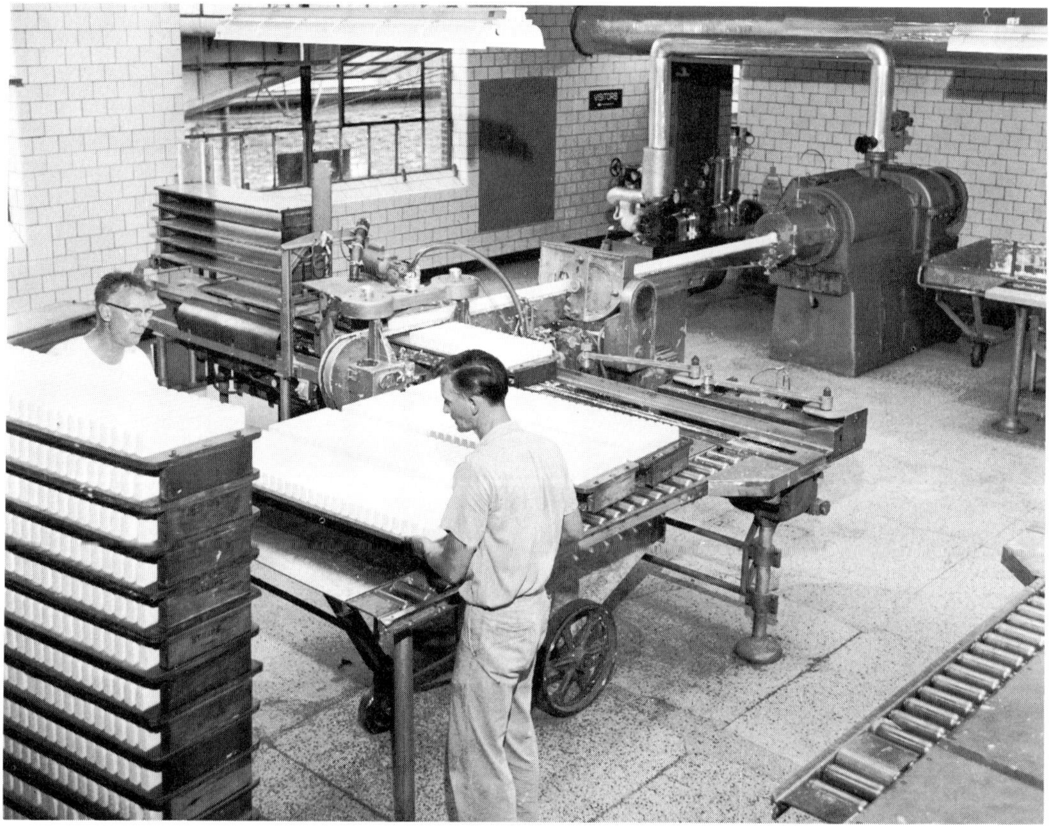

Courtesy of Proctor & Gamble Company

**7.22** Long bars of soap are here cut into cakes.

One major group of plastics becomes soft when heated. They are used to make ice cube trays, squeeze bottles, clear wrappings for food, garden hoses, toys, and phonograph records. Another group of plastics is formed under heat and pressure into permanent shapes. These plastics have such uses as buttons, radio cabinets, and parts for telephones.

As the population of the world increases, our supplies of natural building materials, such as lumber and metal, will be used up. More and more things will be made of plastic, but this is not the only reason for using plastics. They have many characteristics that make them better than other materials. They don't rust as do many metals and they don't rot as do many woods. Many are good insulators because they do not conduct electricity and heat. They can be formed into any shape, thus reducing manufacturing costs.

The age we live in is often called the atomic age, the space age, or the age of computers. True, many advances have been made in these areas of science and technology. If this practice of naming periods of time after scientific advances continues, the age ahead may be called the *Age of Plastics!*

## Have You Learned?

1. What substances are used to make a soap?
2. What advantages do synthetic detergents have over soap when they are being used in hard water?
3. What are two synthetic fibers made by the process of polymerization? Is the formation of a fat or the making of soap more like the making of a polymer?
4. What are plastics? What advantages do plastics have over other materials such as wood and metals?

## REVIEW QUESTIONS

1. Describe the various forms of carbon such as diamond and graphite, and tell how each is used. Explain why the properties of diamond differ so much from those of the other forms of carbon.
2. Draw the structural formulas for methane, ethylene, acetylene, and benzene.
3. What is an isomer? Explain how the existence of isomers increases the number of possible carbon compounds having the same number of carbon atoms.
4. Make a chart listing the following groups of organic compounds, the distinguishing group of atoms in each case, and at least one example of each group of compounds: alcohols, aldehydes, ketones, acids, esters, ethers.
5. Prepare a second chart to summarize the classification of compounds found in foods. The main heading should be carbohydrates, proteins, fats, and vitamins. Show where the following fit in the chart, and give an example of each: monosaccharide, disaccharide, starch, cellulose, acid, sugar.
6. Write the basic or general equations for photosynthesis and respiration. Define each term, and explain the importance of each process in living things.
7. Summarize the chemistry involved in making soap, synthetic fibers, and plastics.

## CAN YOU FIND OUT?

*It may be necessary to use encyclopedias or other reference books in answering the following questions.*

1. Can you find out how organic chemistry is used in the petroleum industry to refine crude oil and in processes such as cracking and polymerization?
2. Investigate the chemistry of drugs. For example, what is the structural formula for aspirin, or acetylsalicylic acid? How is it made?
3. Find out more about photosynthesis and respiration. What are the light and dark reactions in photosynthesis? What methods do scientists use to investigate the chemical processes that occur in a cell of a living organism?
4. During the last few years scientists have learned a great deal about the chemistry of heredity, the process by which characteristics are passed from parent to offspring. Find out how the mystery of DNA was unraveled and how models were used in this work.
5. What new ways are being studied for the production, preservation, and preparation of food? What are the chances of man's someday consuming his food in the form of a pill?
6. What are the possibilities of using materials that we presently call wastes, such as sewage, trash, and leaves, as raw materials for the manufacture of new materials? How many things can you name that once were considered wastes that are now used in manufacturing processes?

## REFERENCES FOR ADDITIONAL STUDY

CHEMISTRY OF LIFE by Katherine Hoffman with activities by Archie Lacey. Scholastic Book Services.
A *Vistas of Science* book that describes many of the important chemical reactions that occur in living things and suggests several interesting activities

THE CHEMISTRY OF LIFE by A. Rae Patton. Random House, Inc.

Presents a good introduction to biochemistry.

GIANT MOLECULES by Herman Francis and the Editors of Time-Life Books, A Division of Time Inc.
One book of the Life Science Library—describes with essays and colorful photographs the science of polymers and other giant molecules

THE LORE OF LIVING PLANTS by Johannes van Overbeek with activities by H. K. Wong. Scholastic Book Services.
A *Vistas of Science* book containing easy-to-understand explanations of some of the mysteries of photosynthesis and other plant processes

MATTER, ENERGY, AND LIFE: AN INTRODUCTION FOR BIOLOGY STUDENTS by Jeffrey Baker and Garland Aleen. Addison-Wesley Publishing Co., Inc.
For those who wish to read more about the chemistry of living things

NUTRITION SCIENCES AND YOU by Olaf Mickelsen. Scholastic Book Services.
A *Vistas of Science* book that discusses the various aspects of food and its uses—types of food, vitamins, minerals, uses of food, and research in nutrition

THE WORLD OF CARBON by Isaac Asimov. Abelard-Schuman Limited.
An account of the part of organic chemistry involved in plants and animals

THE WORLD OF NITROGEN by Isaac Asimov. Abelard-Schuman Limited.
Describes the carbon compounds containing nitrogen that are found in living things

# *Workshop...Unit III*

If you would like to do more chemistry experiments and do not have a source of chemicals, perhaps you can get started by buying one of the many chemistry kits that are available at hobby and toy stores. You should always be very careful to follow directions in doing these experiments. Several experiments are described in this Workshop using materials that can be obtained from drugstores or hobby shops, or that are stocked in most high school chemistry laboratories.

**Experimenting with Light-Sensitive Paper.** Lay opaque objects, such as keys and coins, on a piece of blueprint paper. Expose the paper to bright light until it turns a dark blue, which usually takes about 5 minutes. Wash the paper in cold water. The picture can be made more permanent by also washing it in a dilute solution of potassium dichromate.

You can make your own blueprint paper. Dissolve 10 grams of ferric ammonium citrate in 50 cc of water. Dissolve 10 grams of potassium ferricyanide in 50 ccs of water in another container. In a darkroom mix these two solutions together in a pan. Allow a piece of stiff paper to float on the solution for a few seconds and then hang it in a dark place to dry. Expose the paper to sunlight the same way you did with the blueprint paper that you bought. Can you find out what chemical reactions occur in making and exposing the blueprint paper? Why is the paper washed in water after the exposure is made?

**Developing Photographic Negatives and Making Prints.** Scientists frequently use cameras to detect various kinds of radiation and to record experimental results. In Unit V of this book several experiments are suggested in which photographic film is used in studying radiation given off by radioactive materials. In the Workshop at the end of Unit VI directions are given for making a pinhole camera and for taking pictures with infrared radiation. In doing these experiments, it is very helpful to be able to develop your own film.

To develop photographic film, you will need to work in a dark place with running water. A bathroom or kitchen at night with the windows covered should be satisfactory. Cake pans can be used as trays for holding the solutions and a kitchen measuring cup for measuring the water. Clothespins make good clips to hold negatives and prints while they dry. It will be helpful to have a thermometer to measure the temperature of the water and solutions.

The easiest way to learn how to develop your own negatives is to buy an inexpensive kit that contains all of the necessary chemicals. These chemicals should be dissolved in water according to the directions on the packets and the solutions stored in dark-colored bottles until you are ready to use them. Figure W3.1 on page 256 shows the usual steps in developing black-and-white negatives. If you are going to develop many negatives or rolls of film, you may wish to invest in a developing tank.

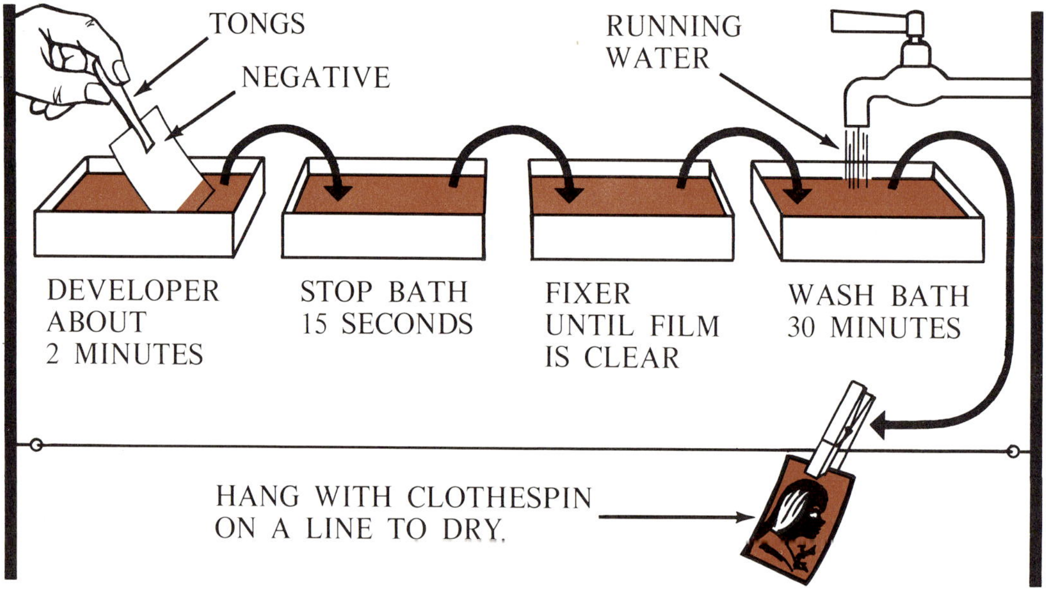


**W3.1** Follow the steps in developing a black-and-white negative film.

To make a print from a negative, the negative is placed on a piece of photographic printing paper and exposed to a source of light. The paper is then developed by a process very similar to that used in developing negatives. NOTE: A more concentrated solution of developer is often used to develop prints than is used to develop negatives; be sure to read the directions on the packet of developer.

There are many kinds of photographic printing paper available. With some you can use a red light, which makes it easier to see what you are doing. One type of printing paper can be used in a partially darkened room and this makes it easy to learn the techniques of making a print.

There are several excellent inexpensive booklets available to help you get started in doing your own darkroom work. These references also tell how to enlarge pictures and how to get special effects in your photography.

**"Raising" a Chemical Flower Garden.** Add about 100 cc of waterglass (sodium silicate), which can be obtained from a drugstore, to 200 cc of water in a beaker. Drop crystals of one or more of the following salts into the solution of waterglass: aluminum sulfate, cadmium nitrate, cobalt nitrate, copper chloride, copper nitrate, copper sulfate, iron chloride, iron nitrate, iron sulfate, nickel nitrate, and nickel sulfate. Structures that look like flowers should form from each of the crystals. Can you explain what happens? Cover the top of the beaker to reduce evaporation if you wish to preserve your chemical garden for several weeks. You also may wish to experiment using other concentrations of waterglass and crystals of other salts.

**Making Rayon.** Dissolve about 25 grams of copper sulfate ($CuSO_4$) in 250 cc of water. Add concentrated ammonium hydroxide ($NH_4OH$) until no more precipitate forms. **CAUTION: Be careful not to**

**inhale any of the vapors!** After the solid material has settled, pour off the liquid. Wash the precipitate with water several times, and then filter it through cotton cloth or a paper towel. Remove the solid material from the filter, and place in a beaker. Add enough ammonium hydroxide to dissolve the material that was formed by the reaction of copper sulfate and ammonium hydroxide. This is a slow process, and the ammonium hydroxide should be added a drop at a time.

Dissolve cellulose, such as cotton or small pieces of facial tissue or filter paper, in the solution. Continue adding cellulose and stir until the solution becomes fairly thick.

Rayon is made by forcing the dissolved cellulose through a small hole into an acid bath. This can be done in the laboratory by forcing it through a tube with a capillary tip as shown in Figure W3.2 given below.

While rayon is made by forcing the dissolved cellulose through tiny holes, sheets of cellophane are made by forcing the dissolved cellulose through long slits into an acid bath.

**W3.2** Did you ever think that you could make rayon? Try it.

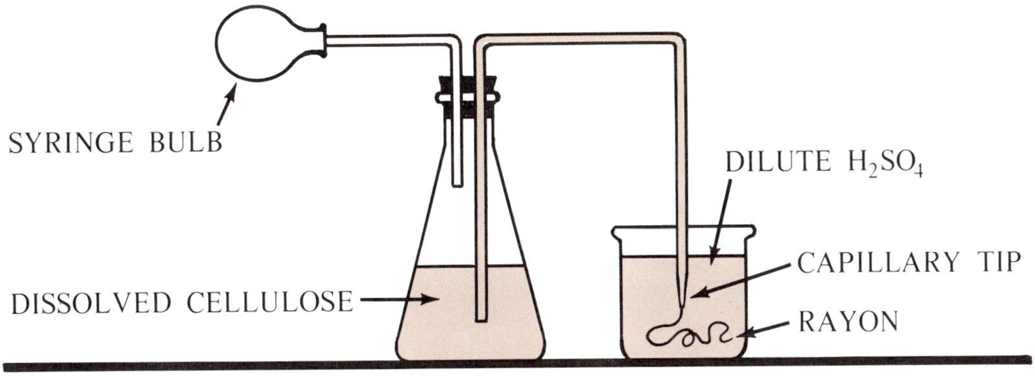

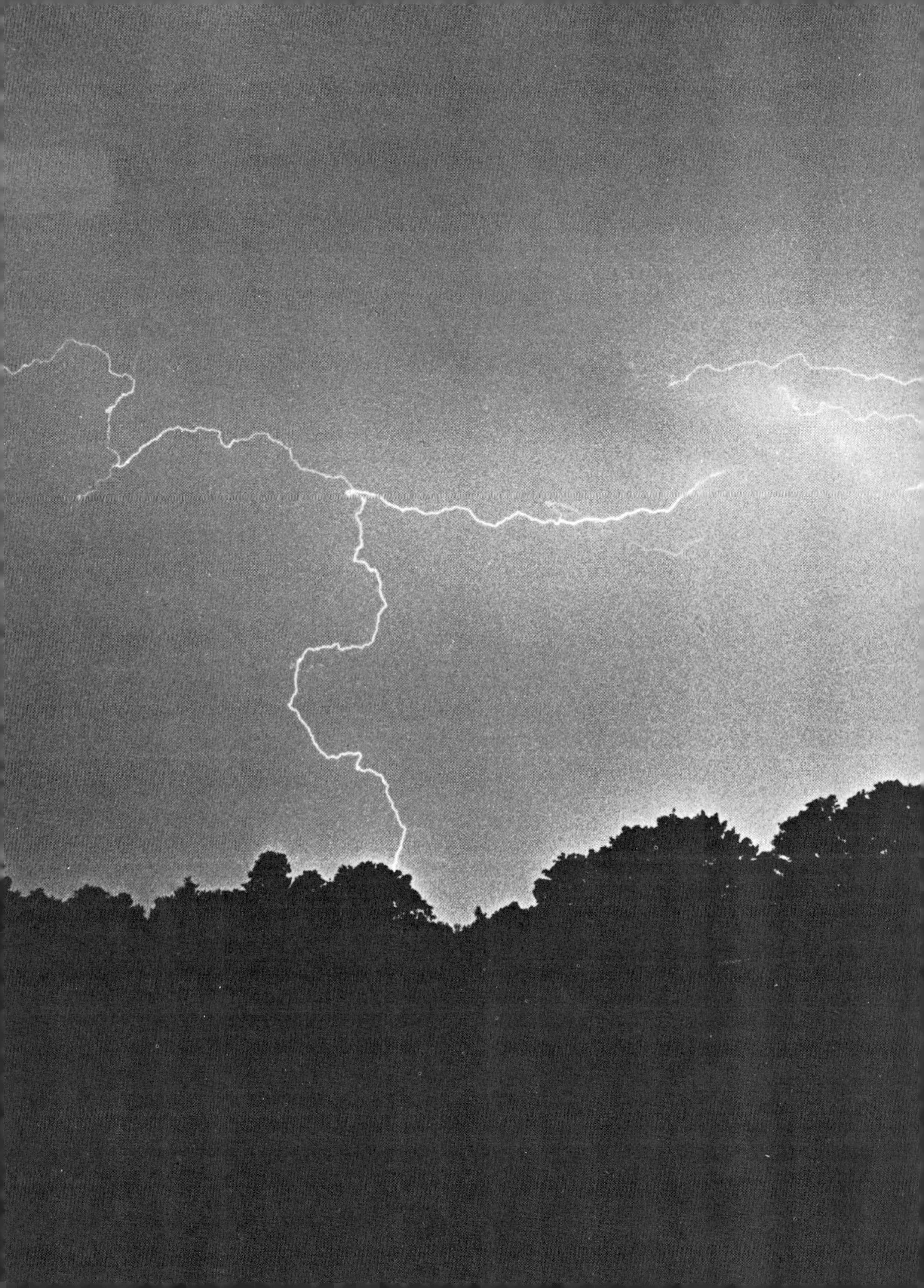

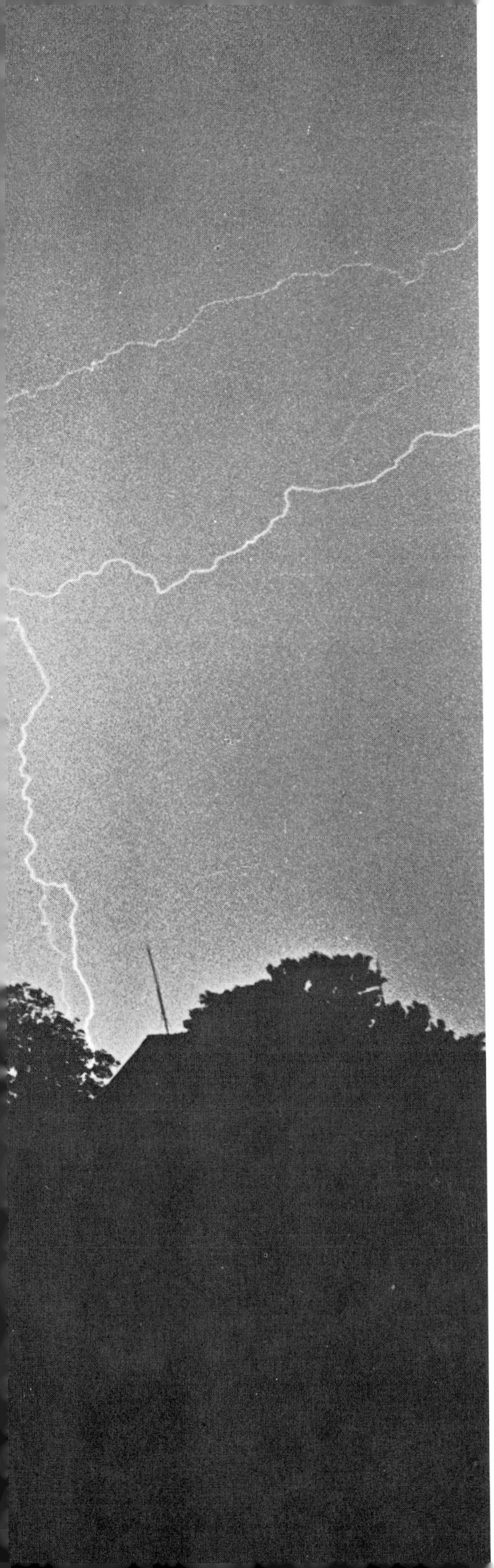

# *unit IV magnetism and electricity*

*Frank Siteman/Stock, Boston*

CHAPTER **8**

# Magnetism

IT WAS ONLY RECENTLY that scientists developed a theory to explain what makes magnets work as they do. No one knows exactly when it was discovered that a certain type of iron ore would attract other rocks. But the Greeks described the strange behavior of magnetite about 2,500 years ago. The Greeks and other ancient peoples learned to use magnets for various practical purposes. Can you name some of these uses? How soon was the magnetic compass developed?

## 1. Magnets Attract Certain Metals

**ARE YOU READY?**

Look up the following words if you are not sure of their meanings:

attract; inverse; magnet; magnetic force; square (mathematical).

Magnets, of course, attract each other. What other types of substances do they attract?

### What Substances Do Magnets Attract?

**MATERIALS:**

A single bar-shaped magnet, a steel paper clip, a pin, various other objects of metal, various nonmetals

**PROCEDURE:**

Slowly bring one end of the magnet close to the paper clip. Describe what happens. Does it make any difference which part of the magnet is placed near the paper clip?

Repeat the above experiment with the pin, which is made of either iron or aluminum, and with coins, paper, wood, and yourself. (CAUTION: **Do not bring the magnet close to a watch or any other delicate instrument.**)

What types of materials do magnets seem to attract?

As you have discovered, magnets strongly attract objects made of iron. Steel is also strongly attracted by magnets. You may not have noticed that magnets also have an attraction for a few other metals, such as nickel and **cobalt** (kō′ bôlt), because in these metals, the attraction is very weak and not generally observable. Indeed, it is now thought that almost all substances are influenced to some degree by magnets, but only iron and steel are strongly attracted.

You probably noticed that as you brought the end of the magnet close to the paper clip, the lightweight piece of iron seemed to jump to the magnet. Therefore, we can conclude that magnetic force can act through air. Materials through which magnetic forces can pass are said to be **transparent** (trans pãr′ ənt) to magnetism. Does magnetic force travel through different materials equally well? To answer this question, try the following experiment.

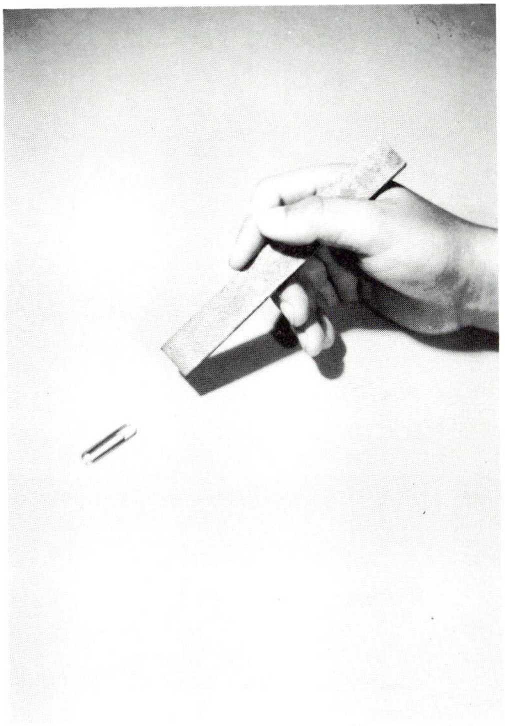

*Norman D. Anderson*

**8.1** From how far away can the magnet attract the paper clip? Try to name the forces involved.

## Making a Magnet Attract Through a Substance

**MATERIALS:**

A bar magnet, a paper clip, several sheets of various materials including cardboard, wood, glass, a thick sheet of iron

Each sheet should be approximately the same thickness.

**PROCEDURE:**

Place the magnet on top of the sheet of cardboard. Place the paper clip under the cardboard in such a way that it is attracted by the magnet. Does magnetic force act through the cardboard? Is cardboard transparent to magnetic force?

Repeat the experiment, using several other types of material in place of the cardboard. Are each of these materials transparent to magnetic force?

You have observed that magnetic force will act through many substances, and that only a few substances seem to have any effect on the strength of this force. If

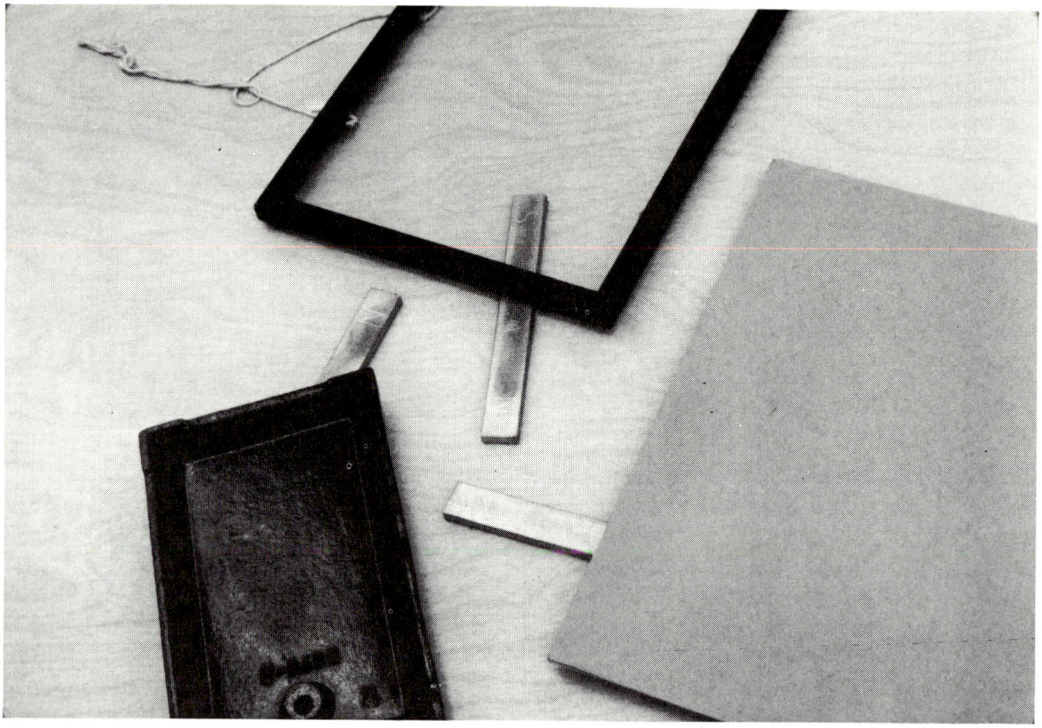

Walter R. Brown

**8.2** Does the magnetic force go through the cardboard, the iron of the ringstand base, and the glass of the picture frame? What is your conclusion about your observations?

you are a careful observer, you may have noticed that the action of your magnet on an iron object depends upon how far apart the two objects are.

To test how the distance between the magnet and an iron object affects the magnetic attraction, perform the following experiment.

## Comparing Distance Versus Magnetic Attraction

**MATERIALS:**

A bar magnet, a book, a paper clip

**PROCEDURE:**

Open the book to its back cover and assemble the equipment as was done in the last experiment, replacing the back cover of the book for the cardboard strip. Is the paper clip attracted by the magnet?

Now remove all of the equipment and turn a few pages of the book. Reassemble the apparatus placing the cover and a few pages of the book between the magnet and the paper clip. If the paper clip is still attracted by the magnet, turn a few more pages to increase the distance between the magnet and the paper clip. Continue to do this until the distance between the two is so great that the paper clip will no longer be held to the bottom of the book.

The strength of a magnet acting through space or any other transparent material varies approximately as the *inverse* of the *square* of the increase in distance. This principle is known as the "Law of the Inverse Square." It simply means that if you double the distance between a magnet and an iron object, the attraction is decreased to $1/2^2$ or $1/4$. If you increase the distance by three times, the force is decreased to $1/3^2$ or $1/9$. In other words, when the distance is increased three times, the force of attraction is only $1/9$ as much as it was before.

### Have You Learned?

On a sheet of paper list the numbers for the questions below. By each number write *T* if the statement is true and *F* if false.

1. A magnet made of aluminum is stronger than an iron magnet of the same size.
2. Metals such as nickel and cobalt are weakly attracted by magnets.
3. Air is transparent to magnetic force.
4. Iron is transparent to magnetic force.
5. If you double the distance between a magnet and an iron object, the magnetic attraction between the two objects is decreased to one-half of what it was before.

## 2. Making Magnets

**ARE YOU READY?**

Look up the following words if you are not sure of their meanings:

iron filings; magnetic force; magnetism; magnetite.

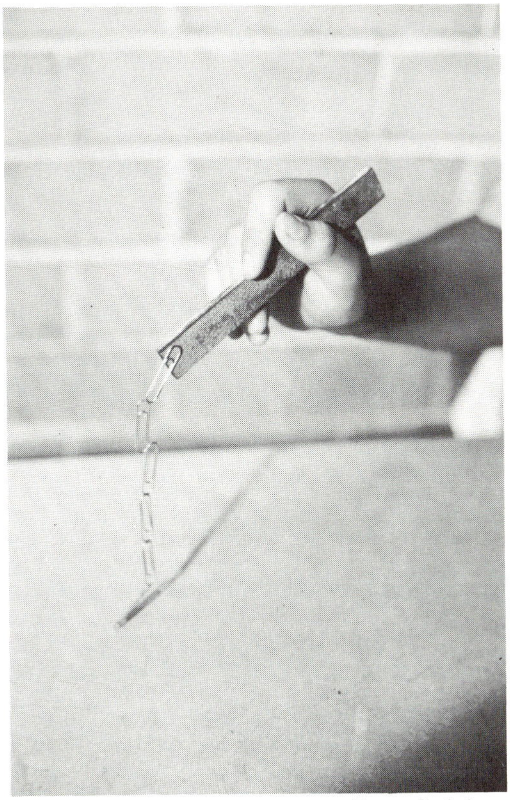

Norman D. Anderson

**8.3** Why do the paper clips attract each other?

The photograph on page 266 shows how magnetite looks. Compare this picture with your magnet. It should be apparent that your magnet is not simply a piece of iron ore. Instead, it is a piece of steel or perhaps an **alloy** (al′ oi), a combination of several metals such as iron, cobalt, and nickel, that has been made into a magnet. The making of magnets of the quality of the one you have is done with the use of electric currents, and will be discussed in the next chapter. However, you can make simple magnets, using the one you already have. These will be weak magnets and will not retain their magnetic power very long, but making them will illustrate several very important things about magnetism.

## Observing Induced Magnetism

**MATERIALS:**

A bar magnet, several paper clips

**PROCEDURE:**

Touch two paper clips together. Describe what happens.

Pick up one paper clip with your magnet in such a way that the paper clip hangs straight down from the end of the magnet. Carefully place another paper clip near the end of the first one. Describe what happens.

How many paper clips can be hung in a chain from the magnet?

The action of magnetic force through a second steel object is called **induced** (in düs′) **magnetism.** The last paper clip in your chain was probably much too far away to be acted upon by the magnet directly. The force of the magnet must have acted on each of the other paper clips in a way that made them act as if they were **magnetized.**

Perhaps after you removed the magnet from the chain of paper clips you discovered that some of the clips remained attached to each other for a brief time. These paper clips had become magnets.

## Making "Permanent" Magnets

**MATERIALS:**

A bar magnet, several paper clips, several straight pins made of steel (How can you tell that your pins are not made of aluminum?)

**PROCEDURE:**

Bend the paper clip until it is as straight as you can make it. Stroke the paper clip with one end of your magnet, moving in only one direction, as shown in the illustration. After giving it about twenty strokes, try to pick up one of the straight pins with the paper clip. Does it make any difference which end you use?

By stroking iron wire with a magnet, you can create a new magnet. Since iron is very soft, it will not retain its magnetism for a very long period of time. Can you measure the effect of increasing the number of strokes on the length of time the paper clip retains its magnetism? A harder piece of iron, such as steel, will hold its magnetic power for a longer length of time. Try magnetizing a steel knitting needle or crochet hook.

The magnet that you have made is called a bar magnet since, like your original magnet, it is in the shape of a bar.

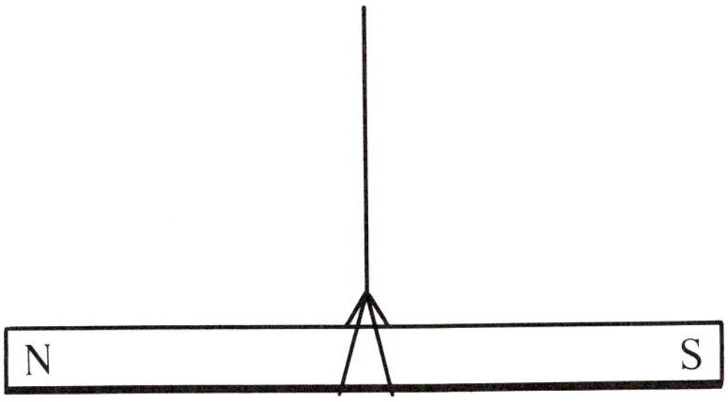


**8.4** Why does this magnet always point in the same direction? What would make it change?

Carefully bend your paper clip magnet until it is in the shape of a U or a **horseshoe.** Pick up a pin with the ends of your horseshoe magnet, and notice that the pin is attracted to both ends of the magnet. Apparently, the shape of the magnet does not affect its magnetic powers. Bringing the ends of the magnet close together, however, increases the effect of the magnet, since both ends are able to act on the attracted objects. Why this is true should be apparent from the next investigation.

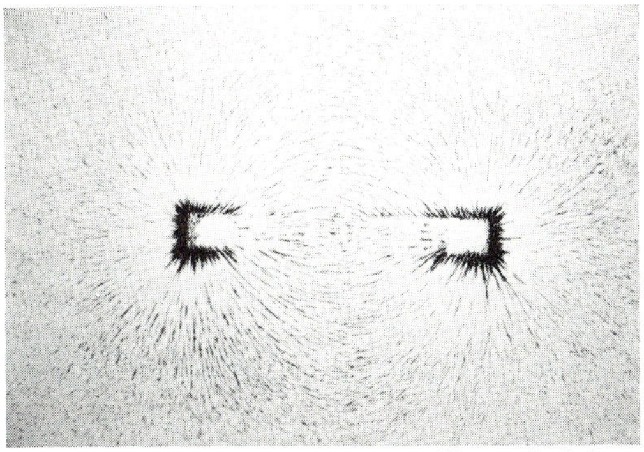

*Norman D. Anderson*

**8.5** Iron filings can be used to show the magnetic field of a bar magnet. Try to explain why.

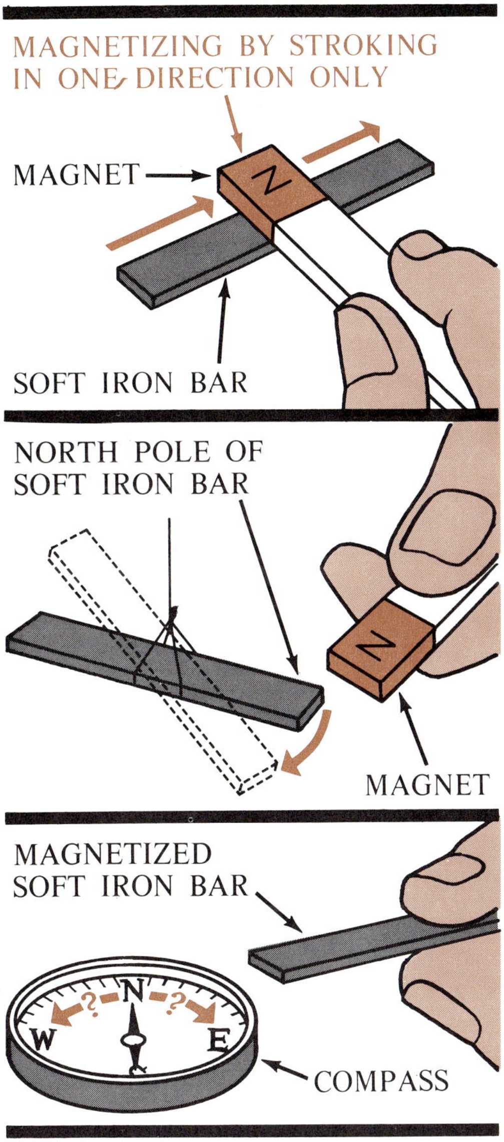


**8.6** Try this method of making a magnet.

## Looking at a Magnetic Field

**MATERIALS:**

A bar magnet, a sheet of stiff paper or cardboard, some iron filings

**PROCEDURE:**

Place the magnet on a table, and place the cardboard sheet on top of it. Slowly sprinkle the iron filings over the surface of the cardboard. Gently tap the cardboard and notice the action of the filings. Can you explain what happens to them?

If you have an overhead projector in your classroom, you may want to repeat this experiment so that the whole class can see it. Place the magnet on the stage of the projector, cover it with a stiff piece of clear plastic, and sprinkle iron filings over the magnet. Can you see on the screen the pattern formed by the iron filings?

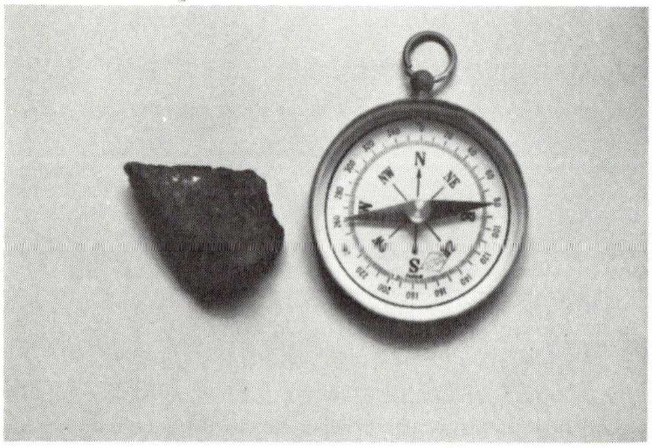

*Norman D. Anderson*

**8.7** A compass needle is affected by the magnetite.

Compare the design made by your iron filings with the photograph on page 265. Are they similar?

The tiny slivers of iron have become attracted by the magnet under the cardboard and have become arranged along certain lines. The whole pattern is known as the **magnetic field** of this particular magnet, and the lines seen in the arrangement of the iron filings are called the **lines of force.**

As you can see, the lines of force seem to run from one end of the bar magnet to the other end. Notice also that the largest number of iron particles accumulated near each end of the magnet, indicating that the magnetic field is strongest here. The ends of a magnet are called the **poles.** Can you predict what the pattern of the field of force of a horseshoe magnet would be? Try it and see.

## Have You Learned?

Select the word from Column B that best corresponds with each definition in Column A. (Do not write in your book.)

| *Column A* | *Column B* |
|---|---|
| 1. A combination of several metals such as iron, cobalt, and nickel is called a(n) _____. | a. alloy<br>b. bar<br>c. center<br>d. force<br>e. horseshoe<br>f. induced<br>g. permanent<br>h. poles |
| 2. If we place an unmagnetized piece of iron in a magnetic field, it will act as if it is magnetized. This is called _____ magnetism. | |

3. A magnet in the shape of a U is called a(n) _____ magnet.

4. The imaginary lines in a magnetic field are called lines of _____.

5. The magnetic field is strongest near the _____ of the magnet.

## 3. Magnets Have Two Poles

**ARE YOU READY?**

Look up the following words if you are not sure of their meanings:

magnetic force; magnetism;
poles (magnetic); poles (of the earth);
repel.

As you have seen, the magnetism of a magnet seems to be concentrated near the ends of the bar. Is the magnetism of the different poles of a magnet the same? The following investigation will help answer this question.

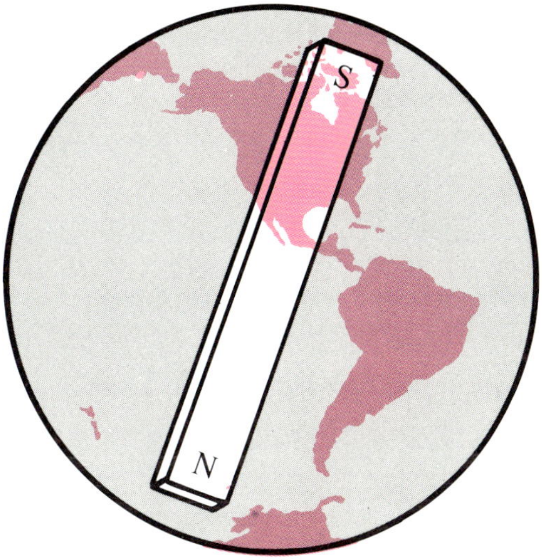


**8.8** The earth acts like a huge bar magnet.

### Investigating the Poles of a Magnet

**MATERIALS:**

A bar magnet, a short piece of string

**PROCEDURE:**

Suspend the magnet from the string, as shown in the diagram. Allow the magnet to swing freely until it stops. (Be sure that there are no iron or steel objects nearby.) Note the direction that each end points. Spin the magnet, and again allow it to swing freely until it stops. Does it point in the same direction each time? In which direction does each end point? (Figure 8.4 page 265)

Since a free-swinging magnet always settles down to point in a generally north-south direction, it is apparent that the poles at the ends of a bar magnet are *not* the same. In order to distinguish between the two different poles, names have been given to them. The pole that points toward the north pole of the earth is called the "north-seeking pole," or north pole for short. The "south-seeking pole" is generally referred to as the south pole. If your bar magnet is not already marked, write *N* on the north-seeking pole and *S* on the south-seeking pole. (Figure 8.8 above)

## Describing the Effect of One Magnet on Another

**MATERIALS:**

Two bar magnets, a short piece of string

**PROCEDURE:**

Mark the poles of each magnet, as described previously. Suspend one magnet from the string, and allow it to settle down and point in a north-south direction. Now slowly bring the *north* pole of the second magnet close to the *north* pole of the suspended magnet. Describe what happens. What happens when the *south* pole of one magnet is brought close to the *north* pole of the other? What happens when the *south* poles of both magnets are brought close together?

Since the poles of your magnets marked *N* both turn toward the north, it is apparent that in some way these poles are alike. Furthermore, the poles marked *S* appear to be similar to each other in some way. The results of the experiments you performed can be summarized by the statement: *Like poles repel; opposite poles attract.*

## Testing for Magnetism

**MATERIALS:**

A bar magnet, a bar of soft iron, a short piece of string, a compass

**PROCEDURE:**

Suspend the piece of iron by the string, as you did with the magnet in previous investigations. Slowly bring the north pole of your bar magnet close to one end and then to the other end of the piece of iron. Describe carefully what you observe.

Magnetize the piece of iron by stroking it, as described on page 264. Now slowly bring the north end of the bar magnet to one end and then to the other end of the piece of iron. Do you observe a different action of the piece of iron in this case?

If the piece of iron was strongly magnetized, the north pole of the iron should have been repelled by the north pole of the bar magnet. In the case of the unmagnetized piece of iron, both ends were attracted to the north pole of the bar magnet. Therefore, the *repelling* of one pole by another is a sure test for magnetism. Can you explain why the attraction of opposite poles is not a good test?

If the bar magnet is so strong that it attracts both ends of the magnetized iron bar, you may wish to use a compass to test for magnetism. Bring one end of the magnetized iron bar near the compass. Does it attract the north-seeking or south-seeking pole of the compass needle? Does the other end of the magnetized iron attract the opposite pole of the compass?

The lines of force, as shown by the iron filings, will also help you to understand the fact that the two poles of a magnet are different from each other.

## Describing the Force Field of Two Magnets

**MATERIALS:**

Two bar magnets, iron filings, a sheet of thin cardboard

**PROCEDURE:**

Place the magnets end to end, leaving a space of about 2-3 cm between them. Place the sheet of cardboard over them, and sprinkle the iron filings onto the cardboard exactly as you did in the activity on page 265. Describe the pattern taken by the bits of iron.

Remove the cardboard, and reverse the position of one of the magnets. Replace the cardboard, and again sprinkle on the iron filings. Is the pattern now different than it was previously?

Can you sketch the fields of force around two magnets whose *similar* poles are near each other? Can you sketch the fields of force around two *opposite* poles?

What would happen if we broke a bar magnet into two pieces? Would we have two pieces of metal, one with a north pole and the other with a south pole?

## Studying a Broken Magnet

**MATERIALS:**

A bar magnet, a steel needle, a short piece of string

**PROCEDURE:**

Magnetize the needle, as described in the activity on page 264. Break it into two parts with a quick bend, or cut it quickly with a pair of wire cutters. Try not to bend the metal back and forth, as this heats the metal and destroys the magnetic properties. Can you explain this? Suspend one half of the needle, using the string as before, and test for the presence of poles at each end of the needle.

If the above experiment was carefully done, you will have discovered that a broken magnet develops poles at its new ends. Therefore, each piece of a broken magnet becomes an entire magnet, complete with opposite poles at each end. What do you think would happen if you could keep on dividing a magnet in half until it reached the size of only a few atoms?

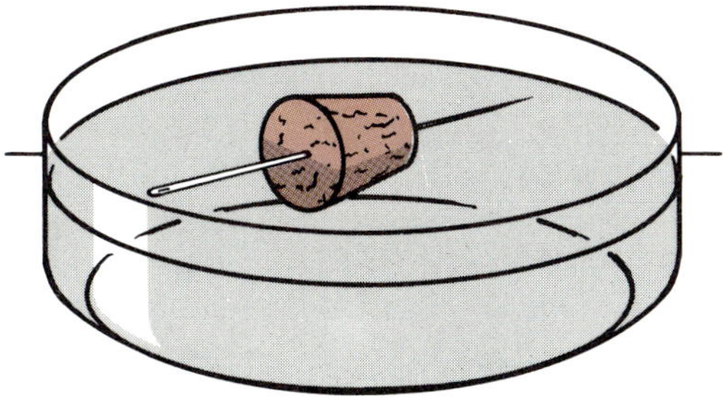

**8.9** You can make a simple compass by floating a magnetized needle on water. Why does it work?

## Have You Learned?

Write a brief answer to each of the following questions, using complete sentences.

1. Why are the poles of a magnet properly called "the north-seeking pole" and "the south-seeking pole"?

2. What evidence do we have to prove that the two poles of a magnet are different from each other?

3. Suppose you have two bars of iron. What experiments could you perform, using only these two bars, to find out whether only one or both of them are magnetized?

## 4. The Earth Is a Magnet

**ARE YOU READY?**

Look up the following words if you are not sure of their meanings:

fluid; poles (of the earth); transparent (to magnetism).

You have already observed that a bar magnet, suspended by a string and allowed to swing freely, will always settle to point in roughly a north-south direction. In this way, the magnet acts as if it were being attracted toward a large magnet lying in the center of the earth, with its magnetic poles near the geographic poles of the earth, as is shown in Figure 8.8 on page 267.

Probably the first practical use to be made of magnetic materials was the construction of magnetic compasses.

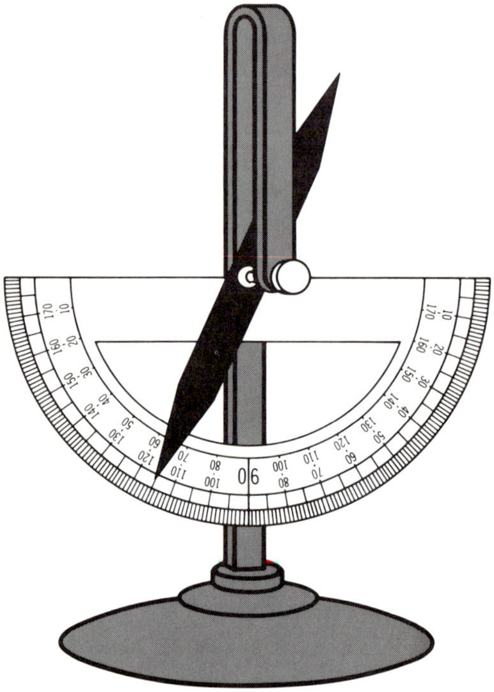

**8.10** Dip needle compass

If you bring the south pole of your bar magnet near the compass needle, you will notice that the end of the compass that pointed north is attracted. Therefore, we can say that the earth acts as if it were a huge magnet, with its *south* pole lying to the *north* of the United States and its *north* pole lying to the *south.* The earth's magnetic poles are continually shifting slightly, which disproves the old theory of a huge mass of magnetic iron buried in the earth. One current idea is that the earth's magnetism is caused by the movement of a metallic fluid that forms the outer half of the center core of the earth. This fluid core is thought to be too hot to be magnetic itself. However, as you will learn in the next chapter, when electric charges move, a magnetic field is produced. Therefore, it is assumed that the

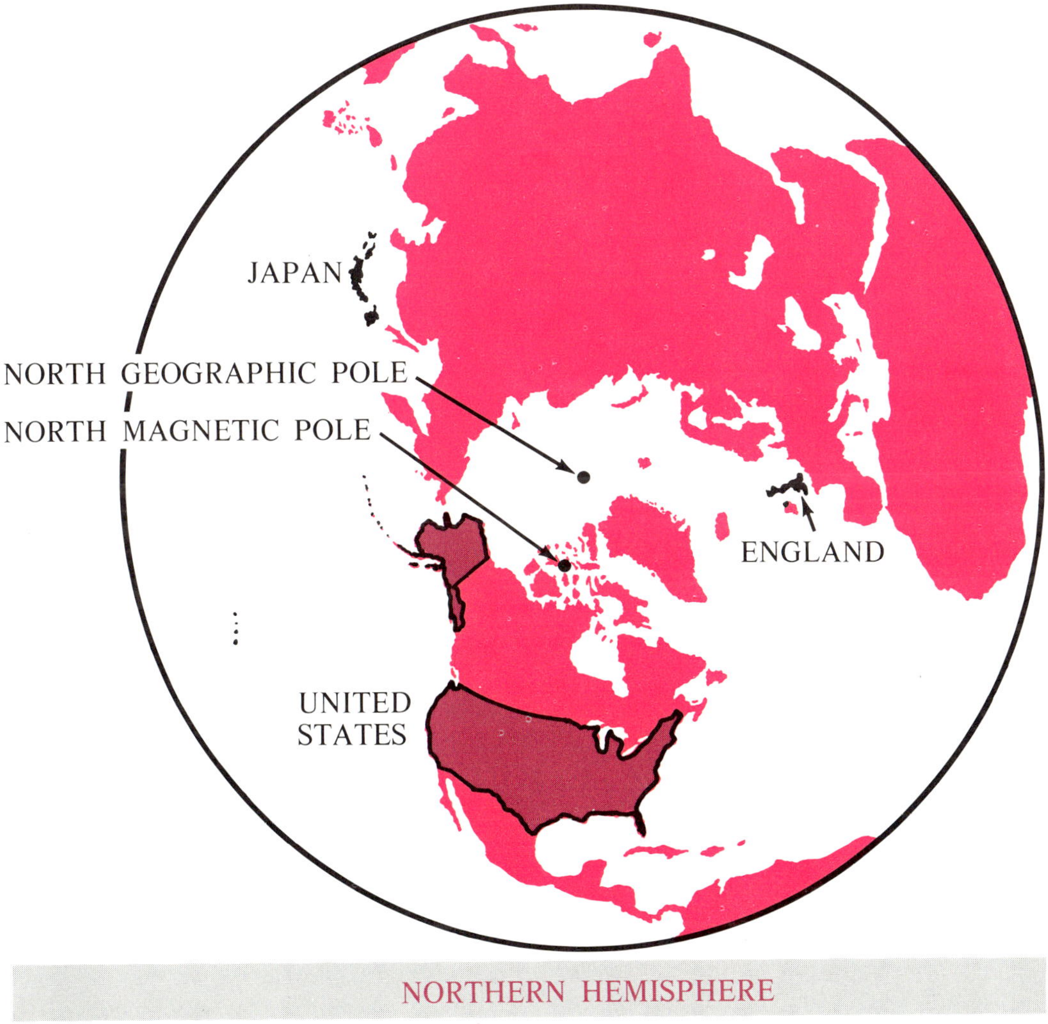


**8.11** The location of the geographic pole and the approximate location of the magnetic pole

**molten** (mōl′ tən) core of the earth is electrically charged.

What would be the action of your compass if you held it in your hand and began walking toward the north, following the direction of the needle? As you moved closer and closer to the magnetic pole, the needle of your compass would dip farther and farther downward. Actually to do this, we would need a special compass, called a **dip needle,** shown in Figure 8.10 on page 270. This compass needle is attached in such a way that it is free to swing downward. Eventually we would find a point, located near Bathurst Island in Northern Canada, where the needle will point straight *down.* This is called the **magnetic pole,** and it lies some 1,600 kilometers away from the north *geographic* pole, as shown above.

## Making a Compass

**MATERIALS:**

A small cork, a long sewing needle, a bar magnet, a cup or shallow container made of a magnetically transparent material

**PROCEDURE:**

Magnetize the needle by stroking it with the bar magnet, as described on page 264. Stick the needle through the cork in such a way that it will float freely on the surface of the water. The needle should turn until it points in a north-south direction. Slowly rotate the cup, first in one direction and then in the other, and observe the action of the needle. Does it always point in a generally north-south direction? (Figure 8.9 page 269)

The map on page 271 shows the northern hemisphere of the earth and the location of the magnetic pole that lies in this hemisphere. Lay a ruler on this map so that it runs from your home through the magnetic pole. This is the direction that a compass needle will point. Now move the ruler so that it runs from your home to the north *geographic* pole. This direction is true north. The difference between *magnetic* north and *true* north is known as **declination** (dek′ lə nā′ shən). What is the declination in England? In Japan? What is the difference between the declination of the East Coast and the West Coast of the United States? Is there any place in the Northern Hemisphere where the declination is zero?

Since the earth acts as if it were one huge magnet, it is surrounded by a magnetic field. If a bar of iron is carefully lined up so that it points toward the magnetic pole, and then heated, it will become a magnet. With soft iron, it is possible to do this simply by hitting the bar with a hammer.

### Have You Learned?

Write on a sheet of paper the word that best completes the statement. (Do not write in your book.)

The first practical use of magnetic materials was in the construction of a (1) _____. It is now generally believed that the magnetism of the earth is due to the movement of a metallic (2) _____ that forms the outer half of the center core of the earth. The (3) _____ north pole lies near Bathurst Island, some 1,600 km away from the geographic north pole. The difference between the direction this pole is from you and the direction true north is from you is called (4) _____. Since the earth acts as if it were one large magnet, it is surrounded by a magnetic (5) _____.

## 5. What Causes Magnetism?

**ARE YOU READY?**

Look up the following words if you are not sure of their meanings:

induced magnetism; iron filings; magnetic field; permanent magnet.

During the study of this chapter you have observed many of the important phenomena of magnetism. Any useful theory as to what causes magnetism should explain all of these observations. Physicists are only now beginning to formulate theories that seem able to do this. However, as you will see in the next chapter, man learned how to use magnetism long before he understood what caused it.

You will recall from Section 3 that when a magnet is broken into two parts, each part becomes a complete magnet. At that time the question was asked: "What do you think would happen if you could keep on dividing a magnet in half until it reached the size of a single iron atom?" Of course, no one has ever been able to do this. However, it is assumed that we would find that *each atom of iron is a magnet.* This assumption forms the basis for the currently accepted theory of magnetism.

Scientists are not at all certain why the atoms of iron, nickel, and cobalt act as tiny magnets. Evidence seems to indicate that the magnetic field of these atoms is caused by the spinning of each electron around its own axis.

These elements that have strong magnetic properties are called **ferromagnetic** (fer′ ō mag net′ ik) metals. It now appears that a sample of a ferromagnetic metal is composed of regions in which the force fields of the magnet atoms are all pointed in the same direction. These regions, called ferromagnetic **domains** (dō mān′), will normally be arranged so that their magnetic fields cancel each other as shown in the photograph on page 274. This arrangement leaves the total sample nonmagnetic. However, under a microscope, the effects of each domain on microscopic bits of magnetite can be seen. These observations show rectangular-shaped areas with magnetic properties, separated by nonmagnetic areas called *walls.* It is assumed that the atoms making up the wall areas are in a scattered arrangement, since they do not exhibit any noticeable magnetism.

When a piece of ferromagnetic material is placed within a magnetic field, the atoms making up the domain walls turn to lie along the lines of magnetic force passing through the metal. As this happens, a layer of the atoms (that were originally lined up in an opposite direction to the magnetic field) becomes scrambled, forming a new wall. The result is that the domain wall shifts to one side, creating a large domain lined up with the outside lines of force, and a smaller domain oriented in the opposite direction. In this way, the piece of ferromagnetic material comes to show magnetic properties of its own. When the outside magnetic field is removed, the forces caused by the smaller domain force the walls to move back to their original positions, leaving the sample nonmagnetic.

In certain alloys, such as Alnico, the induced magnetism remains with the sample, forming a permanent magnet. Alnico magnets are made by mixing aluminum, nickel, cobalt, iron, and copper and heating them until they melt. The alloy is then slowly cooled while inside a magnetic field. The ferromagnetic particles are forced into alignment during the cooling process. These tiny magnets are separated from each other by the nonmagnetic material, which tends to hold them in position.

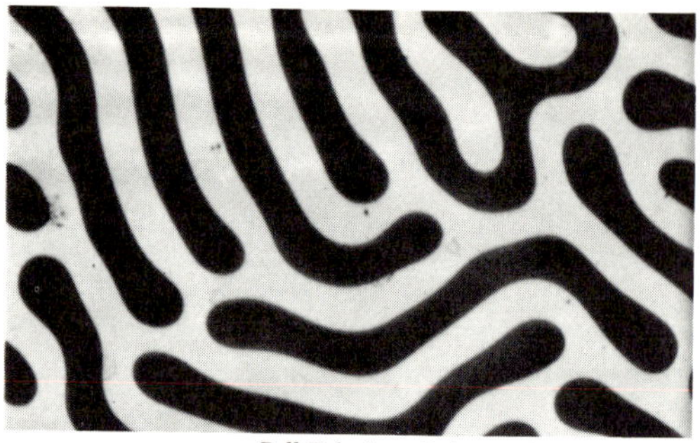

*Bell Telephone Laboratories Incorporated*

**8.12** Ferromagnetic domains

## Arranging Magnetic Particles

**MATERIALS:**

A small test tube, some iron filings, a bar magnet, a small compass

**PROCEDURE:**

Place the iron filings in the test tube, and place it on its side on a table. Gently stroke the tube, in the same manner used to magnetize the soft iron bar in the investigation on page 261. Notice the arrangement of the iron filings. Slowly bring the compass near the end of the test tube. Has the test tube containing iron filings become a magnet? Shake the test tube to disturb the arrangement of the iron filings. Again test it with the compass. Is it still a magnet?

This demonstration is a **model,** used here to show how scientists think the atoms of iron behave. It does not prove the atomic theory of magnetism!

When an object is heated, its atoms move more rapidly. As you might expect, heating may destroy the magnetic properties of a magnet by allowing the atoms to be rearranged. Since the atoms of solids do not normally change their positions, a high heat is required to destroy the magnetism of a permanent magnet. For an iron magnet, a temperature of over 730° C is necessary. Iron, when heated red hot, will not be attracted by even a very strong magnet. Can you explain why?

Hitting an iron bar while holding it in a magnetic field, as described on page 272, apparently shakes the atoms of the domain walls a little and allows them to become rearranged within the bar. The earth's magnetic pole attracts the north-seeking pole of each atom and aligns enough atoms to cause the bar to become a weak magnet.

Liquids and gases are composed of molecules, just as solids are. Experiments have shown that liquids and gases of certain substances have some magnetic properties. Can you explain why a test tube of a liquid could not be made into a strong, permanent magnet?

The atomic theory of magnetism seems to be a valid one. It seems to explain and allow us to predict the phenomena of magnetism. However, to be complete, the theory must explain why the atoms of iron are magnetic. A great deal of experimentation is now going on in this field, and much more information is being gathered. This additional information should result in a better understanding of magnetic phenomena.

## Have You Learned?

On a sheet of paper list the numbers for the questions below. By each number write *T* if the statement is true and *F* if false.

1. A magnet may be as small as a single atom.
2. Elements that have strong magnetic properties are called domains.
3. When a bar of iron is magnetized, its domains change size.
4. Heating a magnet may destroy its magnetism.
5. Test tubes of certain liquids can be made into permanent magnets.

## REVIEW QUESTIONS

Select the answer that best completes each statement. (Do not write in your book.)

1. An iron object is placed 1 cm from a magnet, and the magnetic attraction is measured. Then the object is moved until it is 4 cm from the magnet. At this point the magnetic attraction will be ____ of what it was before.
(a. ⅓; b. ¼; c. ⅛; d. 1/16)
2. All of the following materials are transparent to magnetic force *except* ____.
(a. paper; b. air; c. iron; d. glass)
3. We take an unmagnetized bar of iron, place it close to a magnet, and we find that it will attract small bits of iron. This is an example of ____ magnetism.
(a. induced; b. alloy; c. permanent; d. declination)
4. The lines of force of a bar magnet ____.
(a. lie parallel to the magnet; b. lie at right angles to the magnet; c. run from one end of the magnet to the other; d. begin along the sides of the magnet and run in straight lines in all directions away from the magnet)
5. If the north pole of a magnet is brought close to the north pole of another magnet, ____.
(a. both magnets will attract each other; b. both magnets will repel each other; c. one will attract while the other repels)
6. If a bar magnet is broken into two parts, ____ are formed.
(a. two complete magnets, each with a N and a S pole; b. two magnets, one with two N poles and the other with two S poles; c. two nonmagnetic pieces of iron)
7. The difference between the direction of magnetic north and true north is called ____.
(a. compass direction; b. dip needle direction; c. magnetic field; d. declination)
8. Elements that have strong magnetic properties are called ____.
(a. ferromagnetic; b. alloys; c. induced magnets; d. atoms)
9. Elements that have strong magnetic properties are composed of regions in which the magnetic fields of all of the atoms are pointed in the same direction. These regions are called ____.
(a. domains; b. alloys; c. molecules; d. induced magnets)
10. The magnetic regions of iron are separated from each other by ____.
(a. atoms; b. walls; c. domains; d. alloys)

## CAN YOU FIND OUT?

*It may be necessary to use encyclopedias or other reference books in answering the following questions.*

1. Many of the early discoveries about mag-

nets were made by William Gilbert, an English scientist. Can you find out what he discovered and how?

2. How are the compasses in ships and airplanes fixed so that the metal around them does not affect their accuracy?
3. Where is the south magnetic pole located? Where is the magnetic equator?
4. What is the Aurora Borealis ("Northern Lights")? What effect does the earth's magnetic field have on it?

## REFERENCES FOR ADDITIONAL STUDY

EXPERIMENTS IN MAGNETISM AND ELECTRICITY by Harry Sootin. Franklin Watts, Inc.
Suggests about 200 experiments that can be done with simple equipment

EXPERIMENTS WITH MAGNETISM by Harry Sootin. Grosset and Dunlap, Inc.
Describes many easy-to-do experiments on magnetism

# CHAPTER 9

# Electricity

LIKE MAGNETISM, electricity was apparently discovered first by the ancient Greeks. About 600 B.C., Thales (thā′ lēz) (640?-546 B.C.), a Greek philosopher and scientist, wrote that when a piece of **amber** (am′ bər) was rubbed with wool, it attracted certain lightweight objects. Amber is a **fossilized** form of a substance that comes from trees, and its Greek name is *elektron.* What words do you know that you think may have come from this word?

It wasn't until the late 1500s that people began to learn more about electricity than was known by Thales. During the past four centuries, scientists and engineers have learned how to use electrical energy for thousands and thousands of purposes. How many of these can you name?

## 1. Electricity at Rest

> **ARE YOU READY?**
>
> Look up the following words if you are not sure of their meanings:
>
> attract; electron; evaporate; neutron; nucleus (of an atom); proton.

What Thales discovered over 2,500 years ago was actually electricity. But the type of electricity known to the Greeks is quite different from the electrical energy used to light lamps and run vacuum cleaners. In these appliances a stream of electrons actually move through the wires. This is called **current** (kėr′ ənt) **electricity.** When Thales rubbed a piece of amber with wool, he transferred some of the electrons from

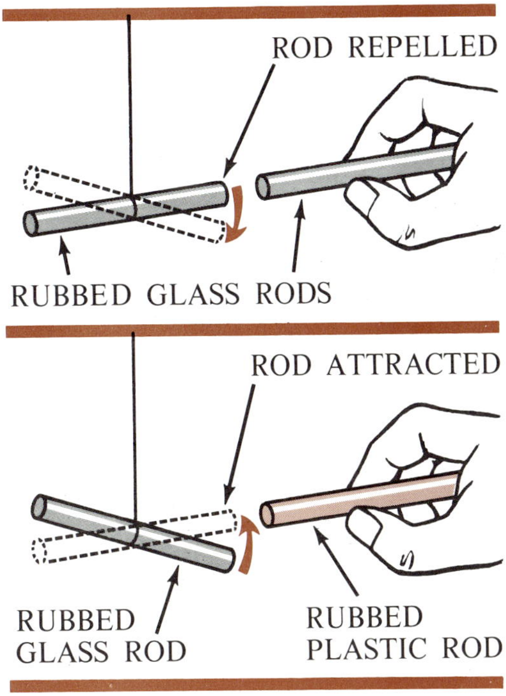


**9.1** Investigating static electricity

the wool to the amber. Since no current actually flows, this phenomena is called **static** (stat′ ik) **electricity.** The word *static* means "stationary," or "not moving."

You are probably well acquainted with static electricity. Perhaps you have received a mild shock when you touched a door handle after walking across a rug. Or perhaps, after sliding across the seat of an automobile, you have been shocked when you touched some metal part of the car. Rub a hard-rubber comb with a piece of cloth, and try to attract small bits of paper with the comb. Lightning is another example of static electricity.

If you can obtain the necessary equipment, try the following activity. If not, read it carefully.

## Investigating Static Electricity

**MATERIALS:**

Two short pieces of solid glass rod, silk thread, a piece of silk cloth, a short piece of plastic rod, a piece of fur or flannel material

**PROCEDURE:**

Tie one glass rod to the end of the silk thread so that it is balanced and free to swing in any direction. (See Figure 9.1.) Rub this glass rod with the piece of silk, and then hang it up, or have a friend hold it for you. Rub the second piece of glass rod with the silk, and slowly bring the ends of the rods close to each other. They should repel each other.

Now rub the plastic rod with the fur or flannel cloth, and slowly bring it close to the end of the glass rod. The plastic rod should attract the free-swinging glass rod.

These objects acted in very much the same ways as the magnets that you experimented with in Chapter 8. Apparently the two glass rods that had been rubbed with silk were *alike* in some way and repelled each other. The plastic rod, on the other hand, apparently was in some way *opposite* to the glass rod and therefore attracted it.

Scientists think that when you rubbed the glass rod with the silk, you *removed* some of the electrons from the atoms on the surface. This resulted in the glass's having a **charge** of static electricity. When the plastic was rubbed, the opposite condition occurred. Electrons from the atoms of the fur or flannel were removed and transferred to the surface of the plastic. This static electrical charge is opposite in nature to the one placed on the glass rod.

You will recall from Chapter 5 that an atom is composed of a nucleus made of protons and neutrons and that electrons revolve around this nucleus. The neutrons do not appear to have any electrical charge, whereas the electrical charges of the protons and the electrons are opposite to each other. To identify these two opposite types, we refer to the electrical charge of the proton as **positive** (+) and to the electrical charge of the electron as **negative** (−).

Normally each atom is composed of an equal number of protons and electrons. Thus, each atom does not show any electrical charge, since each positive particle is balanced with a negative particle. When we removed the negatively charged electrons from one glass rod, we left a positive charge on it. The approach of another positively charged glass rod caused the two to repel each other. By placing more electrons on the plastic rod, we created a negatively charged body that attracted the glass rod. If you accidentally allowed the negatively charged plastic rod to touch the positively charged glass rod, you found that they no longer affected each other. After contact, each rod was neutralized. Can you explain why?

Perhaps the most exciting and dramatic example of static electricity that you have seen is a lightning flash. Benjamin Franklin's famous experiments proved that lightning is actually electrical in nature. But what causes this tremendous release of energy that can destroy trees and buildings and kill people and animals?

The basic cause of lightning is the rise of evaporated water through the air. This dislodges many electrons and causes electrical charges to be formed in different parts of a cloud. For example, a positively charged area will attract electrons, causing them to accumulate in the nearby portions of the cloud and in the ground nearest to the cloud. A negatively charged portion of cloud will drive electrons away from the surrounding clouds and from the nearby ground. Eventually the force between these may become so great that electrons move toward the positively

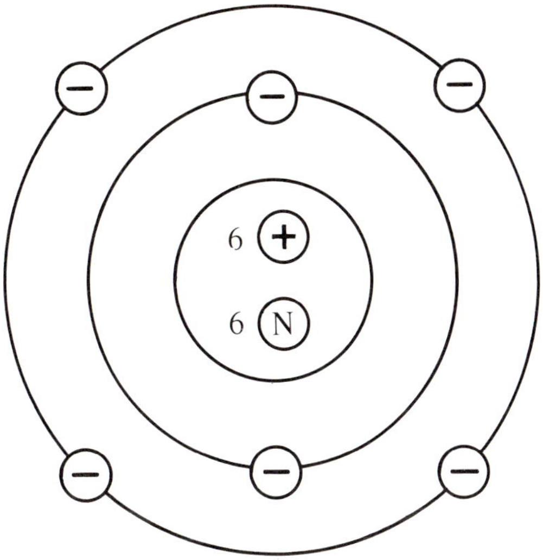


**9.2** Atomic protons and electrons

charged area. This flash is exactly like the spark you sometimes see and feel when you touch a water fountain after walking over a thick rug—except that it involves 20 to 30 million volts!

One practical result of Franklin's experiments was the discovery of a way to protect buildings from lightning damage. By placing metal rods on the top of buildings and connecting them to the ground, most

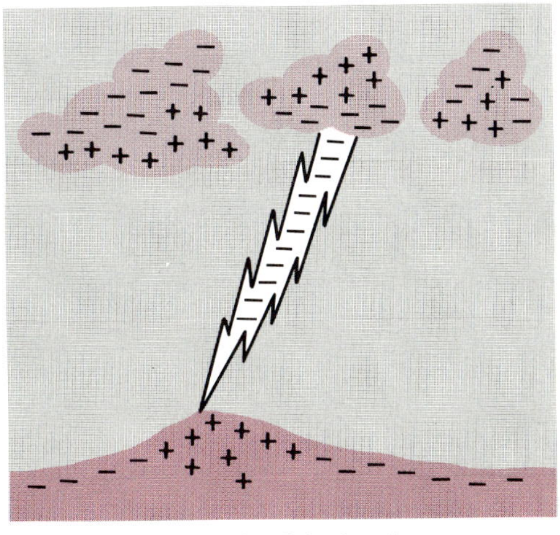

**9.3** Positive and negative lightning charges

of the damage from lightning can be avoided. The lightning rod provides a path for electrons from the ground to be drawn slowly upward to neutralize the positive charges being built up in the cloud. Or, if the cloud is negatively charged, electrons will harmlessly "leak" from it to the ground.

### Have You Learned?

On a sheet of paper list the numbers for the questions below. By each number write *T* if the statement is true and *F* if false.

1. Each of the following is caused by static electricity.
   a. electric lights glowing
   b. lightning flashing
   c. northern lights glowing
   d. electric fan turning
   e. shock you get after sliding across seat of automobile
2. If two objects both contain a surplus of electrons, they will be attracted to each other.
3. Atoms are normally negatively charged.
4. Protons are positively charged, and electrons are negatively charged.
5. A lightning flash is a stream of electrons.

## 2. Experiments with an Electroscope

**ARE YOU READY?**

Look up the following words if you are not sure of their meanings:

charge (electric); electron; induce; negative (electrical charge); repel.

Any device that can detect an electric charge is called an **electroscope** (i lek′ trə skōp). The glass and plastic rods you used in the last section could be called electroscopes.

A great deal can be learned about electricity using the simple instrument described here (Figures 9.4 and 9.5 on the opposite page).

### Building an Electroscope

**MATERIALS:**

A small glass bottle with a rubber or cork stopper, a short piece of copper wire (a copper paper clip will do), a short strip of thin aluminum foil

**PROCEDURE:**

Insert the copper wire through the stopper in such a way that the longer end of the wire hangs into the bottle. Make a right-angle bend about 1 cm from this end of the wire. Hang a short strip of aluminum foil over the wire, as shown in the diagram. Be sure that the foil does not touch the bottom or the sides of the bottle.

The theory that explains how the electroscope works is a simple one. If an electric charge is placed on the copper wire, either by adding or removing electrons, the aluminum foil leaves will become charged. Since both leaves have similar charges, they repel each other. The result is that the two leaves stand away from each other. The angle at which the leaves are to each other indicates the *amount* of electric charge on the electroscope. Can you explain why?

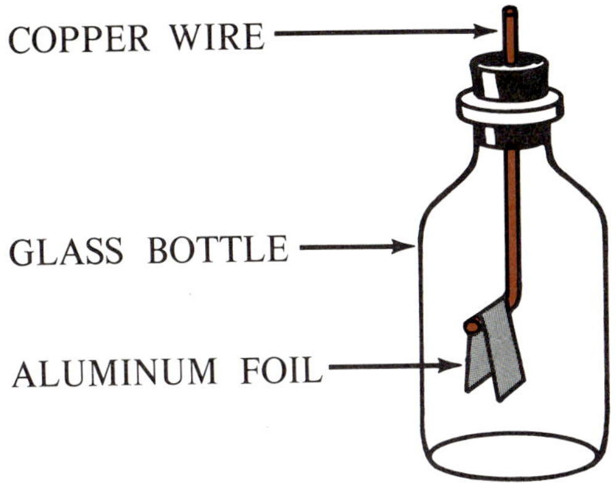


**9.4** An electroscope

**9.5** Charging the electroscope

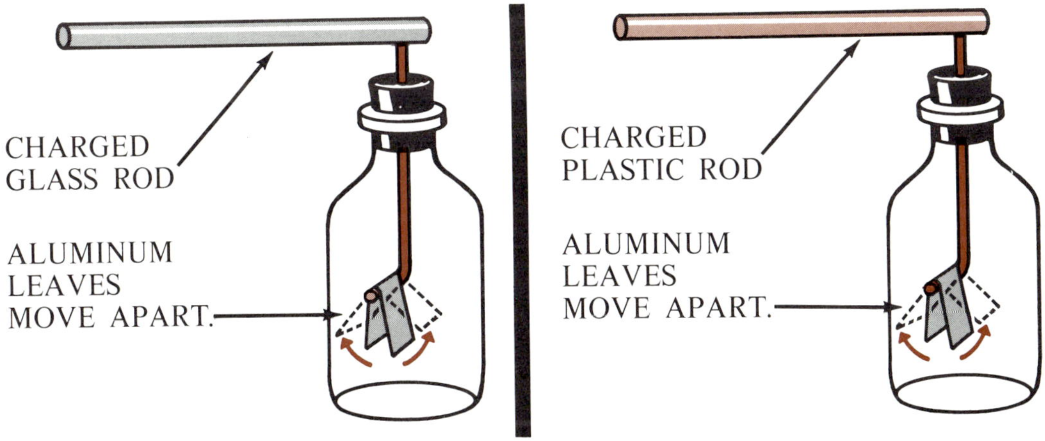


## Charging the Electroscope

**MATERIALS:**

The electroscope constructed in the previous activity, a short piece of glass rod, a piece of silk, a short piece of plastic rod, a piece of fur or flannel material

**PROCEDURE:**

Charge the glass rod by rubbing it with the silk cloth. Carefully touch the top of the copper rod of your electroscope. The aluminum leaves should move apart. Touch the copper rod with your finger. The leaves should move back together.

Now charge the plastic rod by rubbing it with the fur or flannel material, and touch the top of your electroscope rod. The leaves should again move apart. A touch of your finger will allow them to move back together.

The activity on page 281 demonstrates two important principles of electricity. First, it shows the presence of a static electric charge created by rubbing the glass and plastic rods. Can you explain exactly what happens to the electrons and what causes the electroscope leaves to act as they do?

The second important point that you can observe in this experiment is the movement of electrons through a substance. Matter through which electric charges will move is called a **conductor** (kən duk′ tər). The charge placed on the end of the rod travels through the copper wire and through the aluminum leaves. When you touch the rod, the electric charge moves into you. All of these substances are conductors. Recharge your electroscope, and try to discover other conductors. You will discover that some substances, such as wood, are weak conductors. Other substances, such as glass, are very poor conductors.

Since the leaves of your electroscope held their charge for some time, you may have guessed that air is normally a poor conductor. On some days, when the air is very **humid** (hū′ mid), your electroscope may not work at all. Moisture in the air acts as an excellent conductor and allows electrons to flow into or out of your electroscope. When the air is particularly humid, you will find it impossible even to charge the glass or plastic rods.

One excellent way to remove the static electrical charge from an object is to connect it to the earth, since electrons readily flow into or out of the ground. Many electrical appliances in which static charges may develop must be **grounded** if they are to work properly.

While experimenting with magnets you discovered that magnets were able to attract iron objects even though there was a space between them. This is called *induced* magnetism. Induced static electric charges can also be created.

## Making an Induced Electrical Charge

**MATERIALS:**

An electroscope, a plastic rod, a piece of fur or flannel material, a sharp pencil

**PROCEDURE:**

Charge the plastic rod, and bring it *close to* the top of the electroscope rod. Be careful not to touch the rod. The leaves should move apart and remain apart as long as the charged plastic is held close to the top of the electroscope. When the plastic rod is removed, the leaves fall back together.

Again charge the plastic rod, and bring it close to one side of the electroscope rod. With the point of a sharp pencil, carefully touch the electroscope rod on the side *opposite* the plastic rod, and the leaves should fall. Remove the pencil before you remove the plastic rod, and the leaves should again move apart and remain apart.

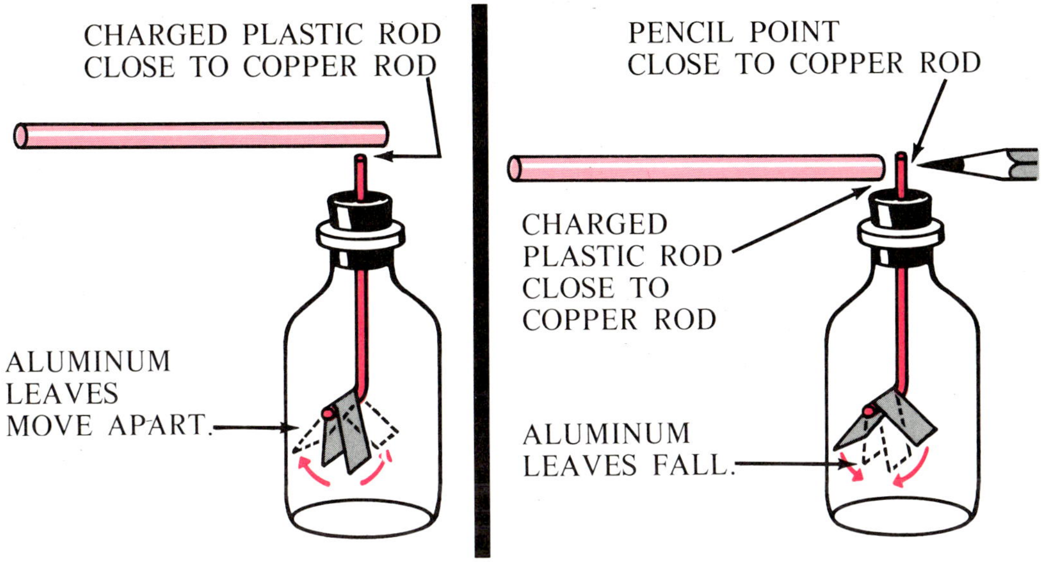


**9.6** Inducing static electrical charges

When the plastic rod that had a negative charge due to an excess of electrons was brought close to the electroscope rod, the electrons of the copper were repelled. As the electrons moved into the leaves, the leaves repelled each other and stood apart. Since the plastic rod did not touch the electroscope, the charge on the electroscope leaves was due to the *displacement* of electrons, not due to the removal or addition of electrons. As soon as the plastic rod was removed, the electrons again flowed into the upper part of the rod, and the leaves fell as they lost their charge. This type of charge is called a *temporary induced charge*.

When the **graphite** (graf′ īt) "lead" of the pencil was touched to the electroscope rod, the electrons that were being repelled by the charged plastic rod flowed out of the copper and into the graphite. At this point the electroscope showed *no charge*. When the pencil was removed, the leaves again repelled each other because of the *shortage* of electrons in the copper rod. Can you predict the action of the electroscope if you repeat the above investigation, using a charged glass rod instead of the plastic rod? Try it, and see if your prediction was correct. Can you explain the movement of electrons in this case?

**9.7** How is the flow of electricity like the water flow in this water-pump system?

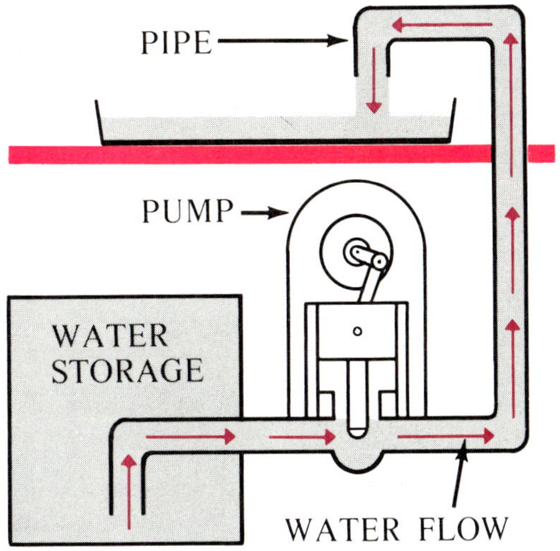

## Have You Learned?

Select the answer that best completes each statement. (Do not write in your book.)

1. An electroscope is a device that can detect electric ____. (charges; current)
2. The leaves of an electroscope repel each other because the charges on them are ____. (opposite; similar)
3. In order to place a charge on an electroscope, it ____ (is; is not) necessary to place more electrons on the copper rod.
4. Types of matter through which electric charges will move are called ____. (conductors; insulators)
5. ____ (Dry; Moist) air allows electricity to flow easily through it.

## 3. Current Electricity

**ARE YOU READY?**

Look up the following words if you are not sure of their meanings:

conductor; dry cell; parallel; series (of objects); static (electricity).

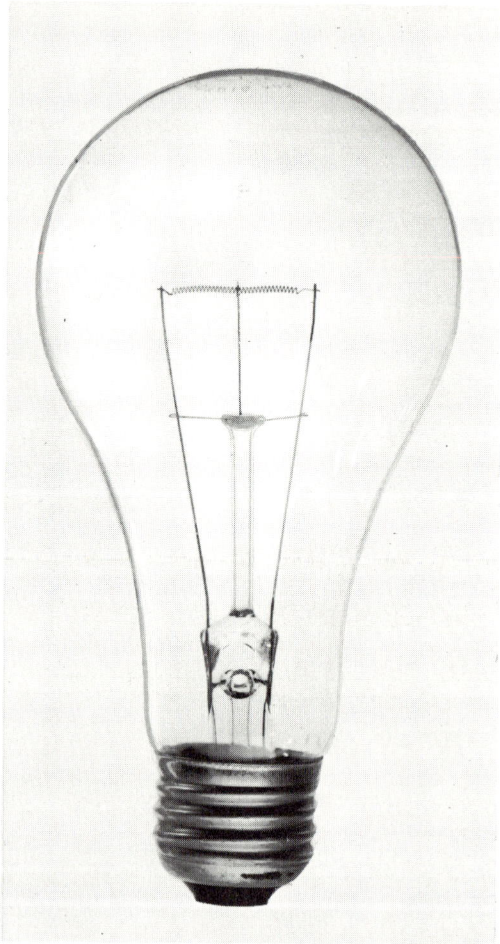

*General Electric Company, Lamp Division*

**9.8** An electric bulb has a fine-wire coil that glows when electricity passes through it.

The electricity that we use in our homes to provide us with light and, in some cases, heat is similar to static electricity in that its energy is caused by the movement of electrons. **Current electrity,** as this more useful form is called, is the flow of a stream of electrons through a conductor. Remember that in static electricity the electrons do not normally move in a stream.

The flow of current electricity has often been compared to the flow of water through a water system like the one in the diagram on page 283. In order for us to get the water to go where we want it to, we need a pipe for the water to flow through and a pump to apply pressure to the water to make it flow. Similarly, in order to get electricity to move as we want it to, we need a conductor for the electrons to flow through and some type of "electron pump." In the next activity, a dry cell forces electrons through a copper wire.

## Making a Simple Electrical Circuit

**MATERIALS:**

A dry cell, a flashlight bulb in a socket, several pieces of copper bell wire

**PROCEDURE:**

Attach one piece of wire to each side of the bulb socket. Attach the opposite ends to the binding posts of the dry cell, as shown in the diagram. The light bulb should light.

Starting at the cell, trace the path of electrons from one binding post, through the wire, through the light bulb (notice carefully the path of the current through the bulb), and back to the cell through the second wire. What happens if the wire is broken at one point? What happens if the bulb is removed from the socket? What do you think would happen if the small wire inside the light bulb were to break?

In this activity you have seen a demonstration of the fact that if electrons are to flow, the wire must form a "closed loop." This loop is called a **circuit** (sėr′ kit), which means a *circle*. If a break occurs anywhere in this circuit, the electric current cannot flow.

In order to keep the electric current traveling within the wires, it is often necessary to wrap the wires with a nonconducting material. Nonconductors, when used in this way, are called **insulators** (in′ sə lā′ tər).

This circuit is a very simple one, consisting of a cell, a bulb, and wire conductors. A more complex circuit might possibly include several bulbs or several cells.

## Using Bulbs in a Series Circuit

**MATERIALS:**

A dry cell, several flashlight bulbs in sockets, several pieces of copper bell wire

**PROCEDURE:**

Arrange the equipment as shown in the diagram. Trace the path of the electrons through the circuit.

What happens if the wire is broken at one point? What happens if one bulb is removed from its socket? Does the light from each bulb seem to be as bright as the light from the bulb in the previous activity?

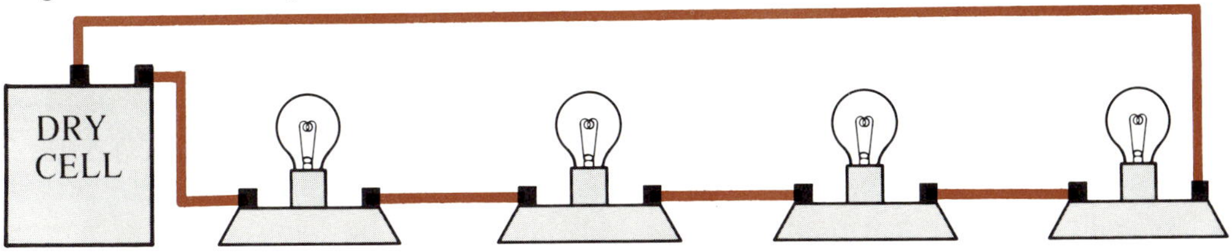

This type of circuit is called a **series circuit,** since each of the bulbs is arranged along the wire in a series. Some strings of Christmas tree lights are arranged in this manner. The major problem with using this type of circuit is that when one bulb burns out, the entire string of lights goes out. Can you explain why this happens?

Another disadvantage of the series circuit is that the lights do not give off so much light as they do in other types of circuits. The reason for this is that each bulb offers **resistance** to the electrons that pass through it. Look carefully at one of the bulbs. The electrons must be forced through the fine wires inside the bulb (Figure 9.8 page 284). When several bulbs are in a series circuit, fewer electrons can be forced through the circuit in a given amount of time.

The following activity shows you how to connect bulbs in another arrangement.

## Using Bulbs in a Parallel Circuit

**MATERIALS:**

A dry cell, several flashlight bulbs in sockets, several pieces of copper bell wire

**PROCEDURE:**

Arrange the equipment as shown in the diagram. Trace the path of the electrons through each bulb and back to the cell.

What happens if the wire is broken at point *A*? At point *B*? At point *C*? What happens if one bulb is removed from its socket? Does the light from each bulb seem to be more bright or less bright than in the previous activity? Can you explain each of these observations?

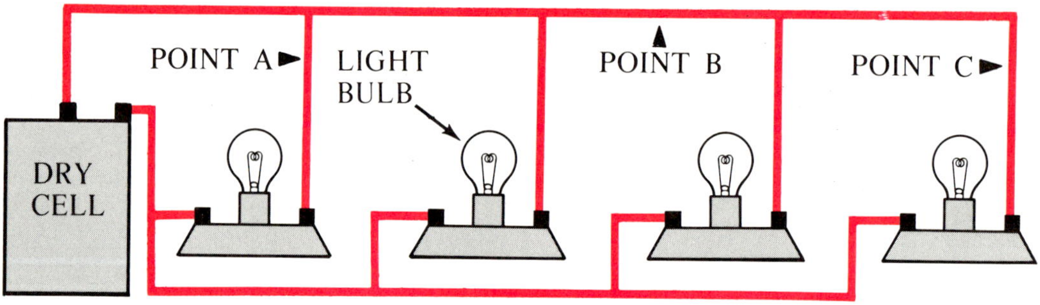


This type of circuit is called a **parallel** (par′ ə lel) **circuit.** House lights are normally wired in this manner. Parallel circuits have several advantages over series circuits. You have already observed most of these advantages.

In the first place, when one bulb of a parallel circuit burns out, the other bulbs in the circuit do not fail. This is because there are several paths for the electrons to take, and a break in one part of the circuit does not affect the other parts. Only if a break occurs between the source of power and the first branch does the entire set of lights go out. Can you explain why this is so?

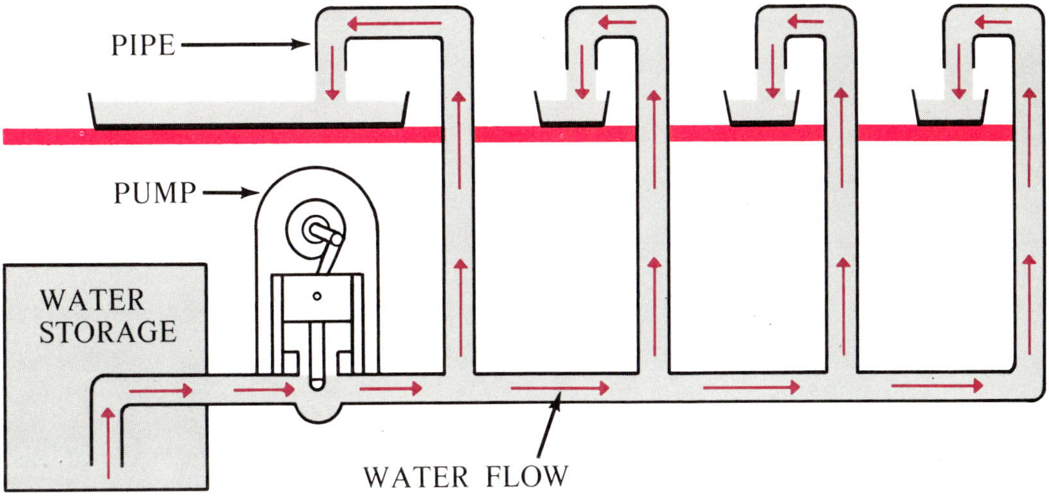


**9.9** You can think of water flowing through parallel pipes as something like a parallel electric circuit.

The second advantage of the parallel circuit is that the more branches there are to the circuit, the *less resistance* the circuit has, and *more electrons* are able to flow through the circuit. Therefore, in a parallel circuit, the addition of new bulbs does not make each bulb burn less brightly, as it does in the case of a series circuit.

To understand this lowering of resistance, consider the water system again. If water is under a certain pressure, its movement is resisted by the pipes through which it flows. If we add more pipes, the total resistance to the flow of water is less. (See Figure 9.9 above.)

Dry cells are often arranged in series as shown in the diagram on page 288. Notice that the binding post on the *center* of each cell is connected to the binding post at the *edge* of the next cell. Several cells connected together in a series such as this form what is known as a **battery** (bat′ ər i). With the cells of a battery connected in series, the pressure on the electrons is increased. Therefore, the number of electrons moving through the circuit per second is greater than the number from a single cell, and, as a result, the light burns more brightly (Figure 9.10 page 288).

A battery may be made by connecting a set of cells in parallel series as shown in the diagram on page 295. In this type of arrangement the pressure on the electrons is the same as it would be for a single cell.

## Have You Learned?

Answer the following questions, using brief complete sentences.

1. In a flashlight what is the "electron pump" that forces the electrons through the bulb?
2. What does the word *insulator* mean?
3. Diagram a series circuit. What will happen if a bulb is removed from its socket? Why?
4. Diagram a parallel circuit. What will happen if a bulb is removed from its socket? Why?
5. How is a battery different from a cell?

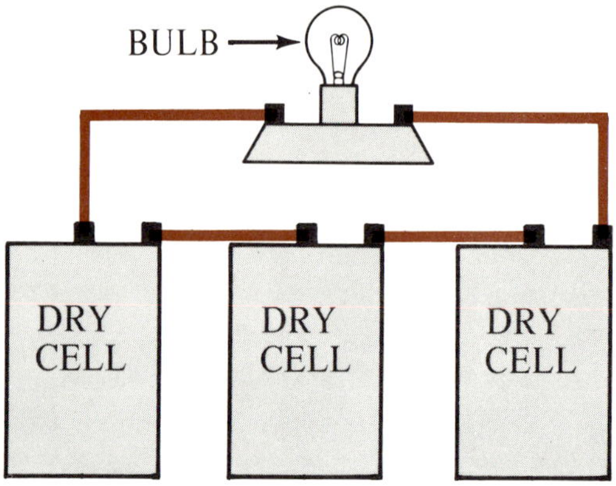


**9.10** Cells in series to form a "battery"

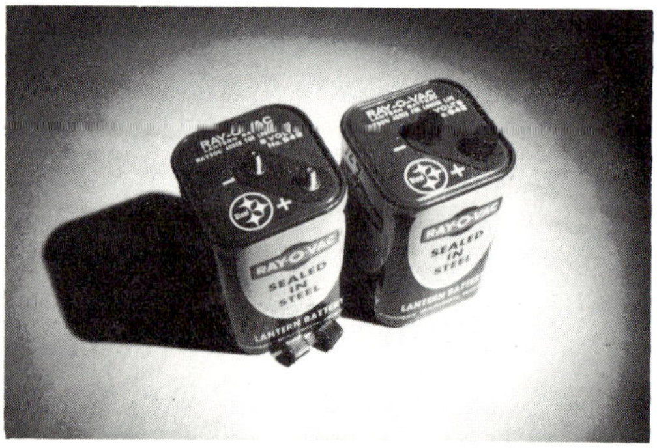

*J. W. McDonald*

**9.11** Dry cells with terminals

## 4. Measurement of Electric Current

> **ARE YOU READY?**
>
> Look up the following words if you are not sure of their meanings:
>
> parallel circuit; potential energy; resistance; series circuit.

You have learned that there are three factors that operate in any electric circuit. These are (1) the pressure on the electrons, (2) the resistance of the parts of the circuit to the movement of the electrons, and (3) the number of electrons that actually move through the circuit. As you have seen, these three factors are related to each other. In order to study them more exactly, they must be measured and represented by numbers.

### Pressure

In the water system pictured in the diagram on page 289, water is caused to flow by pressure. This pressure is caused by the height of the water reservoir. Because the reservoir is higher than the water faucets in the house, the water in the reservoir has *potential energy*. The higher the reservoir is above the faucets, the greater the potential energy of the water and the greater the water pressure in the faucets.

The pressure on electrons of an electric circuit caused by a cell is known as *potential difference*, and the higher it is, the greater the pressure on the electrons. This electric pressure is also known as **electromotive** (i lek′ trə mō′ tiv) **force** and is abbreviated *emf.*

Electromotive force is measured in **volts** (vōlt). The instrument used to measure this force is a **voltmeter** (vōlt′ mē′ tər). To use a voltmeter, we connect it between the two binding posts of the cell. In this way it can measure the difference in potential energy between the two sides of the cell.

The emf of an ordinary flashlight cell is about 1.5 volts. A larger cell will not necessarily have a greater emf, and some very small cells have a greater potential difference than a flashlight cell.

If a voltmeter of the proper size and type is available to you, do the following activities. If this is not possible, read carefully what happens (Figure 9.15).

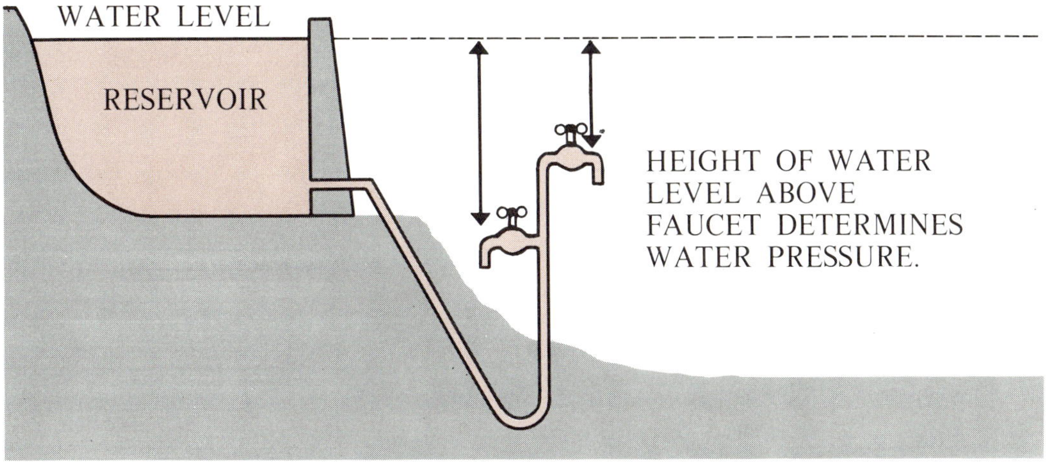


**9.12** In a reservoir the weight of a column of water behind the dam makes pressure.

## Measuring emf in a Series-Connected Battery

**MATERIALS:**

Three 1.5 volt dry cells, a DC voltmeter capable of measuring at least 6 volts, several pieces of copper bell wire

**PROCEDURE:**

Attach short pieces of wire to each of the binding posts of the voltmeter. Touch the wire connected to the positive (+) post of the voltmeter to the center post of the dry cell. Touch the wire connected to the negative (−) post of the voltmeter to the outside post of the dry cell. Does the voltmeter show approximately 1.5 volts of emf?

Connect the cells in series, as shown in Figure 9.13. Again touch the wire connected to the positive post of the voltmeter to the post of one of the last cells in the series. Touch the wire connected to the negative post of the voltmeter to the outside post of the cell at the other end of the series. Does the voltmeter now read about 4.5 volts?

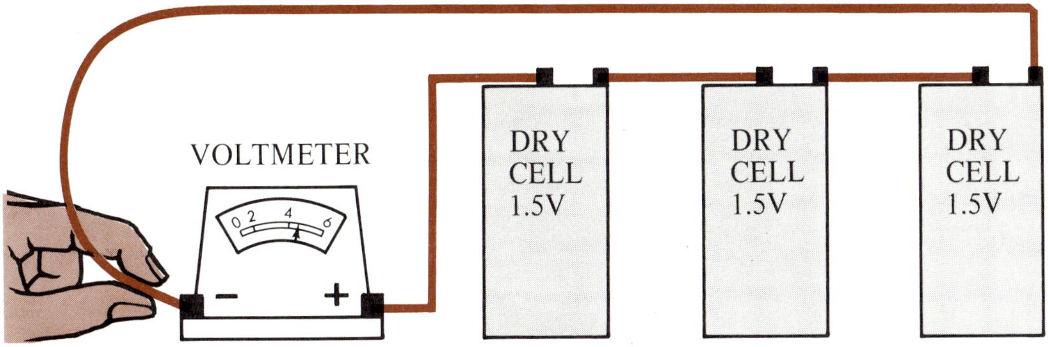


**9.13** Measuring emf in series-connected batteries

Connecting cells in series results in an *increase* in emf over that of a single cell. The emf of such a battery is the *sum* of the emf of each cell in the battery. Thus, three 1.5 volt cells, when connected in series, produce a total of 4.5 volts of emf.

### Measuring emf in a Parallel-Connected Battery

**MATERIALS:**

Three 1.5 volt dry cells, a DC voltmeter capable of measuring at least 3 volts, several pieces of copper bell wire

**PROCEDURE:**

Connect the three dry cells in a parallel circuit, as shown in the diagram. Touch the wires of the voltmeter as in the previous activity. Does the voltmeter show an emf of 1.5 volts?

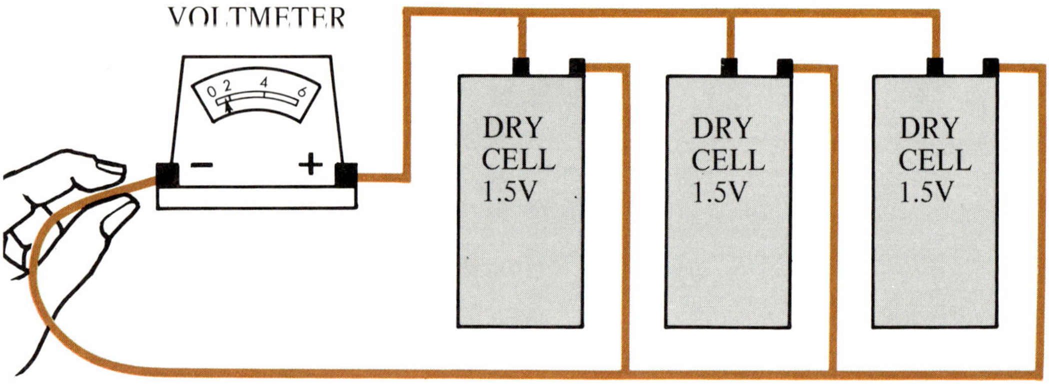


**9.14** Measuring emf in parallel-connected batteries

Cells connected in a parallel series result in an emf that is equal to the emf of only *one* cell. Thus, regardless of the total number of 1.5 volt cells in the set, the emf will not be greater than 1.5 volts.

## Number of Electrons

The water that flows into a house can be measured by a **water meter.** The water meter measures the *gallons of water* that flow through it during the period of time between readings. With an instrument known as an **ammeter** (am′ mē′ tər), the flow of electrons past a certain point can be measured in terms of *the number of electrons per second.*

The number of electrons that flow through most electric circuits is very large. In order to have a smaller number to work with, a special unit called a **coulomb** (kü lom′) is used. An electric charge of $6.28 \times 10^{18}$ (6.28 billion billion) electrons is one coulomb. A current that carries a charge of one coulomb per second past a point is known as one **ampere** (am′ pēr).

Since the ammeter measures the actual flow of electrons, it is always placed *in* the circuit, as shown in Figure 9.16. A reading of one ampere, or **amp** (amp) as it is normally abbreviated, means that 6.28 billion billion electrons are flowing through the ammeter each second.

## Resistance

If the electrons of a circuit are under a certain pressure, the actual number of electrons that will flow in the circuit depends upon the resistance. While resistance is not measured directly, it can be calculated if the **voltage** (vōl′ tij) and **amperage** (am′ pər ij) are both known. The resistance of a conductor is calculated in units called **ohms** (ōm).

If an emf of 1 volt produces a current of 1 ampere, the resistance of the circuit is calculated as being 1 ohm. To give you an idea of what an ohm is, 300 meters of copper wire 0.25 cm in diameter (as is used in most house wiring) has a resistance of 1 ohm.

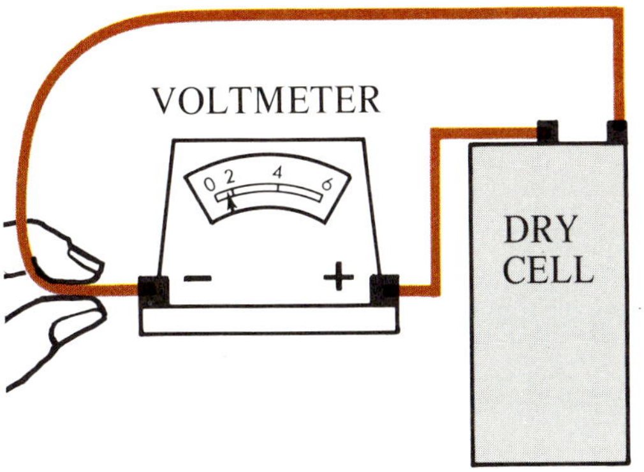


**9.15** Voltmeter

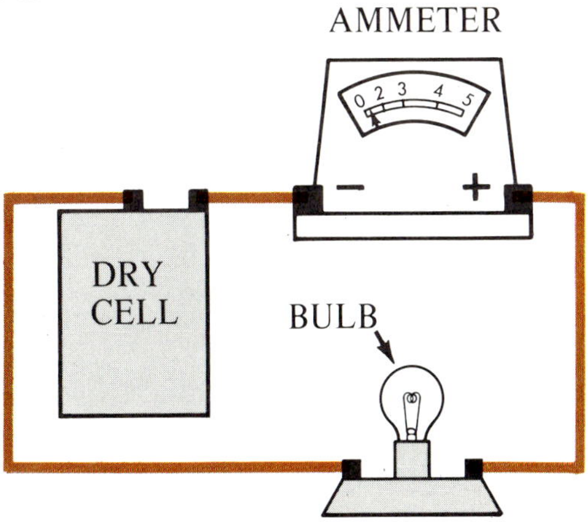


**9.16** Ammeter

## Calculating the Resistance of a Series Circuit

**MATERIALS:**

A 1.5 volt dry cell, two flashlight bulbs with sockets, a DC ammeter, several pieces of copper bell wire

**PROCEDURE:**

Connect the equipment as shown in Figure 9.17 page 292. Touch the wire from the ammeter to the binding post of the cell. Record the reading.

Connect another bulb to the circuit as shown in the diagram. Touch the wire from the ammeter to the binding post of the cell. Is the reading less than before? Can you explain your results?

The added bulb in the series circuit added resistance to the circuit. Did you notice that each bulb burned less brightly in the second experiment than in the first?

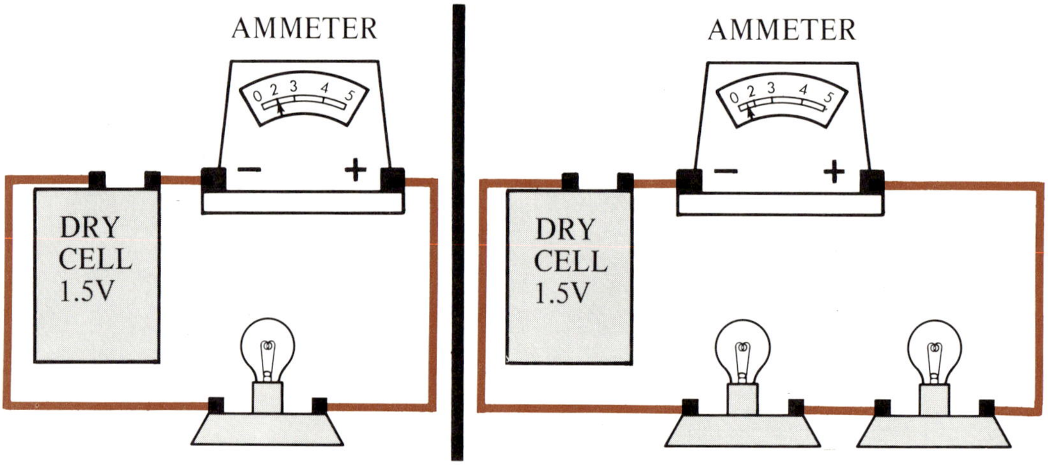


**9.17** What happens to the resistance in a series circuit when you add an electricity user?

Calculate the resistance of each circuit by dividing the number of volts by the number of amps. This may be stated as a formula in this way:

$$\text{Resistance (Ohms)} = \frac{\text{emf (Volts)}}{\text{current (Amps)}} \quad \text{or}$$

$$O = \frac{V}{A}$$

This is known as **Ohm's Law** and can be used to find ohms, volts, or amps if the other two quantities are known.

To find amps, the formula is $A = \frac{V}{O}$ and for volts, $V = AO$.

## Calculating the Resistance of a Parallel Circuit

**MATERIALS:**

A 1.5 volt dry cell, three flashlight bulbs with sockets, a DC ammeter, several pieces of copper bell wire

**PROCEDURE:**

Connect the equipment as shown in Figure 9.18 on page 293. Touch the wire from the ammeter to the binding post of the cell. Record the reading.

Unscrew one bulb in the circuit. Touch the wire from the ammeter to the binding post of the cell. Is the flow of electrons through the circuit greater or smaller now than it was before? Is the resistance of the circuit greater or smaller now than before?

The resistance of parallel circuits *decreases* as more branches are added to the circuit. Calculate how much more resistance this circuit had in each case.

Since some materials are considered to be better conductors than others, you might guess that the resistance of these conductors is different. Copper has less

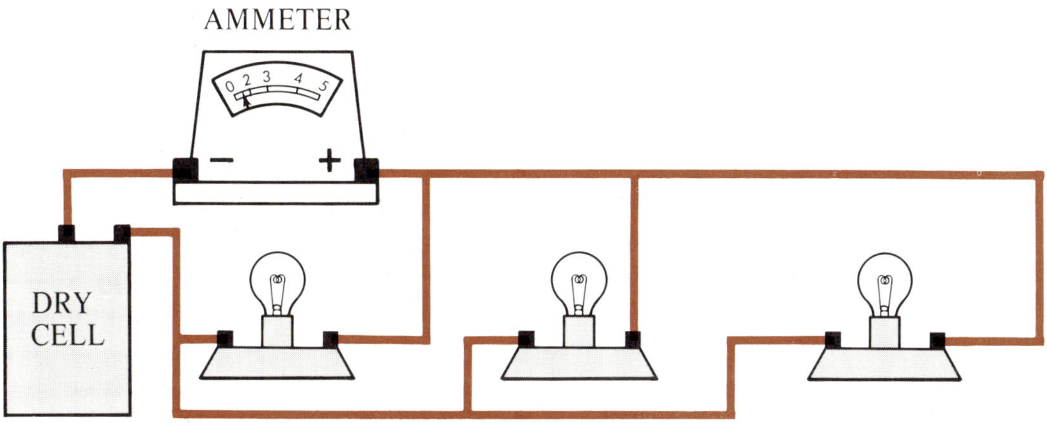

**9.18** Finding the resistance of a parallel circuit

resistance than aluminum, for example, and silver has less resistance than copper has.

## Wire Size and Temperature Also Determine Resistance

The size of the wire used as a conductor also determines the resistance to a great extent. Just as a large water pipe offers less resistance to the flow of water than does a small pipe, a large wire will carry a current of electricity more easily than will a small wire. If 300 meters of wire 0.25 centimeter thick offers a resistance of 1 ohm, a similar wire 0.125 centimeter thick will have a resistance of 4 ohms and will allow only a quarter as much current to flow through it.

The temperature of the conductor determines its resistance too. As the temperature increases, the action of the molecules of the conductor also increases. This increased activity apparently interferes with the flow of electrons from atom to atom, and the resistance increases. Recent experiments with conductors cooled to below

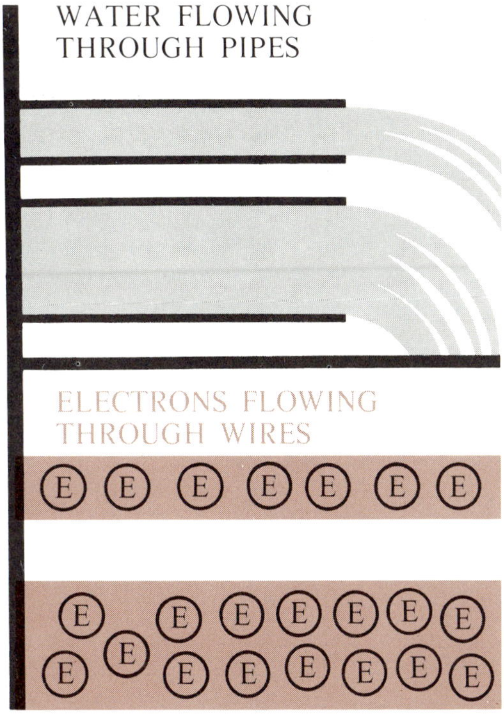

**9.19** Resistance of a pipe and of an electric wire.

−268° C have created superconductors, materials that will carry electric current with no noticeable resistance. In a few cases, a loop has been made of superconductive material, and, once started, the electric current appears to continue to flow around and around without any additional pressure.

### Have You Learned?

On a sheet of paper list the numbers for the questions below. By each number write *T* if the statement is true and *F* if false.

1. A voltmeter measures the electromotive force of a source of electricity.
2. A large cell will usually have a higher voltage than a small cell.
3. Connecting a set of cells in series increases the electromotive force over that of one cell.
4. An ammeter measures the number of electrons flowing through a circuit per unit of time.
5. An ampere is equal to one coulomb per second.
6. The addition of an extra bulb to a parallel circuit adds to the resistance of the total circuit.
7. Some conductors have more resistance than others.
8. A wire of small diameter has less resistance than a thicker wire of the same material.
9. The hotter a wire is, the greater its resistance.

## 5. How Cells Produce Electricity

**ARE YOU READY?**

Look up the following words if you are not sure of their meanings:

conduct; emf; negative charge (electrical); positive charge (electrical); potential difference.

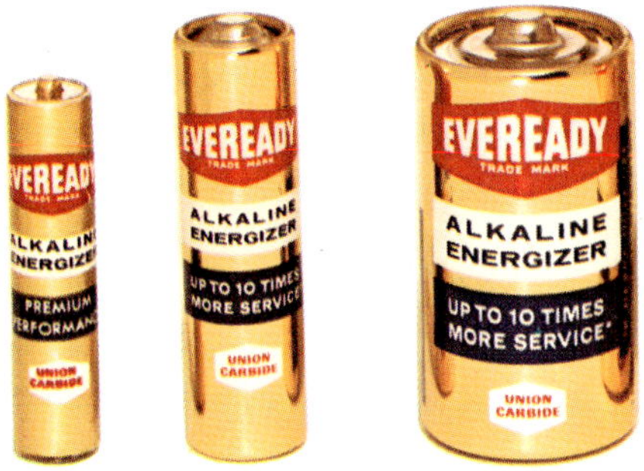


*Union Carbide Corporation*

**9.20** Typical low-voltage dry cells

The cells that you have worked with so far in this study of electricity have all been "dry" cells that produce a low voltage of **direct current.** The term *direct current,* abbreviated DC, means that the electrons flow in only one direction through the circuit. As you will learn later, the electric current used in your home is of a different type.

Low-voltage dry cells are of great use to us. They are used in flashlights, in portable radios, and in many other household appliances. How many other uses can you name?

The electrical systems used in automobiles depend upon another type of direct-current low-voltage cell. In this type, a liquid may be seen by removing the small cap at the top of each cell. These dry cells and the wet cells both produce electricity through a chemical reaction, and neither of them is really "dry."

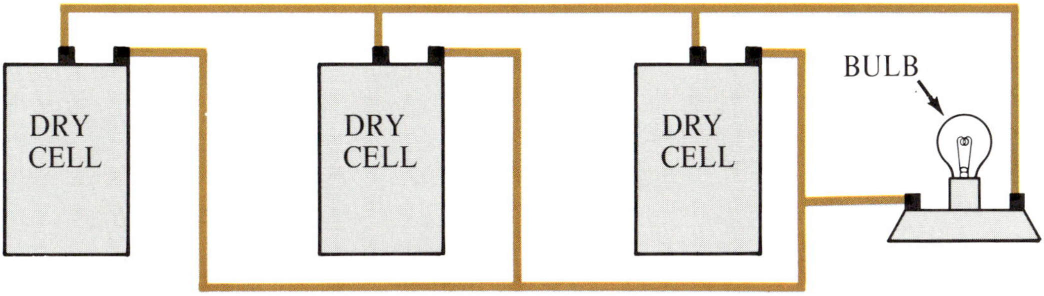


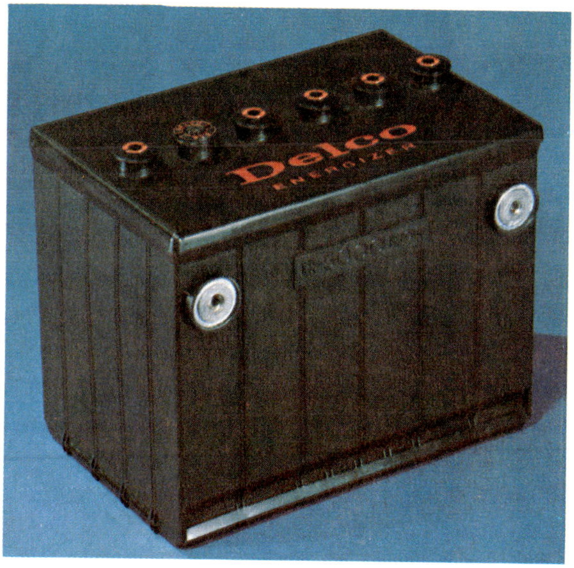


**9.21** (*Above*) A battery can be made by connecting several cells in parallel. (*Left*) An automobile battery

## Making a Simple Cell

**MATERIALS:**

A sensitive **galvanometer** (gal′ və nom′ ə tər), several short pieces of copper bell wire, a variety of fruits (including a lemon), a variety of strips of different metals (including copper, iron, and zinc)

**PROCEDURE:**

Puncture the ends of two strips of metal of different types, and attach to the galvanometer by means of the copper wire, as shown in Figure 9.22 on page 296. Insert the metal strips into various fruits, and record the reading of the galvanometer. Try different metals and different fruits. Do some combinations produce more electricity than others?

Touch the two pieces of clean metal to opposite sides of your tongue. What is the reading on the galvanometer?

Repeat this activity, using various combinations of metals. Describe your results.

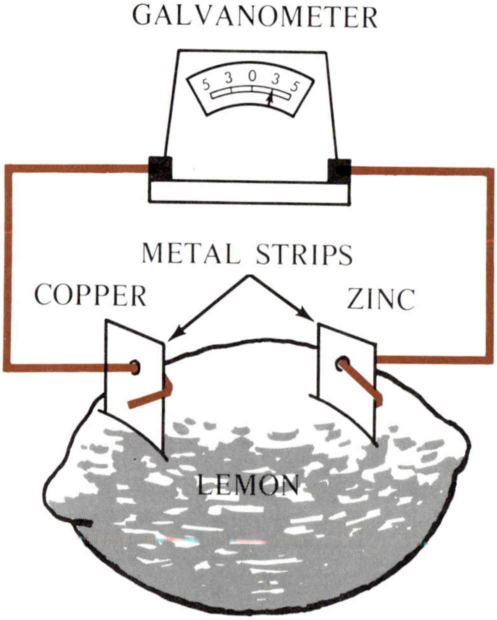


**9.22** What is the electrolyte in this cell? (page 295)

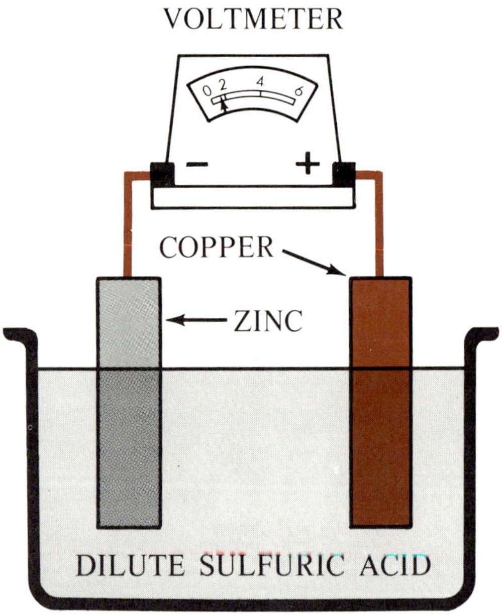


**9.23** Zinc-copper cell

The working of a simple cell of this type depends upon two factors. First, the metals must be dissimilar; that is, they must be of different types. Second, the fluid in which they are placed must be capable of conducting electricity. A fluid of this type is called an **electrolyte** (i lek′ trə līt). A more efficient cell, the zinc-copper cell, will illustrate the chemical reaction that takes place in these cells.

## Making a Zinc-Copper Cell

**MATERIALS:**

A 10-cm strip of zinc, a 10-cm strip of copper, a voltmeter capable of registering at least 2 volts DC, a beaker or other similar glass container, enough dilute sulfuric acid to fill the glass container half full, two short pieces of copper bell wire

**PROCEDURE:**

Connect the metal strips to the voltmeter by use of the copper wire. Place the dilute sulfuric acid in the glass container, and dip the zinc and the copper strips into the acid, as shown in Figure 9.23. Be sure that the zinc strip is attached to the negative post of the voltmeter. What is the reading on the voltmeter? Are bubbles formed around the copper strip?

In this cell the zinc strip dissolves in the acid. As this happens, each zinc atom leaves behind two electrons, and the zinc strip becomes *negatively* charged. It is now

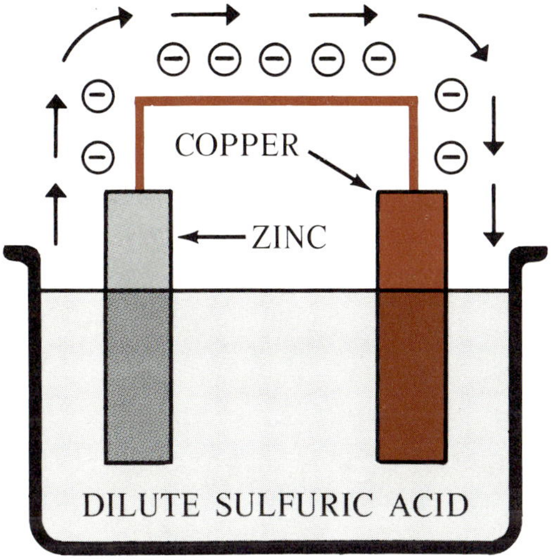


**9.24** Movement of electrons (See below.)

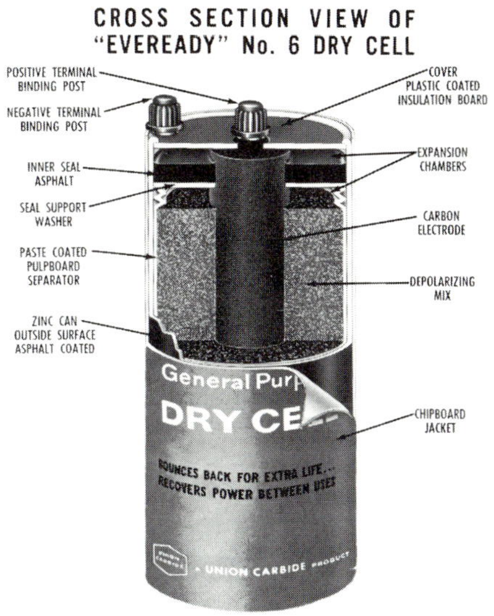


*Union Carbide Corporation*

**9.25** Cross section of typical dry cell

called the **negative electrode** (i lek′ trōd). The zinc atoms, now *positively* charged since losing some electrons, have become zinc ions.

The acid contains ions of hydrogen, which are also positively charged. These ions form when the acid is dissolved in water. The positive hydrogen ions take electrons from the copper strip, form a molecule of hydrogen, and leave the cell in the form of small bubbles. The loss of electrons from the copper strip give it a positive charge, and it is now known as the **positive electrode.**

The collection of electrons on the negative electrode (the zinc strip) and the shortage of electrons on the positive electrode (the copper strip) make up the potential difference between the two. This potential difference, or emf, amounts to about 1 volt. If the two electrodes are connected with a conductor, the electrons flow from the zinc strip to the copper strip.

The so-called "dry" cell is very similar to the cell just described. Figure 9.25 above is of a dry cell cut to show its construction. The outside container is made of zinc, which forms the negative electrode. A carbon rod in the center of the cell is the positive electrode. Between the two is a powder made primarily of carbon, with which the electrolyte makes a moist paste.

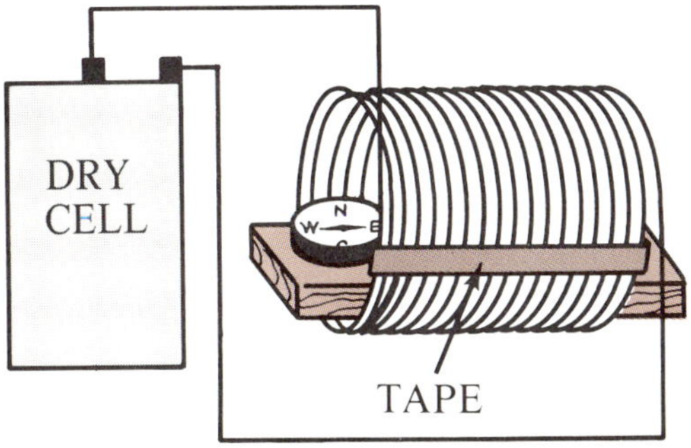


**9.26** Magnetic effects of electric currents (page 299)

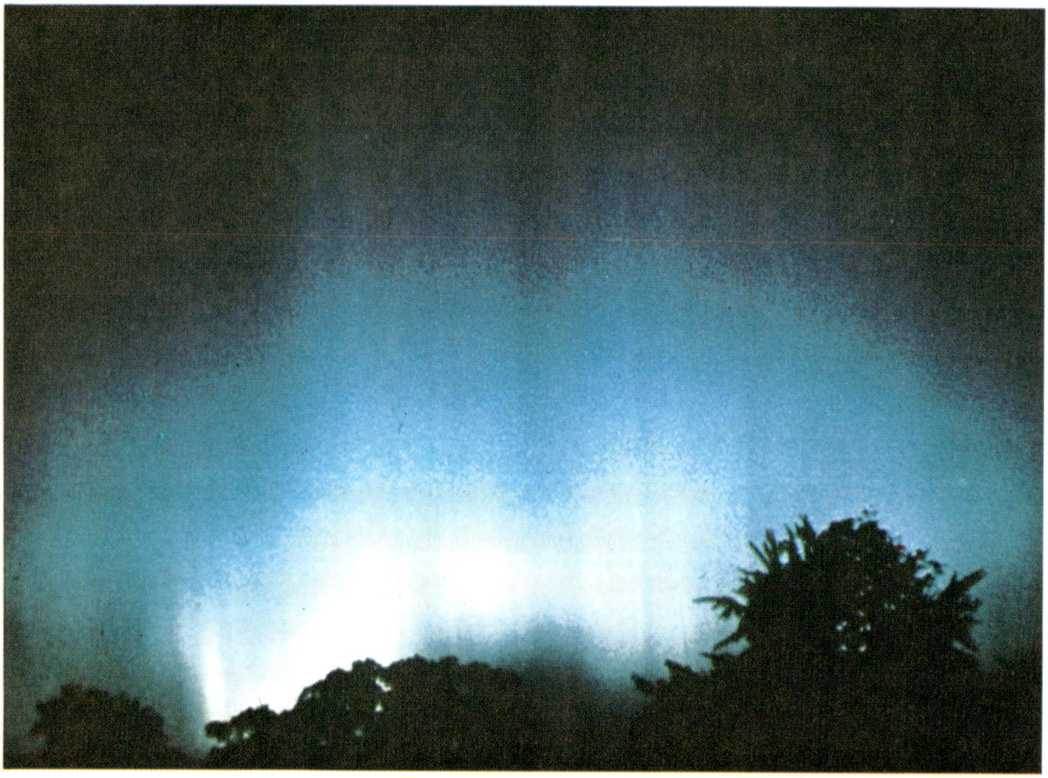

*Official U. S. Naval Observatory Photo*

**9.27** If you live far enough north, you may have seen the "Northern Lights" (*aurora borealis*). Although nothing certain is known to account for auroras, there appears to be some connection with the earth's magnetic poles (page 270, Section 4).

### Have You Learned?

Define the following words, using brief complete sentences.

1. direct current (DC)
2. galvanometer
3. electrolyte
4. negative electrode
5. ion
6. dry cell
7. positive electrode
8. emf
9. conductor
10. voltage

## 6. Magnetism and Electricity

**ARE YOU READY?**

Look up the following words if you are not sure of their meanings:

absolute zero; amperage; attract; electromagnet; magnetic field; meter (electrical); permanent magnet; repel; right angle.

You have already seen that under certain conditions electrically charged substances will attract lightweight objects. As an example, a rubber comb that has been run through dry hair will pick up bits of paper. The relationship between magnetism and electricity is much greater than just this interesting similarity, as you will see from the following activity.

### Observing the Magnetic Effect of an Electric Current

**MATERIALS:**

A dry cell of any size, 15 meters of insulated bell wire, a small compass, a small block of wood

**PROCEDURE:**

Coil the wire into a loop of at least 50 turns by turning it around a small jar or drinking glass. The loop should be about three inches in diameter and can be tied with string or fastened with tape at several points to hold it together. Hold the loop in an upright position, place the wooden block inside the loop, and place the compass on the block, as shown in Figure 9.26 on page 297. Turn the apparatus so that the needle of the compass is lined up directly under the wires on top of the loop. Connect the ends of the wires to the dry cell. Observe the action of the compass needle as you complete and then break the circuit.

Reverse the wires, connecting them to opposite posts of the dry cell. Does this affect the action of the compass needle? Save the coil of wire you have made for use in the next section.

When you allowed the electric current to flow through the loop of wire, the needle of the compass acted exactly as if you had placed a bar magnet over the compass, at right angles to the way the loop of wire was pointing. When you reversed the attachment of the wires to the dry cell, you reversed the flow of current through the wire. As a result of this, the direction of the compass needle was also reversed. Can you make the needle of your compass act in this way by using a bar magnet?

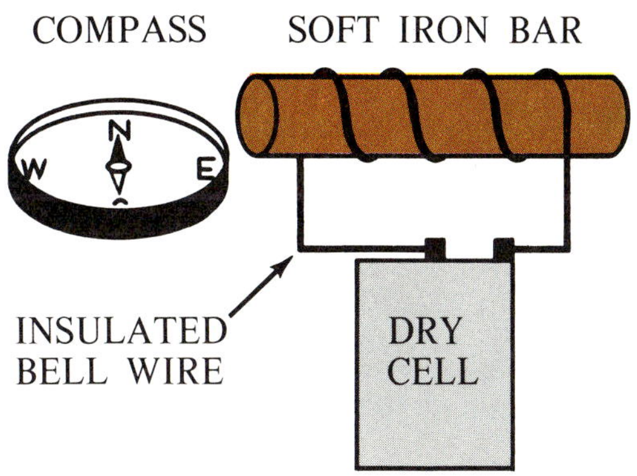


9.28 Electromagnets (page 300)

What can be concluded from this experiment? First, when current flows through a wire, a magnetic field is created around the wire. Second, the magnetic field acts as if it were the result of a magnet's lying at right angles to the wire. Third, the **polarity** (pō lar′ ə ti) of the magnetic field of the wire depends upon the direction of the flow of current through the wire.

The meters that you used to measure the various elements of an electrical circuit in Section 4 are simply modifications of the apparatus you have just constructed. In the meters, however, the pointer is connected to a coil of wire that is free to turn slightly. This coil is placed between the poles of a horseshoe-shaped permanent magnet, and when the current flows through the wire, the coil is attracted and repelled by the permanent magnet. The stronger the current, the stronger the attraction-repulsion, and the further the pointer moves.

The magnetic effects of a current can be increased in several ways. As you might expect, the amount of current flowing through the coil of wire determines the strength of the magnetic field. In the activity above, you made at least fifty turns in the coil. The effect of this was to cause many more electrons to flow past a given point each second. In a coil of 50 turns, the magnetic field will be almost 50 times stronger than in a one-turn coil.

Naturally, anything that increases the amperage in the wire will also increase the magnetic effects of the circuit. You might do this by adding a second dry cell, connected in series with the first, to increase the voltage. Or you might reduce the resistance of the circuit in some way.

The magnetic effects of an electric current can be increased tremendously by placing a bar of soft iron *inside* the coil of wire, parallel to the magnetic field.

## Making an Electromagnet

**MATERIALS:**

Two meters of insulated bell wire, two dry cells, a short piece of soft iron in the shape of a rod, a small compass, a small piece of iron

**PROCEDURE:**

Tightly wrap the iron rod with several turns of the bell wire. Connect one end of the wire to one post of a dry cell. Place one end of the electromagnet close to the compass, and complete the circuit by touching the free end of the wire to the free post of the cell (Figure 9.28). Notice the action of the compass needle.

Reverse the flow of electricity through the wire by reversing the attachment of wires on the dry cell. Does this have an effect on the compass needle different from your first observation?

Complete the circuit, and slowly bring one end of the electromagnet close to a small piece of iron. Notice how far away from the metal your magnet is when you first notice the metal begin to move. Now make several more turns of wire around the iron rod, complete the circuit, and again approach the small piece of iron. Do the additional coils of wire seem to increase the strength of the electromagnet?

Connect the second dry cell in series with the first. Does this seem to increase the strength of the electromagnet?

Again you notice that the flow of electrons through the wire created a magnetic field in the iron bar, with a north pole at one end and a south pole at the other. Reversing the direction of flow of the current reversed the polarity of the electromagnet. A simple rule will help you to remember which pole of an electromagnet will be the north. Wrap your *left* hand around the coil of wire so that your fingers follow the direction of electron flow. You can do this if you remember that the electrons flow from the negative post of the dry cell toward the positive post. With your hand in this position, as shown in Figure 9.29, your thumb lying outstretched along the magnet will point toward the north pole of the magnet.

Electromagnets are used in many of the appliances that you see and use daily. A doorbell or buzzer contains an electromagnet that attracts a metal clapper, making it vibrate. The telephone receiver contains an electromagnet that creates a sound by attracting a metal plate. This creates sounds similar to the voice that originally produced the fluctuations in the electric current. The strength of an electro-

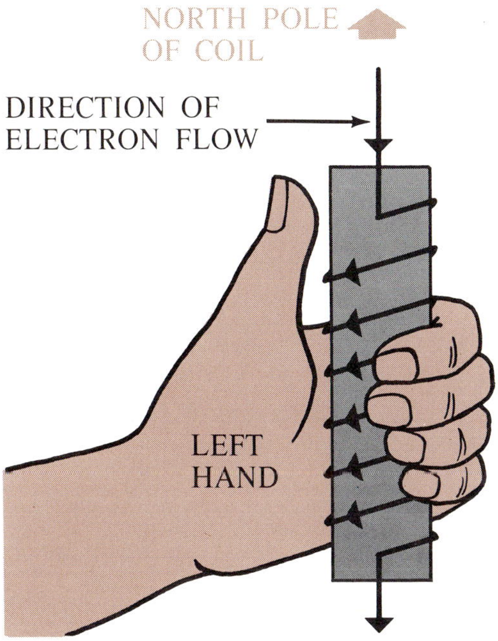


**9.29** In what compass direction is the thumb pointing?

**9.30** Diagram of electric doorbell

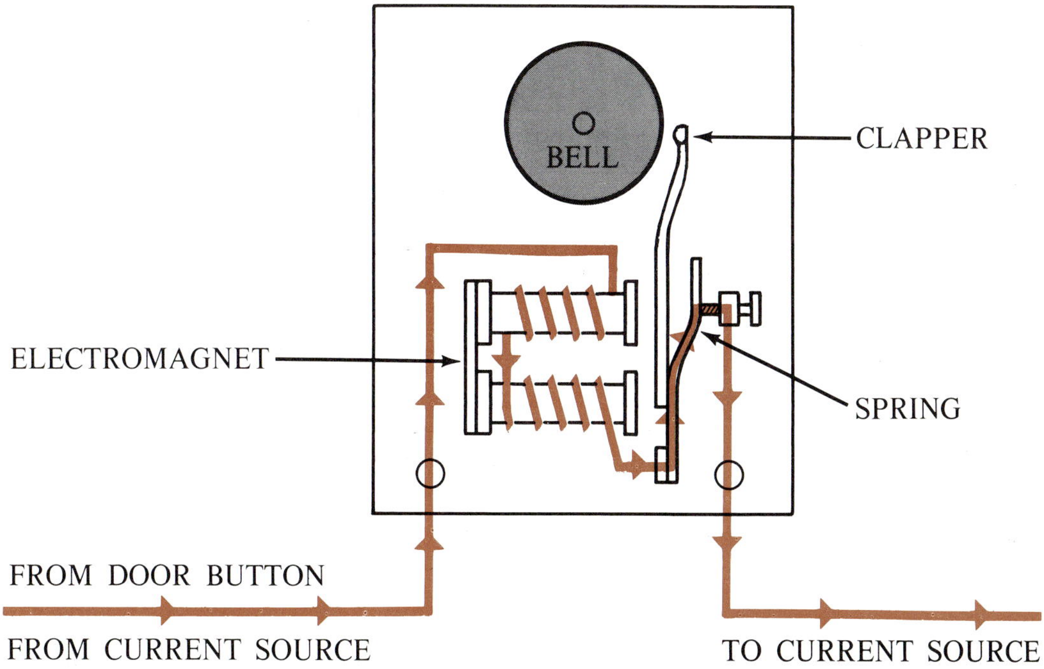

magnet is determined by three factors. You have already observed the effect of increasing the voltage and of increasing the number of turns of wire around the metal core. The third factor is the composition of the core itself. The more **permeable** (pėr′ mi ə bəl) the material of the core is, the stronger the magnet will be.

In Section 4 you learned that when certain materials are cooled to near absolute zero, they become superconductors of electricity. In these materials low voltages are capable of creating tremendously strong currents. When electromagnets are made of these materials and kept at very low temperatures, they can be made to produce very strong magnetic fields.

### Have You Learned?

Write on a sheet of paper the word that best completes the statement. (Do not write in your book.)

When an electric current flows through a wire, a magnetic field is created around the wire. This magnetic field acts as if it were the result of a magnet lying (1) _____ (parallel; at right angles) to the wire. The direction of the flow of current through the wire determines the (2) _____ (polarity; strength) of the magnetic field. If the number of electrons flowing past a given point is changed, the (3) _____ (polarity; strength) of the magnetic field will also be changed. The magnetic effects of an electric current will be (4) _____ (increased; decreased) if the wire is formed into a loop. Placing a bar of soft iron inside the loop (5) _____ (parallel; at right angles) to the magnetic field will increase the strength of the magnetic field.

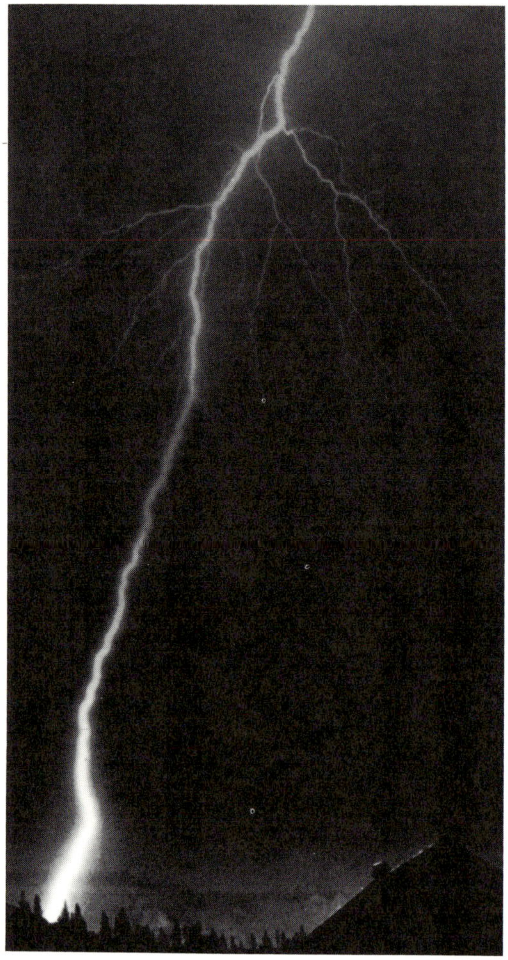

**9.31** What kind of electricity is this? (See page 278.)

## 7. Generating Electricity

**ARE YOU READY?**

Look up the following words if you are not sure of their meanings:

direct current; galvanometer; induce; thermometer.

After the discovery that electric currents produced magnetic fields, the next logical question was "Could a magnetic field create an electric current?" When you have successfully performed the experiment that follows (Electromagnetic Induction), you ought to be able to give your own answer to this question.

## Making Electricity by Using a Magnetic Field

**MATERIALS:**

A sensitive galvanometer, a long length of insulated bell wire, a bar magnet

**PROCEDURE:**

Make a coil of the bell wire so that the loop is about three inches in diameter and contains about 50 turns of wire. Connect the ends of the wire to the binding posts of the galvanometer. Hold the magnet in one hand, and rapidly push it through the loop of wire, as shown in the diagram. Notice the action of the galvanometer needle. Now rapidly withdraw the magnet from the loop of wire. Which direction does the galvanometer needle move?

Hold the magnet stationary, and move the coil of wire over it. Is the action of the galvanometer needle the same as before?

Unwind the loop of wire until only a few coils remain. Move the magnet into and out of this small coil. How far does the needle move compared to the previous experiments? Does moving the coil faster seem to generate more current than when it is moved slowly?

You have observed several important principles of *electromagnetic induction.* Current is generated *only* when the conductor is moving through a magnetic field. When the coil of wire and the magnet are both stationary, no current flows in the wire, and the needle of the galvanometer does not move. As the conductor moves through the magnetic field, current is generated, as you can see by the movement of the galvanometer needle. As the conductor is moved through the magnetic field *in the opposite direction the flow of current is also reversed.* This is shown by the fact that the needle of the galvanometer moves in the opposite direction. These principles hold true whether the coil of wire is moved and the magnet held stationary or the magnet is moved and the wire is stationary.

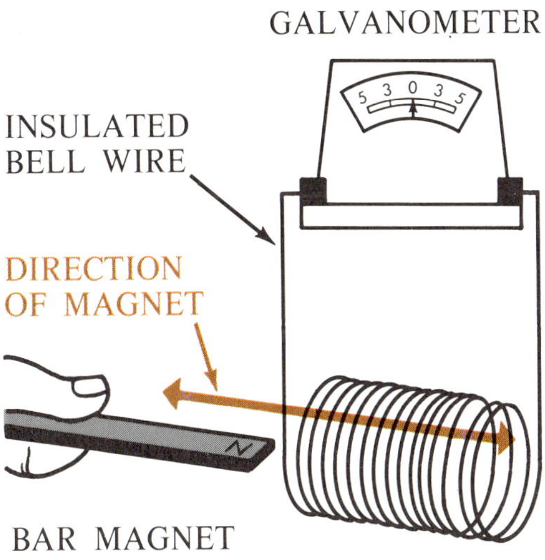


9.32 Electromagnetic induction

If fewer coils of wire are used to make up the loop, less current will be generated. Also, the greater the number of wires that cut through the magnetic field, the stronger the current is. As you might expect, the stronger the magnet, the stronger the current that is generated. You have also noticed that the speed with which the conductor is moved through the magnetic field affects the strength of the current.

In currents produced by chemical cells, the electrons move in only one direction. Currents of this type are called *direct currents*, as you saw on page 294. In currents produced by magnetic induction, the flow of electrons is first in one direction and then in the other. These currents are called **alternating** (ôl′ tər nāt ing) **currents,** which is abbreviated AC. Most of the electricity used in homes in the United States is of this type.

Alternating current is produced by generators (page 58). Generators operate in ways very similar to the coil of wire and magnets that you have just experimented with. In them, insulated copper wire is wound into a form that is called an **armature** (är′ mə chər). The armature may revolve between the poles of an electromagnet, or the armature may form a shell around the outside of the spinning electromagnet. In either case the basic principles are the same. The wires of the armature are cut by the magnetic field of the magnet. Since the direction of movement through the magnetic field changes with each revolution, the current produced is alternating. Each revolution of the generator produces a pulse of electrons in one direction and a second pulse of electrons moving in the opposite direction. This completes a single **cycle** (sī′ kəl). The speed with which the generator is turning determines the **frequency** (frē′ kwən si) of the alternating current produced. The most common frequency in the U.S. is 60 cycles per second.

While most of the appliances that we normally use everyday are made to work on AC, occasionally we need a supply of direct current. A number of different types of **rectifiers** (rek′ tə fī′ ər) are used to make this change.

A special type of rectifier can be built into an AC generator so that direct current is produced. Normally this rectifier is in the form of a **split-ring commutator** (kom′ ū tā′ tər). As shown in Figure 9.34, the commutator reverses the direction of flow of electrons at the exact time that the direction of the current is reversed.

Electromagnetic induction generators produce electric energy from mechanical energy, generally from burning fuel or from falling water. Cells transform chemical energy into electrical energy. Other forms of energy, such as nuclear energy or light energy, may also be changed into electrical energy.

Heat energy may be directly changed to electrical energy with a device called a **thermocouple** (thėr′ mə ku′ pəl).

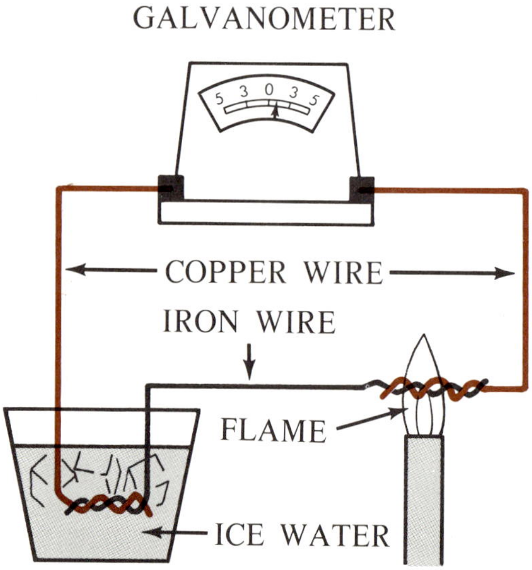


**9.33** Thermocouple

## Building a Thermocouple

**MATERIALS:**

A sensitive galvanometer, two short lengths of copper wire, a single length of iron wire, a glass of ice water, a Bunsen or propane burner

**PROCEDURE:**

Twist each end of the iron wire to one end of each copper wire, forming a long wire consisting of a length of copper, then a length of iron, and finally another length of copper. Connect the loose ends of the copper wire to the galvanometer. Place one of the junctions of the iron and copper wire into the ice water. Place the other junction of the iron and copper wires into the flame of the burner. As the temperature increases, notice the action of the galvanometer needle.

The amount of current created in the thermocouple is directly related to the differences in temperature of the two junctions. That is, the greater the difference in temperature, the greater the amount of current. It depends also upon the type of wires used.

Thermocouples are rarely used to generate electricity. However, they may be found in many industries and laboratories. Here they are used as thermometers, the amount of current produced indicating the difference in temperature between the junctions. Thermometers of this type can be used to measure the temperature in remote places where ordinary thermometers could not be placed or could not be read easily.

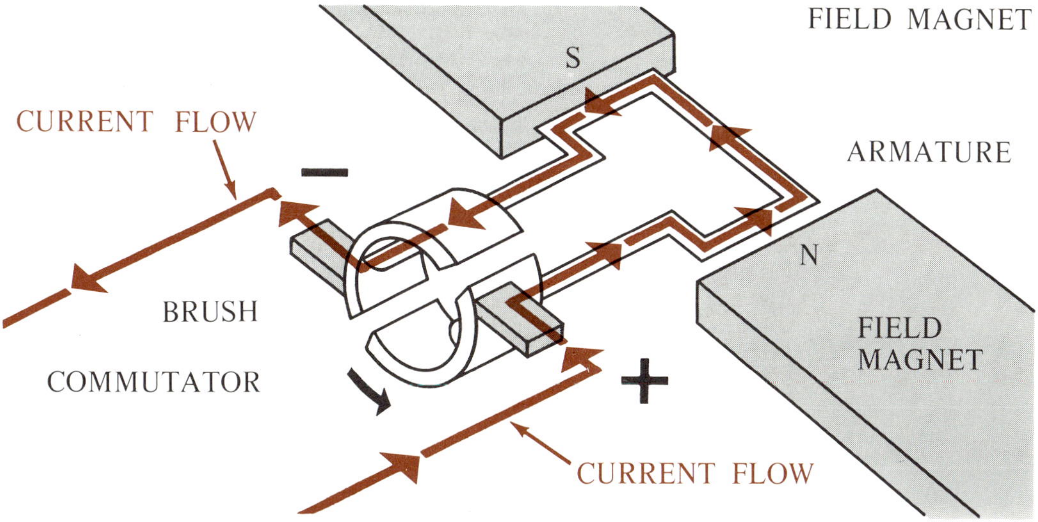


**9.34** Follow the flow of current in this diagram of an electric generator.

### Have You Learned?

Define the following terms, using brief complete sentences.

1. Electromagnetic induction
2. Direct current
3. Alternating current
4. Electric generator
5. Armature (in a generator)
6. Cycle (in alternating current)
7. Frequency (in alternating current)
8. Rectifier
9. Split-ring commutator
10. Thermocouple

## 8. Electric Motors

**ARE YOU READY?**

Look up the following words if you are not sure of their meanings:

armature; commutator; generator.

There are many types of electric motors in existence today, each type used for a specific purpose. All, however, change electrical energy into mechanical energy. This is the reverse of the use of the electric generator, which converts mechanical energy into electrical energy. Like generators, motors use magnetism to accomplish the change.

The type of electric motor described in this section is very similar to an electric generator. In fact, if mechanical energy is put *into* the motor by cranking the shaft, the motor will produce electricity and thus become a generator. Therefore, by careful study of the workings of this motor, one can more easily understand how a generator works.

There are four essential parts to a motor. These are: (1) the two *field* magnets that produce a magnetic field; (2) the *armature*, a coil of wire that also produces a magnetic field; (3) the *commutator* that, as it turns, changes the direction of the current entering the armature, thus changing the polarity of the armature; and (4) two *brushes* that provide a flexible connection between the source of electricity and the commutator.

### Making the Field Magnet

**MATERIALS:**

Two nails 12 cm long, approximately 5 meters of insulated bell wire, a board about 25 cm long and 15 cm wide, a small compass, a dry cell

**PROCEDURE:**

The field magnets of this motor are electromagnets. The top end of one must be a strong north pole, and the top end of the other must be an equally strong south pole. In order to achieve this, a great deal of care must be taken to wind the wire around the magnets in opposite directions.

Drive the nails into the board about 13 cm apart, leaving more than 10 cm of nail above the top of the board. Starting about 8 cm from the end of the bell wire, carefully wrap the wire around the base of one nail.

Be sure that the wire is tightly wrapped and that you always wrap the wire around the nail in the same direction. When you reach the top of the nail, continue winding the wire in the same direction, and again wrap the nail over the first layer of wire. *Be certain that all wires on this nail are wrapped in the same direction.* Continue this process until you have made 100 turns of wire around the nail. Then cut the wire, leaving about 20 cm free.

Now wrap the second nail. Again leave about 8 cm of wire loose, start from the bottom of the nail, but this time wind the wire around the nail in the opposite direction from that of the first nail. Continue winding the wire around the nail, always going in the same direction, until you have made 100 turns.

Connect the short ends of the free wires together.

Using the 10 cm free ends of the wire, connect the field magnets to a dry cell. Test each magnet with the compass to be sure that the head of each nail has an opposite pole. Can you explain why each magnet must be wound in opposite directions?

When connected to a source of electric current, these two powerful electromagnets will create a magnetic field across the gap between them. The lines of force between these magnets are diagramed in the illustration on the right.

We must now place an armature between them. This armature must be made of wire that will cut through the lines of magnetic force.

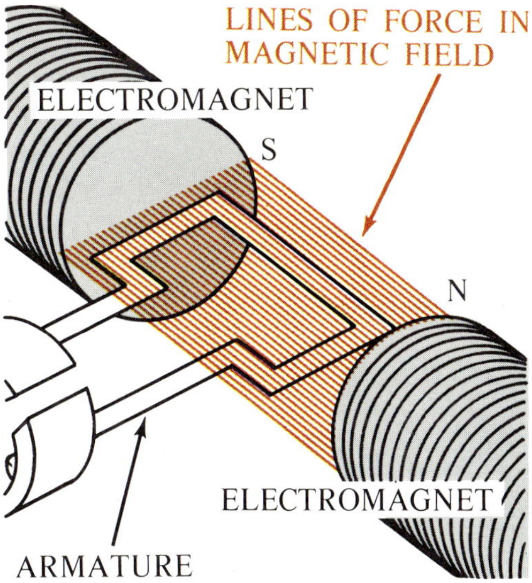


## Making the Armature

**MATERIALS:**

Two nails 12 cm long, about 3 meters of insulated bell wire, one large cork about 4 cm in diameter, one test tube 7.5 cm long, a small compass, a dry cell

**PROCEDURE:**

Carefully force one nail through the cork near the top, as shown in the diagram on page 308. In the bottom of the cork dig a hole large enough so that the closed end of the test tub will fit into it snugly. Drive a nail *up* through the board from the underside, exactly halfway between the two field magnets. Place the test tube over the point of this center nail so that the armature shaft is free to spin easily.

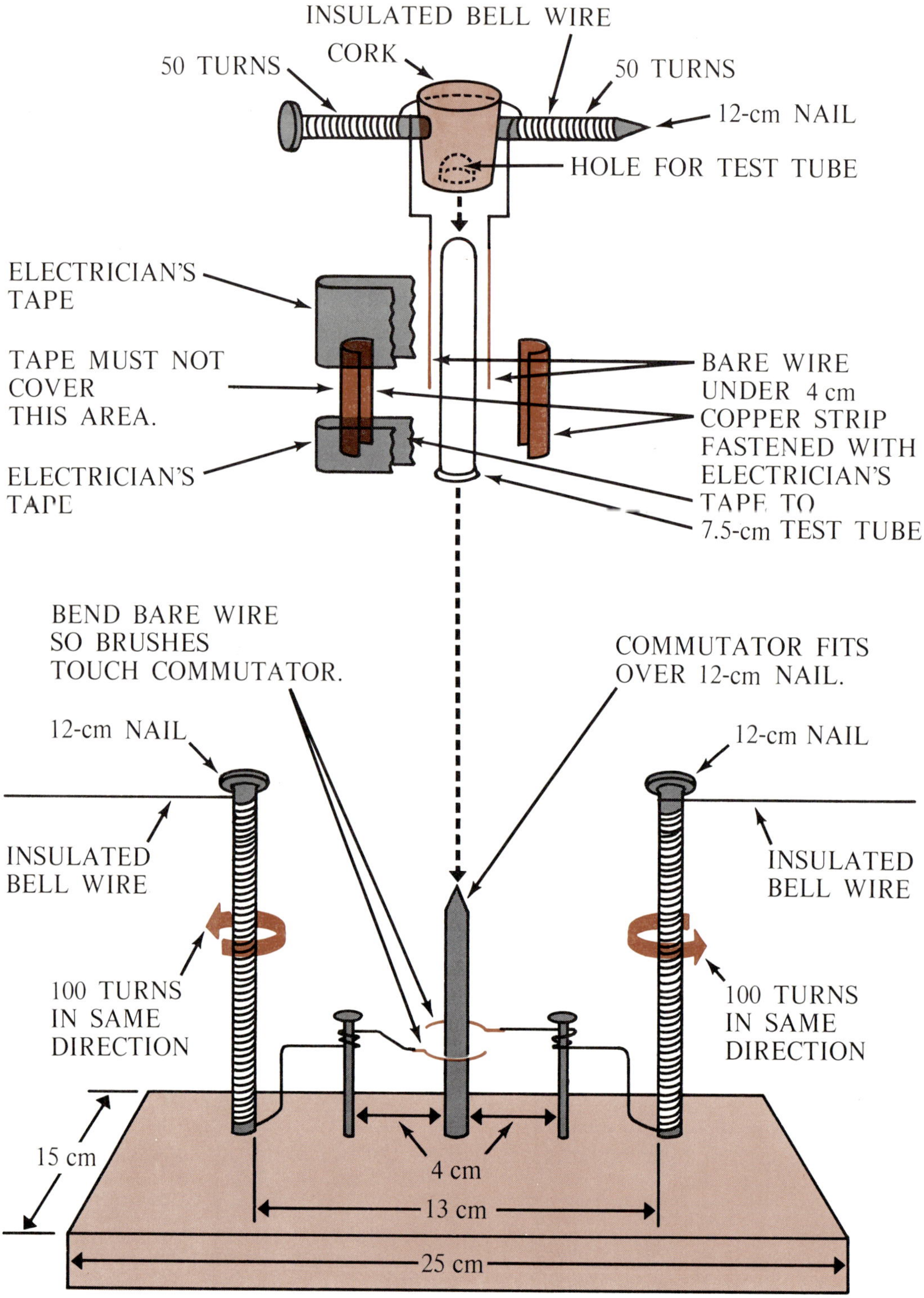


**9.35** Exploded view of the construction of an electric motor

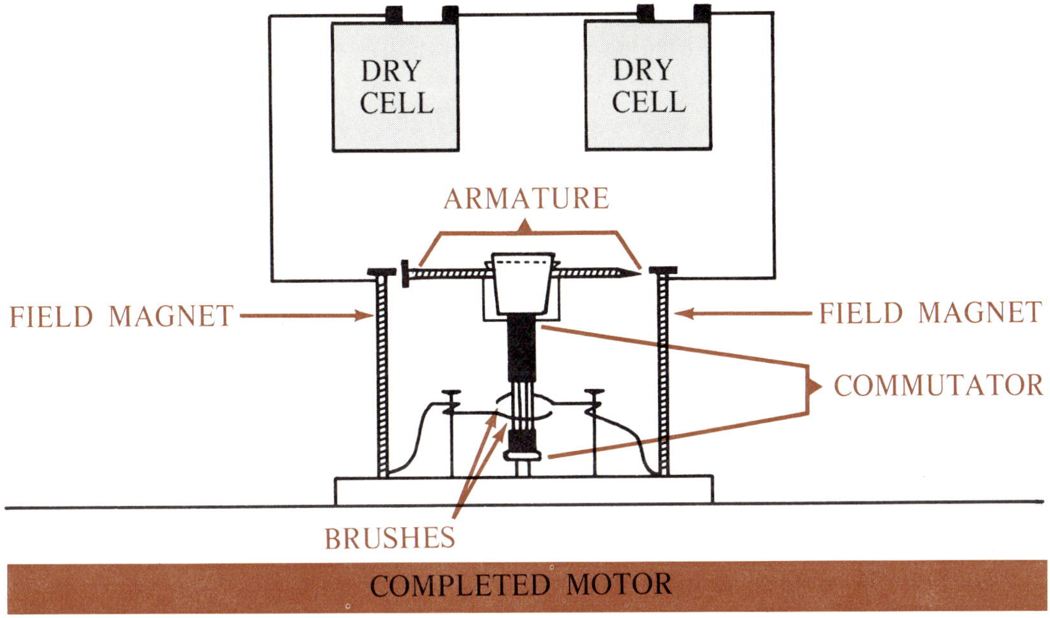


**9.36** View of completed electric motor

Leaving an 8–cm–long end of wire free, begin winding the armature. Start next to the cork, and carefully wind toward one end of the shaft. When you reach the end of the nail, continue winding *in the same direction*, and work your way back to the cork. Continue making windings around one end of the shaft until you have made about 50 turns.

Now drape the wire across the top of the cork, and begin winding the other half of the armature shaft. Start at the end nearest the cork, and *wind in the same direction* that you did previously. Look carefully at the diagram on page 308.

Test the polarity of your armature by connecting the free ends of the wire to the dry cell, and bring the compass close to each end of the shaft. How can you tell if the poles of the armature are opposite?

---

The commutator and brushes are all that are needed to complete the motor.

Your complete motor should look like the picture above.

---

## Making the Commutator and Brushes

**MATERIALS:**

Two small nails, two strips of copper (each 2.5 cm long and each wide enough to reach almost halfway around the test tube of your armature), a small amount of electrician's tape

**PROCEDURE:**

Curve the strips of copper to fit the test tube, near the lower end. Be sure that there is a gap of about 3 mm between each strip. Slip the end of one wire from the armature under one copper strip. Place the end of the other wire from the armature under the other copper strip. Fasten the commutator to the test tube with tape, using pieces at both the top and the bottom of the copper strips.

Drive the two nails about 4 cm away from the commutator. Wrap the 8-cm-long wire end from each field magnet around the nail nearest to it, being sure that the insulation protects the wire from coming into contact with the nail. Strip the insulation from the remainder of the wire, and bend it so that it touches the commutator on opposite sides of the test tube, as shown in Figure 9.35.

Attach a pair of dry cells in series as shown, and spin the armature. If it does not continue to spin, adjust the angle at which the brushes touch the commutator. Always keep the brushes on opposite sides of the test tube. Eventually, you should find one position that seems best, resulting in a rapidly moving armature.

### Have You Learned?

Describe a simple electric motor, naming each important part and telling the function of each part.

## 9. Using Electricity in Our Homes

**ARE YOU READY?**

Look up the following words if you are not sure of their meanings:

amperage; appliance; conduct; friction; grounded; induction; resistance; voltage.

The use of electricity to light our homes has become so commonplace that most of us take such light entirely for granted. However, the development of the **incandescent** (in′ kən des′ ənt) light bulb by Thomas Edison took place less than 100 years ago.

### Using Electricity to Producc Light

Look at a clear light bulb like the one shown in Figure 9.38. Notice that the current must flow through the fine wire, which has a great deal of resistance. The **filament** (fil′ ə mənt) is usually made of **tungsten** (tung′ stən), a metal with a very high melting point. The air has been removed from the bulb to prevent the filament from combining with oxygen and the air replaced with some other gas—generally nitrogen or argon.

As the electrons are forced through it, the filament becomes very hot. Very quickly, it becomes hot enough to glow with a white light. This is the meaning of the term *incandescent*.

The incandescent bulb provides us with a good light, and it is certainly superior to the candles, burning gas, or kerosene that previously provided Americans with light. But it is a very inefficient light. Most of the electrical energy that passes through a light bulb of this type is changed into heat energy. Therefore, new types of light bulbs are being produced.

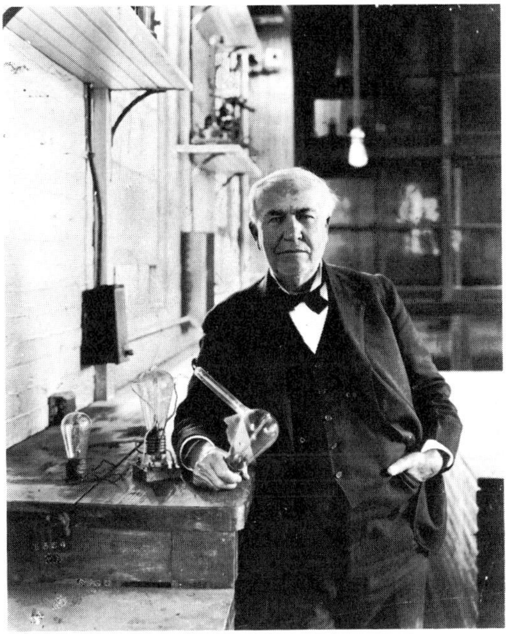

*The Bettmann Archive*

**9.37** Thomas Alva Edison (1847-1931)

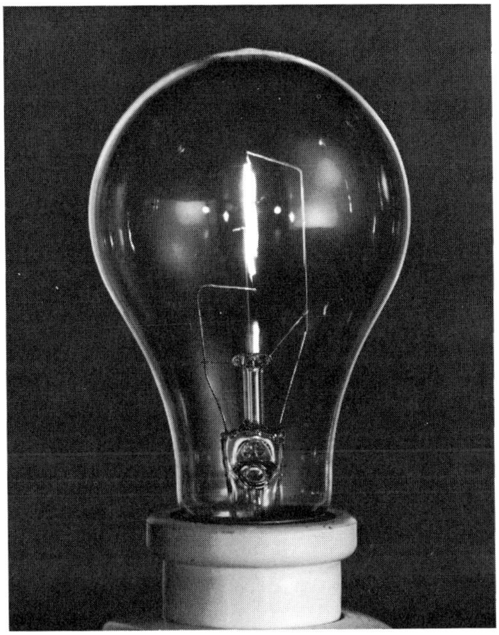

*General Electric Company, Lamp Division*

**9.38** Electric bulb, showing glowing filament

Many gases become fairly good conductors of electricity if they are contained in a bulb at a very low pressure. A current under a high voltage can then be forced through them, causing the gas molecules to give off a glow. The color of the light given off by these types of bulbs depends on the type of gas used. Neon gives off a red color, sodium produces yellow, and mercury glows blue-green. You have seen lights of this type used for advertising signs and street lights (Figure 9.41).

**Fluorescent** (flü′ ə res′ ənt) lamps are similar to these bulbs in that they contain mercury vapor under very low pressure. The ultraviolet light, produced when a current is forced through the mercury vapor, passes through a coating of minerals on the inside of the tube. The energy of the ultraviolet radiation causes these minerals to glow—a process called **fluorescence** (flü′ ə res′ əns). Fluorescent lamps are more efficient than incandescent bulbs, and the quality of light is somewhat better. However, new sources of light are being sought.

## Using Electricity to Produce Heat

A conductor that has a great deal of resistance will become hot as electrons pass through it. This heat is from the friction caused by the electrons as they are forced through the metal. The higher the resistance, the greater the heat given off. The conversion of electric energy into heat energy in the light bulb is a great disadvantage, but in other appliances we use this conversion to our advantage.

How many appliances can you list that convert electrical energy into heat? Each of these works in a similar manner. The heating element consists of a conductor with a high resistance. In most of our heating appliances, this conductor is an alloy of nickel and chromium, called **Nichrome** (nī′ krōm′). The current flows into this element, and the electrons are forced through it. This creates a great deal of friction and thus a great amount of heat.

Three factors determine how hot a heating element will become. The first is the type of conductor used. Copper wire does not have very much resistance to the flow of electrons and, therefore, does not get hot as an electric current flows through it. This explains why the cord attaching an electric heater to the wall socket remains cool even though the heating element becomes red hot. As you have already learned, wires with small diameters offer more resistance to the current than do wires of larger diameter. Therefore, heating elements made of wires with small diameters will produce more heat than those made of larger wires (Figure 9.43).

The second factor that determines the amount of heat produced by a heating element is the amperage of the current. Obviously, the more electrons that pass through a wire the greater the friction caused by their passing. Because of this, some heating elements, such as water heaters, electric stoves, and electric clothes dryers, require a voltage of 230 rather than the normal

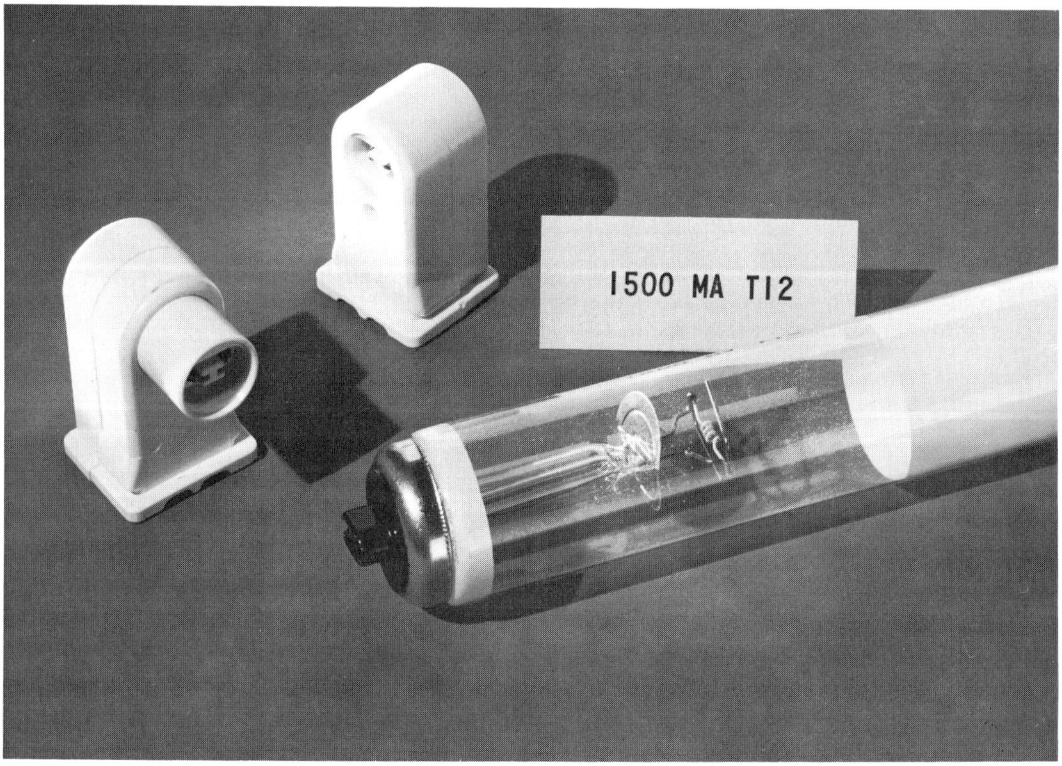


*General Electric Company, Lamp Division*

**9.39** A section of the white coating of this fluorescent tube was removed to show its elements.

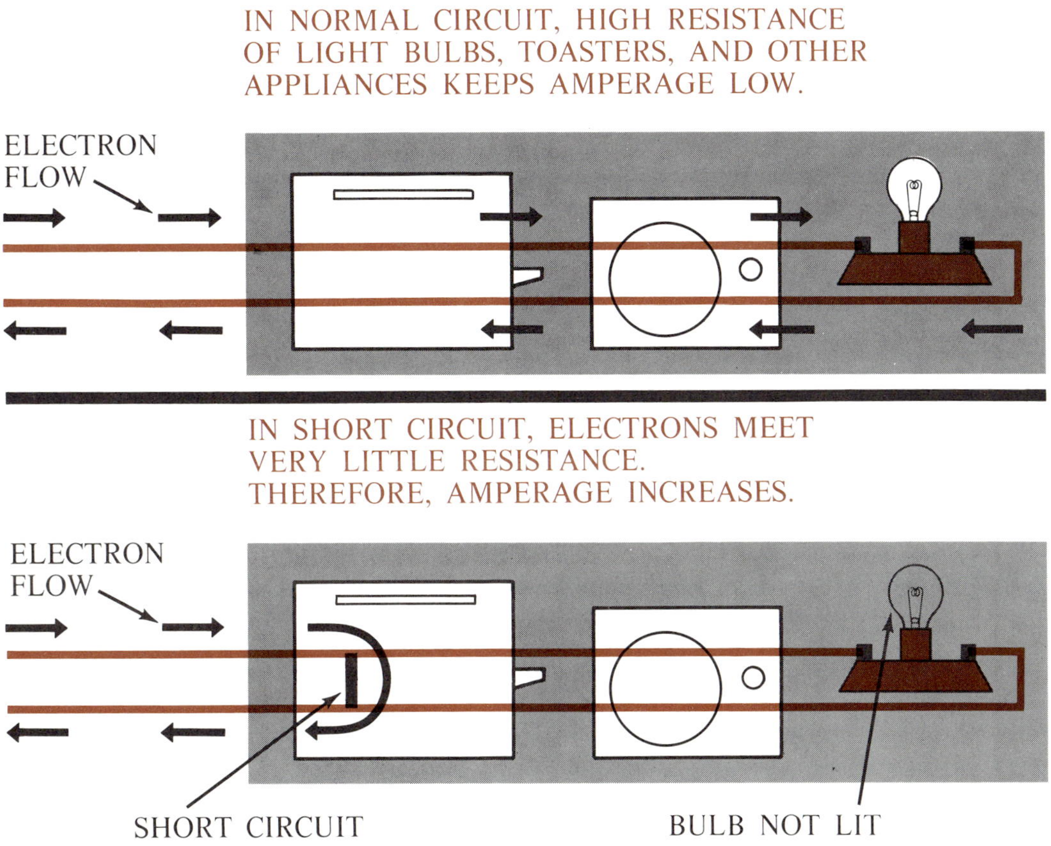


**9.40** Why do you suppose the lower diagram is called a short circuit?

115. The additional pressure forces a higher amperage, and thereby produces more heat.

The third factor is, of course, time. The longer a current is allowed to flow through an appliance, the hotter the element will become. You can notice this effect by comparing the heat produced by an incandescent bulb that has been on for only a brief time with one that has burned for a longer time.

The heat-producing effect of an electric current passing through a resistant conductor is used to protect our appliances, our houses, and ourselves from electricity. The amount of current that will flow through a circuit (the amperage) depends upon the pressure (the voltage) and the resistance of the circuit. In most places in the United States, the pressure is held at a steady 115 volts. Therefore, the amperage of the current flowing through a circuit in our houses depends upon the amount of resistance in the circuit.

## Protecting Electrical Circuits

The electrical system of most homes consists of several separate circuits. Generally, these are designed to carry between 15 and 20 amps of current safely. You will recall that the copper wire used in

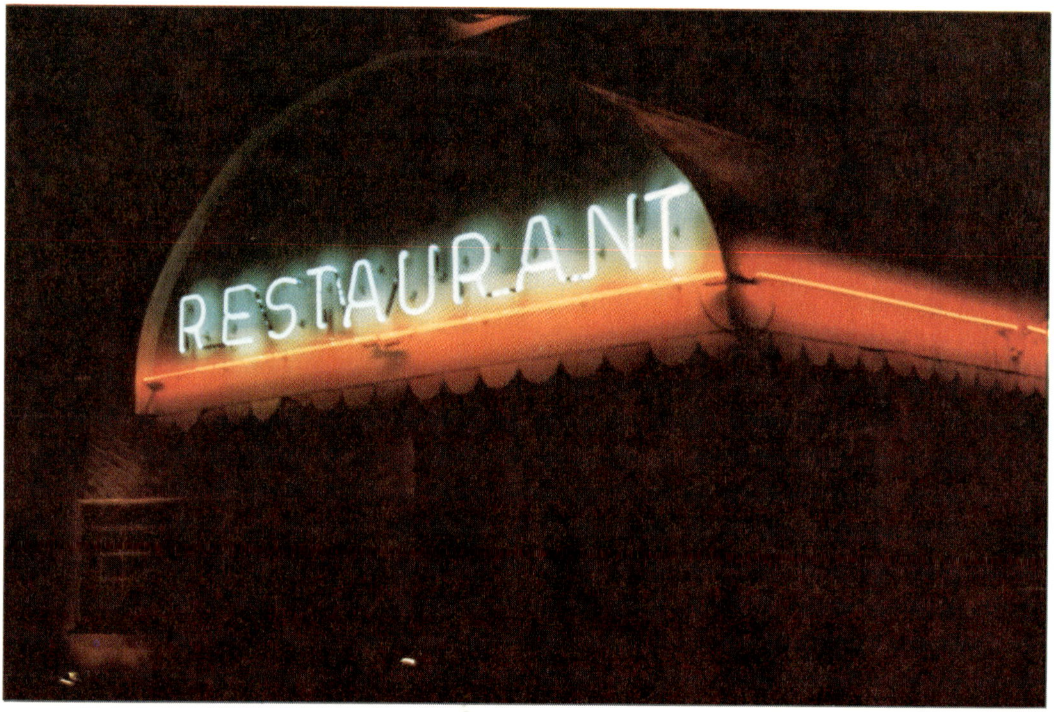


*Norman D. Anderson*

**9.41** Neon gas was discovered in the atmosphere in 1898. *Neon* comes from the Greek word meaning *new*.

your house circuits has a very low resistance—about 1 ohm per 300 meters. If a **short circuit** occurs in this wiring, allowing the current to flow directly from one wire into another, rather than through a high resistance appliance, a tremendous increase in amperage occurs. The heat produced by this flood of electrons can ruin an appliance or set fire to a house.

Normally a person's body and clothing have enough resistance so that they will not be seriously damaged by electricity under a pressure of 115 volts. If, however, the person is well grounded, touching water pipes or standing in water, this flow of electrons can easily kill. The energy that causes our muscles to contract is electrical. A sudden flow of current from outside the body can cause the heart muscle to contract so violently that it stops beating. If it is not started within a minute or two, the interruption of blood circulation will result in badly damaged brain cells, if not in death.

To protect us from these dangerous short circuits, each separate circuit in your house has a **fuse** or a **circuit breaker.** Fuses consist of wires that melt at very low temperatures. When a short circuit occurs and the flow of electrons increases, the heat melts the fuse wire, thereby breaking the circuit and stopping the flow of electricity. The circuit breaker is composed of an electromagnet that opens a switch when the amperage rises above a certain level. Like the fuse, the circuit breaker stops the flow of electricity before serious damage can be done.

## Regulating Current Flow and Voltage

We use the resistance of conductors in other ways than in heating appliances. Perhaps you have seen switches called **rheostats** (rē′ ə stat) that are used to control the brightness of lights or the speed of electric motors. The important parts of these switches are (1) a long, highly resistant wire, generally coiled so that it will not take up too much space, and (2) a control dial that allows you to direct the electric current through any length of the wire you desire. When you set the dial in such a way that the current must travel through the entire length of the wire, it meets a great deal of resistance. Because of this high resistance, little current can flow through the switch; lights dim, or a motor runs at slower speed.

It is more economical to **transmit** (trans mit′) electric current at very high voltages. Thus, **transmission** (trans mish′ ən) lines, which carry current long distances, may carry as much as 400,000 volts. Before the electric current transmitted by such lines is usable in our homes, the voltage must be reduced to 115 volts or 230 volts. The appliance used for this is the **transformer** (trans fôr′ mər).

The principle behind the use of transformers is again induction. A transformer

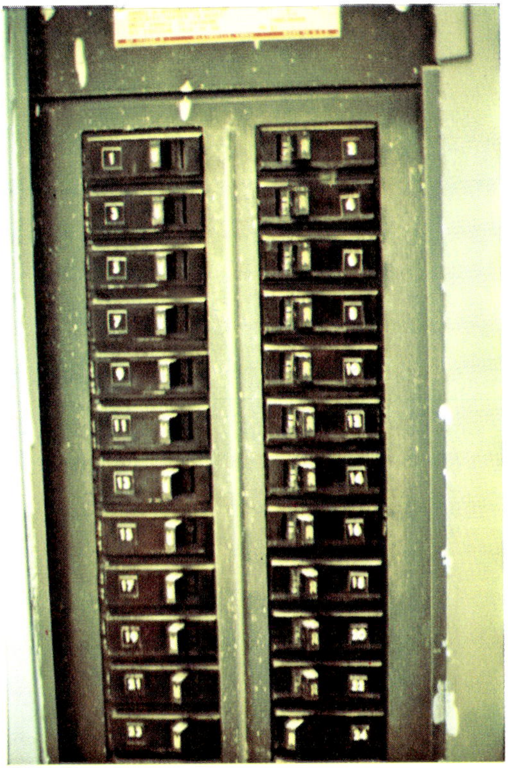

*Walter R. Brown*

**9.42** Circuit breaker

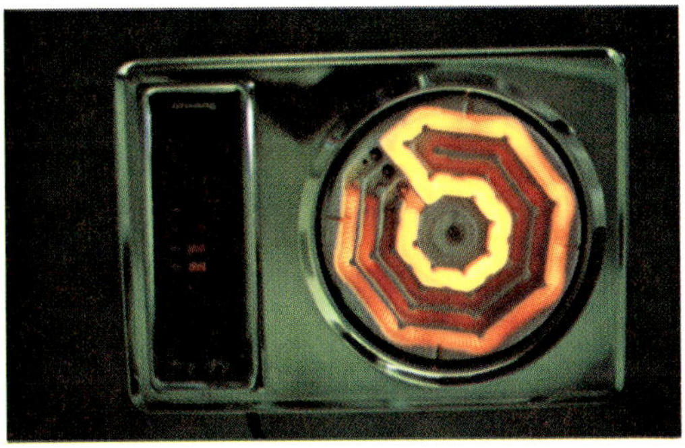

*Norman D. Anderson*

**9.43** The glowing elements of an electric hot plate

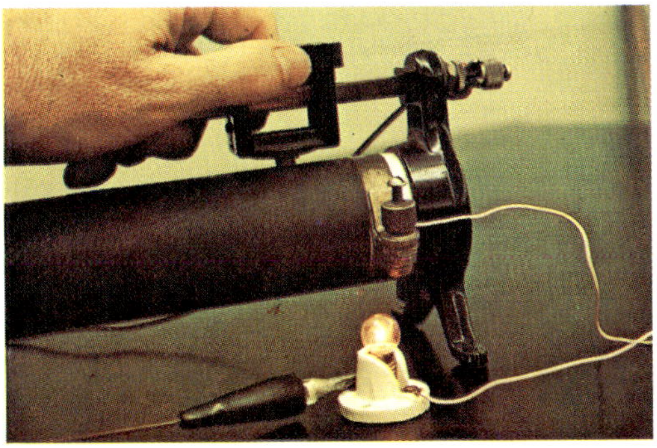

*Walter R. Brown*

**9.44** Rheostat

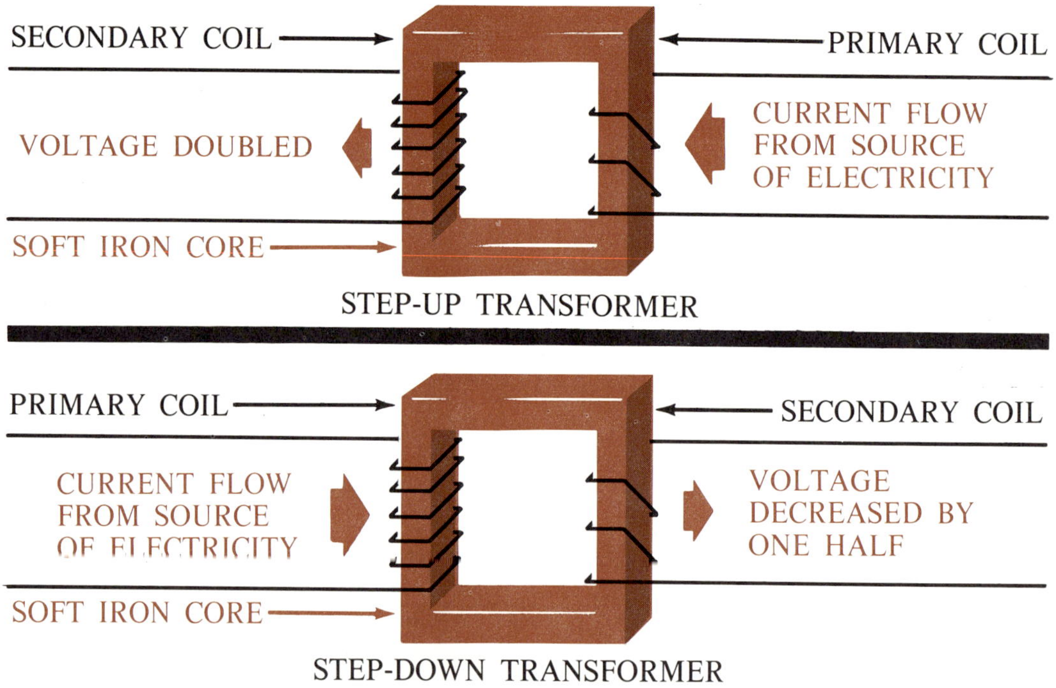


**9.45** What is the difference between these two transformers?

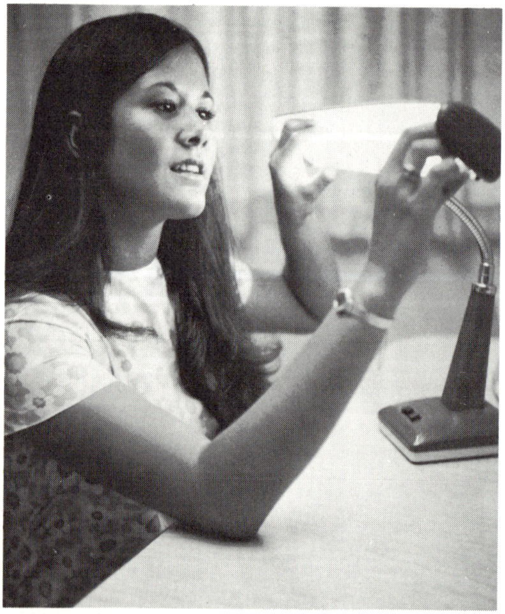

*Alan Cliburn*

**9.46** Will the fluorescent tube burn the girl? (See page 425 in Chapter 14.)

consists of two coils of wire, normally wound around an iron core but insulated from it. The alternating current passing through one coil will induce an alternating current in the second coil. The difference in voltage will depend upon the number of coils of wire in each end of the transformer.

In the **step-down transformer** the coil of wire into which the current flows from the source of electricity (the **primary** coil) has more turns than does the **secondary** coil. If the primary coil has twice as many turns as the secondary coil, the transformer produces electricity at approximately one-half the voltage of the source (Figure 9.45).

In a **step-up transformer** the reverse situation is used. Here the primary coil has fewer turns of wire than does the secondary coil. Therefore, the resulting current has more voltage than did the source.

## Have You Learned?

Select the word from Column B that best corresponds with each definition in Column A. (Do not write in your book.)

*Column A*

1. Something that glows with its own light
2. A glow given off when minerals are struck by radiation
3. A situation in which one wire touches another, allowing the electricity to flow through the wire rather than through the high-resistance appliances
4. A device that consists of wire that melts at low temperatures
5. An electromagnet that opens a switch when the amperage is too high
6. Switches that control the amount of current in a circuit
7. A device that changes the voltage of a current
8. An alloy of nickel and chromium
9. The part of a heating appliance that has enough resistance to get hot
10. Wires that carry high voltage currents over long distances

*Column B*

a. circuit breaker
b. element
c. fluorescence
d. fuse
e. incandescent
f. Nichrome
g. rheostat
h. short circuit
i. transformer
j. transmission lines

## REVIEW QUESTIONS

Answer the following questions using brief, complete sentences.

1. One end of a copper wire is connected to the rod of an electroscope, and the other end is attached to a water pipe. A negatively charged plastic rod is then brought close to the electroscope rod but does not touch it. The leaves of the electroscope do not move. The copper wire is then removed from the electroscope, and the plastic rod is taken away. The leaves then move apart. Explain what happened.
2. List the advantages and disadvantages of series circuits as compared with parallel circuits.
3. What are the advantages and disadvantages of a battery in which the cells are attached (a) in series, (b) in parallel?
4. What are the relationships among voltage, amperage, and ohms?
5. A circuit has an emf of 10 volts, and the total resistance is 2 ohms. How many coulombs per second are flowing in the circuit?
6. Describe how a "wet" cell, made of zinc strips and copper strips placed in sulfuric acid, works.
7. Sometimes a worn-out dry cell can be made to produce electricity again by placing it in a shallow pan of water. Explain why.
8. Describe the electric circuit of a doorbell, and explain why the clapper vibrates.
9. Describe how electricity can be induced by use of a magnet. Explain how the amount of electricity produced in this way can be increased.
10. Describe the difference between an incandescent light and a fluorescent light.

## CAN YOU FIND OUT?

*It may be necessary to use encyclopedias or other reference books in answering the following questions.*

1. Is it possible for lightning to move up-

ward from the ground to a cloud, or does it always go from cloud to ground?

2. What materials are the best conductors of electricity? The poorest?
3. Are the electric circuits in your house in series or in parallel? How can you tell?
4. Are the cells in a flashlight attached in series or in parallel? How can you tell?
5. What are the voltages of the automobile batteries that are most commonly used? How can you tell the voltage of an automobile battery by looking at it?
6. What are the strongest magnets that have been made? How were they made?
7. What are some common uses of electromagnets other than those described in this chapter?
8. What is the source of energy used to generate electricity for your community?
9. What parts of the world use direct current? What parts of the world use AC electric current that is not 60 cycle?
10. Why are thermocouples used, rather than more ordinary types of thermometers?

## REFERENCES FOR ADDITIONAL STUDY

EXPERIMENTS IN MAGNETISM AND ELECTRICITY by Harry Sootin. Franklin Watts, Inc.
Suggests about 200 experiments that can be done with simple equipment

THE MAKING OF THE ELECTRICAL AGE: FROM THE TELEGRAPH TO AUTOMATION by Harold Sharlin. Abelard-Schuman Limited.
Traces the history of electricity with special attention given to the telegraph, electric motor, dynamo, and central power station

THE STORY OF ELECTRICITY AND MAGNETISM by Bernard Seeman. Harvey House, Inc.
An easy-to-read description of electricity and magnetism, including some simple experiments

THE WONDERS OF ELECTRICITY by Hy Ruchlis. Harper & Row, Publishers.
A discussion on the many applications of electricity, including radios, electric motors, and recent advances such as fuel cells

CHAPTER 10

# Electronics and Communication

As you might guess from the name, **electronics** (i lek′ tron′ iks) is the study of electrons. From their understanding of how the electron behaves, scientists and engineers have been able to develop many instruments that make our lives happier and healthier. These include radio, television, RADAR, the X-ray machine, and microscopes that can produce an image that is four-hundred-thousand times the size of the object being studied.

These developments have all taken place only within the last one hundred years. The electron itself was identified only a little before the turn of the century, the X ray was not discovered until 1895, and the first radio signal was sent across the Atlantic Ocean in 1901.

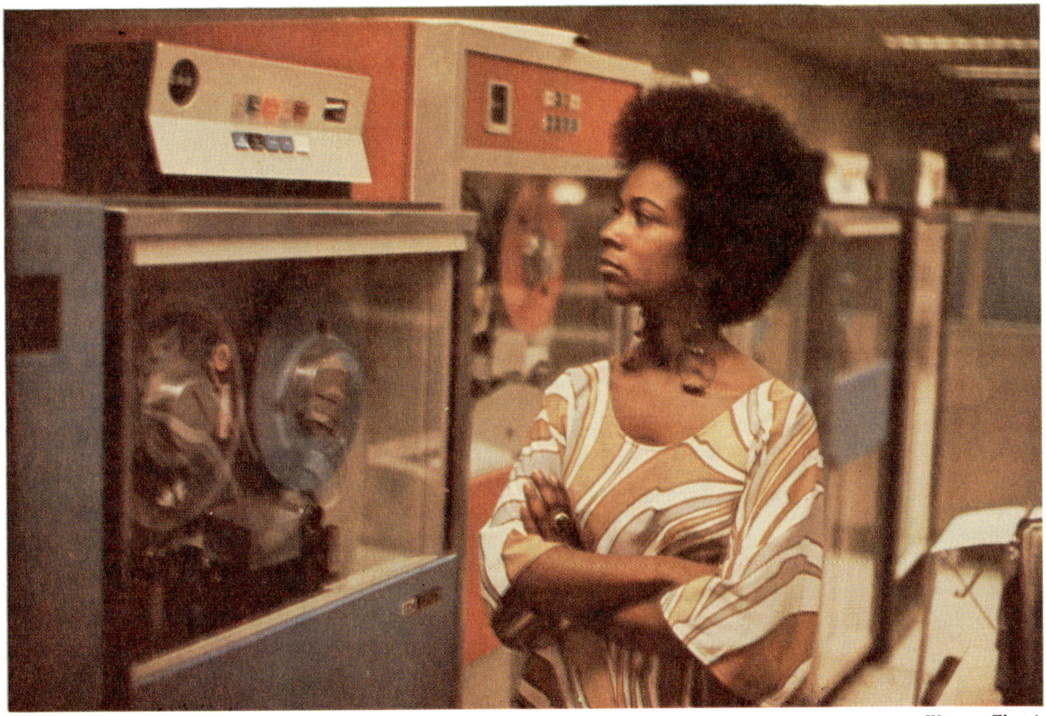

*Western Electric*

**10.1** Electronics has made possible many instruments with far-reaching applications to our lives today.

## 1. Electric Currents into Sound

> **ARE YOU READY?**
>
> Look up the following words if you are not sure of their meanings:
>
> amplitude; conductor;
> DC electric current; electromagnet;
> frequency; microphone; telegraph.

During the last half of the nineteenth century, the only method available for communicating over long distances was the telegraph. As you may already know, the telegraph is a simple arrangement of switches and electromagnets. When the switch is closed, the electric current flows through a wire and around an electromagnet. The activated electromagnet attracts a metal bar, pulling it down with a loud click. In this way, messages are sent in code over long distances.

---

### Building a Simple Telegraph Set

**MATERIALS:**

15 meters of thin insulated copper wire, six large nails, a small tin can, several blocks of wood, a flat piece of wood about 30 cm square, tin snips, hammer, a 1½-volt dry cell

**PROCEDURE:**

Assemble the telegraph set as shown in Figure 10.2. When the key is closed, the electromagnets should attract the sounder. If this does not happen, bend the metal of the sounder until it almost touches the electromagnet.

Can you figure out how to wind the electromagnets so that they will be stronger? Does it make any difference in which direction you wind them?

---

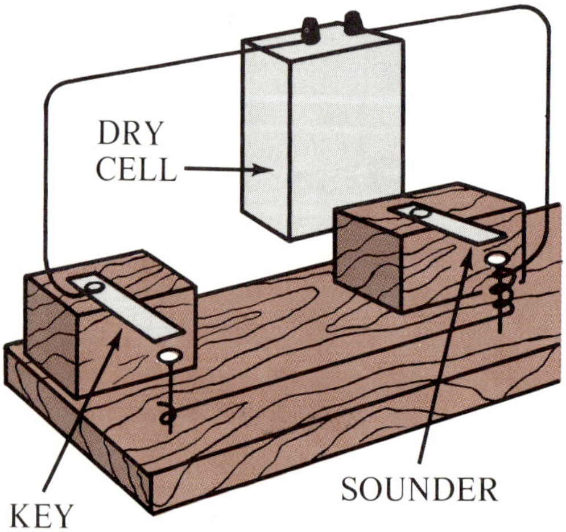


**10.2** Telegraph set, sender and sounder

### The Telephone

In 1876 Alexander Graham Bell succeeded in sending his voice over an electric wire. Since this time, the telephone has improved greatly, but the basic principles are the same as those used by Bell.

In the modern telephone the **transmitter** (trans mit′ ər), or mouthpiece, consists of a thin, flexible **diaphragm** (dī′ ə fram). Under the diaphragm is a small box of small carbon particles through which low-voltage electric current flows. As sound waves strike the diaphragm, it vibrates back and forth. When the diaphragm

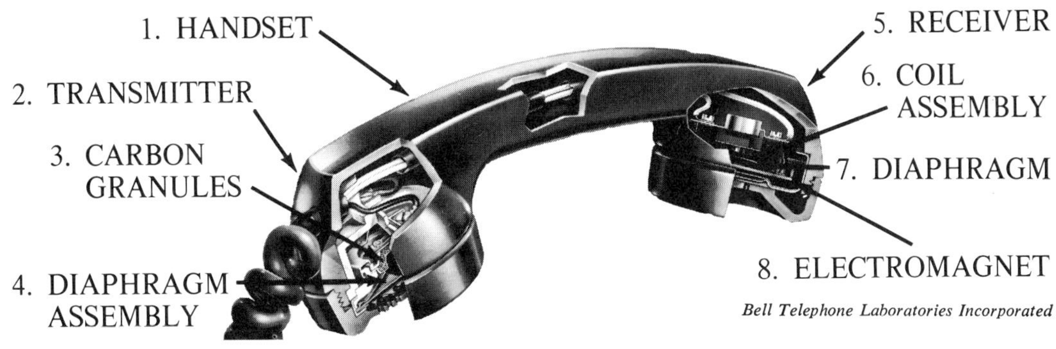


**10.3** Cross section of a telephone handpiece

moves in, the carbon particles are pushed more closely together, making better contact with each other. This increased contact allows a stronger current to flow through the circuit. In this way the exact frequency and amplitude of the sound is changed to variations in the electric current flowing between the two telephones.

The important parts of the telephone receiver are an electromagnet and another diaphragm made of steel. As the varying current passes through the electromagnet, the diaphragm is alternately attracted and released to spring back to its original position. This vibration is tuned exactly to the changes in the electric current and sets up waves in the air that are very similar to the original sound waves that entered the transmitter.

## Microphones and Loudspeakers

One type of **microphone** (mī′ krə fōn) operates exactly like the transmitter of a telephone, with a diaphragm vibrating against a box of carbon particles. In another type the diaphragm is attached to a small coil of wire that lies between the poles of a horseshoe magnet. As the diaphragm vibrates, the coil of wire moves in and out of the magnetic field. This induces a small current in the wire that varies in the same way as do the vibrations of the diaphragm.

In a **crystal microphone,** the diaphragm pushes against a small **quartz** (kwôrts) crystal. As the crystal is squeezed, its surfaces become electrically charged. A large vibration of the diaphragm will generate a larger electric current. A smaller vibration will produce a smaller current. This phenomenon is called the **piezoelectric** (pī ē′ zō i lek′ trik) **effect,** and occurs only in certain kinds of crystals.

Loudspeakers and headphones are the reverse of microphones because they change electric currents back into sound. Some speakers work exactly like the receiver of the telephone, with electromagnets that attract and repel a thin diaphragm. Others are the reverse of the crystal microphone, having a quartz crystal that vibrates as an electric current passes through it.

## Photoelectric Cells

Sound was not added to motion pictures

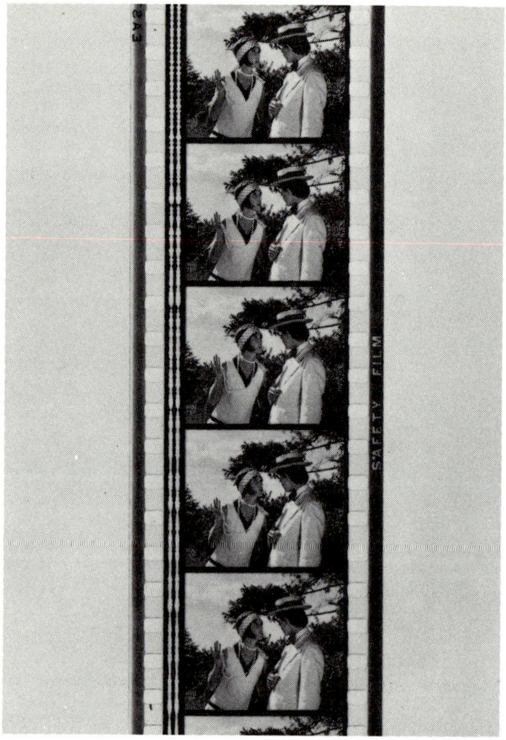


*Courtesy of Eastman Kodak Company*

**10.4** Movie film, showing the sound track at the left

until about 1927. Figure 10.4 above shows a strip of movie film. The irregular pattern along the side of the picture is the sound track. A beam of light shining through the sound track causes the sound that you hear during a film.

This light varies in strength according to the shape of the pattern of the sound track. After passing through the film, it falls on a tube called a **photoelectric** (fō′ tō i lek′ trik) cell that changes the light into electrical energy. A speaker then changes this electrical energy into sound.

The photoelectric effect is an important one in the science of electronics. Certain metals, such as potassium and cesium oxide, have electrons that are so loosely held to the nucleus of the atom that the energy of light is sufficient to move the electrons, thus causing an electric current. This principle is used in the construction of a photoelectric cell.

The photoelectric cell is a glass tube from which most of the air has been removed. Because of this low pressure, this type of tube is called a *vacuum* tube. Within the vacuum tube are two metal parts, or *elements*. One of these is a curved sheet, composed of one of the photoelectric metals. This sheet is attached, through the bottom of the tube, to the negative pole of a source of direct current electricity. This negatively charged element in a vacuum tube is always known as the **cathode** (kath′ ōd).

The other element in a photoelectric tube is a rod made of any good conductor.

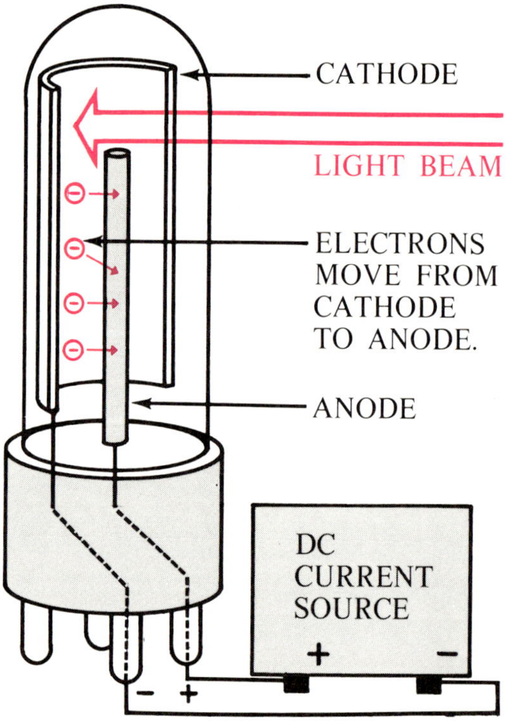


**10.5** Photoelectric cell

This rod is connected to the positive side of a DC source and is called the **anode** (an′ ōd). (See Figure 10.5.)

Since the cathode is separated from the anode by a space, current will not normally flow between them. However, when light strikes the cathode, electrons are thrown from it. Since the anode is positively charged, the loose electrons are attracted to it. The number of electrons on the cathode is renewed from the DC source, and the result is a continuous flow of electricity that stops only when the light stops.

A small amount of light passing through the sound track of a movie film will cause a small amount of current to flow through the circuit. A larger amount of light will cause a larger flow of electrons. These can be used to activate a speaker system in exactly the same way that the current in a telephone line does.

Many uses have been found for the photoelectric cell, other than those in the communication industry. Burglar alarms may be activated by the breaking of invisible beams of energy such as infrared light. Doors can be made to open automatically when a person steps between a source of light and a photoelectric cell. Several types of photoelectric counting machines are now in use. Photoelectric cells can also be seen controlling traffic lights, street lights, and other similar devices.

## Have You Learned?

Select the best answer to each of the following questions. (Do not write in your book.)

1. Which of the following is a part of the telegraph?

   (a) electromagnet; (b) diaphragm; (c) quartz crystal; (d) carbon particles.

2. Which of the following is *not* a part of a telephone?

   (a) diaphragm; (b) electromagnet; (c) photoelectric cell; (d) carbon particles.

3. The piezoelectric effect is a phenomenon that occurs when which of the following is squeezed?

   (a) quartz crystal; (b) diaphragm; (c) carbon particles; (d) vacuum tube.

4. A photoelectric cell is a type of what?

   (a) vacuum tube; (b) telephone; (c) microphone; (d) radio.

5. Which of the following is not involved in the photoelectric effect?

   (a) DC electric current; (b) electromagnet; (c) cathode; (d) anode.

## 2. Radio Communication

> **ARE YOU READY?**
>
> Look up the following words if you are not sure of their meanings:
>
> alternating current; amplitude; discharge; filament; frequency; insulator; piezoelectric crystal; radio station.

Your telephone and your radio are alike in that both instruments allow sound to be sent over long distances. The major difference between the two is that in a radio the broadcast electrical vibrations travel through the air rather than through wires.

### Radio Transmitters and Receivers

At each radio broadcasting station there is an instrument called a *transmitter* that produces alternating current at a very high frequency. Standard radio broadcasts are usually produced by currents that alternate between 600,000 cycles—600 **kilocycles** (kil′ ə sī′ kəl)—and 300,000,000 cycles, or 300 **megacycles** (meg′ ə sī′ kəl), and the UHF (Ultra High Frequencies) between 300 megacycles per second and 3,000 megacycles per second. Television programs are broadcast using VHF and UHF frequencies. (The abbreviation of *kilocycle* is *kc*, that of *megacycle* is *mc*.)

The radio transmitter pumps these AC currents into an **antenna** (an ten′ ə). This produces energy waves with the same frequency. These **radiate** (rā′ di āt) from the antenna. The antenna of a radio receiver is composed of any good conductor of electricity. When the radio waves strike this conductor, the electrons in it are made to vibrate in the same pattern as the waves from the transmitter antenna.

The transmitter waves described above are called **carrier** (kar′ i ər) waves, because they *carry* the radio program to the receiver. To do this, the carrier wave must be changed, or **modulated** (moj′ u̇ lā təd), in some way. Two methods of modulation are common, and you have probably heard radio broadcasts using both methods.

The more common method is called **amplitude** (am′ plə tüd) **modulation,** or AM. Amplitude, you will remember, is the *height* of the wave. As shown in the diagram on page 325, the AM transmission changes the amplitude of the carrier wave so that it resembles the sound pattern.

The second common type of modulation is called **frequency modulation,** or FM. The diagram on page 325 shows how the frequency of the carrier wave is changed to carry the pattern of the sound wave.

The antennas of most radios can be stimulated by waves having a wide range of frequencies. For example, most home radio receivers have built-in antennas that can receive any of the normal frequencies (600 kc to 1,600 kc). Many radio stations within a short distance of our receivers are broadcasting within this range, each on a separate frequency. If we are to hear only one station at a time, we must be able to adjust our receiver so that it will respond to only one frequency.

This is done with a device called a **tuning capacitor** (kə pas′ ə tər). A capacitor is an instrument that will store large electrical charges. It consists of two or more plates

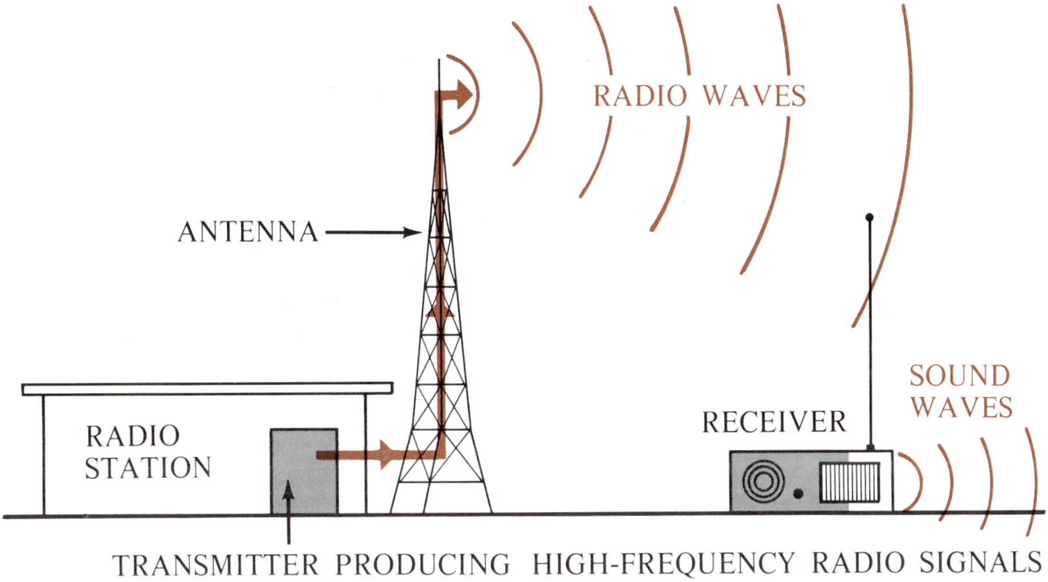


**10.6** Radio transmitter and receiver

of a conducting material, each separated from the others by an **insulator** (in′ sə lā′ tər). A radio tuning capacitor is shown on page 327. In this one the insulating material is the air surrounding the capacitor plates.

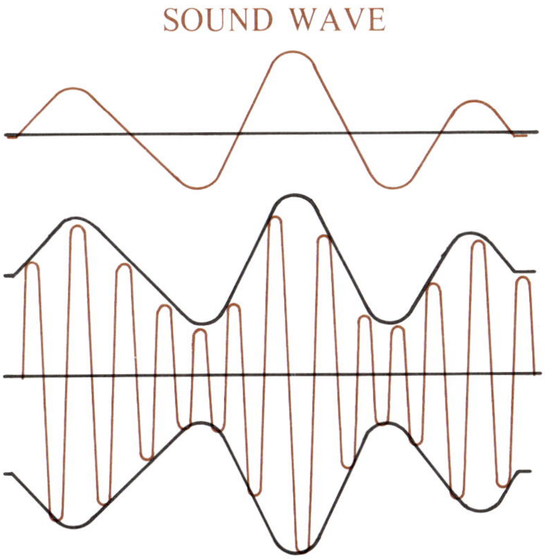


**10.7** AM waves

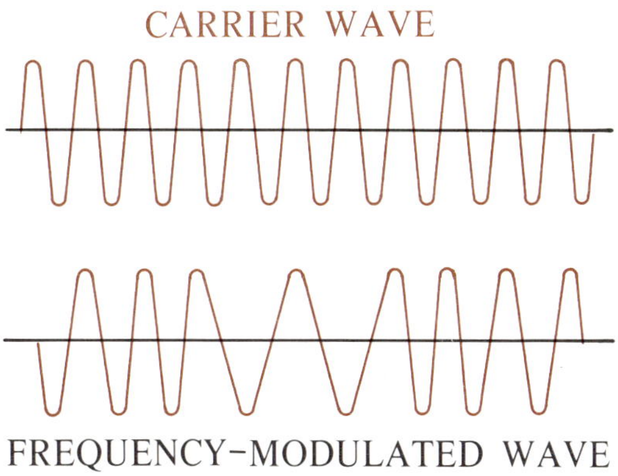


**10.8** FM waves

To tune in a certain frequency, you turn a knob connected to the movable plates of the tuning capacitor. As the plates rotate, the surface area between them increases or decreases and the storage capacity changes. Changes in the storage capacity in turn change the natural frequency of the tuning circuit of the radio. When the capacitor is adjusted so that this natural frequency is the same as that of a particular radio station, you receive that station. You will learn more about what happens when two objects vibrate at the same rate in Chapter 13, which deals with sound.

## Vacuum Tubes

But the radio waves received by the antenna of your radio and tuned by the capacitor are much too weak to operate any type of speaker. Before they can be used, they must be **amplified** (am′ plə fīd). One way to do this is to use a vacuum tube.

The development of this tube began in the year 1883. Thomas Edison was in the process of developing the first electric lamp. After many trials he finally managed to make a lamp that consisted of a carbon filament inside a low-pressure bulb. His filaments, he discovered, burned out after only a few hours of use.

In an attempt to correct this problem, Edison mounted a metal plate near the filament, as shown in Figure 10.9. He first tried to connect this plate to the positive side of a battery, and he noted that his galvanometer indicated that a current was flowing through the circuit, passing from the filament across the empty space to the plate. However, when he connected the plate to the *negative* side of the battery, no current flowed.

Neither of these experiments seemed to increase the life of his filament, so Edison did nothing more with them. However, being a careful scientist, he recorded all of his observations. Fifteen years later, Joseph John Thomson and other investigators were able to explain Edison's observations.

Thomson, who is usually given credit

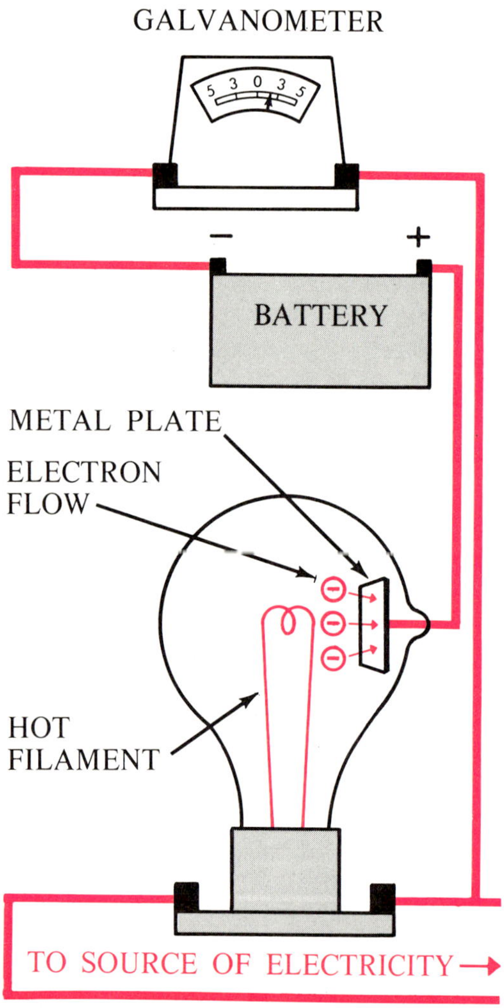


**10.9** Diagram of Edison's tube

for the discovery of the electron, finally guessed that the **Edison Effect** was caused by electrons. Owen Williams Richardson showed that these electrons were "boiling off" from the heated cathode filament and flowing to the positively charged anode plate. In 1904 J. A. Fleming made a vacuum tube similar to the one Edison had made, called a **diode** (dī′ ōd), since it contained two elements. He tried using this diode tube to detect weak radio signals,

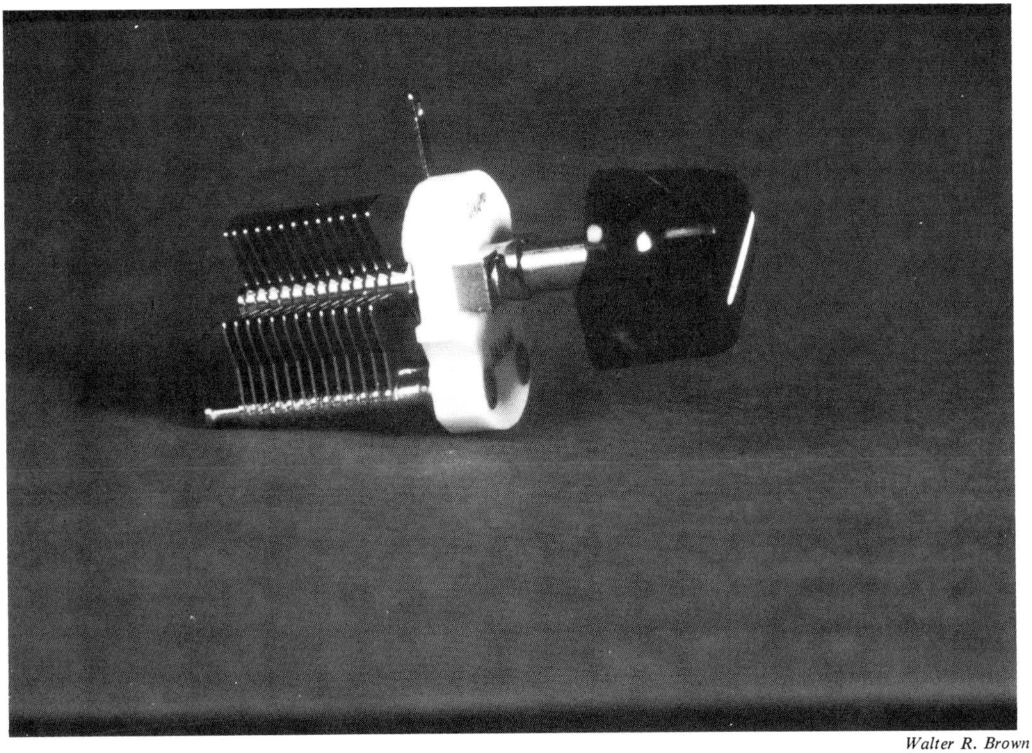

*Walter R. Brown*

**10.10** Radio tuning capacitor

but it proved to be only a little better than the piezoelectric crystals then being used. However, this experiment proved to be a step in the right direction.

Two years later, an American physicist, Lee De Forest, placed a third element in the diode, making the first **triode** (trī′ ōd) vacuum tube. A modified version of De Forest's triode is now used to amplify signals in all radios (Figure 10.11).

The triode consists of a hot, negatively charged cathode, which produces electrons, and a positively charged anode plate, which attracts the electrons. Between the two a third element, called the **grid** (grid), is attached to the antenna.

When the feeble current from the antenna makes the grid negatively charged, the flow of electrons between the cathode and the anode is slowed or stopped completely. When the grid is positively charged, the electrons from the cathode are attracted and pass easily through the screenlike grid to the plate. In this way a very weak current in the grid controls a much stronger current coming from the anode plate. The stronger amplified current from the anode varies with the fluctuations picked up by the antenna. By attaching the anode plate of one triode to the grid of another triode, a series of amplifications can be made.

Vacuum tubes are now available with many more elements than the simple tubes described above. They can be used in many types of electronic instruments.

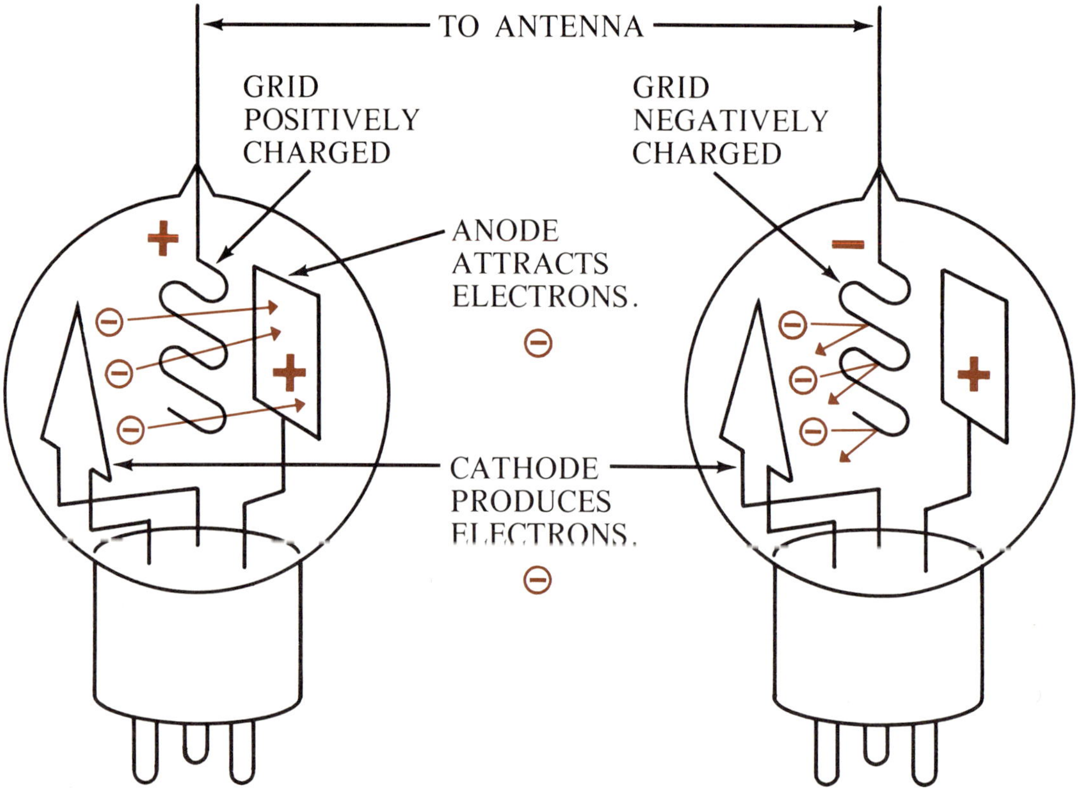


**10.11** Triode tube

## Have You Learned?

On a sheet of paper list the numbers for the questions below. By each number write *T* if the statement is true and *F* if false.

1. One kilocycle equals 1,000 cycles.
2. One megacycle equals 1,000,000 cycles.
3. A VHF broadcast has a frequency that is higher than that of a UHF broadcast.
4. AM and FM radio broadcasts differ only in their frequencies.
5. When a radio signal strikes a receiver antenna, the antenna begins to sway back and forth with the same frequency as the radio signal.
6. A radio receiver must contain several antennas, one for each station that it is to receive.
7. Vacuum tubes may be used to make a radio signal stronger.
8. Edison made the first triode vacuum tube.
9. In a triode vacuum tube, the grid controls the current flowing through the tube.
10. The triode is the most complicated vacuum tube made.

## 3. Transistors—Modified Vacuum Tubes

> **ARE YOU READY?**
>
> Look up the following words if you are not sure of their meanings:
>
> diode; negative side of a battery; Nobel Prize; semi-; triode; vacuum tube; valence.

In 1947 a discovery was made that has changed the entire electronics industry. A simple device called a **transistor** (tran zis′ tər) was developed. Transistors were found to be able to do all of the jobs of the various kinds of vacuum tubes. In addition, they do these jobs more efficiently and require less electricity. Also, transistors produce little heat and do not need the "warm-up time" of vacuum tubes. They also last much longer than vacuum tubes, since they are made of different materials and operate on a different principle.

But perhaps most important, transistors are much smaller than vacuum tubes. Some weigh only $^1/_{100}$ as much as the

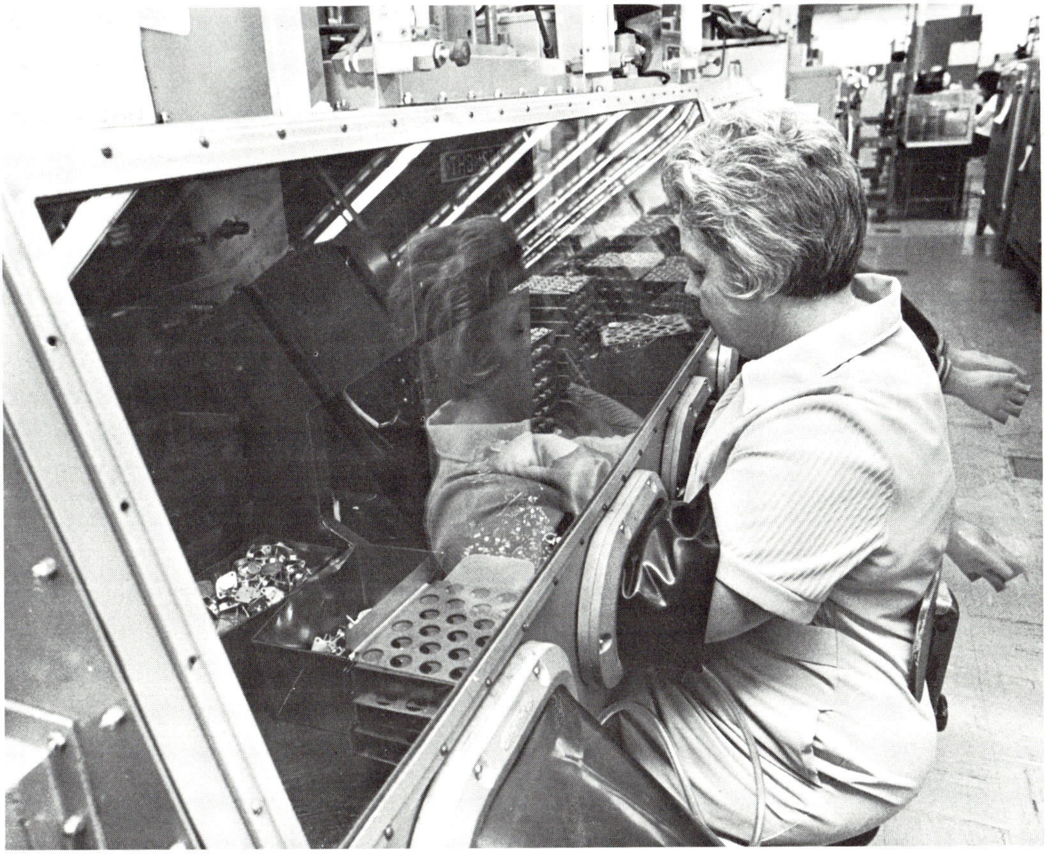

*RCA*

**10.12** This operator is hermetically sealing semiconductors in metal in a dry-nitrogen atmosphere.

glass-and-wire tube that they replace. Because of this and the other qualities of transistors, it has been possible for scientists and engineers to develop a great number of small electronic instruments. Among these are portable radios that can be carried in your pocket, hearing aids that are small enough to fit into the earpiece of eyeglasses, portable television sets, and electronic computers. Perhaps the exploration of space would not have been possible without these useful little devices.

The first successful transistor was developed by three American scientists working at the Bell Telephone Laboratories. As you might guess, the importance of their work was quickly realized, and the three men shared a Nobel Prize in physics.

Transistors are made of crystals of germanium or silicon that contain traces of other elements. In this form the germanium and silicon will conduct small amounts of electricity. Since these materials will not conduct electricity as well as copper yet do conduct some current, they are called **semiconductors** (sem′ i kən duk′ tər).

Germanium and silicon each have valences of *four*. In crystalline form, the atoms form a lattice pattern, similar to the carbon atoms in diamonds, with each atom sharing one electron with each of its four neighbors. In this form the crystal has no free electrons and is therefore a nonconductor.

If to this crystal we add an atom of another element that has *five* valence electrons, a free electron is available to move as an electric current. A semiconductor of this kind is known as an **N-type** (Figure 10.13).

If, on the other hand, an atom of an element with only *three* valence electrons is added, one electron from the germanium or silicon is required to hold the new atom in the lattice pattern. Because of this, there is a spot in the crystal that is short one electron. This spot acts much as if it were a "hole," into which an electron from a neighboring atom can "fall." When this happens, an electric current is created, with the "hole" appearing to move in a direction opposite to that of the flow of electrons. A semiconductor with a "hole" into which electrons can "fall" is known as a **P-type** (Figure 10.14).

If a semiconductor of the N-type is placed next to one of the P-type semiconductors, a simple transistor is formed. If the two semiconductors are attached to a battery with the negative pole of the battery attached to the N-type and the positive pole attached to the P-type, as shown in the diagram on page 331, an electric current will flow. This is because the free electrons in the N-type of semiconductor are repelled by the excess of electrons from the battery while being attracted by the positive charge in the P-type semiconductor. If the poles of the battery are reversed, with the positive side attached to the N-type side of the transistor and the negative pole attached to the P-type, no current will flow. Can you explain why?

In this way the simple **P-N junction transistor** acts in the same way as a diode vacuum tube. Both the transistor and the diode vacuum tube act as a "gate" or a "valve" in the circuit. Electrons are able to flow in one direction only.

It is a simple matter to construct a transistor that will act like a triode vacuum tube. As in the triode, three elements are

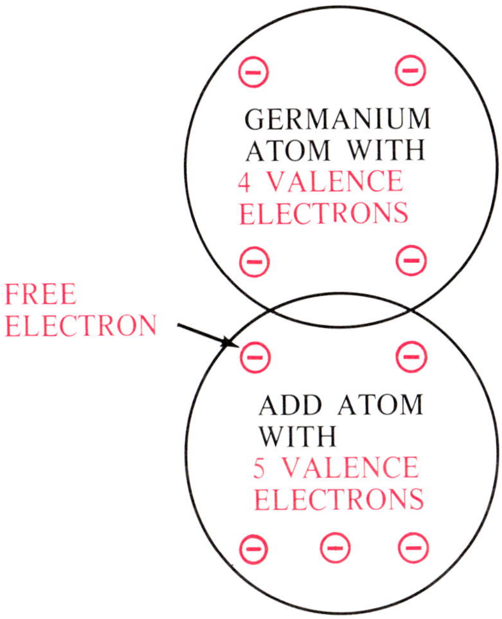


**10.13** N-type semiconductor

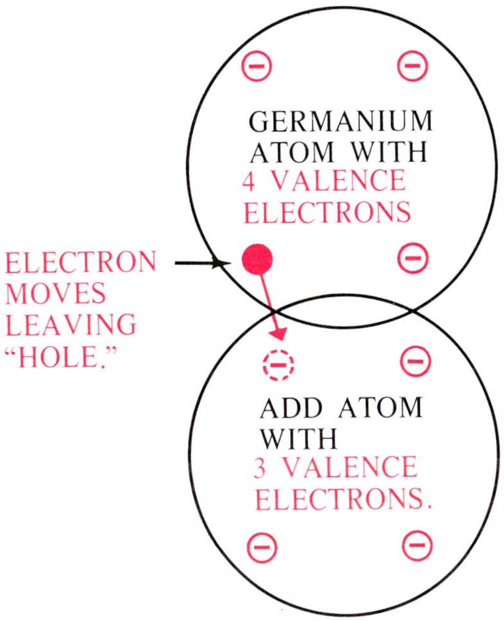


**10.14** P-type semiconductor

needed. One type of semiconductor is sandwiched between two slices of the opposite type of semiconductor. These can be in either order—a P-type in the

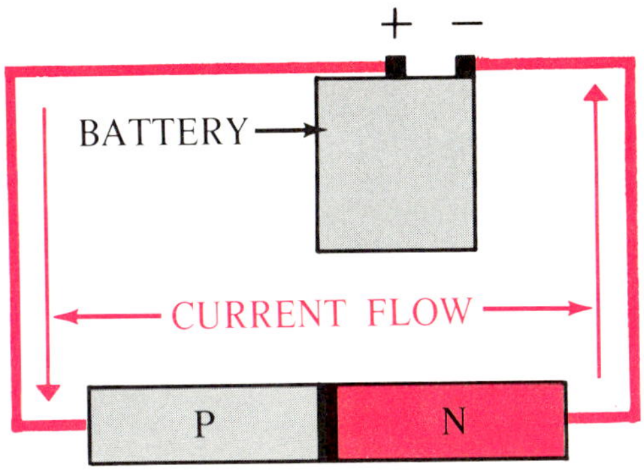


**10.15** P-N junction

center with two N-type semiconductors at either end (a N-P-N junction), or an N-type semiconductor between two P-type semiconductors (a P-N-P junction). In either case the semiconductor in the center of the triode acts as a grid, while the semiconductor at one end acts as the cathode. The semiconductor at the opposite end is, of course, the anode. Like triode vacuum tubes, triode transistors can amplify electric currents.

## Converting Solar Energy

**Solar** (sō′ lər) **batteries** are simply semiconductors made of specially treated silicon. In these the P-N junctions are located at the surface of the crystal, and when light strikes the junction, an electron is knocked from its usual place, and a "hole" is created. As a result, a current of electricity is generated by the energy of the light falling on the battery. (See Figure 10.33 on page 346.)

Present-day solar batteries are able to convert into electricity only about $^1/_{10}$ of the energy that falls on them. Still, they have proven to be very valuable devices. The radios and other electronic equipment of many satellites are powered entirely through energy from the sun. Entire telephone systems now use solar batteries as their main source of electric power. In order to do this, large banks of solar batteries are placed on top of telephone poles where they gather energy from the sunlight (page 60).

As more efficient solar batteries are built, more and more uses will be found.

### Have You Learned?

Answer the following questions, using short complete sentences.

1. What are the advantages of using transistors in place of vacuum tubes?
2. Where were transistors first developed?
3. Why are *impure* germanium and silicon crystals used for transistors?
4. What is the basic difference between an N-type of semiconductor and a P-type?
5. How can a diode transistor be made from N- and P-type semiconductors?
6. How can a triode transistor be made from N- and P-type semiconductors?
7. What are triode transistors used for?
8. How are solar batteries similar to transistors?
9. How efficient are solar batteries?
10. What are solar batteries used for?

## 4. Applications of Cathode Rays

**ARE YOU READY?**

Look up the following words if you are not sure of their meanings:

anode; cathode; microscope; transistor; transmitter; vacuum tube.

About a hundred years ago, a few years before Edison made the observations that eventually led to the development of vacuum tubes and transistors, another observation of the flow of electrons through a vacuum was made. About 1875 an English physicist, William Crookes, was experimenting with the ability of gases to conduct electricity at low pressures. Crookes's discoveries have led to the development of such devices as television, RADAR (rā′ där), and special high-powered microscopes.

Crookes had found that if he reduced the air pressure within a tube, the resistance to electrical energy flow was reduced. He found that at low pressures the air glowed with a faint light as the current passed through it. He then pumped more air from the tube, reducing the pressure more and more. As he did this, the glow became fainter and fainter and finally faded away. Crookes found, however, that the current continued to flow through the tube even though the glow had disappeared. Since the flow of energy came from the negative cathode, Crookes called this phenomenon **cathode rays.** After the discovery of the electron, it was realized that the cathode rays Crookes had found were actually electrons moving at nearly the speed of light.

## The Cathode-ray Tube

The first important use of cathode rays was in the construction of the cathode-ray **oscilloscope** (ə sil′ ə skōp′). The basic part of the oscilloscope is the cathode-ray tube, which is shown in the diagram on page 334. A steady supply of electrons is produced by the heated cathode. Positively charged anodes speed up the electrons and pull them away from the cathodes.

Normally these electrons would travel in a straight line from the anodes. However, they can be controlled by allowing them to pass through two sets of **deflecting** (di flekt′ ing) **plates.** By placing a small electrical charge on these plates, the beam of electrons is deflected up or down by one set of plates and to one side or the other by the second set of plates. In some types of cathode-ray tubes, small electromagnets are used in place of the deflection plates. Whichever method is used, the result is a beam of electrons that moves in a pattern. By studying this pattern we can measure certain characteristics of the current flowing through the deflectors.

In order to make the beam of electrons visible, the front face of the tube is coated with minerals that give off light when they are struck by electrons. This glowing is called **fluorescence.** When the electrons strike atoms of fluorescent minerals, electrons surrounding the atoms are moved away from the nucleus. When they are attracted back by the positive charge of the nucleus, they lose some of their energy in the form of light. In the case of some minerals the glow of light remains for a short time after the electron flow has stopped.

If the electron beam is not affected by the deflectors, it travels in a straight line and forms a glowing dot in the center of the fluorescent screen. If, however, a varying current is applied to the deflectors, the electron beam is caused to move in a characteristic pattern across the face of the screen.

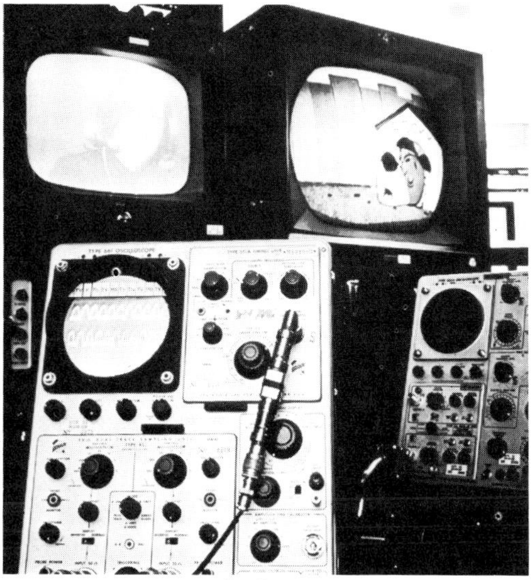

*Bell Telephone Laboratories Incorporated*

**10.16** Oscilloscope

## Television

The picture tube of a television set is a large cathode-ray tube. The electron beam sweeps back and forth across the fluorescent screen, making over 500 sweeps in less than a quarter of a second. The slight phosphorescent quality of the coating of the screen holds the light long enough so that the entire screen glows.

The deflectors of the tube are connected circuits that amplify the TV waves coming from the transmitter. In this way the number of electrons reaching the screen is controlled by the TV transmitter, and a picture appears on the screen.

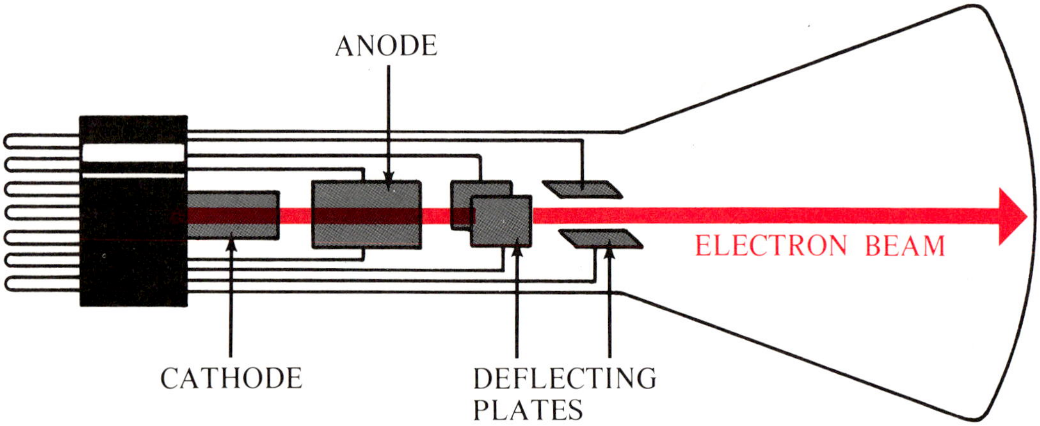


**10.17** Cathode-ray tube

In order to produce a picture in color, the picture tube contains three electron producing cathodes, one for each of the **primary light colors.** The fluorescent screen is composed of tiny dots of three different minerals. One fluoresces with a red glow, another with blue, and the third with green. The electron beam that is following the pattern produced by the red-sensitive camera stimulates only the dots that glow red, reproducing what the studio camera has detected. The blue and green are reproduced in the same manner. A blending of these three colors by your eyes produces the impression of a naturally colored picture. (See Figure 10.18 page 335.)

## RADAR

Another use of the cathode-ray tube is in RADAR, which means "Radio Detecting and Ranging." A RADAR unit consists of a transmitter that sends out high-frequency radio waves, a receiver that is tuned to receive the waves that reflect from various objects, and a cathode-ray tube called a *RADAR screen.* When the radio waves strike an object, they bounce back to the receiver. Since the speed of these waves through the air is known, a measure of the time that elapses between sending and receiving is a measure of the distance the object is away from the unit. The returning radio waves causes a shadow to appear on the RADAR screen, and from this a trained operator can often identify what type of object is being struck by the waves, as well as its direction and distance.

RADAR is commonly used in the navigation of airplanes and ships. Severe storms, such as hurricanes and tornadoes, also can be located and followed by RADAR. Much of our military defense program is based on the ability of RADAR to locate enemy airplanes and rockets in time to allow for a warning to be given. RADAR is even being used to explore the solar system by bouncing radio waves off the moon and planets. Figure 10.19 shows a RADAR detector.

## The Electron Microscope

The electron microscope is another form of the cathode-ray tube. The beam of electrons from the cathode passes

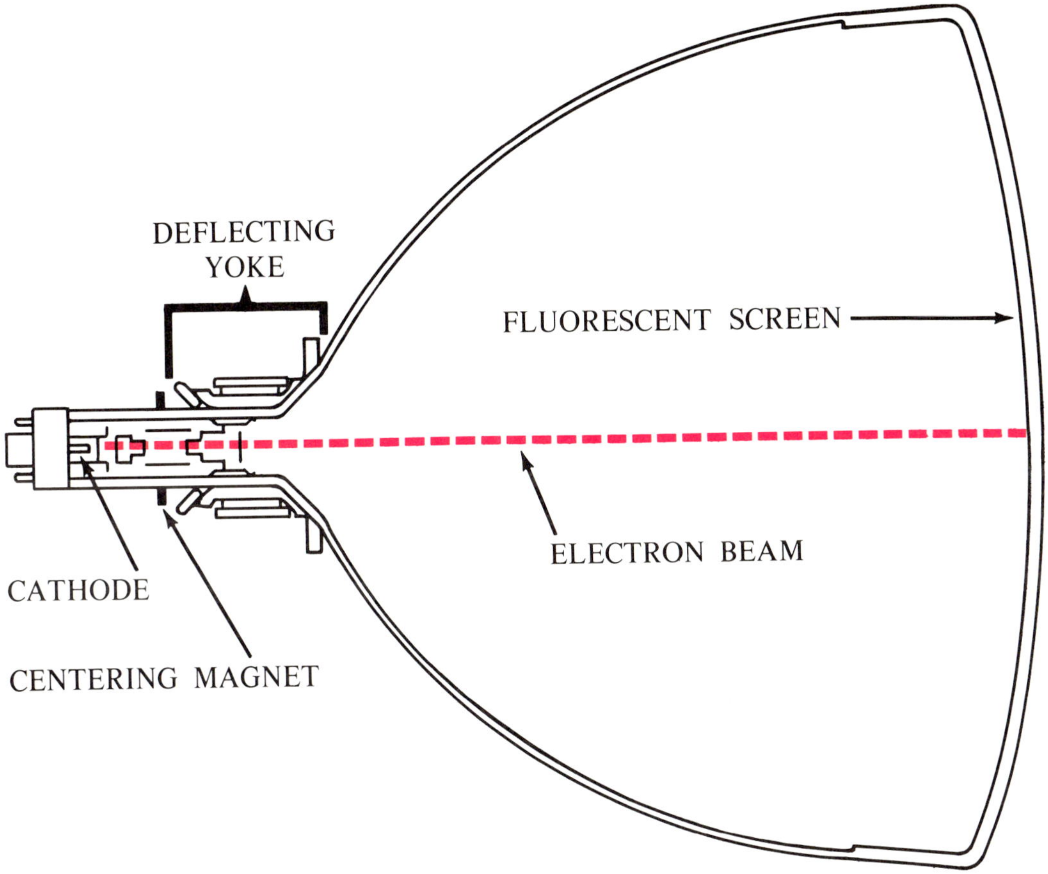


**10.18** Television tube

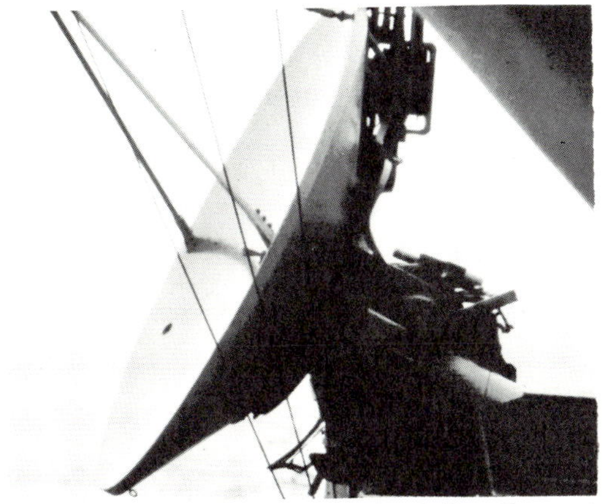

*Official U. S. Navy Photograph*

**10.19** RADAR detector

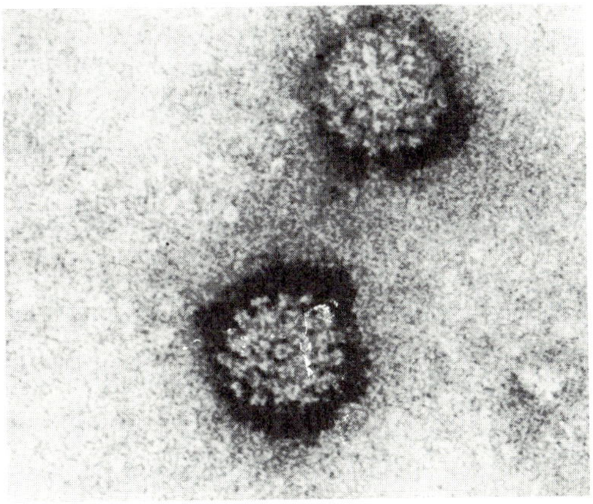

*Parke, Davis & Company*

**10.20** Wart virus magnified 640,000X

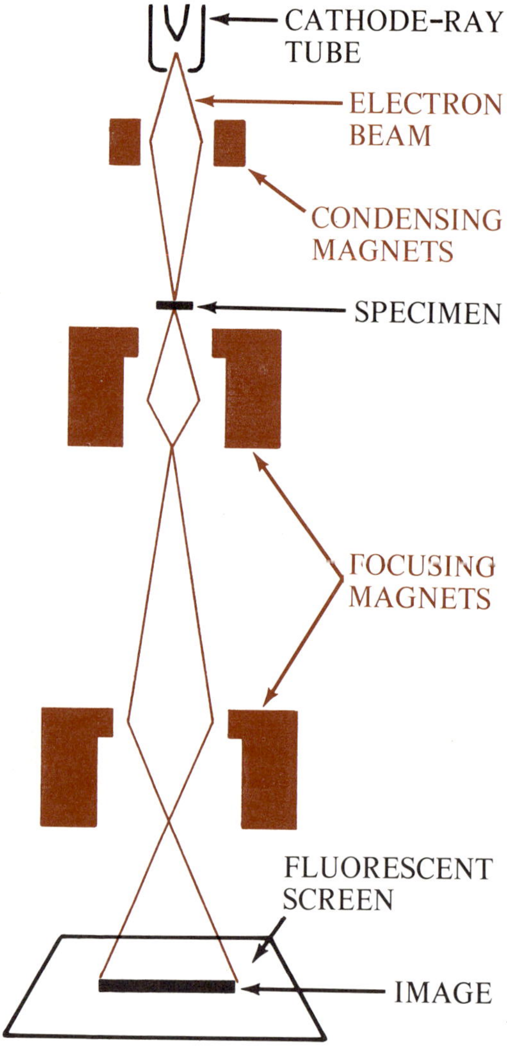


**10.21** Diagram of electron microscope

through and around the object being viewed and onto a fluorescent screen. Focusing is done with electromagnets. A microscope using electrons rather than light is able to magnify objects more than half a million times their actual size. This is about 200 times larger than the magnification of the best light microscopes. Figure 10.20 on page 335 was taken with an electron microscope.

## Have You Learned?

Select the word from Column B that best completes each statement in Column A. (Do not write in your book.)

| *Column A* | *Column B* |
|---|---|
| 1. William Crookes is given credit for discovery of the _____ ray. | a. anode<br>b. cathode<br>c. deflecting plates<br>d. electrons<br>e. fluorescence<br>f. microscope<br>g. oscilloscope<br>h. RADAR<br>i. television tube |
| 2. The first important use of Crookes's discovery was in construction of the _____. | |

3. In using the oscilloscope to study electric currents, the currents are directed through _____.
4. In an oscilloscope the electron beam is made visible by minerals that give off a glow called _____.
5. In a TV set the _____ are connected to circuits that amplify the waves coming from the transmitter.
6. The picture tube of a TV set is a kind of _____-ray tube.
7. In a color TV set, three _____-rays are produced—one for red, a second one for blue, and a third for green.
8. "Radio Detecting and Ranging" is another name for a _____ unit.
9. _____ is used to bounce beams off the moon.
10. An electron microscope uses _____ rather than light to magnify objects.

# 5. X Rays

**ARE YOU READY?**

Look up the following words if you are not sure of their meanings:

absorb; cathode ray; dense; filament; fluorescent.

Perhaps one of the most valuable uses of cathode rays is in the production of very high energy waves called **X rays.** The energy of these invisible waves is so high that they can **penetrate** (pen′ ə trāt) many materials.

## Uses of X Rays

You are probably familiar with the most common use of X rays. Perhaps you have had an X-ray picture taken by a doctor or a dentist. Or perhaps you have stood behind the screen of a **fluoroscope** (flür′ ə skōp) such as the one shown in the photograph below.

When X rays penetrate a part of the human body, they are absorbed by the bones but pass through the less dense muscles and fat. When these rays fall onto a photographic film or onto a fluorescent screen, a shadow of the denser parts of the body is formed. Using these shadow

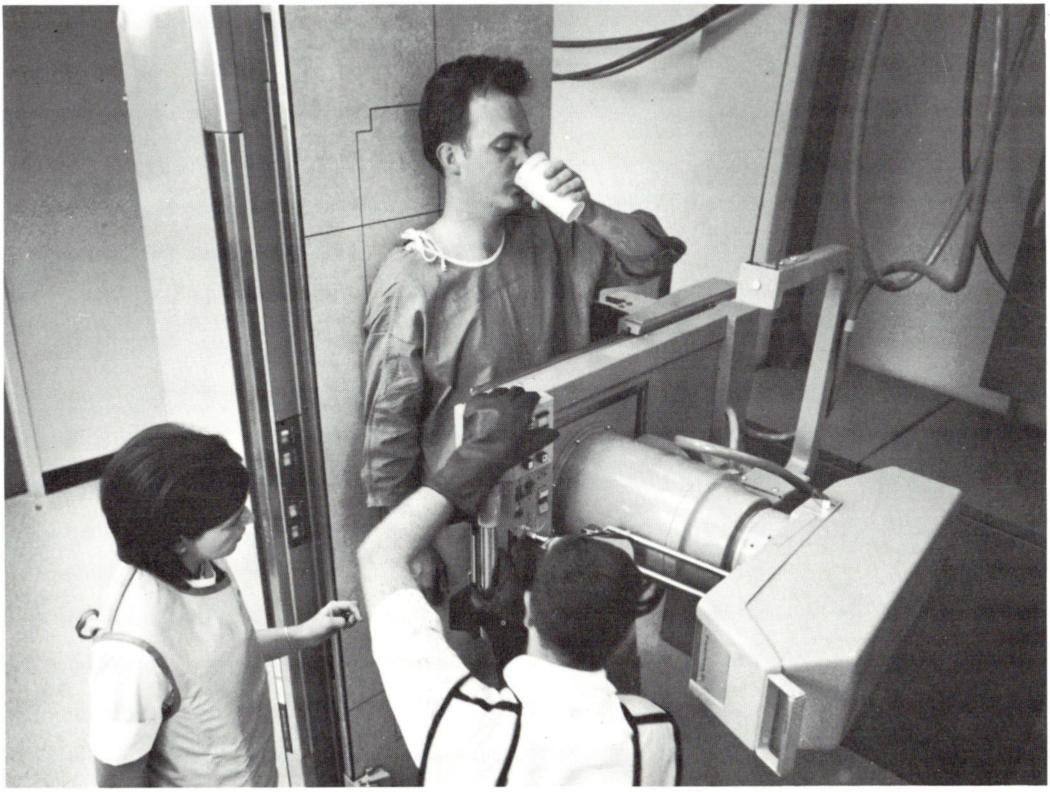

*General Electric Company, Medical Systems Department*

**10.22** The patient is drinking a solution that will be visible through the fluoroscope screen.

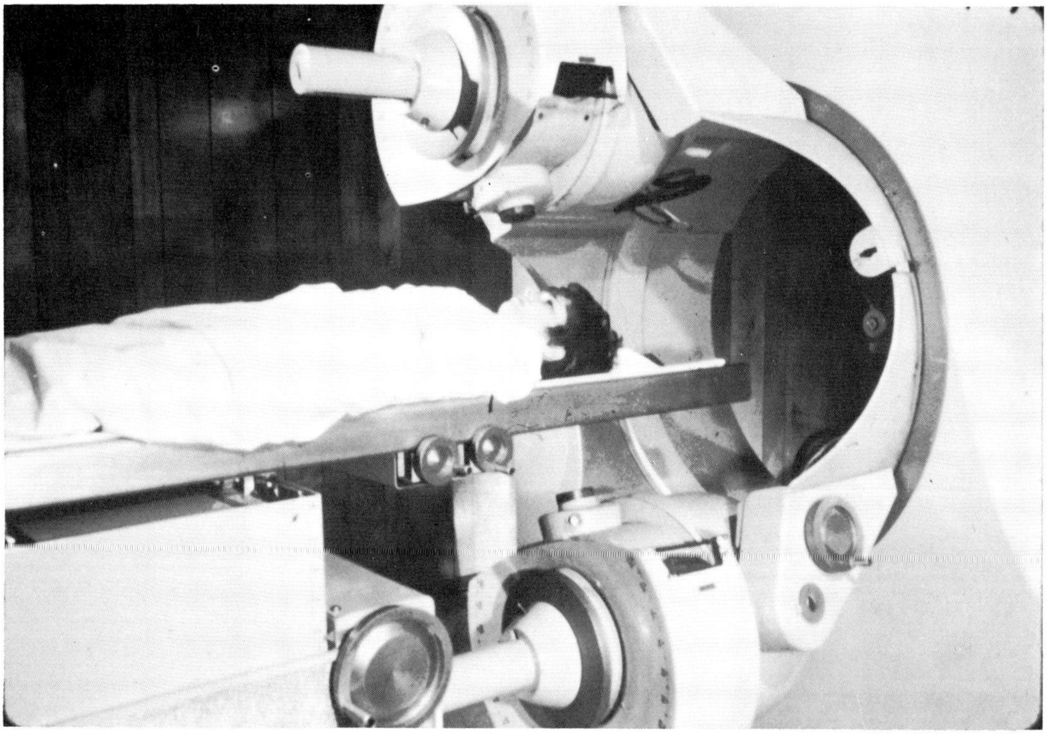

*United States Atomic Energy Commission*

**10.23** A patient about to receive X-ray treatment

pictures, doctors can observe broken bones and other problems before they make a diagnosis or before they operate. The advantage of the fluoroscope is that the doctor does not have to wait for the film to be developed, and he can observe a part of the body in motion.

Many other medical uses for X rays have been found. In the picture above (Figure 10.23), a patient is receiving treatment for cancer. The machine shown produces X rays that kill the cancer cells, but, if carefully controlled, do not harm the healthy cells.

Industry also uses the penetrating power of X rays. The photograph on page 339 shows an X-ray picture of a piece of metal. By directing the rays through it, the scientists can detect flaws deep inside that cannot be seen with the eyes.

The X-ray tube is also a valuable research tool used by many types of scientists. For example X rays can be directed into crystals. The pattern of radiation passing through the crystal will give valuable clues as to how the atoms are arranged.

## Development of X-ray Technology

The effect of X rays was discovered by Wilhelm Roentgen (rent′ gən). The units used to measure X rays are called "roentgens" in his honor. In 1895 Roentgen was working with cathode rays when he noticed that a distant piece of *fluorescent* material was glowing in the dark. He covered the cathode tube with black paper, but the mineral continued to fluoresce. Roentgen knew that cathode rays could not go through the black paper, and neither could they travel through air for such a great distance. He soon learned that he could take photographs of the shadows of the bones in his hand. Roentgen named these mysterious rays "X," since this symbol stands for the unknown.

The X-ray tube is a cathode-ray tube, very similar to the ones you have been studying. The cathode element is in the form of a heated filament. The anode is composed of a block of metal, usually tungsten. As the beam of electrons strikes the metal target, X rays are driven off by the energy of the electrons.

If the voltage difference between the cathode and the anode is increased, the electrons will hit the target with greater energy. Because of this, an increase in the voltage increases the energy of the X rays produced. Using a million or more volts, X rays can be produced that will penetrate a piece of steel over an inch thick.

*U. S. Steel Corporation*

**10.24** X rays reveal the fracture in a piece of steel.

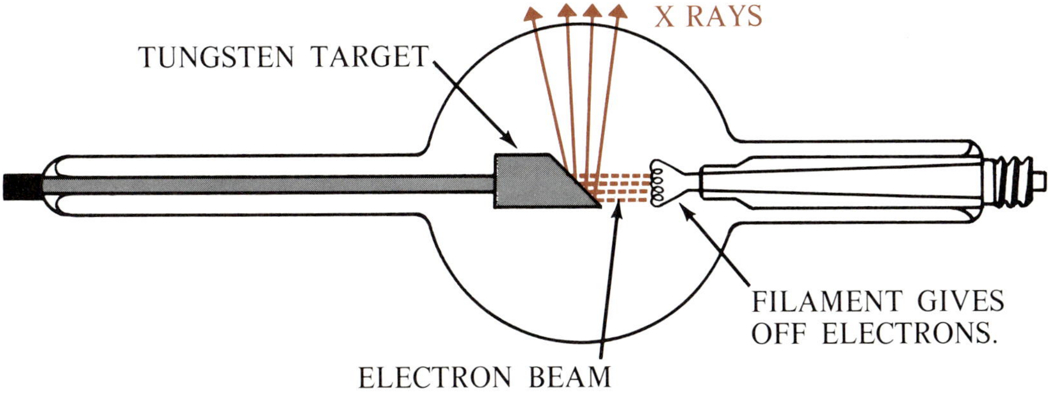


**10.25** X-ray tube

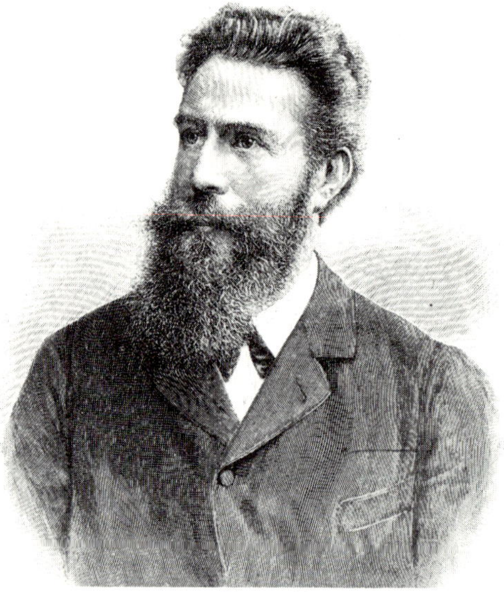

*Historical Pictures Service—Chicago*

**10.26** Wilhelm Konrad Roentgen (1845-1923)

## Harmful Effects of X Rays

X rays can be dangerous. This type of radiation has so much energy that it can damage and even kill living cells, but it can be controlled. The element lead is able to absorb X rays, stopping them completely if it is thick enough. Perhaps you have had your teeth X-rayed recently. If so, the dentist took certain precautions to protect you and himself from the damage caused by too much exposure to the rays. He may have placed a lead-lined apron or sheet over you. Also, he may have left the room or stepped behind a lead wall. Certainly, while his X-ray machine was turned on, he stood behind the X-ray tube to avoid its main ray.

One of the damaging effects of an over-

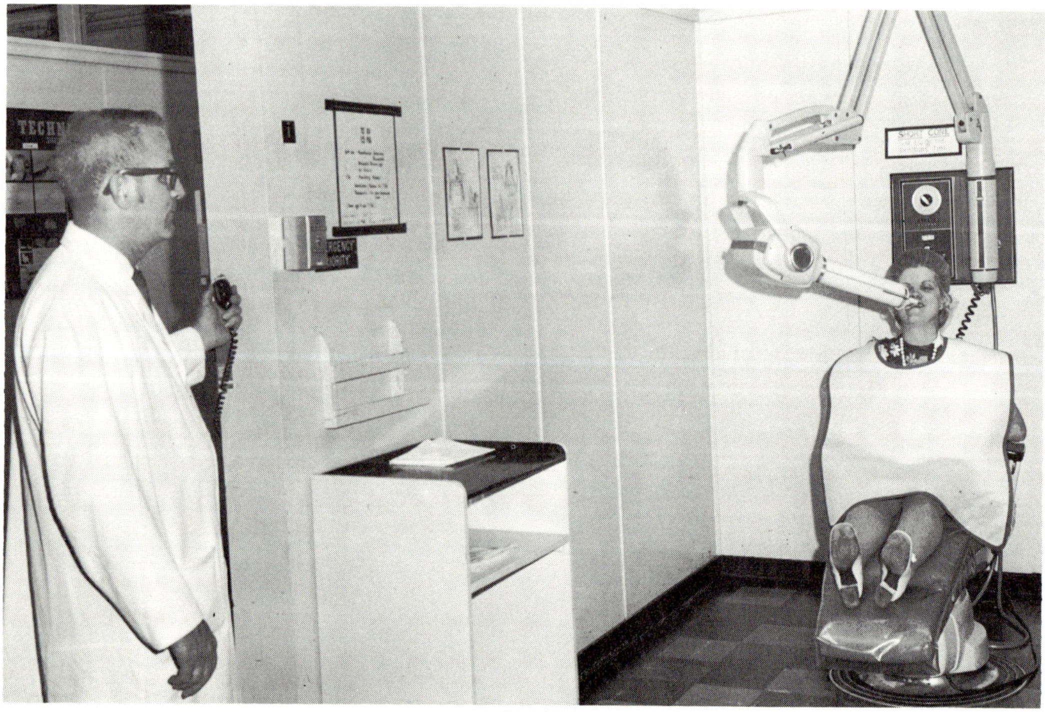

*Temple University School of Dentistry Department of Dental Radiology*

**10.27** The dentist stands well away from the X-ray machine as the patient is X-rayed.

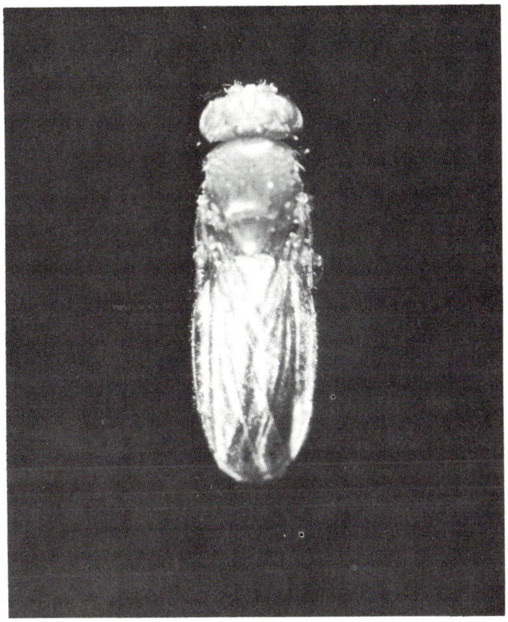

*Courtesy Carolina Biological Supply Company*

**10.28** This photograph shows a normal wild fruit fly.

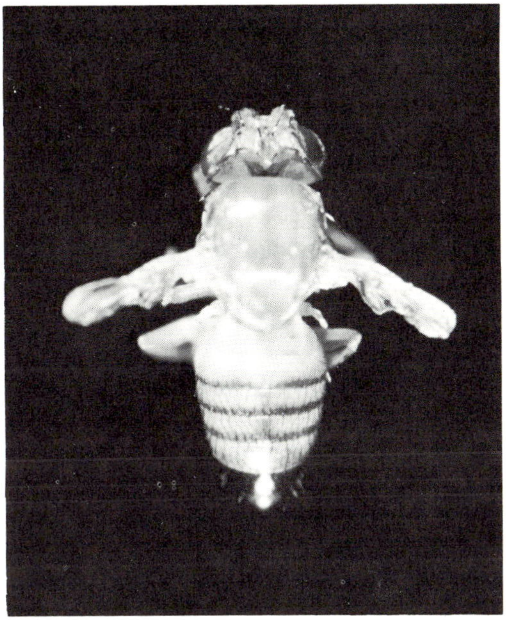

*Courtesy Carolina Biological Supply Company*

**10.29** This fly is a *mutant.* Note that the wings are vestigial and useless.

dose of X rays is the creation of **mutations** (mū tā′ shən). Certain cells of the bodies of all living things are used in reproduction. Within these cells are molecules that determine what characteristics the offspring will have. The arrangement of these molecules sometimes becomes changed, and an offspring that is quite different from its parents is produced. An overexposure to X-ray radiation is one way that these changes can be caused.

Small amounts of exposure to X rays will generally not harm you at all. In fact, it is possible to direct the radiation at certain cells so that these cells are killed, and the other cells are unharmed. In this way, X rays are often used to kill cancer cells.

As you will learn in the next chapter, X rays are not always produced artificially by use of a cathode-ray tube. You are constantly exposed to these naturally produced rays, but the amount that you receive is so small that there is normally no danger from them.

## Have You Learned?

Answer the following questions, using short complete sentences.

1. Who discovered X rays?
2. What are the units used to measure X rays?
3. Why were X rays named "X"?
4. If the voltage of the current going into an X-ray tube is increased, what happens to the X rays?
5. How can X rays be used to help us?
6. How can X rays be dangerous?

## 6. What Is a Computer?

**ARE YOU READY?**

Look up the following words if you are not sure of their meanings:

ammeter; amps; Arabic numerals; digits; ohms; resistance; voltage; voltmeter.

In the last few decades we have come to rely on electronic **computers** (kəm pūt′ ər) to do much of the work of the world. Astronauts depend upon computers, both on the ground and in their capsules, to direct their flights to the moon and back to earth. Scientists use computers to help them solve problems that could be solved in no other way. Banks use computers to keep their records correct. Businesses use them to process orders, to find one item out of millions in their warehouses, and to send out their bills. Manufacturing industries use computers to control many of their machines and arrange for shipment of the finished products. Airlines rely on computers to keep track of the empty seats that may be available on dozens of different flights. Even some schools now use computers to grade papers and assign classes. Can you think of other ways in which we use computers?

### Digital Computers

The most common type of computer is the **digital** (dij′ ə təl) computer. This machine is often referred to as a "data-processing machine" because it is able to take a great deal of data and "process" them mathematically. It is probable that you have come in contact with a digital computer recently. Have you seen cards with rectangular holes punched in them? Or have you seen bank checks with numbers printed on them with special ink? Or have you taken a test in which you were required to mark your answers on a special sheet of paper with a certain type of pencil? All of these pieces of paper are processed by digital computers.

How can a machine do all of these complicated jobs? Actually, the basic idea of a digital computer is not very complex. When you were younger, you probably added numbers by counting on your fingers. When you did this, you were using a very simple digital computer. And this is a good way to remember the name of this machine, since the word "digit" can mean a finger as well as one of the ten Arabic numerals that we use in our system of arithmetic.

But you have 10 fingers to count on, and our Arabic system has ten numerals: 0,1,2,3,4,5,6,7,8, and 9. The digital computer has only an electric circuit on which to count, and there can be only two conditions—*off* and *on*. For this reason, the digital computer can count on only two "fingers."

Therefore, a different system of arithmetic is used. It is called "base 2." (Our Arabic system is called "base 10." Can you see why?) Perhaps you have studied base-2 mathematics in school. If not, you may want to read more about it in an encyclopedia or other reference book.

The base-2 system is shown below, using the numerals 1 through 10. In a digital computer the symbol "0" can mean that that particular circuit is "off," and "1" can mean that the circuit is "on."

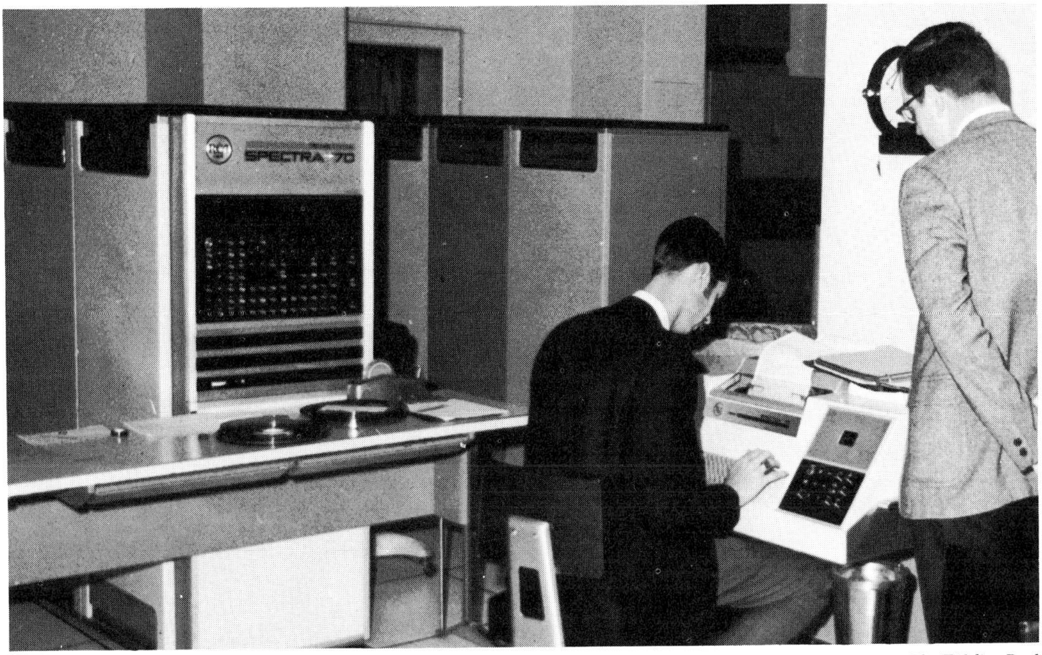


The Fidelity Bank

**10.30** Computers are used today in most banks and in many other businesses.

| *Base 10* | *Base 2* |
|---|---|
| 0 | 0 |
| 1 | 1 |
| 2 | 10 |
| 3 | 11 |
| 4 | 100 |
| 5 | 101 |
| 6 | 110 |
| 7 | 111 |
| 8 | 1000 |
| 9 | 1001 |
| 10 | 1010 |

## How Do You Solve Problems?

Suppose that your teacher sets up an electric circuit consisting of some dry cells and light bulbs connected in series. He then gives you a voltmeter and an ammeter and asks you to find the resistance of the circuit. How would you go about solving this problem?

Your first step would be to gather the data that you will need to solve the problem. So, you would put your meters into the circuit and measure the voltage and the amperage of the circuit. Your second step would be to consult your memory in an attempt to remember the relationship between volts, amps, and ohms that you learned in Chapter 9. Then, after you remembered that "$\text{Ohms} = \frac{\text{Volts}}{\text{Amps}}$," you would decide that you must divide the reading of your voltmeter by the reading of the ammeter in order to arrive at the correct answer. The fourth step would be to perform this division. As a last step you would record your answer in the form

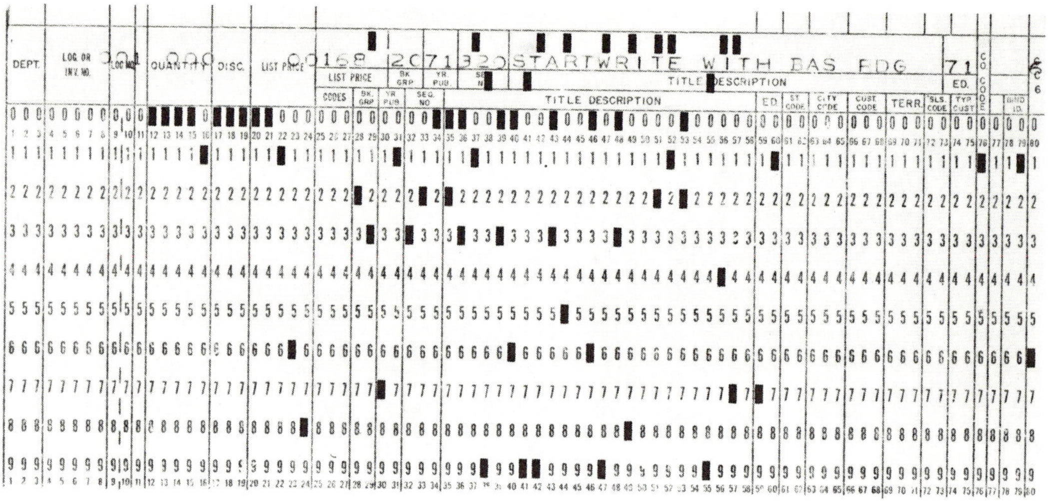


**10.31** The information on this computer card is in the form of rectangular holes.

required by your teacher and turn it in to be checked.

## How Do Digital Computers Solve Problems?

Digital computers are used by many scientists and businessmen to solve problems that are much more complicated than that given above. However, their digital computers solve their problems by using the same steps that you used.

The first step—the collection of data—is performed by human beings. The data and a series of instructions called a **program** are written in a **code** that the machine can "read." The data and the program are then fed into the computer. Sometimes this information is in the form of holes punched in cards, sometimes it is on magnetic recording tape, or it may be in the form of magnetic ink on paper.

All the data are stored in the **storage** or **"memory" unit** of the computer. When the computer is asked a question, it is able to recover this information from its "memory." The **control unit** selects instructions from the memory unit and directs the rest of the computer as to how it must solve the problem. This is actually done by the **arithmetic unit.** Once the problem is solved, the answer is sent to the **output unit** where it is given a form that the operator can read and use.

A digital computer basically can do only addition and subtraction. To multiply, the computer must add. For example, to multiply 6 times 3, the computer adds 6 + 6 + 6. Can you see how this will give the right answer? How can a computer manage a division problem?

## Analog Computers

A second type of computer is the **analog** (an′ ə lôg) computer. This computer is used for solving many scientific problems. Although there are general-purpose analog computers, very often an analog computer is built to solve only a specific kind of problem and cannot be used for other kinds of problems. Thus, it is limited.

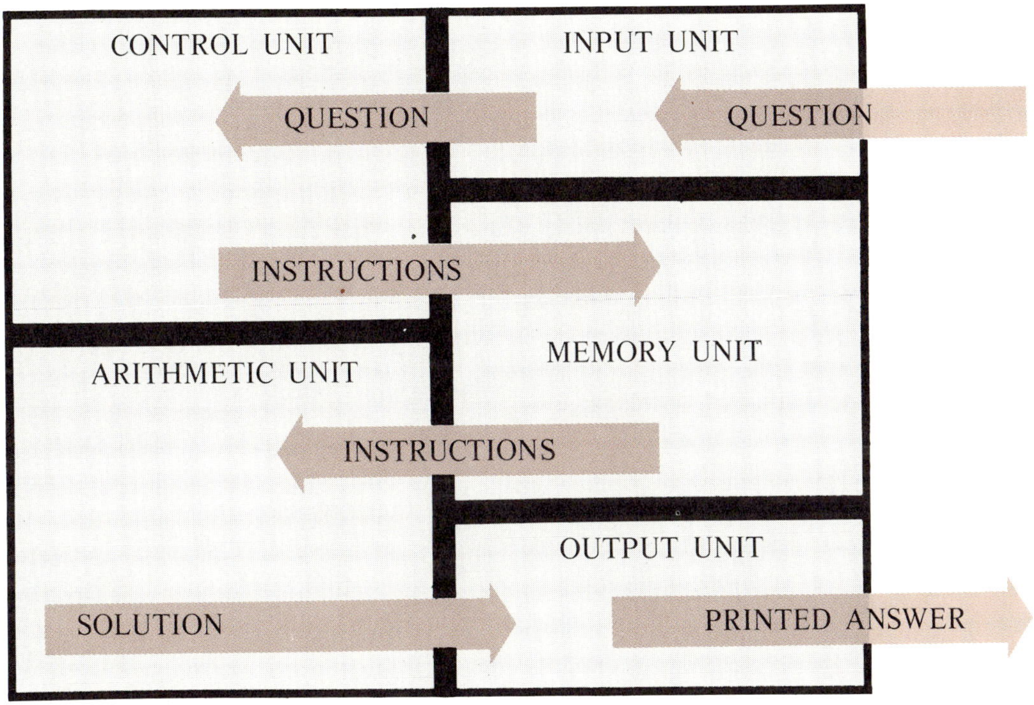


**10.32** Schematic drawing of a computer system

Scientists and engineers use analog computers to study situations in which conditions are constantly changing, such as an airplane in flight or a rocket during blast-off. In order to do this, the computer must be designed to act as a model, or **analogy** (ə nal′ ə ji), of the real situation. We have used many analogies in this book. For example, in Chapter 9 you read that an electric circuit was similar to a water system in many ways. Because of this similarity, the water system is said to be **analogous** (ə nal′ ə gəs) or *similar to* an electric circuit.

A simple example will show how an analog computer might be used. Suppose that we want to design a water system, and that we can vary both the pressure on the water and the resistance. In order to determine the flow of water at a number of different pressures and resistances, we could feed a great deal of data into a digital computer and get accurate answers. Or we could build a simple analog computer in which we could vary both the voltage (pressure) of the current and the ohms (resistance). By adjusting these two characteristics of the circuit, we could determine their effects directly by reading an ammeter. Since $\text{Amps} = \dfrac{\text{Volts}}{\text{Ohms}}$ and since $\text{Flow of Water} = \dfrac{\text{Pressure}}{\text{Resistance}}$, the readings of the ammeter would be analogous to the flow of water through the system. These results would not be so accurate as those of the digital computer, but we could get them very rapidly and by using a very simple instrument.

## Have You Learned?

On a sheet of paper list the numbers for the questions below. By each number write *T* if the statement is true and *F* if false.

1. Scientists are the only people who use computers.
2. The most common type of computer is the digital computer.
3. The "data-processing machine" is another name for a digital computer.
4. Digital computers solve problems by analogies.
5. The cards we often see that have rectangular holes punched in them are probably used with digital computers.
6. Digital computers use "base-10" arithmetic.
7. The digital computer has very limited use.
8. A water system is somewhat analogous to an electric circuit.
9. The analog computer is simpler than the digital computer.
10. Analog computers can be used only for problems involving water pressure.

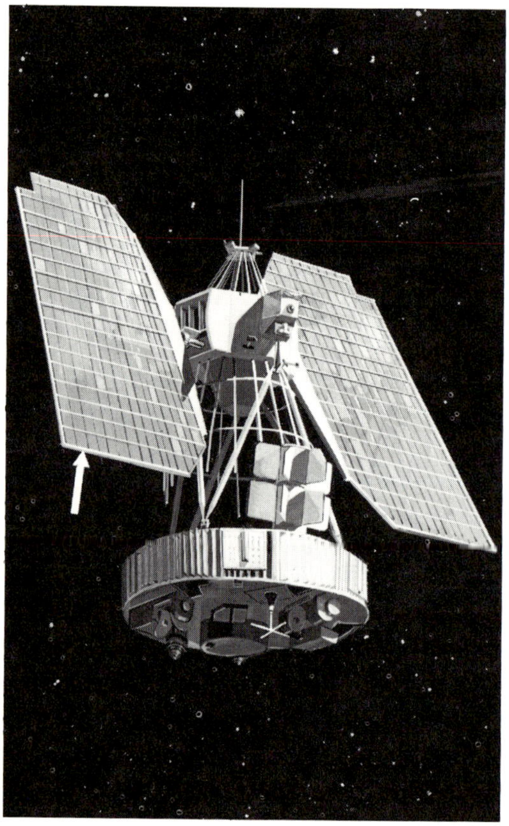

*NASA*

**10.33** Nimbus B experimental weather satellite. The arrow indicates one of the solar paddles that power the electronic information-gathering equipment of the satellite. (See page 331.)

## REVIEW QUESTIONS

1. Discuss the piezoelectric effect. Explain what it is and what it can be used for.
2. Telephones and some microphones and loudspeakers contain a part called a diaphragm. Explain what this part is for and how it works.
3. Draw a diagram of a photoelectric cell, and explain how it works.
4. Explain in detail how a telegraph set works.
5. Explain the difference between UHF, VHF, and Standard radio broadcasts.
6. Explain the difference between AM and FM broadcasts.
7. Explain how we can tune a radio so that it receives only one station.
8. What are the major differences between a diode and a triode vacuum tube?
9. Explain how the use of the grid element in a vacuum tube controls the strength of the current passing through the tube.
10. What is a semiconductor?
11. Why does an electric current move in only one direction through a transistor?
12. In what ways are TV picture tubes similar to oscilloscopes?
13. Name four instruments having cathode-ray tubes as important parts of them.
14. How does an X-ray tube differ from the usual cathode-ray tube?

15. Explain the difference between a digital computer and an analog computer.

## CAN YOU FIND OUT?

*It may be necessary for you to use encyclopedias or other reference books in order to answer the following questions.*

1. How did Alexander Graham Bell invent the telephone?
2. What improvements have been made in the telephone over Bell's first model?
3. In what ways other than those mentioned in this chapter is the piezoelectric effect used?
4. Photoelectric cells are very widely used. Some of these uses are listed on page 323. Describe in detail how one of these devices works.
5. Is there any relationship between the height of a radio transmitter antenna and the frequency of the signals it broadcasts?
6. What are the advantages and disadvantages of the various frequency bands (Standard, VHF, UHF)? What use is made of each?
7. What types of vacuum tubes other than diodes and triodes are used in communication instruments?
8. In what kinds of communication instruments are transistors now being used?
9. What are some uses for oscilloscopes other than those mentioned in this chapter?
10. When was RADAR invented, and how was it first used?
11. Why is an electron microscope able to magnify objects more than a light microscope?
12. How much exposure to X rays is necessary before they become dangerous?
13. What are some of the uses for computers in your community?

## REFERENCES FOR ADDITIONAL STUDY

CAREERS AND OPPORTUNITIES IN ELECTRONICS by John Carrol. E. P. Dutton & Co., Inc.
Includes facts about electronics in general and also describes the work of the scientist and electronics engineer in fields such as broadcasting and industrial electronics

COMPUTERS: TOOLS FOR TODAY by Claude J. De Rossi. Childrens Press.
An excellent introduction to how computers work and the kinds of tasks they are used to perform

SCIENCE PROJECTS IN ELECTRONICS (Second Edition) by Edward M. Noll. Howard W. Sams & Co., Inc. Publishers.
A helpful guide for doing projects in electronics

TRANSISTORS AND CIRCUITS: ELECTRONICS FOR YOUNG EXPERIMENTERS by W. E. Pearce and Aaron E. Klein. Doubleday & Company, Inc.
Contains many interesting ideas for projects in electronics

THE TELEPHONE: HOW IT WORKS by Jermone J. O'Connor. G. P. Putnam's Sons.
Tells how the telephone works, both as a transmitting-receiving instrument and as part of a transmission system

# *Workshop... Unit IV*

**Building a Simple Radio Receiver.** Inexpensive kits containing the parts and directions for building a radio receiver are available from many hobby stores and radio shops. If you would like to build a receiver from scratch, you will need the following materials:

Block of wood, about 20 cm × 30 cm × 2 cm
Spool of insulated No. 27 copper wire
1N34 transistor
Variable condenser (can be obtained from an old radio)
Four stove bolts 4 cm long with two nuts each
Two clips (see picture of receiver)
Pair of earphones
Cardboard tube 4-5 cm in diameter by 15 cm (from roll of paper toweling)
30 cm of wire for outside antenna

A diagram using electrical symbols is frequently used to show how to wire an electrical circuit. The drawing below is a schematic diagram of a radio receiver. Refer to both as you assemble your receiver.

The first step in assembling the receiver is to wind about 80 turns of wire on the cardboard tube. The wire should be wound neatly, with each turn just touching the one next to it. Allow about 15 cm of wire on each end and pull these ends through the holes in the cardboard tube, as shown in the picture. This will keep the coil from coming loose. The coil can be held on the board by thumb tacks. Be sure to scrape the insulting varnish off the ends of the wire before fastening it to the stove bolt terminals.

Assemble the rest of the receiver, following the wiring diagram and consulting the picture. Connect one of the coil terminals to a ground (water pipe or metal stake in the ground). Connect the other coil terminal to an antenna, which is a wire stretched between two insulators. The longer and the higher the antenna, the better; however, if there is a radio station nearby, you may be able to get by with only a few meters of antenna.

While listening with your earphones, slowly turn the variable condenser until

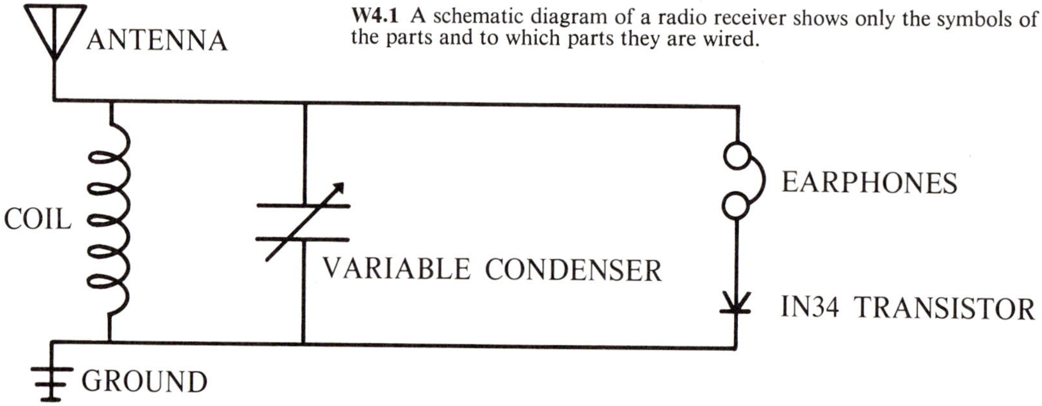


**W4.1** A schematic diagram of a radio receiver shows only the symbols of the parts and to which parts they are wired.

you hear a station. If you cannot get a station, check the connections to make sure all wires have the insulation removed and that electricity can flow through the circuit. If any of the plates on the variable condenser are bent and touch each other, the condenser should be replaced.

If you would like to build a more powerful radio that has a loudspeaker and that can receive more stations, check a book on radios for plans and consider assembling one of the many kits available.

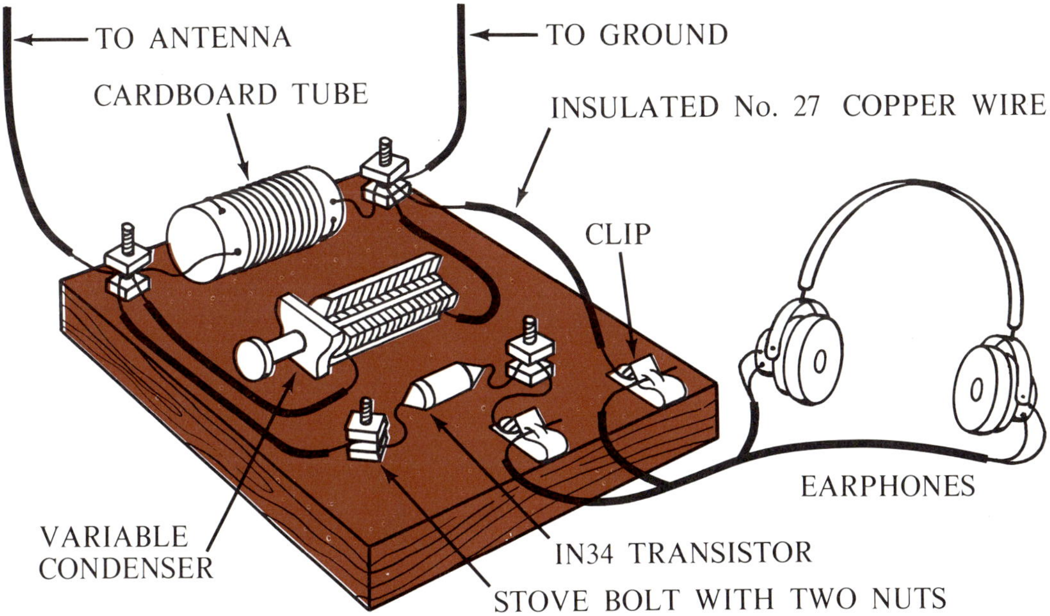


**W4.2** You will have fun making this transistor radio. Why don't you get into it?

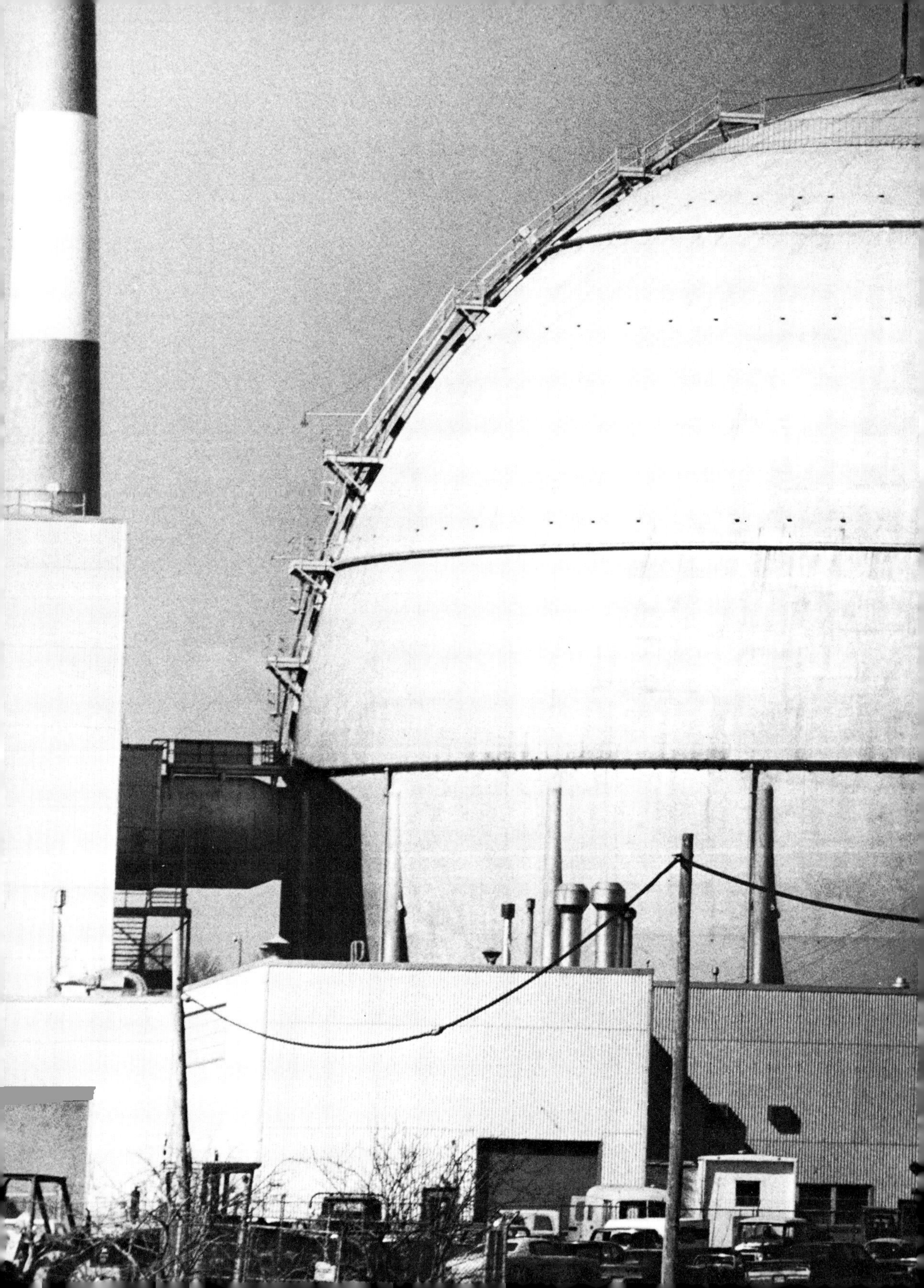

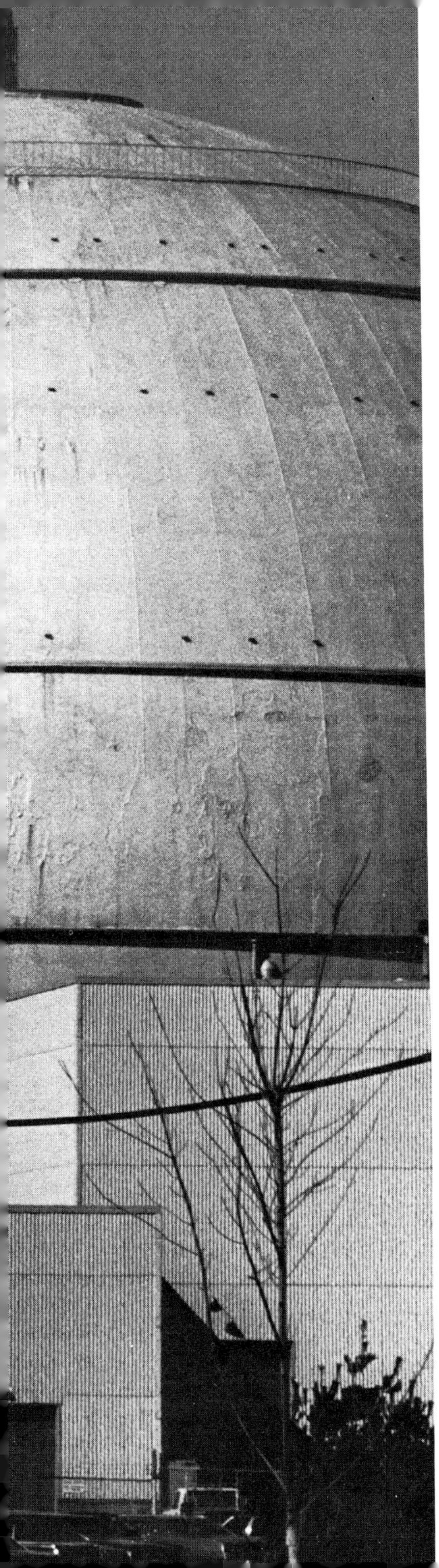

# unit V
# the energy of the nucleus

Roger Malloch/Magnum Photos, Inc.

CHAPTER **11**

# Natural Radioactivity

ON AUGUST 6, 1945 a 4,050-kilogram device was dropped on Hiroshima, Japan. This new weapon exploded with a force of 18,000 metric tons of TNT, and "atomic bomb" and "atomic energy" became household words. After the war scientists turned their attention to the development of peaceful uses of atomic energy. To understand the many applications of atomic energy that have since been developed, we must first know something about the inside of the atom—the nucleus. It is also necessary to know what happens in the nucleus when radioactive atoms fly apart.

## 1. Early Work on Radioactivity

**ARE YOU READY?**

Look up the following words if you are not sure of their meanings:

artificial; electroscope; fluorescent; piezoelectric effect; ultraviolet; X ray.

In science one researcher often builds on the work of other investigators. So it was in the case of Roentgen's discovery of the X ray, which was described in the last chapter. Antoine Henri Becquerel (bek′ ə rel′), like his famous scientist father, was interested in fluorescent materials. These are materials, such as certain minerals, that glow when they are exposed to sunlight or to ultraviolet light.

When Becquerel learned of Roentgen's work, he began to wonder if the fluorescence he was studying contained some of the X rays described by Roentgen. He decided to experiment to find out. He placed a crystal of a **uranium** (ūr ăn′ i əm) compound on a photographic plate that had been wrapped in black paper. He placed these in the sunlight, reasoning that the sunlight would make the fluorescent crystal glow, and any X rays given off would expose the plate. The black paper would keep the plate from being exposed by the sunlight.

When the plate was developed, he found it to be partially exposed, or fogged. It appeared that the uranium was giving off X rays. Before Becquerel could repeat his experiments, the weather turned cloudy for several days. He placed an unexposed photographic plate and uranium in a desk drawer and waited for the sunlight that he needed for his experiments.

While he waited, he decided to develop some of the plates stored in the drawer. He wondered if perhaps a little of the fluorescence continued and if the plate would be slightly exposed. To his amazement the film was exposed as much as when the uranium compound had been exposed to the sunlight. He continued to experiment and found that the uranium compound gave off *radiation* regardless of whether it was in the sunlight or not. He also found that the radiation discharged an electroscope and that some of the radiation was even more penetrating than X rays.

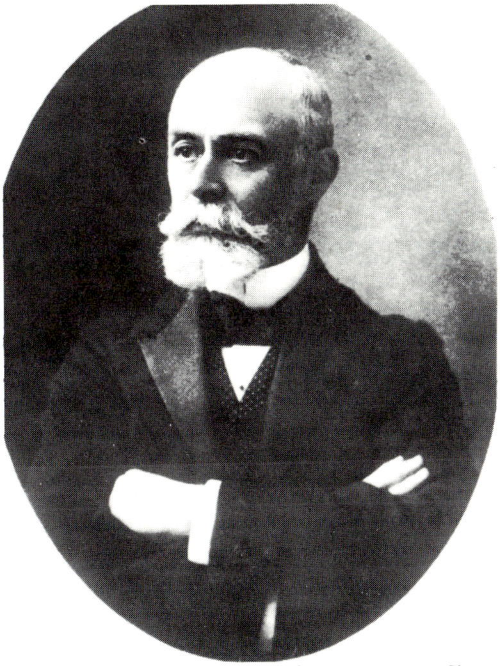

*Historical Pictures Service—Chicago*

**11.1** Antoine Henri Becquerel (1852-1908)

## Duplicating Becquerel's Work

You can easily duplicate some of Becquerel's work by exposing photographic film with radioactive materials. In a *completely dark* room, cut a roll of black-and-white film into several pieces. Place objects that are thought to contain radioactive materials on the film, and store the objects and the film in a dark place for several days. For example, you may wish to use radioactive minerals or the hands or dial from a clock or watch that glows in the dark. Also try a new mantle, which is the sack used in gas lanterns. A mantle contains radioactive thorium.

Develop the film, and examine the negative for evidence that the radioactive materials have exposed or fogged the film. Packages of chemicals needed for developing black-and-white film are available in kit form at camera stores and many drugstores. An alternate method of doing this experiment is described in the Workshop at the end of this Unit.

**11.2** Duplicating Becquerel's experiment

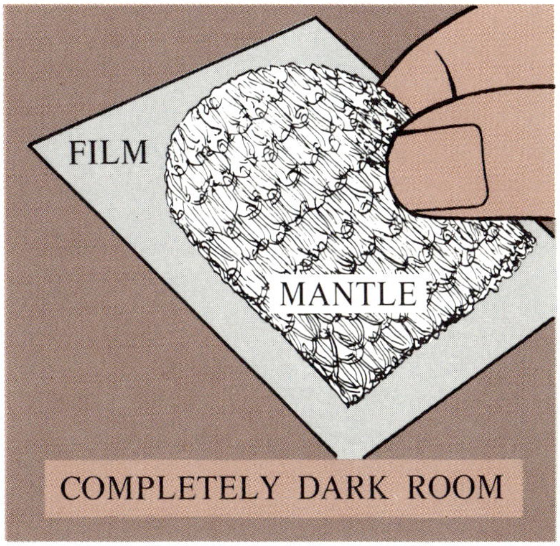

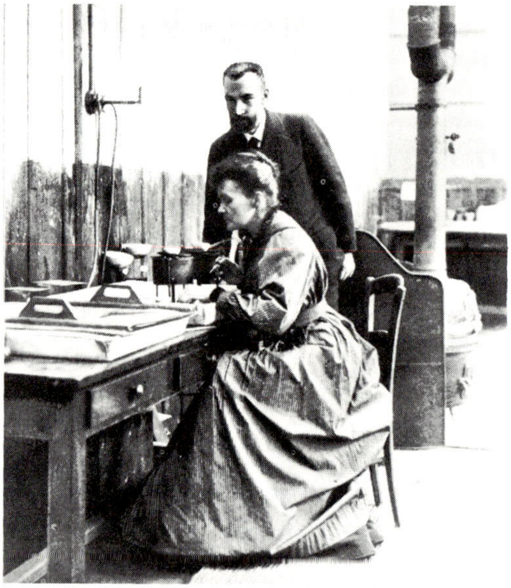

*Historical Pictures Service—Chicago*

**11.3** Marie and Pierre Curie in their laboratory, 1903

## The Work of the Curies

At about the same time Becquerel was doing his work, two other Frenchmen also made an important discovery. Pierre Curie (pē ãr′ kū ri′) and his brother discovered the piezoelectric effect. As was explained in Chapter 10, if a force is applied to certain crystals, its surfaces become electrically charged. The Curie brothers used this principle to build an **electrometer** (i lek′ trom′ ə tər), which could be used to measure very small amounts of electricity.

In 1895 Pierre Curie married a student from Poland who had come to France to study science. Marie Curie, who was doing research for her doctor's degree, decided to use her husband's electrometer to measure the amount of radiation given off by certain substances. She soon found that the amount of radiation given off varied with the number of uranium atoms present. It did not make any difference how the uranium atoms were combined with other elements. She also discovered that the element **thorium** (thôr′ i əm) gave off radiation like that given off by uranium.

Pierre Curie realized the importance of his wife's findings and joined her in the investigation of radioactivity. They used an ore named **pitchblende** (pich′ blend′) as their source of uranium. One day they found a piece of pitchblende that was more radioactive than usual. In fact, their measurements and calculations showed that it was more radioactive than pure uranium. They concluded that the piece of pitchblende must contain another element even more radioactive than uranium.

The Curies set about to isolate this unknown element. They dissolved pieces of pitchblende in acid and then carried out many chemical reactions to separate the unknown element. In a few months they were able to isolate an element about 400 times more radioactive than uranium. They named it **polonium** (pə lō′ ni əm) in honor of Marie's homeland, Poland.

But something else in the pitchblende was giving off even more radiation than was given off by polonium. In a few months they were able to isolate traces of this mysterious substance. It took them four years of hard work to reduce a ton of pitchblende to three-hundredths of an ounce of the white powder that gave off so much radiation. They called their new element **radium** (rā′ di əm).

In 1903 Pierre and Marie Curie shared the Nobel Prize in physics with Henri Becquerel in recognition of their study of the radiation of uranium. In 1911, Marie Curie received the Nobel Prize in Chemistry for the discovery of polonium and radium and for studying the properties of radium. She did not share the second Nobel Prize with her husband, since Pierre Curie had been killed in a traffic accident some five years earlier (in 1906).

The Nobel Prize, the world's highest honor in science, was established by Alfred Nobel, the Swedish inventor of dynamite. The prizes are awarded to those making important discoveries in physics, in chemistry, and in medicine and **physiology** (fiz′ i ol′ ə ji). In addition to the awards in science, Nobel Prizes also are given to authors of outstanding works of literature and to those who work for international peace. Check an encyclopedia for a list of the scientists who have received the Nobel Prize. You will find listed many of the names and many of the discoveries you have read about in this book.

The work of the Curies was continued by a daughter, Irène Curie. She and her husband, Frédéric Joliot (zhô lyō′), discovered a way to produce artificial radioactive elements. For this important contribution, they received the Nobel Prize in Chemistry in 1935. Another daughter, Eve Curie, became an author and wrote a biography of her famous mother. This book is listed in *References for Additional Study* at the end of this chapter on page 374.

As is true of most advances in science, the credit cannot be given entirely to a few. Hundreds of scientists have contributed to our knowledge of radioactivity. However, much of their work is based on the work of Roentgen, Becquerel, and the Curies, and these are important names in the history of science.

### Have You Learned?

Match the definition in Column A with the names in Column B. (Do not write in your book.)

| *Column A* | *Column B* |
|---|---|
| 1. Codiscoverer of artificial radioactive elements | a. Roentgen |
| 2. Discovered X rays | b. Becquerel |
| 3. Codiscoverer of the piezoelectric effect | c. Irène Curie |
| 4. Discovered that uranium gives off radiation | d. Marie Curie |
| 5. Coinventor of the electrometer | e. Pierre Curie |
| 6. Received two Nobel Prizes | |
| 7. Discovered polonium and radium (two answers) | |

## 2. Three Kinds of Rays

**ARE YOU READY?**

Look up the following words if you are not sure of their meanings:

deflect; detect; electron; ionize; magnetic field; nucleus; radiation; radioactivity.

Henri Becquerel discovered natural radioactivity in 1896. This was at a time when we still did not know much about atoms. It wasn't until 1913 that Niels Bohr (nēls bōr) suggested that electrons are arranged in shells around the nucleus of the atom. The proton wasn't identified until 1920 and the neutron until 1932. As you shall see, the early studies of radioactivity contributed a great deal to our understanding of atoms.

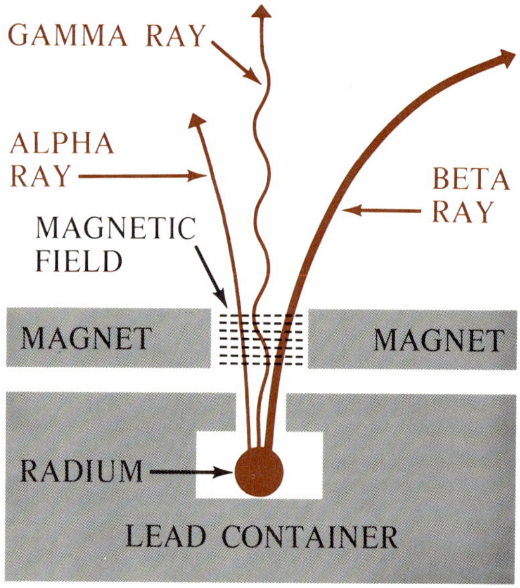


**11.4** Rutherford's experiment

Ernest Rutherford (ruᴛʜ′ ər fərd), a British scientist, showed that a radioactive substance may give off three kinds of radiation. He placed a small amount of radium in a lead container as shown in Figure 11.4. Lead is a substance that stops most radiation, and the only radiation leaving the container was that going out of the hole on the top. Rutherford placed a magnet at the top of the container to see if a magnetic field affected the stream of radiation.

Rutherford found that a magnetic field bent some of the radiation to the left. These he called **alpha** (al′ fə) **rays.** Some of the radiation was bent to the right, but more than in the case of alpha rays. This radiation was named **beta** (bā′ tə) **rays.** The remainder of the radiation did not appear to be affected by the magnetic field and continued to travel in a straight line. This was named **gamma** (gam′ ə) **rays.** Alpha, beta, and gamma are the first three letters of the Greek alphabet, which is often used for scientific symbols and in formulas.

Rutherford reasoned that alpha rays and beta rays were made up of particles with electrical charges and thus were deflected, or bent, by the magnetic field. The fact they were bent in opposite directions indicated that they had opposite charges. Furthermore, he reasoned that *alpha particles* had more mass than *beta particles* since they were not affected as much by the magnetic field. Gamma rays were found to be similar to X rays and not affected by the magnetic field.

## Properties of the Three Types of Radiation

1. *Alpha Particles.* An alpha particle is the nucleus of a helium atom. It is made up of two protons and two neutrons and thus has a positive charge of two and an atomic weight of four. Do you see why this is so?

Alpha particles travel at speeds of about 19,000 kilometers per second, or about one-fifteenth the speed of light. Since they are relatively large compared to other kinds of particles, they do not pass through materials as easily as other particles. They can be stopped by a sheet or two of paper and usually do not travel farther than about 9 centimeters through air. When they strike other atoms or molecules, electrons are often knocked off, causing ions to be formed.

2. *Beta Particles.* Beta particles are fast-moving electrons with speeds ten or more times faster than those of alpha particles. Beta particles have negative charges, and their paths can be deflected by electrically charged bodies or magnetic fields. Because

of their size and speed they can pass through thicker materials than can the slower-moving and heavier alpha particles. However, most beta particles can be stopped by a thin sheet of metal.

3. *Gamma Rays.* Gamma rays are a form of high energy radiation much like X rays. They have no weight and travel at the speed of light, or about $3 \times 10^{10}$ cm per second. Like X rays they can penetrate, or go through, very dense materials such as wood, flesh, and metal. Experiments have shown that gamma radiation can penetrate 30 cm of concrete.

## How Can Radiation Be Detected?

There are several ways used to detect the presence of radiation from radioactive materials and to measure the amount.

1. *Photographic Film.* Early investigators such as Becquerel and Rutherford used photographic plates or film to detect radiation, and this method is still used. People who work in hospitals, research laboratories, nuclear power plants and other places where radioactive materials are used wear **film badges.** These are small pieces of film, enclosed so that light will not expose them, that are clipped to a coat or other clothing. Periodically the film is developed to see if the wearer has been exposed to excessive radiation.

2. *Electroscopes and Similar Devices.* Becquerel learned that radiation causes an electroscope to discharge. The radiation causes the air around the leaves to ionize, and the ionized air is a good conductor of electricity. The charge on the leaves of the electroscope leaks off more quickly if the surrounding air is ionized. A **dosimeter** (dō sim′ i tər) is a device based

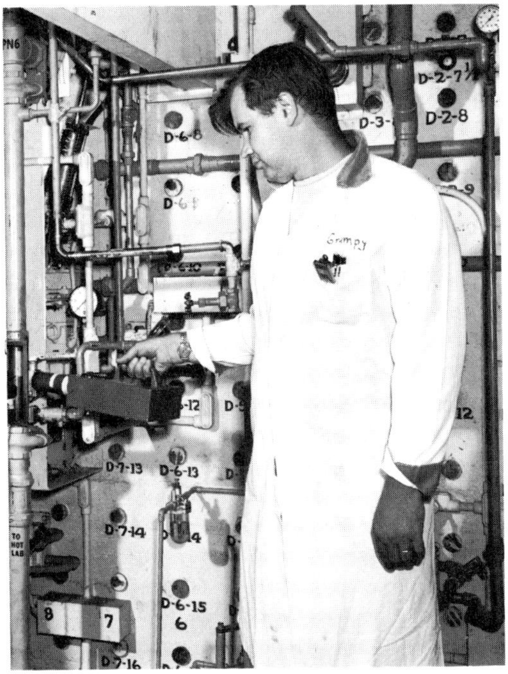


*Brookhaven National Laboratory*

**11.5** Health physicist wearing film badge

on this principle that is used to measure the amount of radiation. One type of dosimeter is about the size and shape of a fountain pen. This pocket dosimeter can be checked at any time, and thus a worker does not have to wait, as in the case of the film badge, to see how much radiation he has been exposed to (Figure 11.6).

3. ***Geiger*** (gī′ gər) ***Counters and Scintillation*** (sin′ tə lā′ shən) ***Counters.*** These are electrical devices that are used to detect and measure the amount of radiation. The Geiger counter works on the same principle as the dosimeter. Radiation causes the gas in a tube to ionize, and an electrical current flows through the tube of ionized gas. The current is amplified and used to light a bulb, to make a click on a loudspeaker, or to run a counter much like the mileage indicator on an automobile.

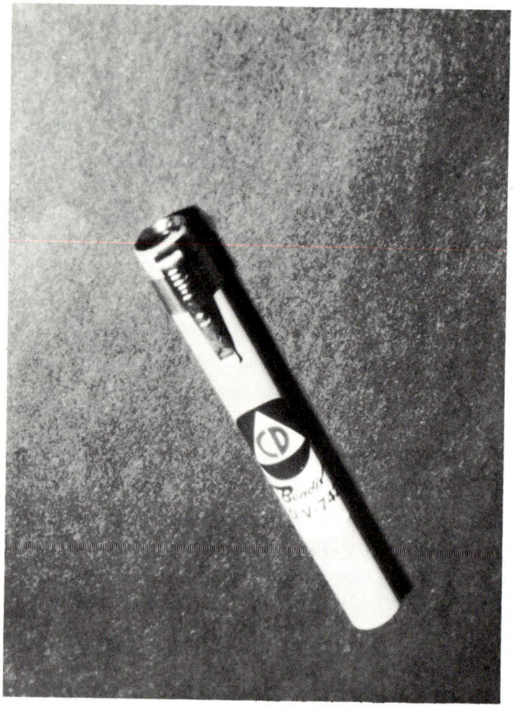


*Walter R. Brown*

**11.6** Dosimeter

In the case of the scintillation counter, radiation strikes a crystal. This causes a small flash of light to be given off. This is similar to what happens when electrons strike the inside coating of a fluorescent light tube and cause it to glow. The light given off is detected by a photoelectric cell, and the small electrical current produced is amplified. As in the case of the Geiger counter, the results can be reported to an observer as flashes, clicks, or numbers on a counter.

## Detecting Radioactivity

If your school has a Geiger counter, set it up, and perform the following demonstrations. If not, perhaps your teacher can borrow one or arrange for a demonstration by a Civil Defense official, fireman, or prospector.

(1) Without any radioactive materials nearby, adjust the Geiger counter so that an occasional click is heard or flash is observed. Does this *background radiation* vary from day to day? Is it the same throughout the day?

(2) Bring a radioactive source near the Geiger counter. Does the number of clicks or flashes increase? What other objects, such as watches and clocks with luminous dials, make the number of clicks or flashes increase?

(3) Try placing different materials between the detecting tube of the Geiger counter and a radioactive source. Would a piece of cardboard, a sheet of glass, or a sheet of lead make the best shield?

4. *Cloud Chamber.* Radiation passing through vapors such as alcohol causes the alcohol gas to condense. This is because the radiation produces ions, and tiny droplets of alcohol condense on these ions. These tiny droplets appear as trails and can be observed or photographed for future study. For directions on how to build a cloud chamber and more about how they work, see the Workshop at the end of this Unit.

## Units Used to Measure Radioactivity

One of the units used to measure the amount of radioactivity is called the **curie**, in honor of Marie and Pierre Curie. A curie is the amount of a radioactive substance in which $3.7 \times 10^{10}$ disintegrations are occurring per second. Since this is a rather large number, a smaller unit called the **millicurie** (mil′ ə kū′ ri) is often used.

Another unit is used to measure the amount of radiation absorbed by living materials exposed to radiation. It is the **roentgen,** which was named after the discoverer of X rays. One roentgen is the amount of radiation that produces $1.6 \times 10^{12}$ ions when gamma radiation passes through one gram of air. The **milliroentgen** (mil′ ə rent′ gən), which is equal to $^{1}/_{1,000}$ of a roentgen, is a smaller unit used to measure the amount of radiation absorbed.

## Have You Learned?

1. Explain how Rutherford separated the radiation from radium into three parts.
2. Identify and describe some of the properties of alpha particles, beta particles, and gamma rays.
3. Name several ways that radioactivity can be detected and measured. What are two devices frequently worn by people working near radioactive materials?
4. What are the two basic units used to measure the amount of radioactivity? How do they differ?

## 3. How Radioactive Substances Decompose

**ARE YOU READY?**

Look up the following words if you are not sure of their meanings:

decompose; emission; isotope; neutron; radioactivity; valance.

By now you may be wondering what happens to a radioactive atom when it breaks down and one or more particles or rays are given off. To understand, let us first review what we know about the structure of atoms and about isotopes.

### A Review of Atomic Structure

In Chapter 5 a model of the atom was described that had a nucleus consisting of protons and neutrons with electrons traveling around the nucleus in a definite pattern. The *atomic number* of an element was defined as the number of protons in the nucleus and also is equal to the number of electrons. Since radioactivity involves changes that occur within the nucleus, we won't have to worry about these electrons circling the nucleus. Do you see how chemistry differs from nuclear science? To give you a hint, what part of the atom was studied to determine the combining power or valence of an atom?

The atomic weight of an element is equal to the number of protons plus the number of neutrons. Atoms of some elements contain varying numbers of neutrons and thus have different atomic weights. These atoms of the same element that have different atomic weights are called *isotopes.* The element carbon has three isotopes: carbon-12 (6 protons and 6 neutrons), carbon-13 (6 protons and 7 neutrons), and carbon-14 (6 protons and 8 neutrons).

Scientists have identified over 1,500 different isotopes of the 103 known elements, and about 1,200 of these are radioactive. Only about 50 of the radioactive isotopes are found in nature, and the rest have been made in the laboratory.

To see how a radioactive atom breaks down, let us use uranium-238, which is a

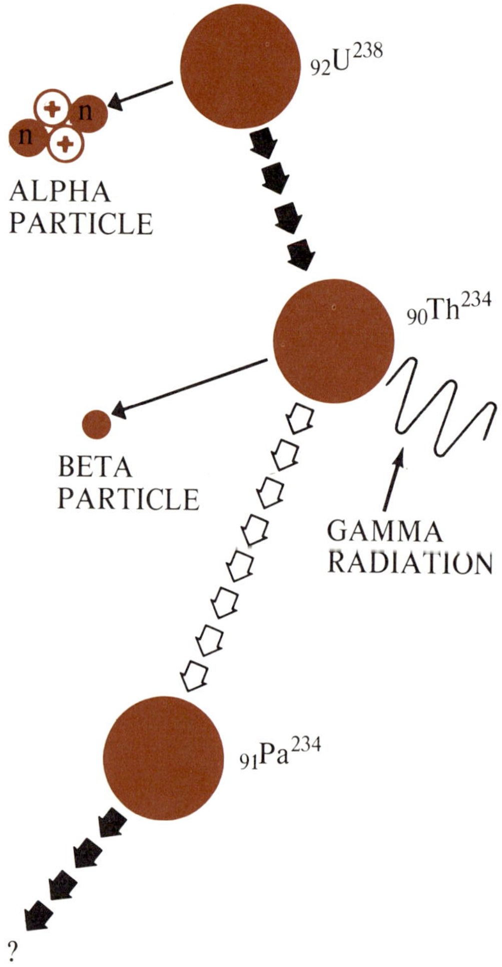


**11.7** Disintegration series

radioactive isotope of uranium found in nature. Uranium-238 breaks down in a regular series of steps that is called a **disintegration** (dis in′ tə grā′ shən) **series.** (*Disintegrate* means *to break down* or *to decompose.*)

In the first step of the series, uranium-238 gives off an alpha particle and becomes thorium-234. This can be written as an equation. A special way is used to note atomic numbers and atomic weights, or **mass numbers** as they are called when working with nuclear changes. The *mass number* is defined as the whole number nearest the actual weight of the isotope in atomic weight units. The atomic number is written below and to the left of the symbol for the element, and the mass number is written above and to the right of the symbol.

$$_{92}U^{238} \longrightarrow {}_{90}Th^{234} + {}_{2}He^{4}$$

(alpha particle)

An alpha particle is shown as helium in the equation. Remember that we are interested only in the nucleus when we are talking about radioactivity. An alpha particle is composed of two protons and two neutrons as is the nucleus of the helium atom. In the next step of the uranium-238 disintegration series, thorium-234 decomposes to form **protactinium-234** (prōt′ ak tin′ i əm) and a beta particle and gamma radiation.

$$_{90}Th^{234} \longrightarrow {}_{91}Pa^{234} + \text{Beta} + \text{Gamma}$$

Notice that the mass number remained the same but that the atomic number increased by one. This indicates that the atom of protactinium formed has one more proton than the atom of thorium that decomposed. A beta particle, which is an electron, is given off when a neutron turns into a proton and a **neutrino** (nü trē′ nō). A neutrino has no charge, as the name suggests, and zero rest mass.

The important thing to remember is that when a beta particle is given off, the number of protons in the nucleus increases by one, and the number of neutrons decreases by one. Thus the mass number, which is the sum of the number of protons and neutrons, remains unchanged. The emission of gamma radiation, which sometimes accompanies an alpha or beta particle being given off, does not affect either the atomic number or the atomic mass number.

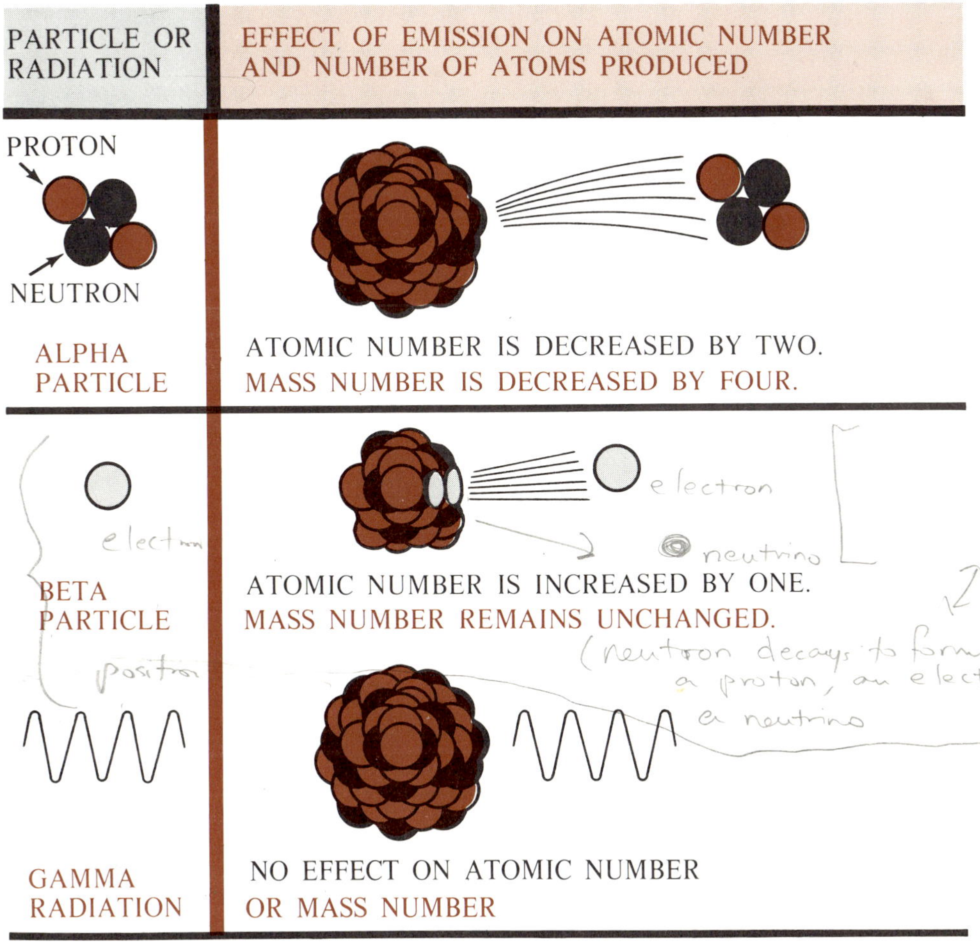


**11.8** This is another model to represent what is shown in Figure 11.7.

| *Particle or Radiation* | *Effect of Emission on Atomic Number and Mass Number of Atom Produced* |
|---|---|
| Alpha Particle | Atomic number is decreased by two and mass number decreased by four. |
| Beta Particle | Atomic number is increased by one and mass number remains unchanged. |
| Gamma Radiation | No effect |

The first two steps of the uranium-238 disintegration series have been shown in equation form. Can you write the equations for the next three steps? You probably will have to check the Periodic Table of the Elements on page 160 for the atomic numbers of the various elements. In the third step the protactinium-234 gives off a beta particle and gamma radiation. In the following step an alpha particle is given off. In the fifth step of the series, another alpha particle and gamma radiation are emitted. If you have written the equations correctly, the product of the third equation, or the fifth step, should be $_{88}Ra^{226}$. What element is this?

The disintegration of uranium-238 continues from $Ra^{226}$ through a series of nine more steps. The final product is lead-206, which is not radioactive.

**Have You Learned?**

Complete the following summary of the section by writing on a sheet of paper the word (or words) that best completes each statement.

The __(1)__ of an element indicates how many protons there are in the nucleus. The number of protons plus the number of neutrons is the atom's __(2)__. __(3)__ are atoms of the same element that have different atomic weights or masses. When __(4)__ are given off during disintegrations, the atomic number of the atoms formed is decreased by two and the mass number is decreased by four. The atomic number is increased by one and the mass number is unchanged when __(5)__ are emitted. The emission of __(6)__ has no effect on the atomic number and mass number. A __(7)__ is a particle with no charge and zero rest mass that is formed when a beta particle is emitted. The regular series of steps involved in the breakdown of an isotope such as uranium-238 is called a __(8)__. The last isotope formed in the $U^{238}$ series is __(9)__.

## 4. The Rate of Radioactive Decomposition

**ARE YOU READY?**

Look up the following words if you are not sure of their meanings:

decompose; disintegrate; disintegration series; isotope; photosynthesis; radioactive decay.

It is not possible to say when a certain atom of a radioactive substance, such as thorium-234, will decompose and give off radiation. This would be like trying to predict when a certain kernel of popcorn in a hot skillet was going to explode. We can, however, make some fairly accurate predictions about how long it will take for 50 percent of the kernels in a cup of popcorn to pop. Likewise, scientists have learned how to predict how long it will take for one half of a large number of atoms of a radioactive isotope to decompose.

Thorium-234 is the first product formed in the uranium-238 disintegration series. It takes about 24 days for half of one gram of thorium-234 to change to protactinium-234. The length of time it takes for half of a radioactive isotope to decompose is called its **half-life.** Would the remaining

**11.9** Try to interepret this half-life curve of thorium.

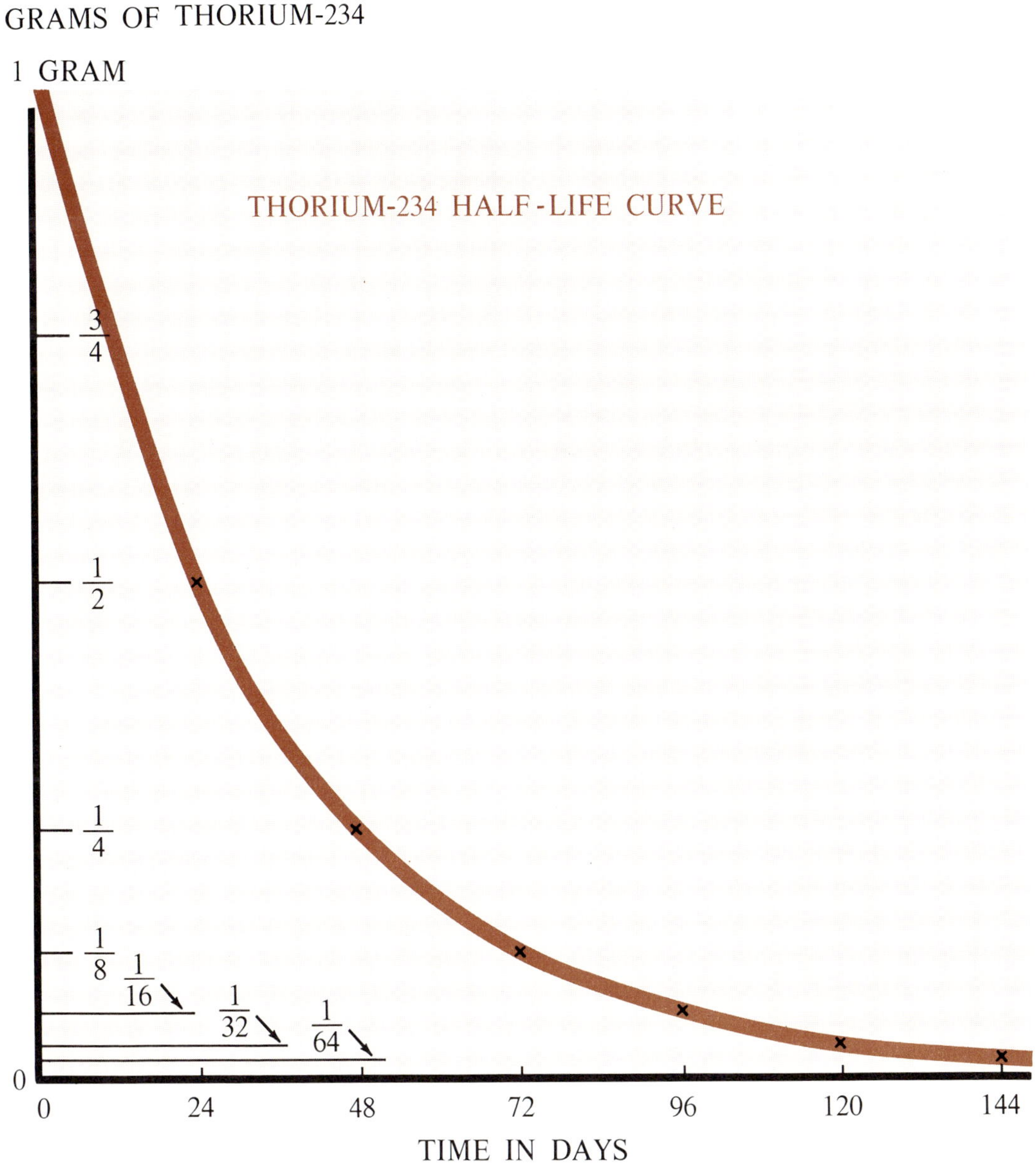

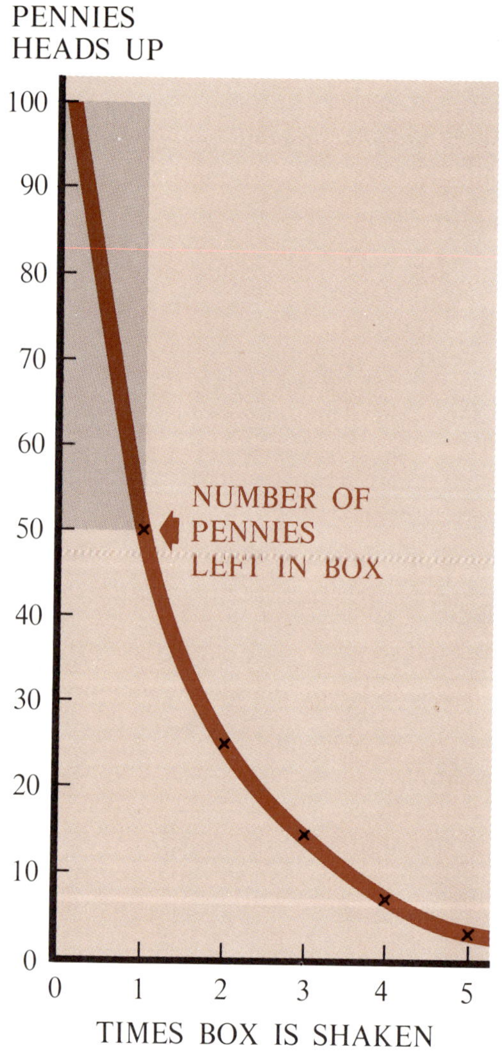


**11.10** Heads up versus number of times shaken

thorium-234 decompose during the next twenty-four days? No, only one half of the remaining one half, or one fourth, of the thorium-234 would decompose during the second 24-day period. How much do you think would decompose during the third 24-day period? The fourth 24-day period? How long do you think it would take for all of the thorium-234 to decompose?

The half-life of a radioactive isotope can be plotted on a graph. Figure 11.8 shows the half-life curve for thorium-234. The amount of radioactive thorium-234 is shown on the vertical axis and the time in days on the horizontal axis. Can you use the graph to answer the above questions about how much thorium-234 would decompose during the third and fourth 24-day periods?

### Plotting a Half-life Graph

Place 100 pennies "heads up" in a shoe box. Shake the box in all directions for a few seconds. Remove the pennies that have turned tails up, and record the number of pennies remaining in the box. Think of the pennies that are heads up as being radioactive atoms and those that have turned tails up as products of radioactive atoms that have decomposed.

Shake the box again for a few seconds and again remove the pennies that have turned tails up. Record the number remaining. Continue shaking the box and removing pennies that turn tails up until all the pennies have been removed.

Plot your results on a graph like the one in Figure 11.10. The dark line is the expected results for the first five tries. Does the line you have drawn vary from the dark line representing the expected results? If so, how do you explain this? Can you explain how the line on the graph is like the line on a graph representing the half-life of a radioactive element?

The half-life of different isotopes varies

from very long periods of time to periods only a small fraction of a second long. The half-life of several isotopes is given in Table I.

TABLE I

| *Isotope* | *Half-life* |
|---|---|
| Uranium-238 | $4.5 \times 10^9$ years |
| Uranium-234 | $2.5 \times 10^5$ years |
| Carbon-14 | 5,760 years |
| Radium-226 | 1,622 years |
| Radon-222 | 3.8 days |
| Bismuth-214 | 19.7 minutes |
| Polonium-214 | $1.6 \times 10^{-4}$ seconds |

## Using Half-life to Determine Age

The atmosphere of the earth contains very small amounts of carbon dioxide made up of carbon-14. Carbon-14 is a radioactive isotope that has a half-life of 5,760 years. Although some of the $C^{14}$ in the atmosphere is decomposing, the total amount of $C^{14}$ remains about the same. This is because nitrogen atoms are continually being bombarded by radiation from outer space and changed to $C^{14}$ atoms.

Plants take in $CO_2$ during photosynthesis, and thus a living plant also contains about the same amount of $C^{14}$ as the atmosphere. Animals eat plants or other animals, and thus they, too, contain about the same amount of $C^{14}$ as plants and the atmosphere.

When a plant or animal dies, it no longer takes in carbon, and the amount of $C^{14}$ it contains begins to decrease because of radioactive decay. At the end of 5,760 years, the organism would contain only about one-half as much $C^{14}$ as when it was alive. If the remains of an organism contains only one-fourth as much $C^{14}$ as living things do, one would suspect that they were about 11,520 ($5{,}760 \times 2$) years old. Do you see why?

This method of determining the age of the remains of once living things, such as a mummy or a piece of wood, is called **carbon dating.** This method can be used to determine the age of the remains of living things up to about 46,000 years. In material older than that, so much of the $C^{14}$ has disintegrated that it is not possible to make accurate estimates.

The presence of uranium-238 and lead-206 in rocks is used to predict the age of the rocks. Earlier it was explained that $U^{238}$ disintegrates through a series of steps to $Pb^{206}$. The time it takes for this to happen is known, and since the half-life of $U^{238}$ is so long (4.5 billion years), this is a slow process. The older the rock, the more of the $U^{238}$ one would expect to have been converted to $Pb^{206}$. Some rocks found in Canada and Africa have been dated using this method and are believed to be about $3.3 \times 10^9$ (3.3 billion) years old!

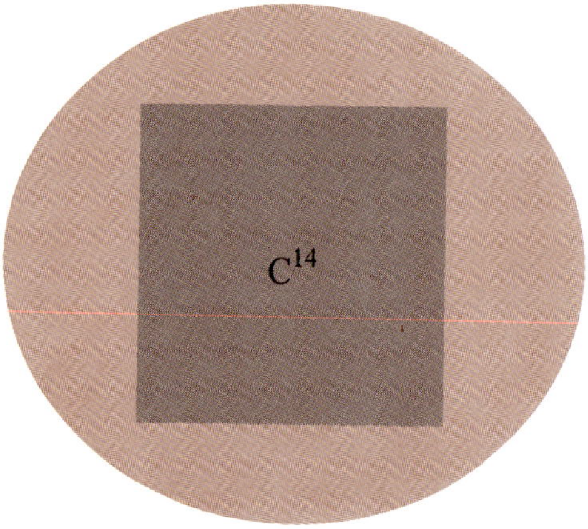


DEAD ORGANISM FIRST DAY

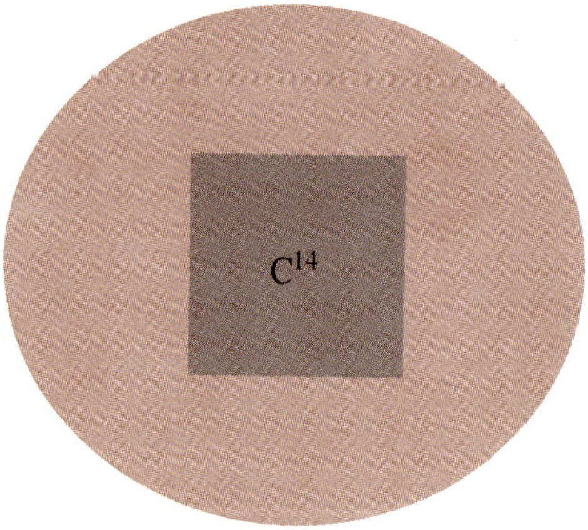


AFTER 5,760 YEARS

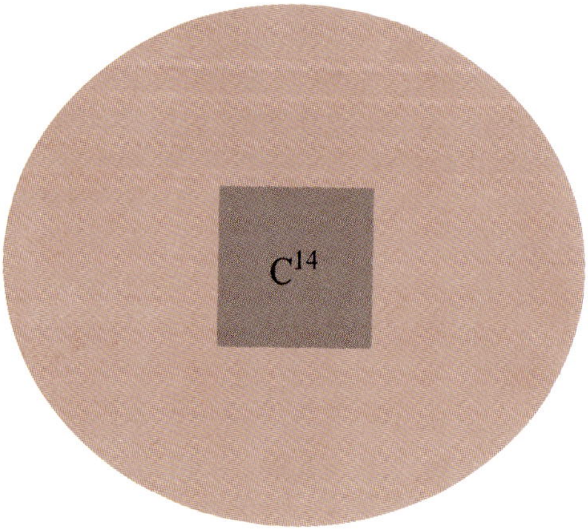


AFTER 11,520 YEARS

**11.11** Carbon dating

## Have You Learned?

1. Assume that you have 1,000 grams of a radioactive isotope that has a half-life of 6 days.
   (a) How much of the material would you expect to be still radioactive at the end of 6 days?
   (b) At the end of 12 days?
   (c) How long would you predict it would take for all but 1/16 of the material to lose its radioactivity?
   (d) How long do you think it would take for all of the material to lose its radioactivity? Explain your answer.
2. Explain how the age of an object can be determined by carbon dating. Can the age of any object be determined? How old would you predict an object to be if it had only 1/8 as much carbon-14 as is found in the atmosphere and in living things?

## 5. Bombarding the Nucleus

**ARE YOU READY?**

Look up the following words if you are not sure of their meanings:

alchemist; alpha particle; bombard; positron.

After Rutherford had discovered that radium gives off three kinds of radiation, he experimented with the effects of radiation on substances. In one series of experiments, he noticed that when particles pass through a thin metal sheet, the spot formed on a photographic film was fuzzy.

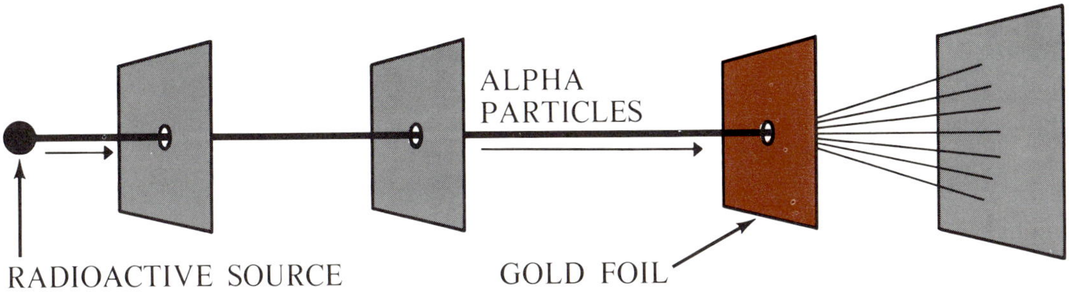


**11.12** Rutherford's experiment

It appeared that some of the particles had been slightly deflected, or pushed to one side, as they passed the metal sheet.

Further experiments showed that when a thin sheet of gold foil was bombarded, most of the alpha particles went right through the metal. However, some of the particles were deflected, and a few were reflected almost back on their original source. In Rutherford's own words, "It was almost as incredible as if you fired a 15-inch shell at a piece of tissue paper and it came back and hit you."

The results of the experiment indicated that atoms are mainly empty space with a very compact nucleus in the center. This would explain why most of the alpha particles passed through the gold foil. In a positively-charged nucleus, the alpha particle would be reflected backward just as a ball bounces off a wall. Alpha particles passing near the nucleus would be deflected because bodies having like charges repel each other.

## Bombarding the Nuclei of Atoms

This way of studying atoms has been described as shooting buckshot into a chicken house and observing what flies out. In 1919 Rutherford bombarded nitrogen atoms with alpha particles. He found that some of the alpha particles were absorbed by the nitrogen and oxygen and protons were formed.

$$_{2}He^{4} + {_{7}N^{14}} \longrightarrow {_{1}H^{1}} + {_{8}O^{17}}$$

alpha particle   nitrogen   proton   oxygen

Rutherford had accomplished what the alchemists had dreamed of but had failed to do. He had managed to change one element to another. The process in which one element is changed to another is called **transmutation** (trans′ mū tā′ shən). Knowledge of how to bring about transmutation was used to make several important discoveries following Rutherford's bombardment of nitrogen with alpha particles.

Scientists found that when lightweight elements were bombarded with alpha particles, a radiation was produced that had much greater penetrating power than alpha particles. This lead to the discovery of the neutron. The following equation shows how neutrons and carbon atoms are formed when **beryllium** (bə ril′ i əm) is bombarded with alpha particles.

$$_{2}He^{4} + {_{4}Be^{9}} \longrightarrow {_{6}C^{12}} + {_{0}n^{1}}$$

alpha particle   beryllium   carbon   neutron

In 1934 the husband-wife team of Frédéric Joliot and Irène Curie bombarded magnesium with alpha particles. When they removed the source of alpha particles, they found that something in the magnesium continued to give off radiation. The following equation shows what happened.

$$_{2}He^{4} + {}_{12}Mg^{24} \longrightarrow {}_{14}Si^{27} + {}_{0}n^{1}$$

alpha particle, magnesium, silicon, neutron

Some of the alpha particles were captured by magnesium atoms, and silicon atoms were formed and neutrons emitted. Silicon-27, however, is a radioactive isotope and decomposes to form aluminum and positrons.

$$_{14}Si^{27} \longrightarrow {}_{13}Al^{27} + \text{positron}$$

The Nobel Prize in Chemistry was given in 1935 to the Joliots for their discovery of a way to make elements radioactive. Scientists have since made all the elements radioactive. These radioactive isotopes are called **radioisotopes** (rā′ di ō ī′ sə tōp) and many of the ways they are used are described in the next section.

## Machines for Bombarding the Atom

The early experimenters used alpha particles from a radioactive source to bombard the material being studied. These alpha particles were rather slow-moving compared to other particles. What was needed was a way to bombard targets with faster-moving particles.

Ernest Lawrence, an American scientist, invented a way to speed up protons. He used electromagnets to make protons travel in circles and each time around the protons were made to go faster. They then were allowed to shoot out of the machine and strike a target. Lawrence called the machine a **cyclotron** (sī′ klə tron), since it made the particles move in circular paths while they were being speeded up.

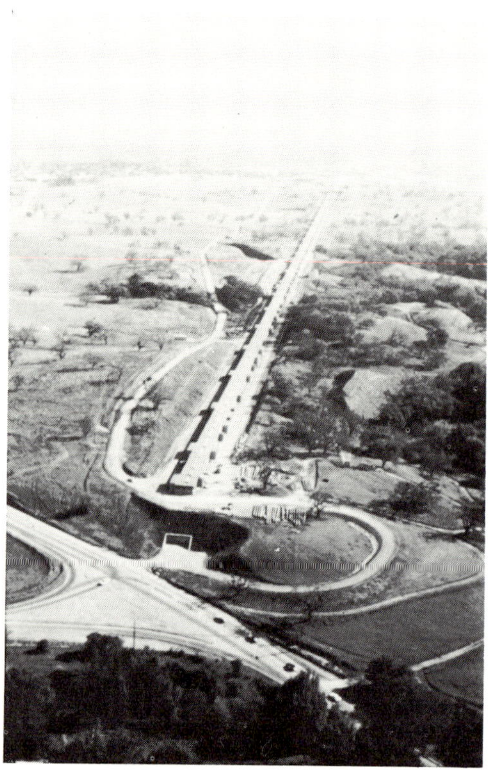

*Stanford University*

**11.13** Linear accelerator at Stanford University

Other **particle accelerators** (ak sel′ ər ā′ tər), or "atom-smashers" as they sometimes are called, have been developed since the invention of the cyclotron. The **betatron** (bā′ tə tron′) is used to accelerate electrons. The **synchrotron** (sing′ krə tron′) accelerates atomic particles to speeds approaching the speed of light. In a synchrotron at the Brookhaven National Laboratory on Long Island, protons travel in circular orbits for distances of about a

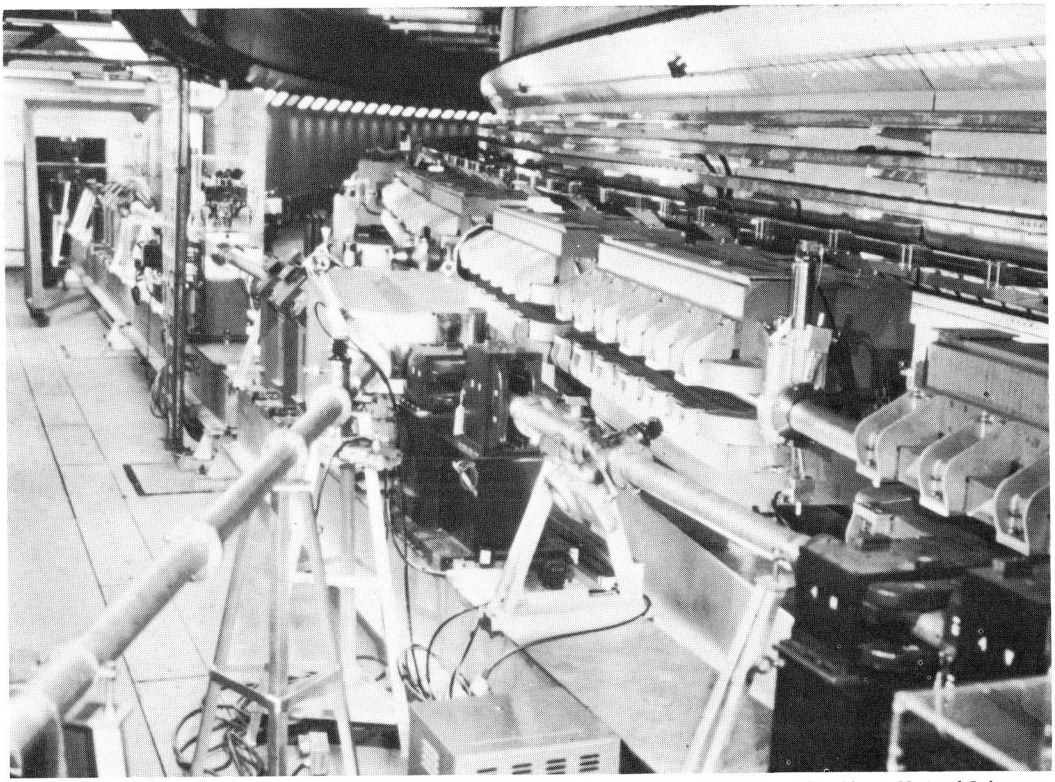

*Brookhaven National Laboratory*

**11.14** Part of the 800–meter–circumference ring of the alternating-gradient synchrotron at Upton, New York. Why do atomic particles have to be speeded up?

quarter of a million miles before they reach these fantastic speeds (see above).

## Man-made Elements

The development of the Periodic Chart of the Elements was described in Chapter 5. Several of the spaces in the chart remained vacant until scientists used particle accelerators such as the cyclotron to bombard other elements. The elements having atomic numbers 43, 61, 85, and 87 were made in this way. They are still classified as natural elements even though they have not been identified in nature.

Elements having atomic numbers larger than 92 also have been made by bombarding other elements. These elements are all radioactive and decompose to form one of the 92 natural elements. Three of the elements, **Berkelium** (bėr kē′ li əm), **Californium** (kal′ ə fôr′ ni əm), and **Lawrencium** (lô ren′ sē əm), were named in honor of Ernest Lawrence and the University of California at Berkeley where much of this research was done. Glen Seaborg, a scientist at Berkeley, shared the Nobel Prize in Chemistry in 1951 for the discovery of plutonium and his work in making several of the other man-made elements.

## Have You Learned?

Match the definitions in Column A with the names and terms in Column B. (Do not write in your book.)

| *Column A* | *Column B* |
|---|---|
| 1. Invented the cyclotron | a. betatron |
| 2. First particle accelerator | b. cyclotron |
| 3. Discovered way to make radioisotopes | c. Joliot and Curie |
| 4. Did experiments that lead to discovery of the nucleus of the atom | d. Lawrence |
| 5. Honored for working in making man-made elements | e. Rutherford |
| 6. Accelerates protons to speeds near that of light | f. Seaborg |
| 7. First to demonstrate transmutation | g. synchrotron |
| 8. Accelerates electrons | |

**11.15** Coleus is a useful plant for studying the movement of tracer radioisotopes in a plant.

*David Greene*

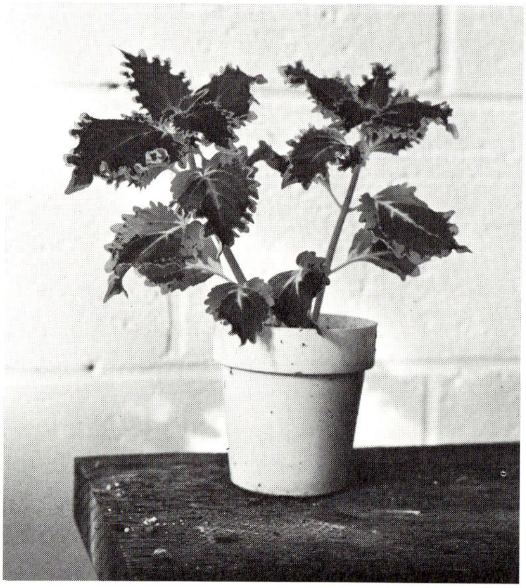

# 6. Uses of Radioisotopes

**ARE YOU READY?**

Look up the following words if you are not sure of their meanings:

cancer; glucose; photosynthesis; radioisotope.

Radioisotopes have been described as one of the most important research tools that scientists have obtained during this century. Several of the ways they have been used are described in the section that follows.

## Tracers

An atom of a radioisotope is the same as other atoms of an element except in two ways. First, the radioisotope contains fewer or more neutrons and thus has a different atomic weight. Second, since it is radioactive, it decomposes and gives off radiation in the process. An important way that radioisotopes and other isotopes of the elements are alike is that all of the atoms of an element act the same way during a chemical reaction. It doesn't make any difference if some atoms are radioactive or if some weigh more than others.

Because radioisotopes behave the same way as other atoms but give off radiation, they can be used to trace what happens during a chemical reaction. This can be illustrated by the process—photosynthesis—used by green plants to make food, which was described in Chapter 7. The general equation for the reaction that takes place in photosynthesis is

$$6\ CO_2 + 6\ H_2O \xrightarrow[\text{Chlorophyll}]{\text{Sunlight}} C_6H_{12}O_6 + 6\ O_2$$

Looking at the equation you might get the idea that the process is a fairly simple chemical reaction. Using radioisotopes, however, scientists have discovered that many, many reactions take place before glucose is formed. For example in some experiments plants were placed in carbon dioxide containing radioactive carbon-14. Once some of the carbon-14 has been absorbed into the plant, the chemicals in the plant containing the carbon-14 are relatively easy to identify. Using the knowledge of what chemicals are formed, scientists have been able to piece together a picture of the series of reactions making up photosynthesis.

Radioisotopes, or "tagged atoms" as they sometimes are called, have been used to trace the movement of atoms through animals. For example, when food containing a radioisotope of iodine, $I^{131}$, is eaten, it has been found that most of it will move to the **thyroid** (thī′ roid) gland in the neck after a short period of time. Careful measurements of the amount of $I^{131}$ that accumulates in the thyroid gland can be used to determine how healthy it is. Tagged atoms also have been used to determine the life span of different kinds of cells. Human red blood cells, labeled with atoms of radioactive iron-59, were found to have an average life span of about 120 days.

Extensive use has been made of radioisotopes in investigating how plants use the various elements in fertilizer. Researchers have found that tobacco plants do not use phosphate fertilizers put on the surface of the soil during the growing season. Other investigators found that crops grown in rows produce more when phosphorus fertilizer is placed *in* the ground near the seeds instead of being spread *on* the ground. Other experimenters have shown that some plants, such as fruit trees and pineapples, can absorb fertilizer faster when it is sprayed on their leaves instead of being placed on the ground. With this new knowledge, farmers are able to produce more food with less expense.

## Using a Radioisotope as a Tracer

A radioisotope, phosphorus-32, can be used to trace the movement of phosphorus through a plant. $P^{32}$ is safe to handle in small amounts and can be obtained from scientific supply houses without any special permits. Since it has a rather short half-life of 14.3 days, it should be used as soon as it arrives.

Place at least two cuttings of a plant such as a **coleus** (kō′ lē əs) in a beaker containing a solution of $P^{32}$. If a Geiger counter is available, use it to see if you can detect when the $P^{32}$ reaches the leaves. You may wish to use some of the $P^{32}$ solution to water a coleus potted in soil. Does the $P^{32}$ reach the leaves faster in the case of the cuttings or the potted plant? (See Figure 11.15.)

After the cuttings have been in the $P^{32}$ solution for 48 hours, remove 2 of the leaves. Place these, in the dark, on pieces of unexposed X-ray or black-and-white photographic film. Develop one piece of the film after 24 hours and the other after 48 hours.

Remove 2 more leaves after the cuttings have been in the $P^{32}$ solution for 96 hours. Expose these leaves to film, one for 24 hours and the other for 48 hours. The pictures that are made this way are called **radioautographs** (rā′ di ō ô′ tə graf′). Look at the word and see if you can explain what each part means. From the results of your investigations, how long should the cuttings be left in the $P^{32}$ solution, and how long should the film be exposed to get the best radioautographs?

## Other Uses of Radioisotopes

The harmful effects of too much radiation have already been pointed out. Excessive amounts of radiation cause cancer and change the characteristics of an organism's offspring. Strange as it may seem, small amounts of radiation can be used to treat cancer. In the case of cancer of the thyroid gland, radioactive iodine is placed in the body. Tracer experiments have shown that most of the radioactive iodine is soon concentrated in the thyroid gland. The gamma rays given off by the radioactive iodine kill the cancer cells but do not harm

**11.16** A radioactive tracer was first injected into the patient. This tracer gradually reached the kidneys of the patient. The radioactive tracer gives off low-energy gamma rays, which are detected by the instrument above the patient. The instrument beside the patient changes the gamma-ray signals into a kind of picture of the kidney. Doctors then study the picture to understand the condition of the kidney.

*Brookhaven National Laboratory*

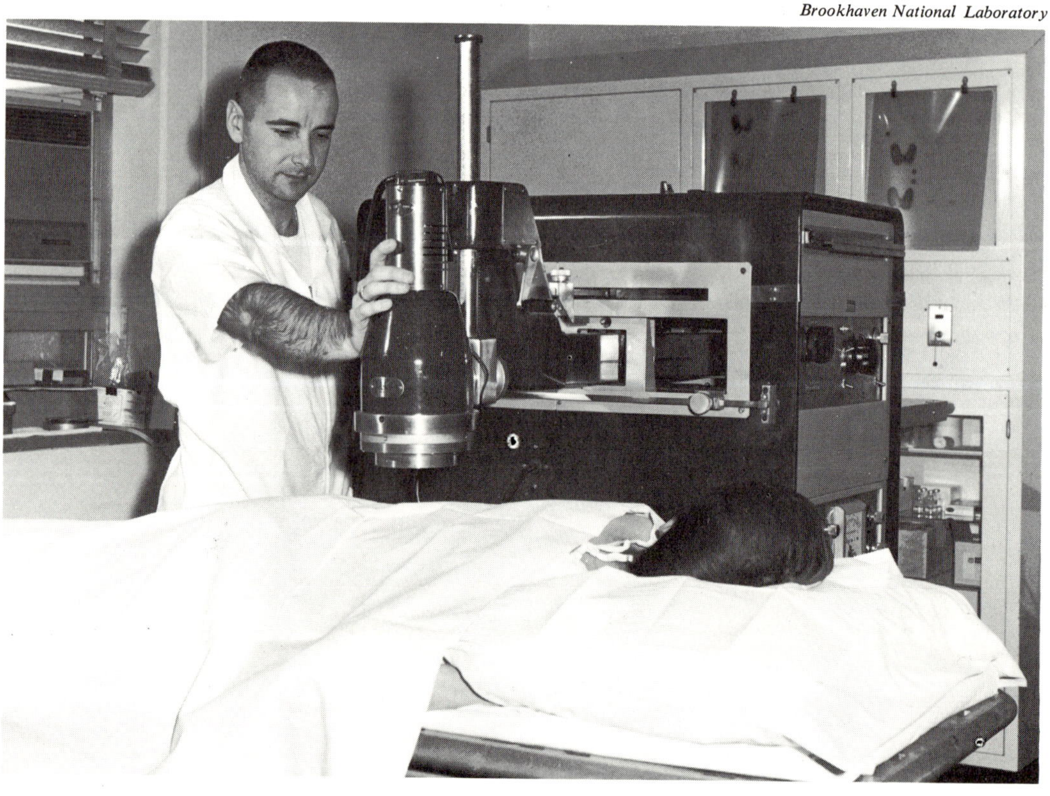

the healthy ones. In like manner, radioactive phosphorus moves to the bones and can be used to radiate the material inside the bones.

## Observing the Effects of Radiation on Seeds

Seeds which have been exposed to various amounts of radiation are available from several scientific supply houses and seed companies. They usually have been exposed to gamma radiation given off by cobalt-60. Plant some of these seeds and when plants come up, observe how the plants are different from plants grown from seeds that have not been exposed to radiation. Check characteristics such as size, leaf color, flower color, etc.

Industry uses radioisotopes in many ways. Radioisotopes placed in floor wax and in the rubber of tires are used to measure how these materials wear. Radiations from radioisotopes are used to measure the thickness of materials such as paper or metal as they roll by at speeds of several miles per hour. A piece of radioactive cobalt the size of a pebble can replace an X-ray machine weighing several hundred pounds in finding the flaw in a piece of metal. A small amount of radioactive material is placed in gas or oil being pumped through pipelines and used to find the leaks.

These are just a few of the many ways radioisotopes are used. What is amazing is that these applications have been developed in this century and most of them are products of the last twenty-five years.

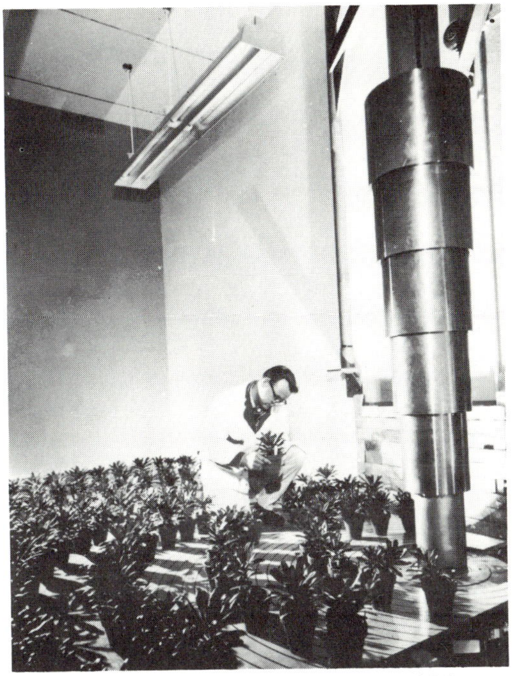

*Brookhaven National Laboratory*

**11.17** Simulation of the effects of fallout on plants.

### Have You Learned?

On a sheet of paper list the numbers for the questions below. By each number write *T* if the statement is true and *F* if false.

1. Since radioisotopes are either heavier or lighter than other isotopes of an element, they act differently in chemical reactions from isotopes that are not radioactive.
2. Radioactive carbon-14 was used to investigate the series of reactions involved in photosynthesis.
3. Radioisotopes are used to treat cancer.
4. Radiation from radioisotopes can cause cancer.
5. The characteristics of an offspring are never affected by a parent's being exposed to radiation.

## REVIEW QUESTIONS

1. Describe the work of Becquerel and Pierre and Marie Curie.
2. What is the Nobel Prize? Name some scientists who have received the Nobel Prize, and describe the contributions of each.
3. What are the three kinds of radiation discovered by Rutherford that are given off by radium? What are some of the characteristics of each of the different kinds of radiation?
4. Name at least four devices that are used to detect radiation, and explain how each works.
5. Explain what happens to the atomic number and mass number of an atom when an alpha particle is given off; when a beta particle is given off; when gamma rays are given off.
6. What is the half-life of a radioisotope? How is the half-life of $C^{14}$ used to determine the age of once living things?
7. Name at least three things that were discovered by bombarding atoms with alpha particles.
8. Tell how radioisotopes are used as tracers and in other ways.

## CAN YOU FIND OUT?

*It may be necessary to use encyclopedias or other reference books in answering the following questions.*

1. What methods and instruments are used in prospecting for ores containing radioactive elements? From what parts of the world are radioactive ores now obtained?
2. Explore how particle accelerators work and the kinds of experiments that are done with them. What is a betatron? a cosmotron?
3. Investigate how radioisotopes are made, include their manufacture in atomic reactors.
4. Find out as many ways as you can that radioisotopes have been used in a certain field such as medicine or agriculture.
5. Read about how the elements with atomic numbers larger than 92 have been made.

## REFERENCES FOR ADDITIONAL STUDY

ATOMIC RADIATION AND LIFE by Peter Alexander. Penguin Books, Inc.
Describes the effects of radiation on living things such as hereditary changes and cancer, and uses of radiation in working with living things

BREAKTHROUGHS IN SCIENCE by Isaac Asimov. Scholastic Book Services.
Describes twenty-six far-reaching discoveries made by twenty-nine scientists, including the contributions of Roentgen, Becquerel, the Curies, Einstein, Rutherford, and Lawrence

INSIDE THE ATOM (Second Edition) by Isaac Asimov. Abelard-Schuman Limited.
Discusses many aspects of atomic energy —isotopes, radioactivity, particles, and future uses of atomic energy

MADAME CURIE by Eve Curie. Doubleday & Company, Inc.
A biography, by her daughter, of one of the most famous women of science

RADIOISOTOPES by John Woodburn. J. B. Lippincott Company.
Discusses many uses of radioisotopes, including applications in determining the age of objects and in medicine, farming, industry, and research

CHAPTER **12**

# Fission and Fusion

THE TWENTIETH CENTURY is often called the Atomic Age. Most of what we know about the atom has been discovered since 1900, and harnessing the energy of the atom was accomplished during the second half of this century. Atomic energy is used to generate electricity, power ships and submarines, and research is underway to develop atomic power for automobiles, airplanes, and space vehicles. As you know there is another side to the story of atomic energy, because the development of the atomic bomb came before many of these peaceful uses of atomic energy.

## 1. Releasing the Energy of the Atom

> **ARE YOU READY?**
>
> Look up the following words if you are not sure of their meanings:
>
> alpha particle; bombard; convert; energy; Law of Conservation of Energy; Law of Conservation of Matter; mass; matter; nuclei.

Earlier in this book you read about the Law of Conservation of Energy and the Law of Conservation of Matter. These laws state that neither matter nor energy can be created or destroyed. For example, more energy cannot be obtained from a machine than is put in. On the other hand, when less energy is obtained than was put in, heat or light produced by friction accounts for the difference. In chemical reactions, the number of atoms of an element on one side of the equation must equal the number of atoms of the element on the other side of the equation. Can you explain how this is an example of the Law of Conservation of Matter?

In 1905 Albert Einstein (al′ bert īn′ stīn) proposed that matter and energy are really different forms of the same thing. He believed that it might be possible to change matter to energy and energy to matter. Furthermore, he developed an equation, $E = mc^2$, to show how much energy could be obtained by converting matter to energy.

If Einstein was right, it meant revising the Law of Conservation of Energy and the Law of Conservation of Matter to say that the total amount of matter and energy in the universe cannot be changed. In other words, if energy is increased, mass is decreased, and vice versa.

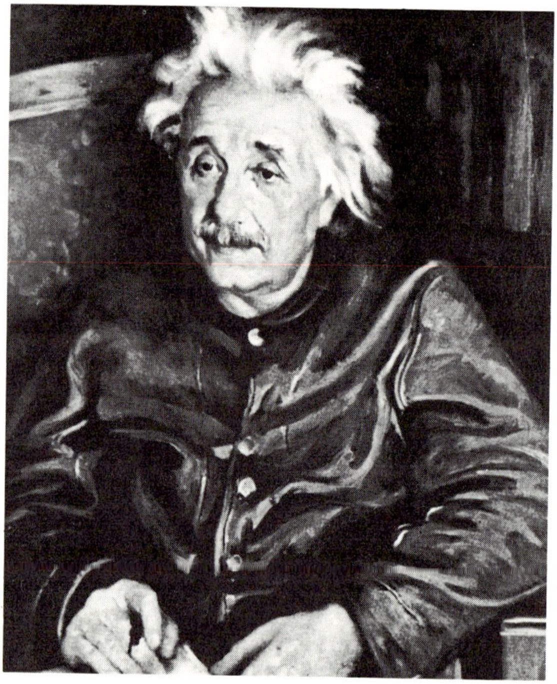

**12.1** Albert Einstein, painted for *Time* by S. J. Woolf

*Historical Pictures Service—Chicago*

ALBERT EINSTEIN—1879-1955

A few years ago a building was being constructed in New York City. On the walls of this building the builder wished to place statues of the scientists who had done the most to change our way of life. In order to determine who were the most famous scientists of all time, he sent a letter to a group of this country's best-known scientists and asked them to send nominations for this honor. Each of the lists varied, but on *every* list was Albert Einstein. Of the fourteen geniuses of science who were finally selected, Einstein is the only one who lived during this century.

He was born in Germany in 1879, but he was educated primarily in Switzerland. After completing his undergraduate college work in 1900, he worked at the Swiss Patent Office and, in his spare time, wrote four of the most important scientific papers in history. One of these was the first statement of his Special Theory of Relativity.

Because Einstein worked entirely with higher mathematics and the logic of a great mind, it is difficult for us to understand all of the details of his theories. In his first relativity theory, written in 1905, he suggested that light waves and other similar forms of energy *always* travel at the same speed, regardless of the speed of their source or the speed of the person observing them. In other words, whether we travel *toward* the sun or *away* from it, our measurement of the speed of light will be the same. Basing his theories on this idea, Einstein suggested that many surprising observations of rapidly moving objects could be made. You may enjoy reading about these in an encyclopedia or some other reference book.

After he published these papers, Einstein was recognized as a great scientist and, at the age of 30, he returned to Germany as a professor of physics. There he continued to work on his theories, and in 1916 he published the General Theory of Relativity. In this paper, he suggested that the old ideas about gravity were not quite accurate. Several experiments have shown that his ideas are probably correct.

In 1932 Einstein left Germany and eventually settled in the United States. He became a citizen in 1940. Here he lived in Princeton, New Jersey, and continued to work on theories of the nature of magnetism and gravitation until his death in 1955.

In Einstein's now-famous equation, $E$ represents energy in **ergs** (ėrg), $m$ is mass in grams, and $c$ is the speed of light in centimeters per second. To show how this equation works, let us calculate the amount of energy that could be produced by converting 1 gram of matter to energy. Remember that a gram is a small amount of matter—a dime weighs about 2.5 grams.

$$E = mc^2$$
$$E = (1)(3 \times 10^{10})(3 \times 10^{10})$$
$$E = 9 \times 10^{20}$$
*or* 900,000,000,000,000,000,000 ergs

The erg is a very small amount of energy, equal to about the amount of energy required to lift a postage stamp the distance equal to the thickness of five sheets of paper. However, $9 \times 10^{20}$ is a very large number. Expressed in calories, 1 gram of matter converted to energy would produce $2 \times 10^{13}$ calories. This is about the amount of energy produced by burning *3,000 tons of coal!* As you can see, a small amount of matter could be converted to a tremendously large amount of energy.

## Experimental Work

As is often the case in science, a new theory suggests a great deal of experimental work. Although Einstein had proposed his theory of how matter and energy were related in 1905, no one was able at that time to convert matter to energy in the laboratory. It wasn't until 1932 that the first experimental evidence was obtained that indicated that matter could be converted to energy.

Cockcroft (kok′ krôft) and Walton (wôl′ tən), two British scientists working in Rutherford's laboratory, bombarded lithium with fast-moving protons to form

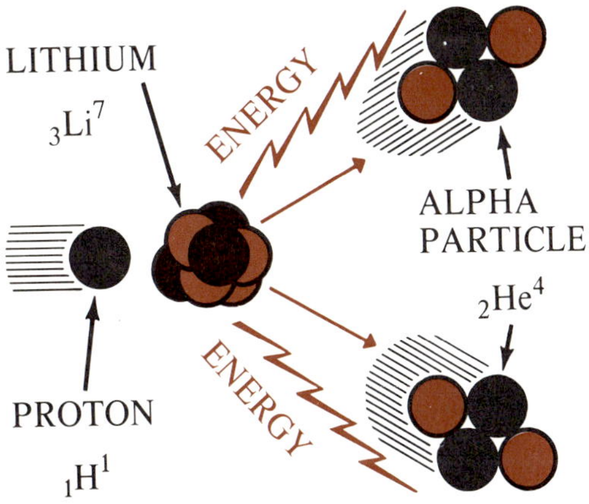


**12.2** Lithium bombarded with protons

alpha particles. The alpha particles were found to have energies about 100 times greater than was expected. Where did this energy come from?

Cockcroft and Walton compared the mass of the lithium atom plus the mass of the proton with the mass of the two alpha particles produced. They found that the alpha particles had slightly less mass than the combined masses of the lithium atom and the proton. They used Einstein's equation, $E = mc^2$, and found that the very small amount of mass lost would produce enough energy to accelerate the alpha particles to the speeds at which they had been observed. Thus we had the first experimental evidence that mass could be converted to energy (Figure 12.2).

In 1939, Hahn (hän) and Strassmann (shträs′ män) bombarded uranium-235 with neutrons. They were repeating an experiment that Fermi (fer′ mi) of Italy had done a few years earlier. Fermi had learned that neutrons could be slowed down by passing them through paraffin. The slow neutrons were absorbed better by the nuclei of $U^{235}$ atoms than were neutrons moving at faster speeds. Can you suggest why this might be so? Fermi con-

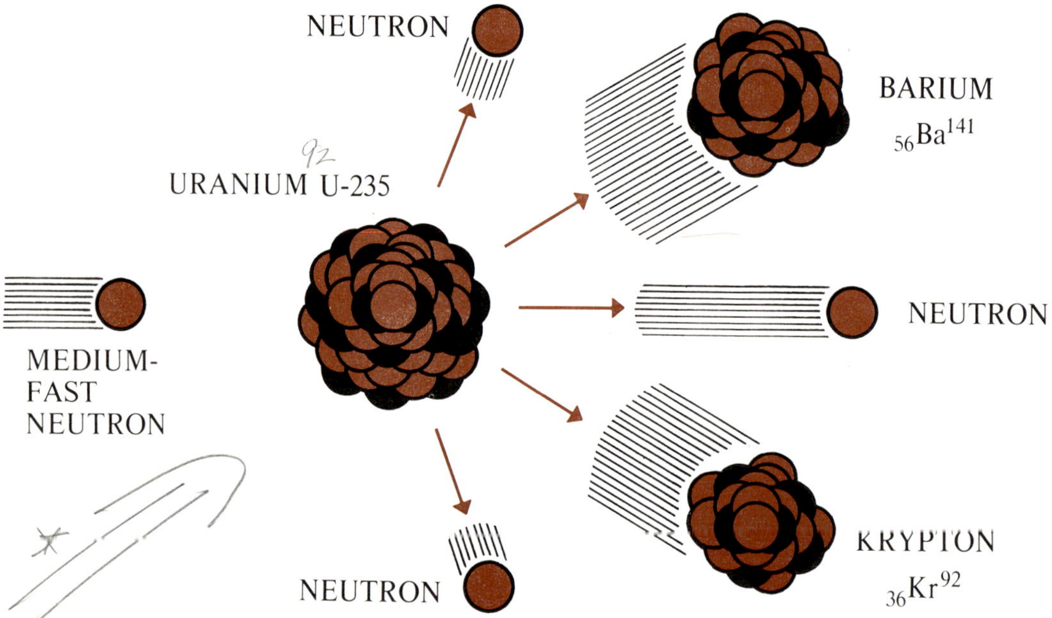


**12.3** A neutron at the left bombards an atom of uranium-235. What happens?

cluded incorrectly that the element having an atomic number of 93 was formed. (See Figure 12.3.)

When Hahn and Strassmann repeated Fermi's experiment, they found that $U^{235}$ bombarded with neutrons produced atoms of **krypton** (krip′ ton) and **barium** (bãr′ i əm) plus a great deal of energy. Not certain as to what had happened, they published the results of their experiment without an explanation. It was Meitner (mīt′ nər), a famous woman scientist, and her nephew, Frisch (frish), who suggested that the uranium atom splits apart to form two lighter atoms. They named this process **fission** (fish′ ən), because they thought it was like the way that cells in a living organism divide. Frisch has written an interesting book about this discovery and some of the work that followed. It is listed in the *References for Additional Study* at the end of this chapter.

## Have You Learned?

1. State the famous equation developed by Einstein. Explain what each letter represents and how the Law of Conservation of Energy and the Law of Conservation of Matter had to be revised as a result of Einstein's ideas and the experimental work that followed.

2. Who was the first to show that mass can be changed to energy? Describe the experiment that was done to show this.

3. Describe the contributions of each of the following scientists:

   a. Fermi
   b. Hahn
   c. Strassmann
   d. Meitner
   e. Frisch

## 2. Finding Out More About Fission

> **ARE YOU READY?**
>
> Look up the following words if you are not sure of their meanings:
>
> disintegrate; fission; graphite.

Shortly after the discovery of fission, a group of scientists suggested that when neutrons cause $U^{235}$ atoms to split to form barium and krypton, perhaps one or more neutrons are also given off. If this were the case, these neutrons could cause more $U^{235}$ atoms to split. This would then produce more neutrons that would cause more $U^{235}$ atoms to split, and so on.

It would be necessary for each fission of a $U^{235}$ atom to produce more than one neutron if a **chain reaction** was to take place. To understand why this is so, imagine several stick matches stuck in a piece of clay about 2 centimeters apart and arranged in a row. If the match at one end is lighted, it lights the next match which lights the next match and so on. This would be like a $U^{235}$ atom giving off one neutron when it splits, and the neutron striking another $U^{235}$ atom, causing it to split and so on. Since some of the neutrons probably would not be absorbed, each fission of a $U^{235}$ atom would have to produce more than one neutron in order to keep the chain reaction going.

Additional research soon revealed that the fission of $U^{235}$ produced on the average about 2.5 neutrons. Thus the possibility of a chain reaction's taking place looked good. Remember that scientists already knew that each fission of a $U^{235}$ atom produced a great deal of energy. In a chain reaction, millions of atoms of $U^{235}$ would split in less than a second, and an almost unbelievable amount of energy would be produced.

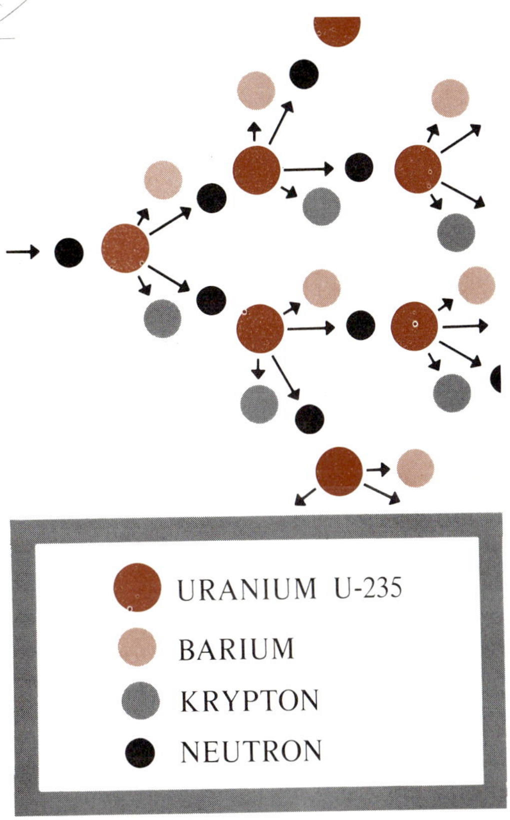


**12.4** Chain reaction

### Demonstrating a Chain Reaction

Place a row of stick matches about one centimeter apart in a piece of clay or in holes drilled in a board. Light the match at one end, and time how long it takes the flame to reach the match at the other end.

Arrange another group of matches as shown in Figure 12.5 on page 380.

Light the match in the middle, and time how long it takes for the flame to reach all

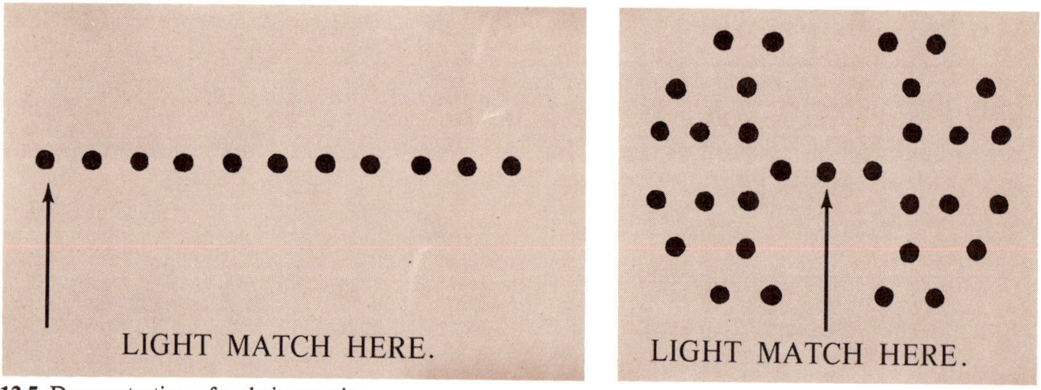


**12.5** Demonstration of a chain reaction

of the matches. (**CAUTION: Hold in a pair of long-handled tongs the match being used to light the middle match.**) Does it take more or less time than when the matches are arranged in a row? Explain how matches arranged as shown in the diagram are like a chain reaction in which each atom that disintegrates gives off enough particles to cause two more atoms to fly apart.

Because of their religious beliefs and the possibility of war, a number of European scientists fled to the United States in the 1930s from Germany, Italy, and other countries. Toward the end of the decade some of these scientists and their American colleagues became worried by what they had learned of the atomic research being conducted in Nazi Germany. They persuaded Albert Einstein (see page 376) to support an appeal to the American government, and in August of 1939 Einstein wrote a letter to President Franklin Roosevelt, suggesting that the Administration establish contact with the atomic scientists in the United States and suggesting, also, that funds be provided to speed up the experimental work (Figures 12.7A, B pages 382-383). Money was soon forthcoming, and the scientists went to work on the many problems that had to be solved before an atomic bomb could be made.

Fermi was an Italian scientist who, after going to Sweden to receive the Nobel Prize, fled to this country. He and his co-workers performed the experiment that proved a chain reaction was possible. The experiment involved building the first **atomic pile,** or **nuclear reactor** as they are usually called now (opposite page).

Fermi's experiment was carried out with great secrecy under the stands of the football field at the University of Chicago. The first atomic pile consisted of 256 metric tons of graphite, 36 metric tons of uranium compounds, and strips of cadmium, all arranged in layers. Each of these three kinds of materials had an important role in making the atomic pile work.

The uranium was the **fuel.** The atoms of $U^{235}$ split to produce neutrons and energy. Such a large amount of uranium was necessary because it was a mixture of about one $U^{235}$ atom to each 140 $U^{238}$ atoms. The $U^{238}$ atoms do not split in the same manner as do the $U^{235}$ atoms.

The graphite acted as a **moderator** (mod′ ər ā′ tər). The moderator slows down the neutrons so that they can be more readily absorbed by the atoms of $U^{235}$. Without the moderator, the neutrons would go flying out of the reactor, and a chain reaction would not be possible.

The cadmium was used to control the rate of the reaction. Cadmium absorbs neutrons, and when the strips of the metal were in place, some of the neutrons were absorbed by the cadmium rather than the uranium-235. In later models of nuclear reactors, the cadmium was shaped in the form of rods and called **control rods.**

On December 2, 1942, Fermi and his fellow researchers tested the first atomic pile. When the cadmium strips were

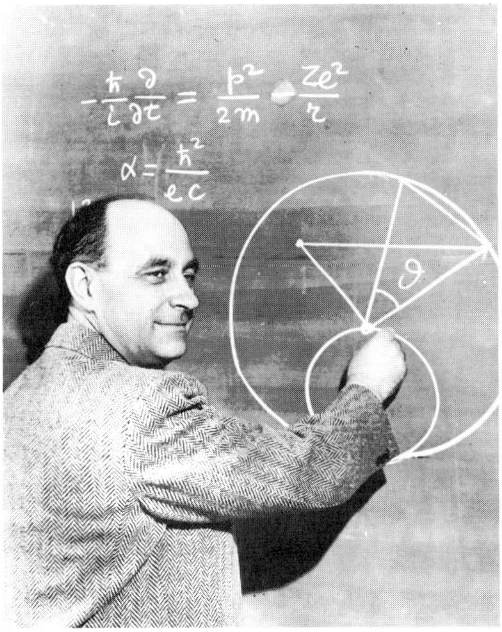

**12.6** (above) Enrico Fermi (1901-1954); (below) model of the first atomic pile at the University of Chicago

*Argonne National Laboratory*

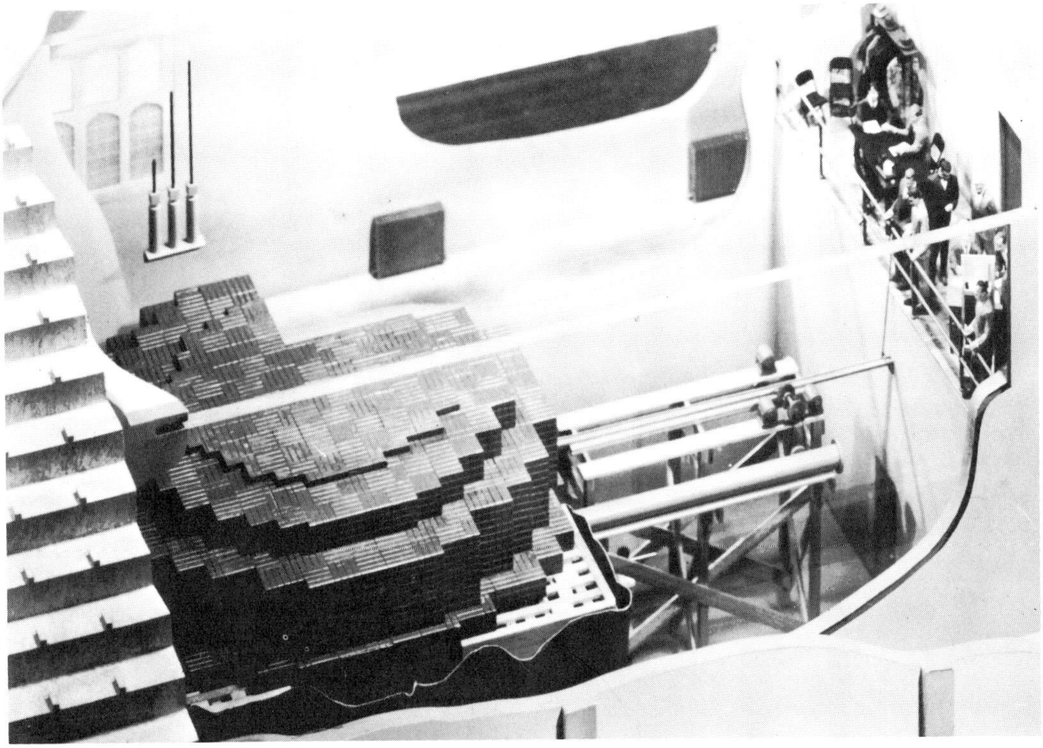

Albert Einstein
Old Grove Rd.
Nassau Point
Peconic, Long Island

August 2nd, 1939

F.D. Roosevelt,
President of the United States,
White House
Washington, D.C.

Sir:

Some recent work by E.Fermi and L. Szilard, which has been communicated to me in manuscript, leads me to expect that the element uranium may be turned into a new and important source of energy in the immediate future. Certain aspects of the situation which has arisen seem to call for watchfulness and, if necessary, quick action on the part of the Administration. I believe therefore that it is my duty to bring to your attention the following facts and recommendations:

In the course of the last four months it has been made probable - through the work of Joliot in France as well as Fermi and Szilard in America - that it may become possible to set up a nuclear chain reaction in a large mass of uranium,by which vast amounts of power and large quantities of new radium-like elements would be generated. Now it appears almost certain that this could be achieved in the immediate future.

This new phenomenon would also lead to the construction of bombs, and it is conceivable - though much less certain - that extremely powerful bombs of a new type may thus be constructed. A single bomb of this type, carried by boat and exploded in a port, might very well destroy the whole port together with some of the surrounding territory. However, such bombs might very well prove to be too heavy for transportation by air.

**12.7** Einstein's famous letter to President Franklin D. Roosevelt

-2-

The United States has only very poor ores of uranium in moderate quantities. There is some good ore in Canada and the former Czechoslovakia, while the most important source of uranium is Belgian Congo.

In view of this situation you may think it desirable to have some permanent contact maintained between the Administration and the group of physicists working on chain reactions in America. One possible way of achieving this might be for you to entrust with this task a person who has your confidence and who could perhaps serve in an inofficial capacity. His task might comprise the following:

a) to approach Government Departments, keep them informed of the further development, and put forward recommendations for Government action, giving particular attention to the problem of securing a supply of uranium ore for the United States;

b) to speed up the experimental work, which is at present being carried on within the limits of the budgets of University laboratories, by providing funds, if such funds be required, through his contacts with private persons who are willing to make contributions for this cause, and perhaps also by obtaining the co-operation of industrial laboratories which have the necessary equipment.

I understand that Germany has actually stopped the sale of uranium from the Czechoslovakian mines which she has taken over. That she should have taken such early action might perhaps be understood on the ground that the son of the German Under-Secretary of State, von Weizsäcker, is attached to the Kaiser-Wilhelm-Institut in Berlin where some of the American work on uranium is now being repeated.

Yours very truly,

A. Einstein

(Albert Einstein)

*Courtesy of Franklin D. Roosevelt Library, Hyde Park, New York*

slowly removed, it was found that the $U^{235}$ gave off enough neutrons that were absorbed by other atoms of $U^{235}$ to keep the chain reaction going. With the demonstration of a chain reaction, the construction of an atomic bomb appeared possible.

### Have You Learned?

1. What is a chain reaction? Why must more than one neutron be produced for each fission of an atom in order for a chain reaction to take place?
2. Explain how an atomic pile works. What are the functions of the fuel, moderator, and the cadmium sheets or rods?
3. How did Fermi's success in building an atomic reactor indicate that an atomic bomb was possible?

## 3. The Atomic Bomb

**ARE YOU READY?**

Look up the following words if you are not sure of their meanings:

atomic pile; beta particle; debris; diffuse; fissionable material; half-life; ionize; moderator; reactor; research and development; uncontaminated.

Although Fermi's success in building an atomic pile indicated that an atomic bomb was possible, much work had to be done before the first bomb was made. The *Manhattan Project* was organized to carry out the necessary research and development. As a result of an agreement between President Roosevelt and Prime Minister Churchill of Great Britain to cooperate on the development of an atomic bomb, scientists from both countries, plus those of other countries who had fled to the United States, were available to work on the project.

### Obtaining Fissionable Material

A major task was to obtain enough fissionable material. Uranium, as it is mined from the earth, contains only 0.7 percent $U^{235}$, and the remaining 99.3 percent is $U^{238}$. Two methods were worked out to separate the $U^{235}$ from the $U^{238}$. In one method, the uranium was ionized and the ions accelerated to very fast speeds. A magnetic field was used to separate the two kinds of ions, since the slightly lighter $U^{235}$ ions were deflected more than the $U^{238}$ ions.

In the other method, the uranium was combined with fluorine to form gaseous $UF_6$. The gaseous uranium fluoride was forced through a long tube containing

**12.8** Gas-diffusion process

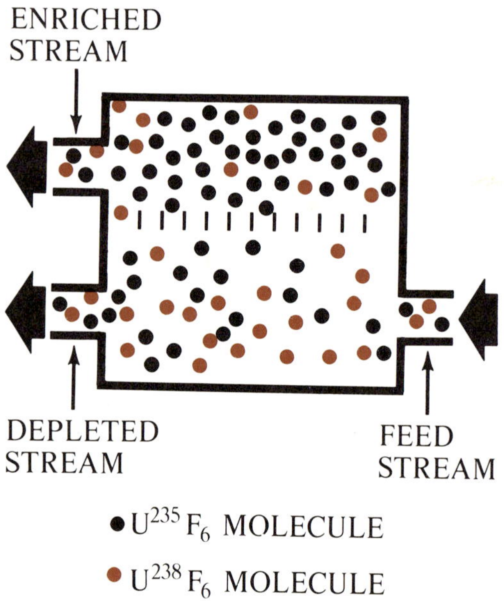

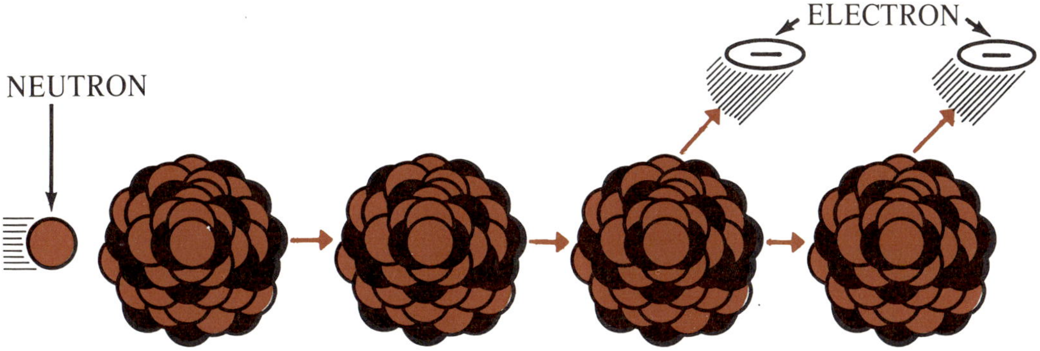


**12.9** Production of plutonium in a breeder reactor

holes that was enclosed in another tube. The lighter molecules of $U^{235}F_6$ diffused through the holes at a slightly faster rate than the molecules of $U^{238}F_6$, and this could be used to separate the $U^{235}$ from the $U^{238}$. See Figure 12.8 on page 384. A huge plant was built at Oak Ridge, Tennessee, to obtain a supply of $U^{235}$ using these two processes.

Scientists made an important discovery when they learned that $U^{238}$ absorbs neutrons to form $U^{239}$. This isotope has a short half-life of 23 minutes and decomposes by giving off a beta particle to form **neptunium-239** (nep tü′ ni əm). Neptunium-239, with a half-life of about 2 days, gives off a beta particle to form plutonium-239. The reason that this discovery was so important is that plutonium-239, like uranium-235, is fissionable and can be used to make a bomb.

Plutonium-239 can be made in a reactor containing a mixture of $U^{235}$ and $U^{238}$. The $U^{238}$ atoms are converted to $Pu^{239}$ when they absorb a neutron given off during the fission of $U^{235}$. Reactors used to make fissionable materials like plutonium-239 are called **breeder reactors**. A plant containing breeder reactors for the production of plutonium-239 was built at Hanford, Washington.

In Fermi's atomic pile, 256 metric tons of graphic were used to slow down the neutrons. Obviously it was not practical to build a bomb that contained that much graphite. Scientists studying the problem suggested that if enough fissionable material such as $U^{235}$ was brought together, a moderator would not be needed. The $U^{235}$ atoms would act as a moderator to slow down the neutrons, and most of the neutrons would be absorbed before they escaped. The smallest amount of $U^{235}$ that would keep the chain reaction going was called the **critical mass.**

## The First Atomic Bombs

By 1945 enough $U^{235}$ had been separated from $U^{238}$ to make a bomb, and a supply of $Pu^{239}$ also had been produced. Scientists and engineers, many working in a large government laboratory at Los Alamos, New Mexico, had worked out the many problems involved in the design of the

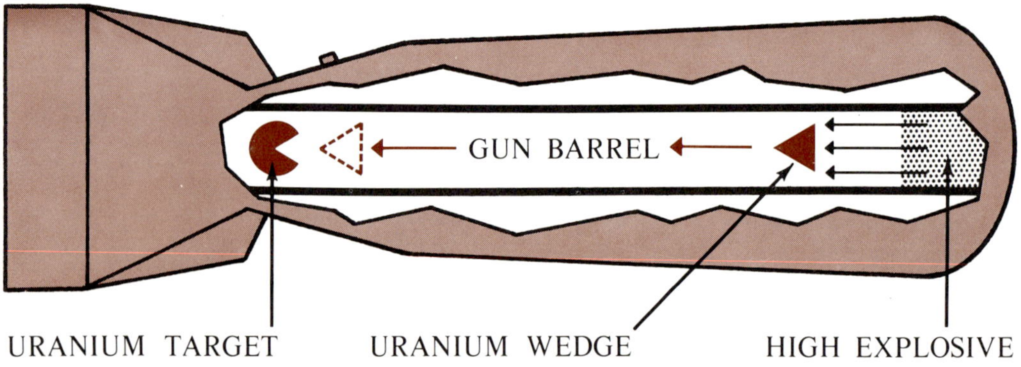

**12.10** Atomic bomb

bomb. The first atomic bomb, using plutonium-239, was exploded on July 16, 1945 in the southern part of New Mexico.

On August 6, 1945, an atomic bomb containing uranium-235 was dropped on Hiroshima, Japan. The diagram of the bomb in Figure 12.10 shows how simple it really was. A wedge of uranium-235 at the front of the bomb was shot into a ball of uranium-235, about the size of a baseball, at the rear of the bomb. The ball of uranium-235 had a notch into which the wedge of $U^{235}$ fitted. With the wedge of uranium in place, the total amount of uranium was greater than the critical mass, and the chain reaction began.

A second atomic bomb was dropped on Nagasaki, Japan, on August 9. It was a plutonium bomb like the one that had been tested earlier in New Mexico. A few days later World War II ended.

## Effects of Atomic Explosions

Atomic bombs like those dropped on Japan produced an explosion equal to that produced by 18,000 metric tons of TNT. Temperatures of several million degrees were produced near the center of the explosion, temperatures that melted rocks and metals. A blast of compressed air caused by the heat moved outward from the center, crushing buildings and causing much damage.

The explosion of an atomic bomb also produces much harmful radiation. Neutrons and gamma radiation are produced by the fission of the uranium or plutonium in the bomb. When the bomb explodes, dirt and other materials are sucked up into the mushroom-shaped cloud. This debris, which is made radioactive and falls back to the earth, is called **fallout.**

An atomic bomb explosion may produce as many as 200 different radioisotopes. About two-thirds of these have a half-life of less than one day. This is one of the reasons why *fallout shelters* have been recommended. By staying in a fallout shelter for several days with a supply of uncontaminated food and water, it is possible to escape most of the harmful effects of the radioisotopes with short half-life.

Some of the debris from an atomic explosion may be carried high into the atmosphere and not fall out for months or even years. In the case of radioisotopes that have relatively long half-life, such as strontium-90 and cesium-137, fallout from

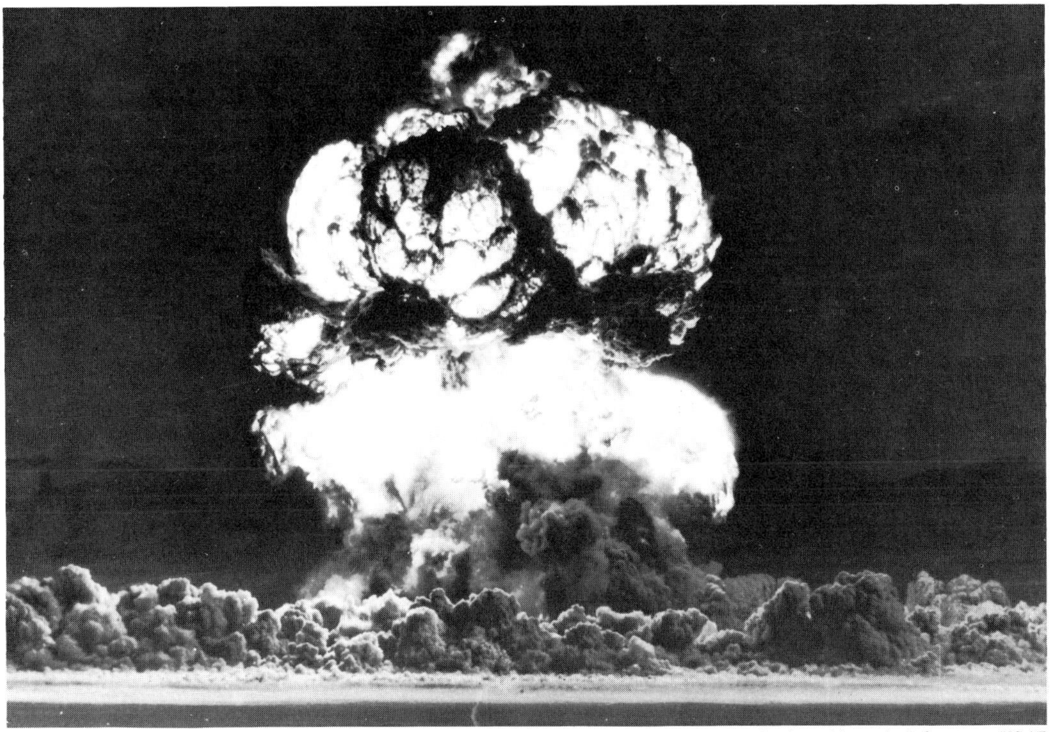

*Lookout Mountain Laboratory, USAF*

**12.11—12.12** (above) an atomic explosion; (below) steel works at Nagasaki after the atomic explosion of August 9, 1945

*United States Atomic Energy Commission*

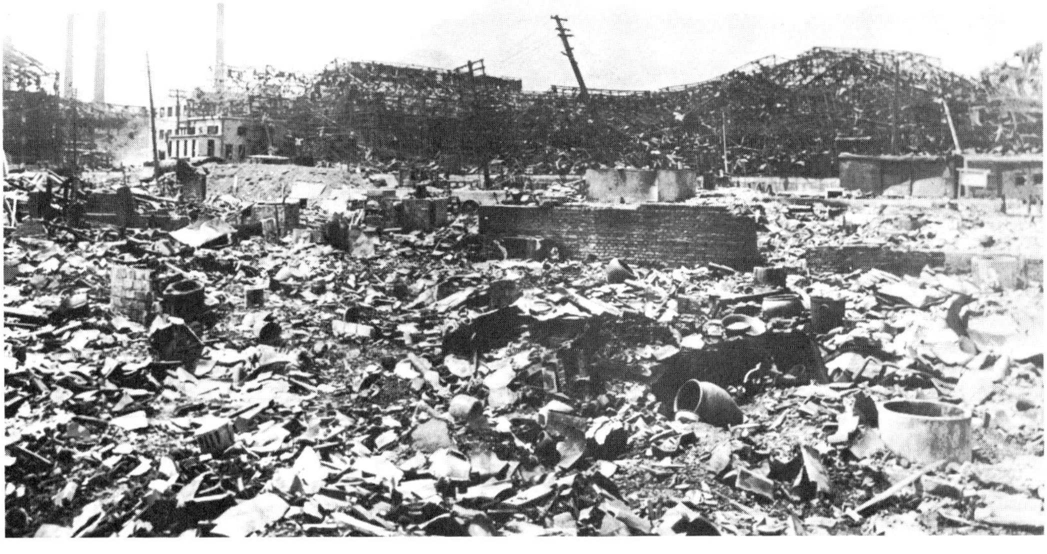

an atomic explosion can be a hazard years after the explosion occurs. When strontium-90 is consumed in foods by human beings, it concentrates in the bones, and the beta particles it gives off can be harmful.

In the 1950s many people, including several famous scientists, became concerned about the harmful effects of fallout produced by atomic explosions. In 1963 the United States, Great Britain, and Russia agreed to stop testing nuclear devices on the ground, in the air, and under water. Since underground explosions produce little or no fallout, these were not banned.

### Have You Learned?

1. Describe the two methods that were used to separate uranium-235 from uranium-238. Why was it necessary to separate these two isotopes?
2. What is a breeder reactor? How is it used to make plutonium-239?
3. Explain how the uranium-235 bomb works. Why is it necessary to keep the two pieces of uranium-235 separated until the time of explosion?
4. What is fallout, and why is it harmful? What can people do to protect themselves from fallout?

## 4. Using the Energy of Fission

**ARE YOU READY?**

Look up the following words if you are not sure of their meanings:

atomic pile; breeder reactor; control rods; diesel engine; moderator; radioisotope; reactor; tracer; turbine.

Since the end of World War II in 1945, thousands of uses have been made of atomic energy. Many of the applications involve the use of nuclear reactors. Although many different kinds of reactors have been built, they all contain the same basic parts, and they are similar in many ways to Fermi's first atomic pile.

The source of energy is the *fuel,* which is a fissionable material such as uranium-235 or plutonium-239. Graphite is still used in many reactors as a *moderator* to slow down the neutrons so they will be absorbed by atoms of the fuel. In the *swimming-pool* type of reactor, the fuel is placed in a large tank of a special kind of water that acts as the moderator. *Control rods* are made of cadmium or other materials that absorb neutrons but are not changed by them.

As atoms of the fuel split, neutrons and energy are produced. The fast-moving neutrons are slowed down by the moderator. When the control rods are in place, most of the neutrons are absorbed by the rods of cadmium. As the control rods are removed from the reactor, more of the neutrons are absorbed by the fuel, and the rate of the reaction increases. Moving the control rods in and out speeds up or slows down the reactor just as the speed of a car is changed by moving the accelerator pedal up and down. (See Figure 12.13 on page 389.)

The heat energy produced by a reactor is removed by the use of a **coolant** (kül′ ənt). Depending on the type of reactor, the coolant may be water, liquid sodium, a gas such as carbon dioxide, or some other material. The coolant surrounds the core of the reactor and removes the heat as the coolant in the radiator system of an

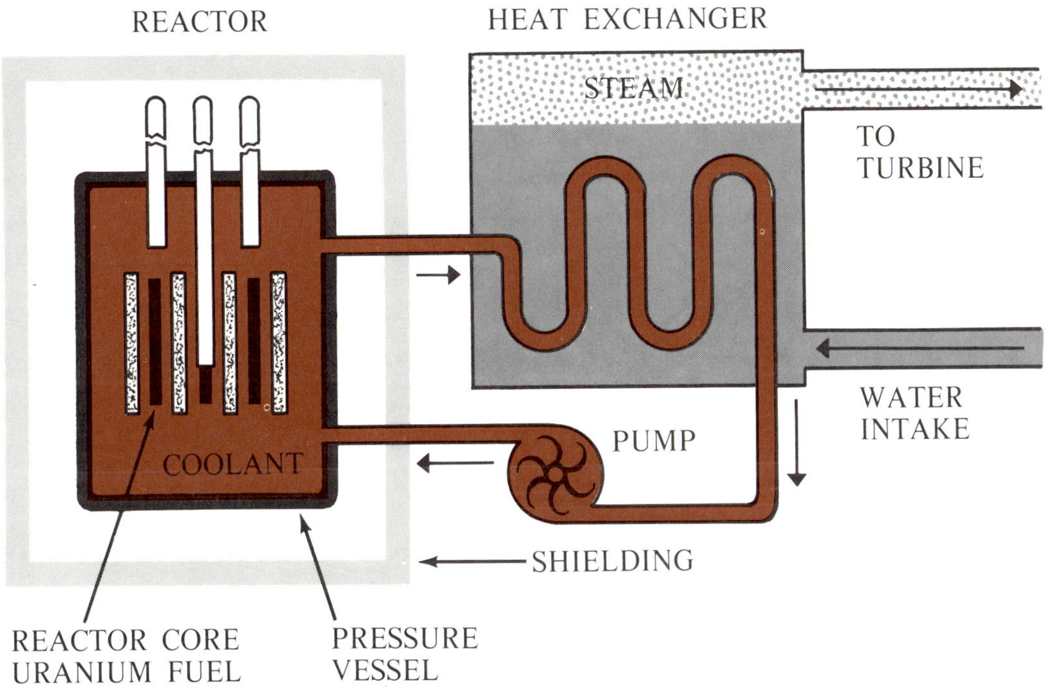


**12.13** Nuclear reactor

automobile removes the heat produced by the car engine.

Since neutrons and gamma radiation are given off during the fission of the fuel, the reactor must be shielded to protect the operators. Reactors are surrounded with thick concrete walls and lead plates to stop the dangerous radiations. In order for reactors to be used to power automobiles and aircraft, shields must be developed from lightweight materials.

## Using Reactor Energy as a Source of Power

The heat energy produced by the reactor can be used to boil water or other liquids, which are then used to turn a turbine. In the case of reactors used to generate electricity, the turbine drives an electrical generator. The first nuclear power plant in the United States began operations in 1957, and since then many larger plants have been built. At the present time it costs about the same amount to generate electricity using coal or other conventional fuels as it does to use nuclear energy. However, it is expected that more and more electricity will be generated using nuclear power as ways are found to do it less expensively and as our coal supplies decrease. (See Figure 12.14 page 390.)

The heat energy from a reactor is also used to propel submarines and ships. In this case the turbine drives the propellor of the vessel. The first nuclear-powered submarine, the *Nautilus*, was launched in 1954. Unlike submarines powered by diesel engines and batteries, nuclear-powered submarines can stay under water

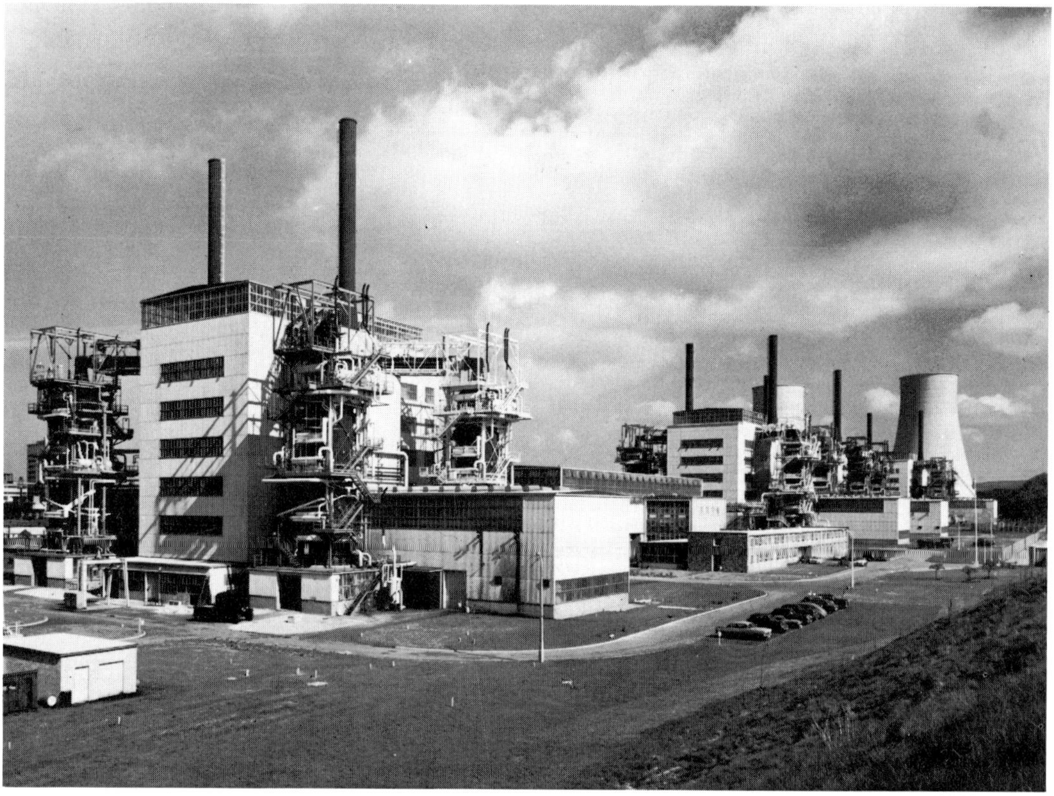

U. K. A. E. A.

**12.14** The world's first large-scale nuclear power plant at Calder Hall in the northwest of England

for long periods of time. In 1958 the *Nautilus* was the first submarine to sail under the ice cap covering the North Pole. Two years later another nuclear-powered submarine traveled around the world under water. The *Savannah,* the first merchant ship to use nuclear power, began operations in 1962. About 45 kilograms of uranium-235 provides enough energy to propel the *Savannah* around the earth 14 times without stopping for fuel. (See Figures 12.15A, B on page 391.)

## Other Uses of Reactors

The use of the *breeder reactor* to make plutonium-239 for the first atomic bomb was discussed in the previous section. Research continues on the use of breeder reactors to make fissionable materials. Since it is possible to change all the world's supply of uranium-238 into plutonium-239, which can be used as the fuel in a reactor, scientists believe that there will not be a shortage of atomic fuels for a long time.

The radiations produced in a reactor are used to make hundreds of different radioisotopes. As was described in Chapter 11, these are used as tracers, in the treatment of disease, and in many other ways. The reactor also is used as a source

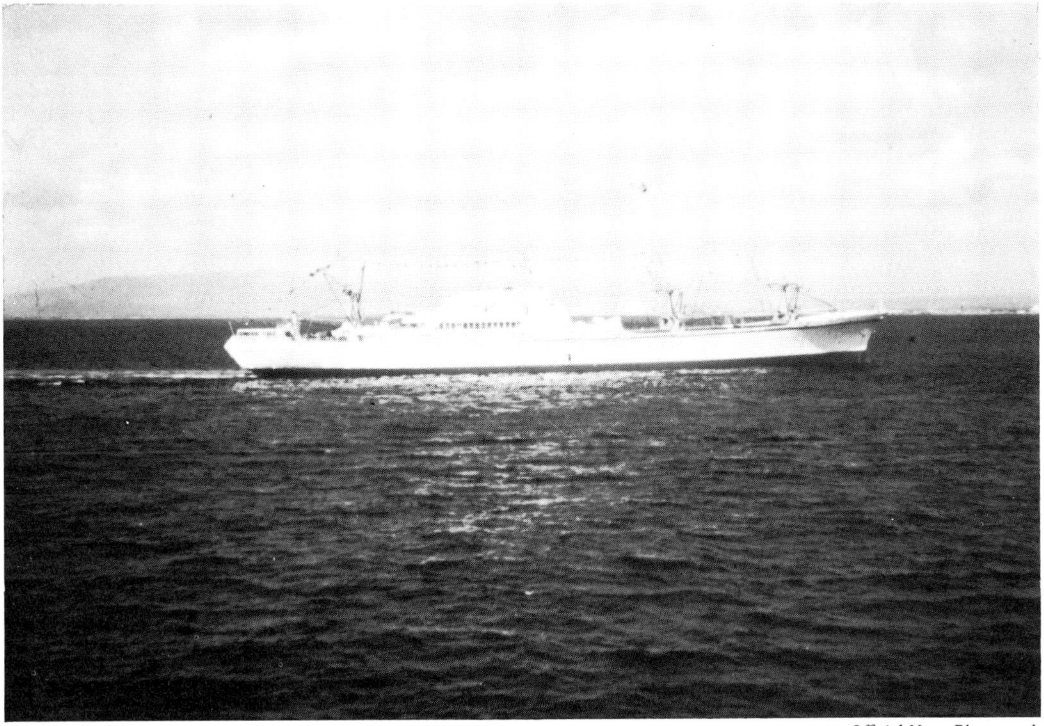

*Official Navy Photographs*

**12.15** (above) the *Savannah*; (below) the *Nautilus*; the first merchant ship and the first submarine to use atomic power

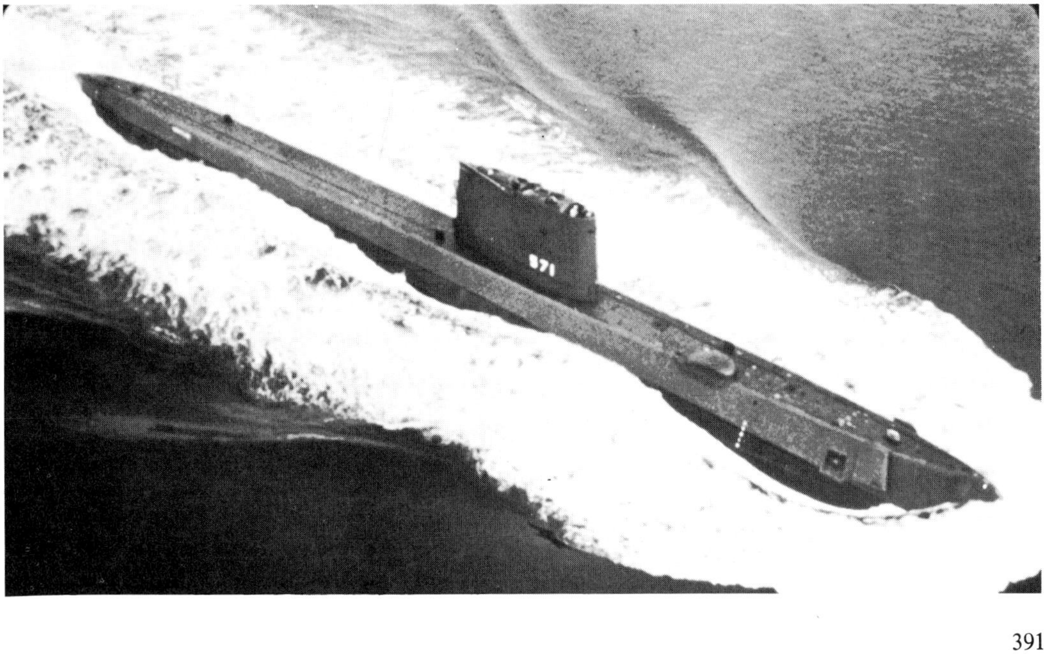

of radiation for research projects of various kinds.

## Controlled Atomic Explosions

Research continues on how to use atomic explosions for peaceful purposes. It has been suggested that atomic explosions can be used to move large amounts of earth to build canals or to make harbors. There are plans to blast a canal across Panama to replace the one now in use, which is too small for today's supertankers. Tests have been conducted to determine how much energy is needed, where the explosion should take place, and how the amount of fallout from the explosion can be reduced.

In 1962 an atomic explosion was used to blast a hole over 360 meters wide and 90 meters deep. About 12 million tons of earth were moved, and only a small amount of radioactive material escaped. Atomic explosions have been used to make huge underground rooms over 45 meters across and 24 meters high. How many ways can you suggest that these underground rooms could be used?

Other proposals have been made to use nuclear energy to remove the salt from seawater and to control the world's weather. One such proposal involved exploding atomic bombs over the Arctic to produce clouds. The clouds would act as a blanket to trap radiation from the sun, and the entire Arctic region would be warmed. Of course if the weather were changed enough to melt the polar ice cap, the level of the oceans would rise, and many of the seaports of the world would be covered by water.

### Have You Learned?

Complete the following summary of this section by writing on a sheet of paper the word or words that best complete each statement.

The fissionable material used in a reactor is called the (1) _____. The (2) _____ slows down the neutrons, and the rate of the reaction is regulated by the (3) _____. The heat produced by the reactor is removed by the (4) _____ and can be used to make steam to turn a (5) _____. Reactors are shielded to protect the operators from harmful (6) _____. The (7) _____ was the first submarine powered by nuclear energy, and the (8) _____ was the first nuclear-powered merchant ship. A (9) _____ reactor is used to make fissionable materials. (10) _____ also are made in a reactor and can be used as tracers.

## 5. Combining the Nuclei of Atoms

**ARE YOU READY?**

Look up the following words if you are not sure of their meanings:

electrolysis; fission; fragment; isotope; nuclei; radioactive.

The fission of atoms involves splitting atoms of heavy elements into smaller parts. As you have seen, scientists learned how to control this process and have used it in many ways. Scientists suspected that a process that was the opposite of fission also could be used as a source of energy. In this process, lightweight elements would be made to combine to form heavier elements.

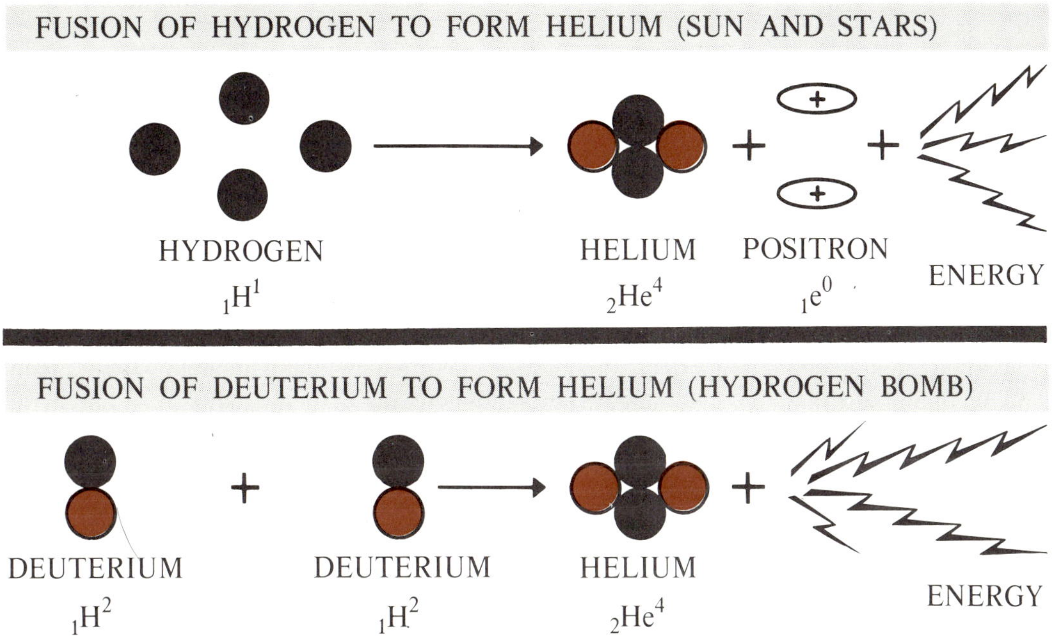


**12.16** These two models show two types of fusion.

This process is called **fusion** (fū′ zhən), which means to join together. Fusion takes place at temperatures of many millions of degrees and the atoms are without their shells of electrons at these temperatures. This is why we speak of nuclei instead of atoms when describing what happens during fusion.

The energy of the sun and stars is produced by the fusion of hydrogen nuclei. Four hydrogen nuclei, under conditions of high temperature and pressure, combine to form one helium nucleus. The total mass of the four hydrogen nuclei is slightly greater than the mass of the helium nucleus, and the mass lost in the reaction is converted to energy. On the sun $3.6 \times 10^{10}$ metric tons of hydrogen are converted to helium and energy each minute. However, there is little danger of the sun's running out of hydrogen. Scientists estimate that the sun contains enough hydrogen to last billions of years.

The atomic bomb using a fission reaction provided scientists with one way to obtain the high temperatures needed for a fusion, or **thermonuclear** (thėr′ mō nü′ kli ər), reaction. The hydrogen on the sun is the isotope with one proton in its nucleus, thus having an atomic mass of one. Scientists found that this isotope of hydrogen would not combine to form helium even at the high temperatures produced by the atomic bomb. However, two heavier isotopes of hydrogen called **deuterium** (dü tēr′ i əm) and **tritium** (trit′ i əm) could be used.

Deuterium has an atomic mass of two and is written $H^2$. It can be obtained by the electrolysis of water since small amounts of deuterium exist in nature. Tritium, $H^3$, is a radioactive isotope of hydrogen that is made artificially by bombarding lithium with neutrons.

## Hydrogen Bomb

Scientists in the United States first tested the fusion of hydrogen on a small scale in 1951. Since then several hydrogen bombs have been exploded. In 1954, one such bomb was exploded by the United States on a small coral island in the Pacific Ocean. The explosion produced a force equal to the force that would be produced by exploding 13,500,000 metric tons of TNT. Compare this with the force produced by the first atomic bombs, and you will find this hydrogen bomb to be 750 times more powerful. Since 1954 more powerful hydrogen bombs have been made.

In a hydrogen bomb, an atomic bomb is exploded to produce high temperatures and pressures. The deuterium and tritium in the bomb fuse to form helium. Energy is produced both by the fission of the atomic bomb and by the fusion of the hydrogen. In one type of hydrogen bomb, part of this energy is used to split atoms of uranium-238, producing even more energy.

The effects of a hydrogen bomb explosion are similar to those of an atomic bomb's except the hydrogen bomb produces more energy and causes more damage. An important difference, however, is

**12.17** Stellarator at Princeton University

*Plasma Physics Laboratory, Princeton University*

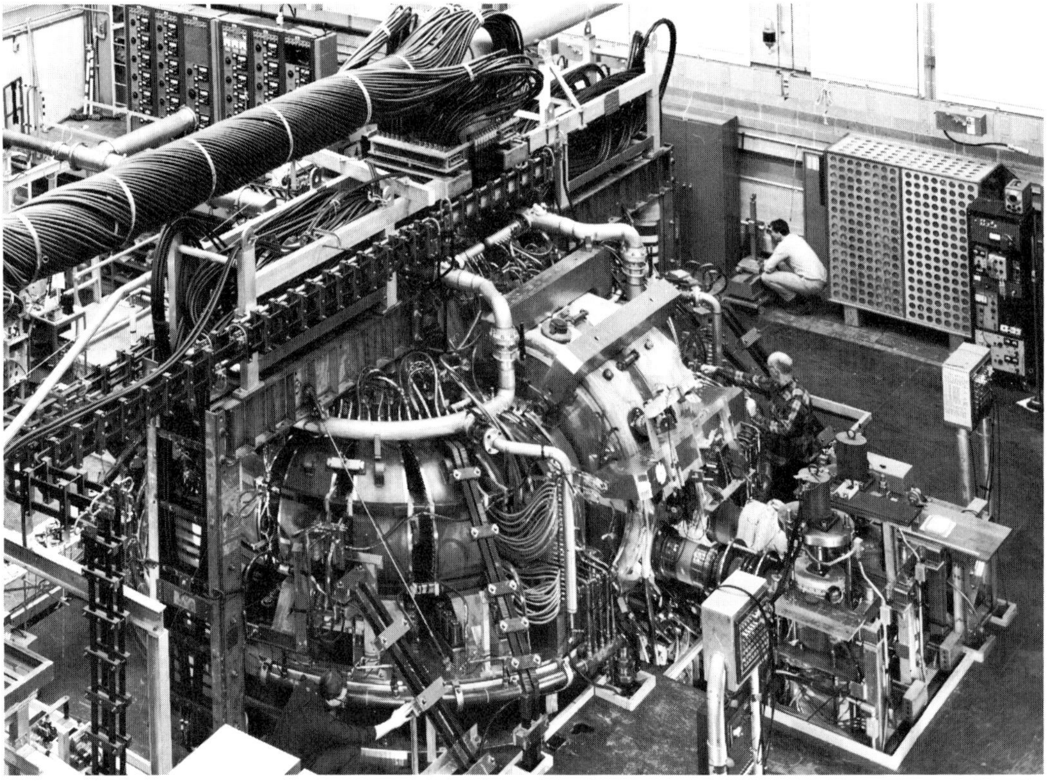

the amount of radioactive material produced by the explosions. In the atomic bomb, the fissionable material splits to form many radioactive fragments. On the other hand, the fusion of hydrogen into helium does not produce any radioactive material. The only radioactive material produced by the hydrogen bomb is that resulting from the explosion of the atomic bomb used to get the fusion started. Scientists have tried to develop a "clean bomb" by building one in which most of the energy is produced by fusion.

## Controlling the Energy of Fusion

There would be several advantages to using fusion as a source of energy. Hydrogen, the basic fuel, is an abundant element and does not cost much compared with uranium and other atomic fuels. The fusion of hydrogen produces helium, which is a harmless gas, instead of the dangerous radioactive materials produced by fission. But how could something be made to hold a reaction that produces temperatures of the sun and stars? And how can temperatures of hundreds of millions of degrees be produced to cause fusion to take place?

The **Stellarator** (stel′ ər ā′ tər) (see Figure 12.17 page 394) is one of the devices that have been built in an attempt to find answers to these questions. Ions of hydrogen are accelerated in a doughnut-shaped tube from which all the air has been removed. As the speed of the ions increases, so does the temperature. Although temperatures of over 6,000,000° C. have been produced, this is far short of the estimated 100,000,000° C. needed to make fusion take place.

### Have You Learned?

Select the word from Column B that best corresponds with each definition in Column A. (Do not write in your book.)

| *Column A* | *Column B* |
|---|---|
| 1. Produces the energy of the sun and stars | a. fission |
| 2. Thermonuclear reaction | b. fusion |
| 3. Used to set off a hydrogen bomb | |
| 4. Stellarator used to explore possibilities | |
| 5. Hydrogen combines to form helium | |
| 6. Produces radioactive fragments | |
| 7. Atomic bomb | |
| 8. Deuterium and tritium | |

### REVIEW QUESTIONS

1. Explain why it was necessary to revise the Law of Conservation of Energy and the Law of Conservation of Matter. What part did Einstein play in this?
2. Define *fission* and *fusion*. How are these processes alike, and how do they differ?
3. Use the following terms to explain how a reactor works: fuel; chain reaction; moderator; control rods; coolant; shield.
4. Make a diagram of the atomic bomb and the hydrogen bomb, and explain how each works.
5. List as many uses of atomic energy as you can. Also suggest ways that atomic energy may be used in the future.

### CAN YOU FIND OUT?

*It may be necessary to use encyclopedias or other reference books in answering the following questions.*

1. How are fallout shelters designed to protect people from the harmful effects of a nuclear explosion? For example, how is

fresh air, free from radioactive material, provided?

2. How are radioactive wastes disposed of? What reasons can you suggest for not burying them in the ocean?
3. Find out about different types of reactors, and how they are constructed and used. What research is being done to find new ways to build and use reactors?
4. Look into the research being done to find a way to control fusion.
5. Can you find out more about the nuclear reactions that take place in the sun and stars?

## REFERENCES FOR ADDITIONAL STUDY

ATOMIC ENERGY: THE STORY OF NUCLEAR SCIENCE by Irene Jaworsky and Alexander Joseph. Harcourt Brace Jovanovich, Inc. Describes atomic particles and nuclear reactions, including experiments that can be done with simple equipment

THE HISTORY OF THE ATOMIC BOMB by Mikael Blow and the Editors of American Heritage. American Heritage Press. The complete story of the atomic bomb, from Democritus's suggestion of the atom to the explosion of the first bomb, and some of the events that have followed

PIONEERS IN SCIENCE by Frank Siedel and James Siedel. Houghton Mifflin Company. Two-page biographies and one-page portraits of 48 great scientists, ranging from Aristotle and Archimedes to modern greats such as Einstein, Lawrence, and Fermi

KNOWING THE ATOMIC NUCLEUS by R. Hobart Ellis, Jr. Lothrop, Lee & Shepard Company. A simple but clear presentation of the structure of the atom, including some "home-spun" examples of the structure of the nucleus and the effects of radioactive atoms

# *Workshop... Unit V*

**Making an Alpha Source.** Several of the experiments on radioactivity require a source of alpha particles. A source can easily be made by burning a gas mantle in a crucible. The ash of the mantle contains thorium, which gives off alpha particles as it disintegrates.

Coat the head of a pin with rubber cement or model cement, dip it in the ashes of the mantle, and let it dry. Repeat the procedure until you have collected a ball of cement and ashes about the size of a large match head on the end of the pin.

**Building a Spinthariscope** (spin thar′ i skōp′). A spinthariscope is a device used to observe the flashes of light produced when alpha particles strike a fluorescent substance. All that is needed to build one is a box, ruler, lens, cardboard tube, fluorescent screen, and an alpha source. The spinthariscope is assembled as shown in Figure W5.1. The fluorescent screen can be made by coating a piece of paper with clear cement and sprinkling zinc sulfide dust on it.

**W5.1** Even you can make a spinthariscope.

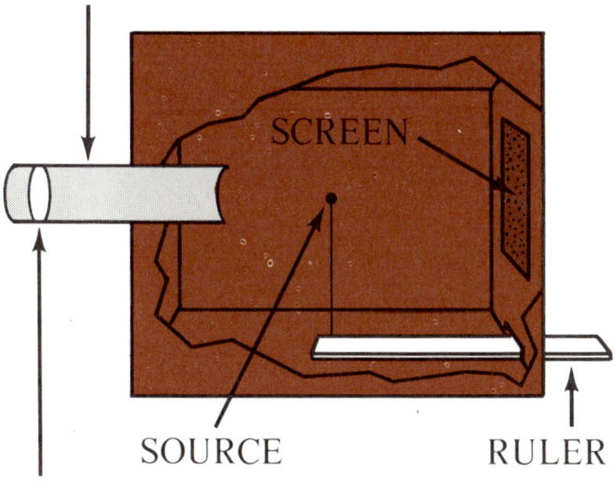


The lens should be a convex one, shaped like the one in the diagram, thicker in the middle than on the edges. Use the lens to focus sunlight on a sheet of paper, and measure the distance from the lens to the paper. You should use a lens for which this distance is from 5 to 12 cm. Both the cardboard tube and the box should be slightly shorter than the distance from the lens to the spot of sunlight on the paper. After the spinthariscope has been built, move the tube and lens in or out until you see a mark on the screen clearly.

The spinthariscope is used in a completely dark room. After allowing several minutes for your eyes to become adapted to the darkness, look through the lens toward the screen. To begin with, pull the ruler out so that the source is close to the screen. You should be able to see flashes of light caused by the alpha particles striking the zinc sulfide. Once you have observed these flashes, see if you can determine how far alpha particles travel through air by moving the source away from the screen until you no longer can see the flashes of light.

**Constructing a Cloud Chamber.** A small jar such as those used for peanut butter can be used to construct a cloud chamber. Use rubber cement to glue black velvet inside the lid and the bottom of the jar. The piece in the bottom of the jar should have a hole in the center about the size of

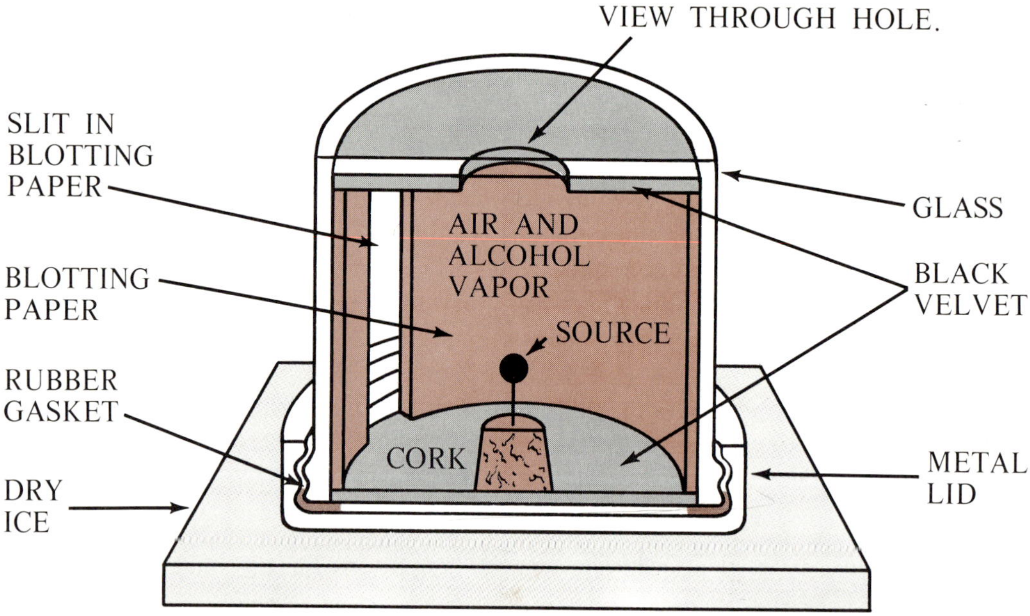


**W5.2** You can build a cloud chamber out of a peanut butter jar by following the directions below.

a dime. Also glue a small piece of cork inside the lid to hold the radioactive source. Cut a piece of blotting paper to fit inside the jar. It should touch the velvet on the top and bottom when the lid is in place. There should be a slit about one-half inch wide on one side. (Figure W5.2.)

Push the pin with the alpha source into the cork. Pour rubbing alcohol into the lid until it is about 1 cm deep and then screw the inverted jar on the lid. The alcohol will quickly travel through the blotting paper and the inside of the jar will be filled with alcohol vapor. Place the jar, lid downward, on a piece of dry ice. CAUTION: Do *not* handle the dry ice with your hands, use gloves or a pair of tongs.

Shine a bright light through the slit, and look down through the hole in the velvet. As the dry ice cools the alcohol vapor, some of the vapor will condense around dust particles in the air to form a mist. After a few minutes the mist should clear, and you will be able to see trails left as an alpha particle moves through the alcohol vapor. An alpha particle ionizes the air, and tiny droplets of the alcohol condense around the ions to form the trails.

**Making Radioautographs.** In Chapter 11 directions were given for using radioactive materials to expose photographic film that had been cut into pieces. An alternate method involves the use of a black-and-white film cartridge like those used in Instamatic cameras. Place a film cartridge in a camera, and advance the film to take the first exposure. In a completely dark room, remove the cartridge. Place a radioactive source such as a mantle or a luminous watch dial on the film. Store it in a completely dark place for several days. The film then can be put back in the camera and advanced to the next picture. All this must be done in the dark to keep light from exposing the film. Keep a record of what is used to expose each part

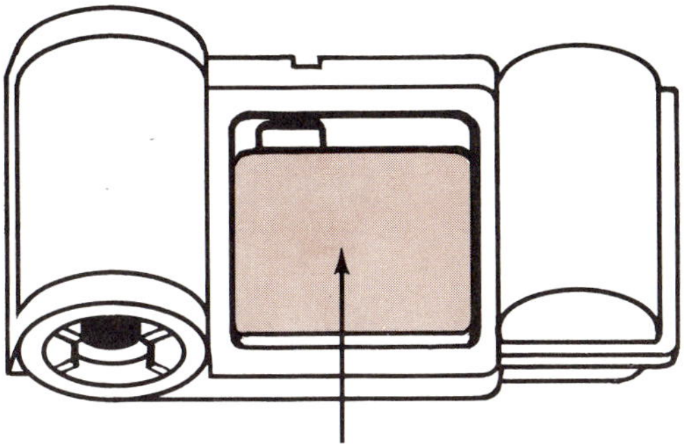

**W5.3** Making an audioradiograph

of the film and the length of each exposure. Once all of the exposures have been made, have the film developed as usual. Do not order prints made as you will want to examine the negatives first (Figure W5.3).

**Discharging an Electroscope.** Place a radioactive source near a charged electroscope, and measure how long it takes the electroscope to discharge. Compare this time with the time it takes the charge to leak off the electroscope when a radioactive source is not nearby.

**Demonstrating a Chain Reaction.** Arrange 40 to 50 mousetraps in rows in a box about 30 cm high. Set the traps, and place two rubber stoppers. to represent neutrons, on the loop of each trap. Throw a rubber stopper in the box to get the reaction started and quickly cover the box with a piece of glass. This will allow you to observe what happens. Notice that some of the traps usually are not set off just as some atoms of a fissionable material are not split during a chain reaction. (Figure W5.4.)

**W5.4** A mousetrap chain reaction

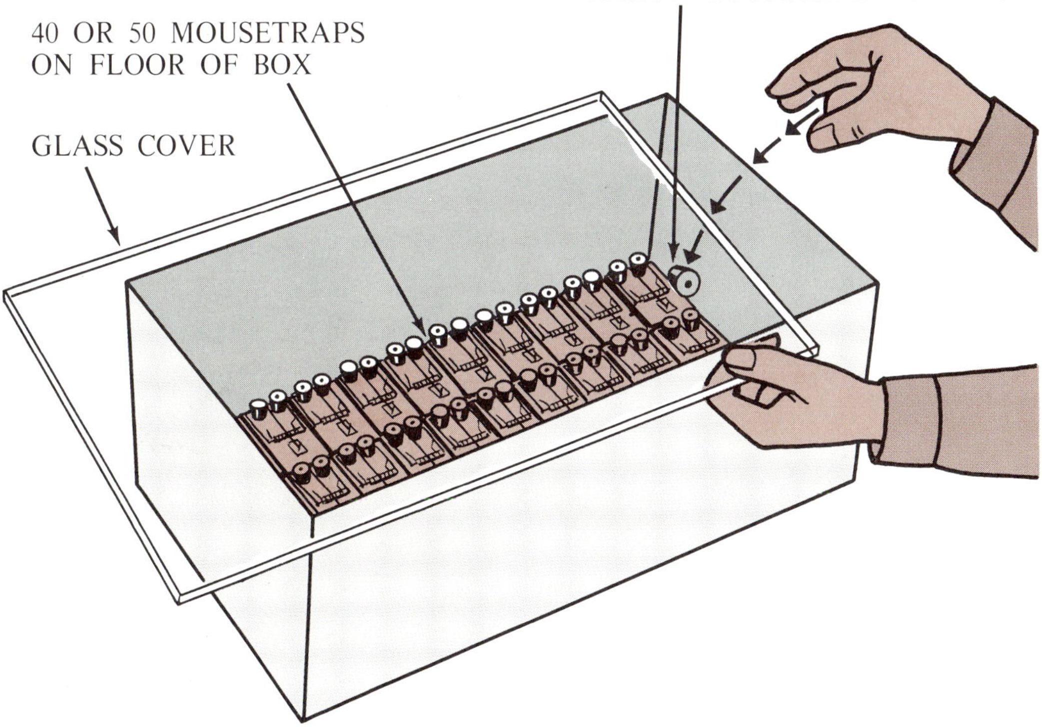

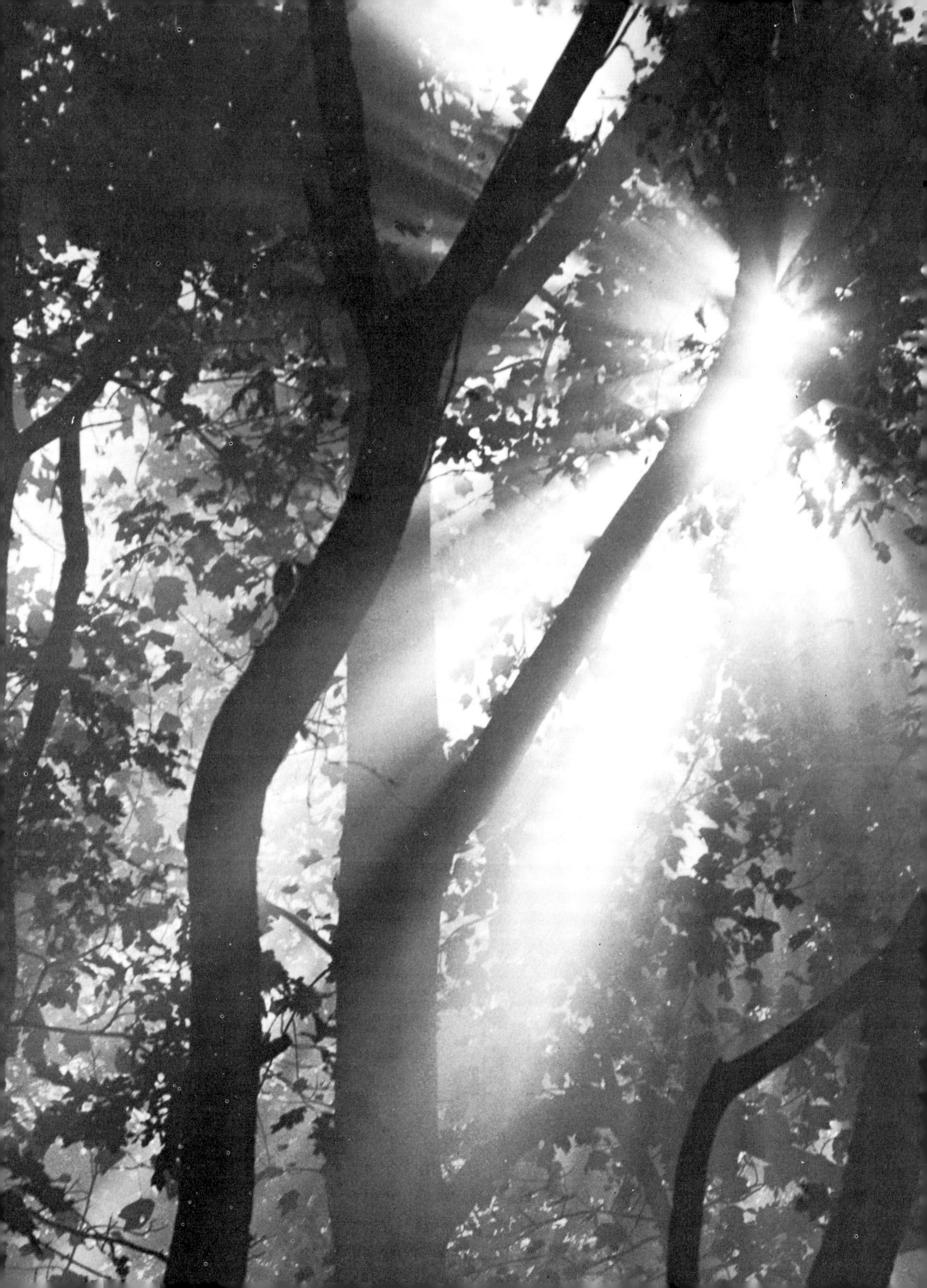

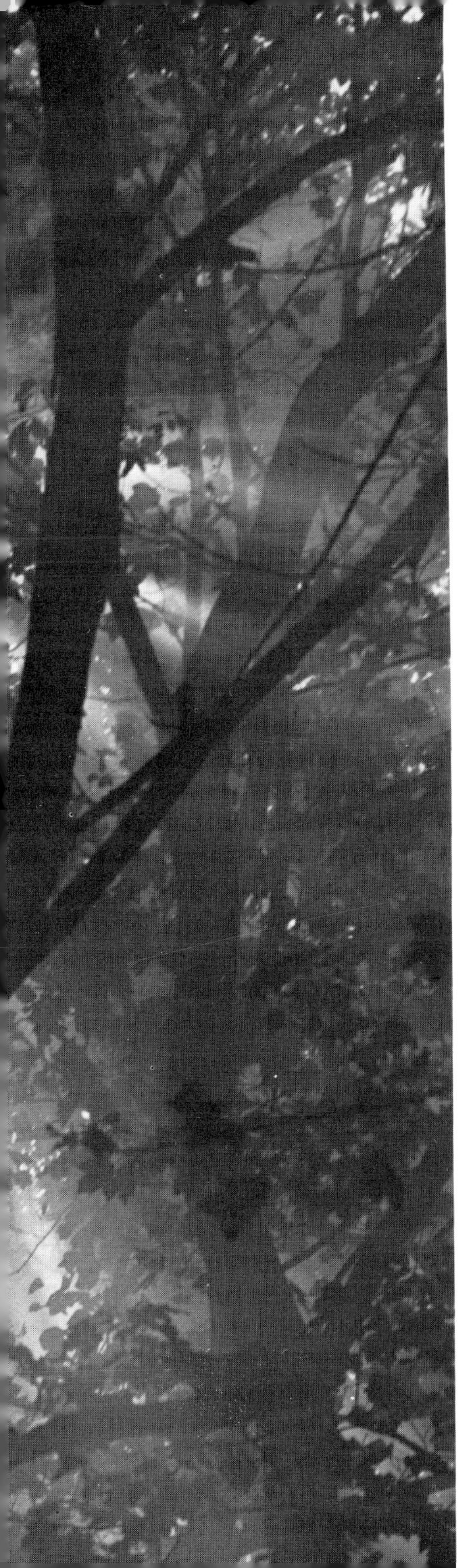

# *unit VI*
# *energy in waves*

*Grant Heilman*

CHAPTER **13**

# Sound

All of our lives we have enjoyed listening to and playing music. Understanding how sounds are made and how we hear them can make these experiences even more enjoyable.

But, before we begin the scientific study of sound, we must first understand the waves that we often see in water.

## 1. Energy Through Wave Motion

**ARE YOU READY?**

Look up the following words if you are not sure of their meanings:

crest; cycle; kinetic energy; right angle; transmitted; velocity.

You have already learned that energy in the form of heat can be transferred through the motion of molecules (conduction) or through the movement of a large mass of matter from one place to another (convection). Heat energy can move from one end of an iron bar to the other through the action of molecules of the iron. Or heat energy can circulate throughout a room by currents of air.

### Waves on Water

But you may have also observed that energy can be transmitted through or across the surface of matter by another means. You have undoubtedly watched a toy boat or a bit of wood floating in water. A rock dropped in the water some distance from the boat creates a disturbance on the

**13.1** Waves move outward in all directions.

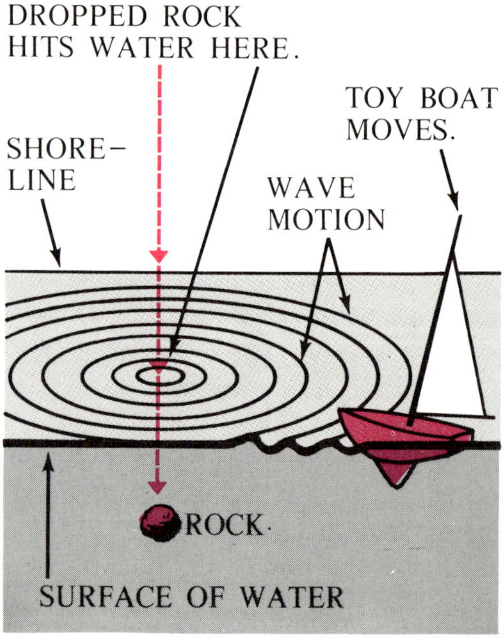

surface of the water that eventually causes the boat to move. The kinetic energy of the falling rock was transmitted by the motion of the water to the boat. This energy traveled from the point at which the rock hit the water to the boat in the form of **waves** (Figure 13.1).

If you are a careful observer, you noticed that the boat did not move very far. Instead of moving away from the source of the disturbance, it simply bobbed up and down. If we could watch a particular particle of water in a wave, we would see that it moved almost straight up and down and eventually returned to a point near that from which it started.

Because of cohesive forces between the water molecules, the movement of one molecule causes a similar up-and-down movement in the nearby molecules. In this way, the energy wave moves across the surface of the water, even though the individual particles return close to their original positions. Near the shore, of course, the wave may "break" and allow the particles of water to move toward and away from the land.

Waves such as these, in which the individual particles move mostly at right angles to the movement of the wave, are called **transverse** (trans vėrs′) waves. The motion of such waves is difficult to observe in water, but a model can be easily constructed.

**13.2** Preparing for observing transverse waves

*Norman D. Anderson*

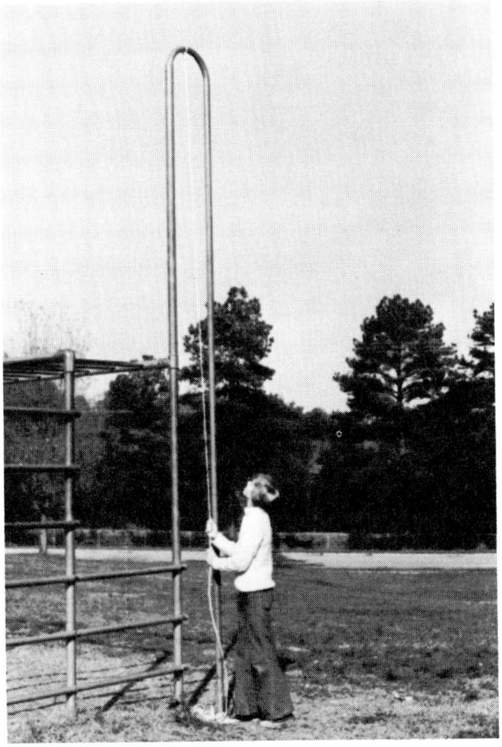

**13.3** Formation of wave

*Norman D. Anderson*

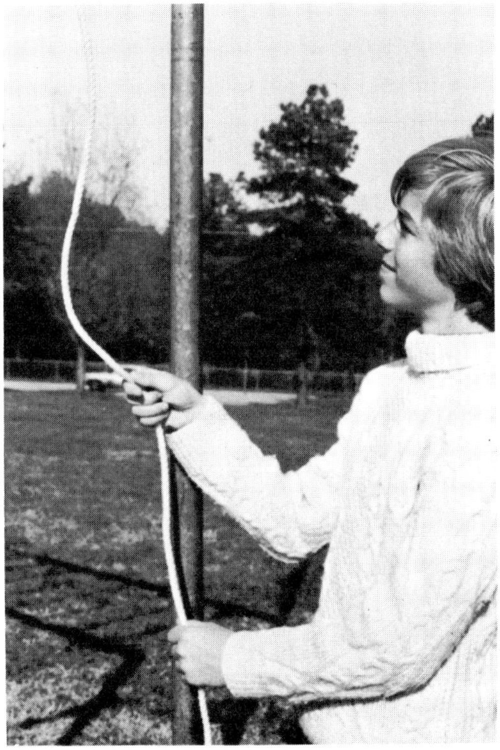

## Observing Transverse Waves

Figures 13.2 and 13.3 show a girl in the process of shaking one end of a rope so that it forms transverse waves. Try doing this yourself. You will see that a rope wave will travel away from your hand and up the rope. It might start down again.

## Characteristics of Waves

Like all transverse waves, the particles of the rope actually move from side to side, while the energy from the movement of your hand moves upward along the length of the rope. Several quick jerks of the rope will send several waves traveling up the rope, one after the other, as shown in the diagram (Figure 13.4) below. From these, you can identify several characteristics of waves.

First, each wave has a *length.* If we measure the distance from the top of one wave to the same point at the top of the next, we will have measured the **wavelength.**

Actually, the length of a wave need not be measured from crest to crest, as described above. In a series of waves, such as in the rope model, there are a number of particles that are moving in the same direction and that are the same distance from their normal positions. These particles are said to be in **phase** (fāz) with each other. Several particles that are in phase with each other have been identified in the diagram below. One wavelength may be defined as the distance between two particles that are in phase with each other. Notice that in any one wave, there can be only two particles that are in phase with each other. In the same wave there is one *other* particle that is the same distance from its normal position as the in-phase particles, but that is moving in the opposite direction. This particle is out of phase with the other two.

The height of the wave, from the midpoint to the top (or from the midpoint to the bottom) of the wave, is called the amplitude. It is a measure of the maximum distance a particle of the rope moves from its starting position. You can vary the amplitude of the rope waves by increasing

**13.4** The wavelength is a characteristic of waves. And the frequency of a wave is the number of full waves that pass a fixed point every minute.

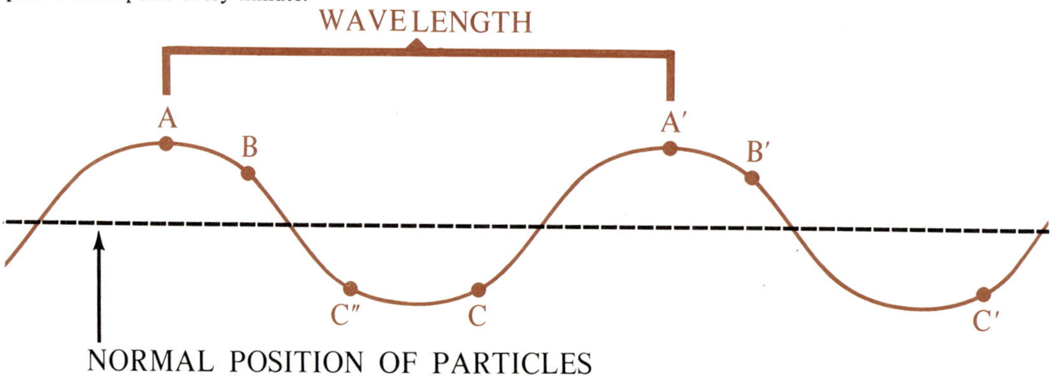

the amount of energy you put into the wave. Therefore, the amplitude of the waves in a given bit of matter is a measure of the energy of the wave.

The number of waves that pass a given point each second is a measure of the **frequency** (frē′ kwən si) of the wave. The units usually used to express frequency are **vibration** (vī brā′ shən) *per second* (vps) or *cycles per second* (cps). The word vibration means back-and-forth motion. The word **cycle** refers to a complete circle. Can you explain what makes up one complete cycle in the case of the waves traveling through the rope in the activity on page 403?

Waves also have a definite **velocity.** With the proper instruments, you could measure the rate at which the energy wave travels from your hand to the end of the rope. The velocity of a wave depends upon its frequency and its wavelength. Suppose that a wave source is producing waves that are 15 cm long and that their frequency is 10 vps. During the first second, 10 waves, each 15 cm long, will leave the source. Therefore, at the end of the first second, the front of the first wave will be 150 cm ($15 \times 10$) away from the source. As you can see, the velocity of a wave (V) can be calculated by multiplying the wavelength (L) times the frequency (F). The formula is $V = L \times F$.

Transverse waves have several other measurable characteristics, but these four —wavelength, amplitude, frequency, and velocity—are the important ones for you to learn at this time.

## A Second Type of Wave

Not all energy waves are transverse waves. Most energy waves are **longitudinal** (lon′ jə tü′ də nəl) waves. In these types of waves, the particles of the **medium** (mē′ di əm) through which the energy travels moves *back and forth in the same direction that the wave* is moving.

### Observing Longitudinal Waves

**MATERIALS:**

A metal spring, made of loose coils (The toy known as Slinky will do nicely.)

**PROCEDURE:**

Attach one end of the spring to a solid support, or have a friend hold it. Holding the other end, stretch the spring to almost its full length. Squeeze a few coils of the spring together, and release them. A longitudinal wave should travel away from you through the spring.

Can you set up a series of waves in the spring?

When you squeezed the coils of the spring together, you created the form of the longitudinal wave. In one area, the particles were packed more closely to-

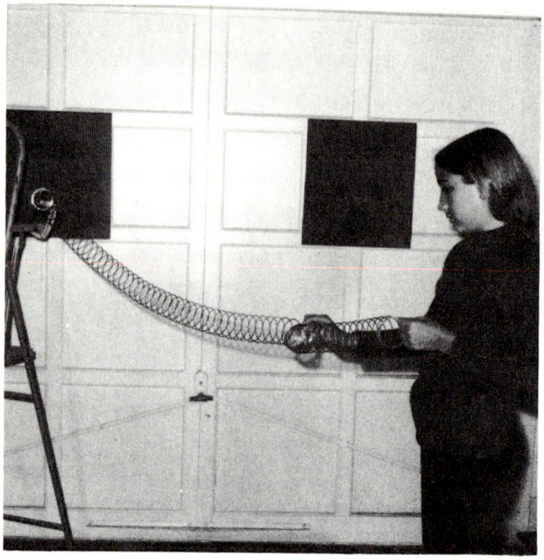

J. W. McDonald

**13.5** Observing longitudinal waves (procedure)

gether than was normal. This part of the longitudinal wave is known as the **compression** (kəm presh′ ən) area. On either side of the compression were areas in which the particles were farther apart than normal. These areas are called **rarefactions** (rãr′ ə fak′ shən).

The wavelength of a longitudinal wave is the distance between two particles that are in phase, just as it was in the case of the transverse wave. It is easiest to measure between two areas of maximum compression or between two areas of maximum rarefaction.

The amplitude of a longitudinal wave can be measured by finding the maximum distance one particle (one coil, in the case of the spring) moved from its normal position. The frequency of this type of wave can be found by measuring how many times a second a specific particle moved from its normal position, through a complete back-and-forth cycle, and returned to its normal position. The same figure can be obtained by counting the number of compressions that passed a certain point in one second. Velocity, as in the transverse wave, is a measure of the time it takes the compression to travel a certain distance in a certain direction.

## Have You Learned?

Select the word from Column B that best corresponds with each definition in Column A. (Do not write in your book.)

| *Column A* | *Column B* |
|---|---|
| 1. Waves in which individual particles move at right angles to the movement of the wave | a. amplitude |
| 2. A measure of the distance between two wave particles that are in phase with each other | b. compression |
| 3. A measure of the height of a wave | c. frequency |
| 4. A measure of the number of waves that pass a given point each second | d. in phase |
| 5. A measure of the rate at which wave energy travels | e. length |
| 6. Waves in which individual particles move back and forth in the same direction that the wave is moving | f. longitudinal |
| 7. The opposite of rarefaction | g. transverse |
| 8. The type of waves observed in water | h. velocity |
| 9. Two particles that are moving in the same direction that are the same distance from their normal position | |
| 10. The product of wavelength times wave frequency | |

## 2. How Sound Travels

> **ARE YOU READY?**
>
> Look up the following words if you are not sure of their meanings:
>
> density; hypothesis; instantaneous; longitudinal wave.

Sound waves are longitudinal waves of energy that move through matter in very much the same way that energy moves through the spring (see page 406). The fact that sound travels through matter can easily be demonstrated by use of the equipment shown in the diagram on page 408.

If an electric bell is placed inside a large container, and the air is slowly pumped out forming a partial *vacuum*, the sound of the ringing bell becomes fainter and fainter until it can no longer be heard. When air is allowed to flow back into the container, the sound of the bell becomes louder and louder.

Perhaps you can demonstrate this for yourself.

### Listening for Sound in a Vacuum

**MATERIALS:**

A heat-resistant, round-bottomed flask, a rubber cork to fit the flask, a small bell (such as those used on Christmas packages), a short piece of stiff wire, a source of heat, a small quantity of water

**PROCEDURE:**

Place the water in the flask, and heat until it is boiling. Attach the bell to the wire, and insert the wire into the underside of the stopper. When a quantity of steam is seen coming from the mouth of the flask, remove the heat, and quickly insert the stopper in such a way that the bell hangs down into the flask, as shown in Figure 13.6 on page 408.

The flask is now full of water vapor (steam). As the steam cools, it turns back into water, leaving the flask nearly empty of air. This vacuum is not very complete, but when the flask is shaken gently, you may be able to tell that there is less sound than when the flask is full of air.

### Speed of Sound

Perhaps you have noticed that you see the flash of lightning before you hear the thunder it creates. Or perhaps you have seen someone far away hit a nail with a hammer and a moment later heard the sound of the blow. From these observations you should have hypothesized that sound travels much more slowly than light.

The speed of light is 299,792 kilometers per second. Light from the sun, some 149,600,000 km miles away, reaches the earth in only about 500 seconds—a little more than 8 minutes. Over the distances that we use in our everyday lives, we see light within fractions of a second after it leaves its source. The light from a flash of lightning that is 10 kilometers away, for

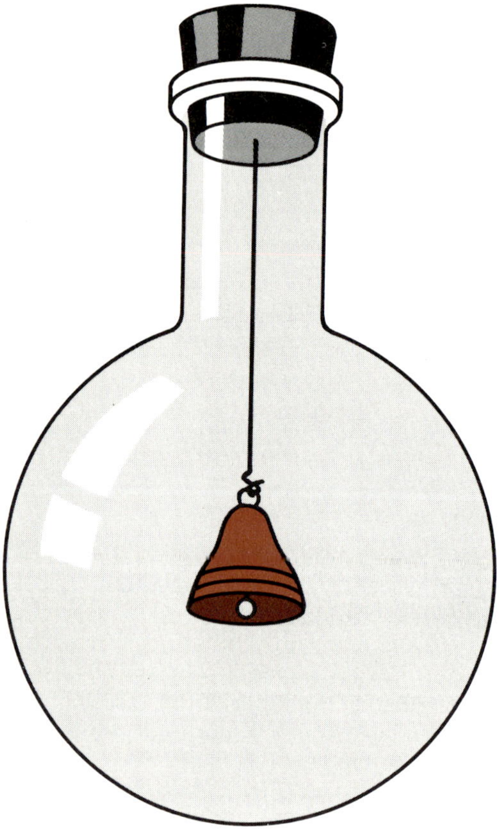

**13.6** Sound in a vacuum

example, reaches your eye in approximately $^{1}/_{30,000}$ of a second—almost instantaneously!

Sound travels at a much slower speed than this. If you were to stand 175 meters from a large building, you would discover that the sound of your voice would travel to the wall and the echo would bounce back to you in about one second. From this, we can calculate that the sound traveled about 350 meters per second (175 meters back to your ear). This is only about $^{1}/_{1,000,000}$ as fast as light! Anyone can make a rough measurement of sound.

Assuming that the speed of light is instantaneous, can you calculate how far away a lightning flash is if you hear the thunder 10 seconds after you see the flash? Five seconds?

## Factors Affecting the Speed of Sound

The figure 350 meters per second, used here for the speed of sound, is only approximate. The time that it takes for sound to pass through a substance depends upon two characteristics of the matter itself. These characteristics are **elasticity** (i las′ tis′ ə ti) and *density.* Elasticity is the ability of matter to resume its original shape after it has been distorted. Density is the weight of a unit volume of matter, and therefore indicates how closely packed the molecules of the substance are.

Imagine two different substances. In substance *A* the molecules move back to their original position much more slowly than in substance *B.* In other words, *A* is less elastic than *B.* If you set up a series of longitudinal waves through both substances, through which would the energy be able to move more rapidly?

Now imagine that you have another substance that is very dense, and that you are able to move its molecules so that they are farther apart. Will sound energy travel through the substance more rapidly or less rapidly than before? Remember that in its less-dense form, each molecule is freer to move, since it is not affected as much by other molecules around it. Also remember that in less-dense substances the mass of the matter moved by the wave will be somewhat less.

Your last hypothesis is easy for scientists to test. Using accurate instruments, they can measure the speed of sound through cold air, and later the same day, through warmer air. They have found that, since warm air is less dense than cold air, the speed of sound increases with the temperature. This increase amounts to about 60 cm per second for each 1° C of increase in temperature.

The speed of sound through a certain substance depends upon the *ratio* of the elasticity to the density of the substance. In substances in which this ratio is large—that is, in substances in which the elasticity is high and the density is low—the speed of sound will be high. In substances in which the ratio is smaller—a low degree of elasticity and a high density—the speed of sound will be low.

The elasticity-to-density ratio of solids is generally higher than in liquids. Therefore, sound travels through most solids more rapidly than through most liquids. All liquids have higher elasticity-to-density ratios than do gases; so sound travels through liquids faster than through gases. At 20° C sound travels through air at 334 meters per second, through water at about 1,251 meters per second, and through steel at 4,999 meters per second.

## Have You Learned?

Select the answer that best completes each statement. (Do not write in your book.)

1. Sound waves are ____ (longitudinal; transverse).
2. Normally sound travels ____ (faster; more slowly) than light.
3. Sound travels through air at approximately ____ (350; 3,500) meters per second.
4. The speed of sound through a substance depends upon the ____ (elasticity-to-density; density-to-elasticity) ratio of the substance.
5. The speeds of sound through water and steel are ____ (equal; different).
6. Sound moves ____ (faster; slower) through warm air than through cold air.
7. Sound ____ (will; will not) travel through a vacuum.
8. Normally sound travels through steel ____ (faster; more slowly) than it travels through air.
9. If you hear the thunder 4 seconds after you see the lightning flash, you know that the lightning was (less than; more than) 1 kilometer away.

**13.7** Through which substance does sound travel the fastest?

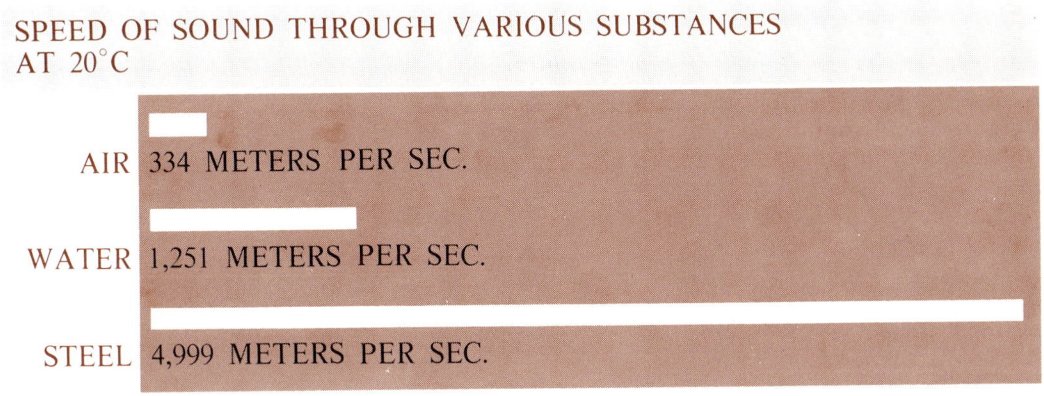

## 3. How Sounds Are Produced and How We Hear Them

**ARE YOU READY?**

Look up the following words if you are not sure of their meanings:

anti–; compression; longitudinal wave; out of phase; rarefaction; vibration.

Sound is a form of energy that travels through matter in longitudinal waves. Therefore, sound must be produced by something that produces compression and rarefaction of the particles of the matter through which it passes. (*Rarefaction*, which means *that which is rarefied*, is a section of minimum pressure in a substance through which compression waves are traveling.)

### Observing Sound-producing Objects

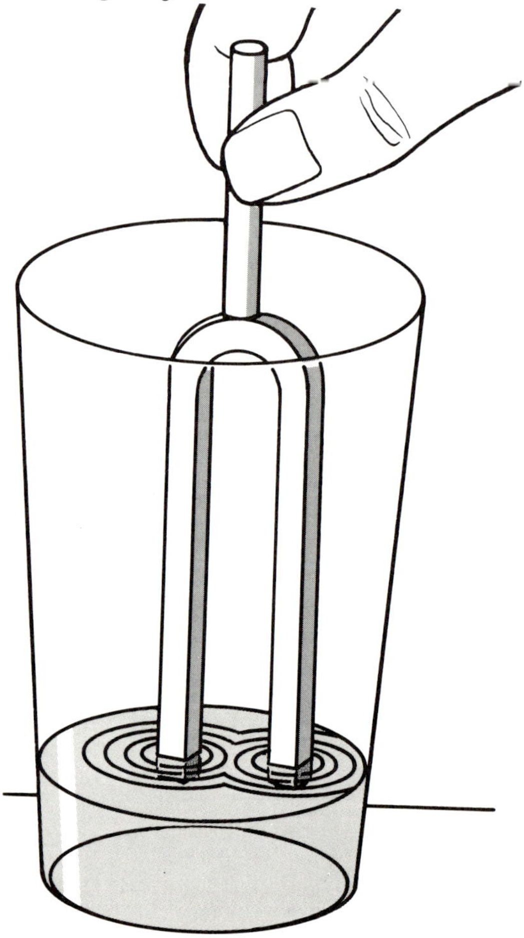

**MATERIALS:**

A large rubber band, a drum, a tuning fork, and a variety of other sound-producing objects

**PROCEDURE:**

Stretch the rubber band as tightly as possible. Pull it to one side, and release it. Can you hear a sound?

Place a wad of paper, a paper clip, or any other lightweight object on the head of a drum. Strike the drumhead sharply. Describe the action of the objects that you placed on the drumhead.

Strike the tuning fork against the rubber heel of your shoe or against the palm of your hand. Do *not* hit the tuning fork against a solid object such as the edge of the table, because it may break the fork. Touch the fork with your finger, or put it into a glass of water while it is still making a sound. Describe the motion of the tuning fork.

Place your fingers on your throat as you talk. Can you feel movement?

Can you see or feel movement in other objects that produce sound waves?

## Vibrations Cause Sound

The movement that you observed in the above activity is always a back-and-forth movement. A careful observation of a tuning fork will illustrate how these vibrations cause sound.

As the arms of the tuning fork move away from each other, work is done on the molecules of the air around them. The molecules closest to the fork receive energy as they are forced away (Figure 13.8).

This movement causes the compression part of the wave, which passes through the air as the energy is passed from molecule to molecule. As the arms of the fork move together, they leave behind an area containing fewer molecules than normal. As surrounding air molecules move into this **rarefied** (rãr′ ə fīd) area, they lose energy. In this way, each movement of the fork produces alternating compression and rarefaction of the air molecules around it.

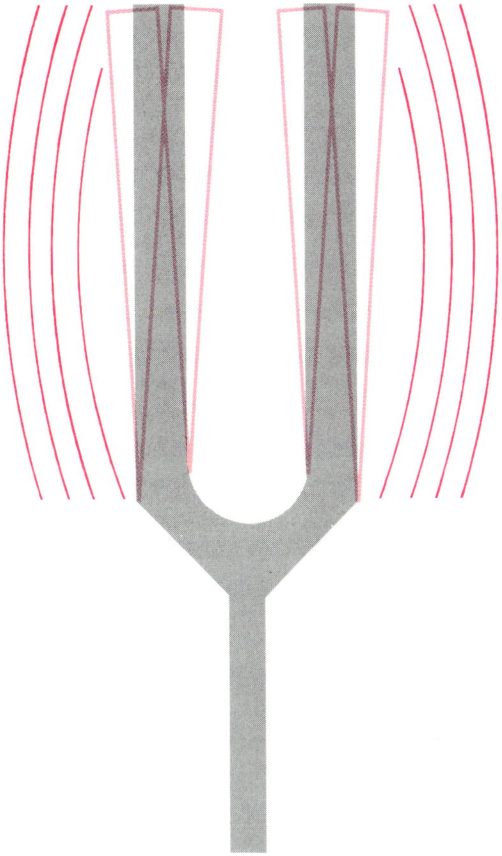

**13.8** Sound waves are produced by a tuning fork.

## How We Hear

But not all vibrating objects produce sound. You cannot hear a person waving his hand back and forth, although you realize that one is alternately compressing and rarefying the air molecules around one's hand. To most of us, sound is not produced unless we can hear it, but to the scientist, sound is waves in the air, whether it can be heard or not.

Figure 13.9 on page 412 shows the structure of the human ear. The sound waves enter the passageway of the outer ear. They strike the **eardrum,** making it vibrate. Inside the eardrum are three tiny bones that conduct the vibrations to the **cochlea** (kok′ li ə), or the inner ear. The last bone, the **stirrup,** is attached to the cochlea at a thin bit of tissue called the **oval window.**

The cochlea consists of many cavities, each containing a fluid. In this fluid float many nerve endings that lead to the brain. The vibration of the oval window causes the fluid to vibrate, and this stimulates the nerves. Our brains have learned to interpret these vibrations as sound.

## Nodes and Antinodes

Sometimes sounds interfere with each other in such a way that we cannot hear them. If two identical sounds are created

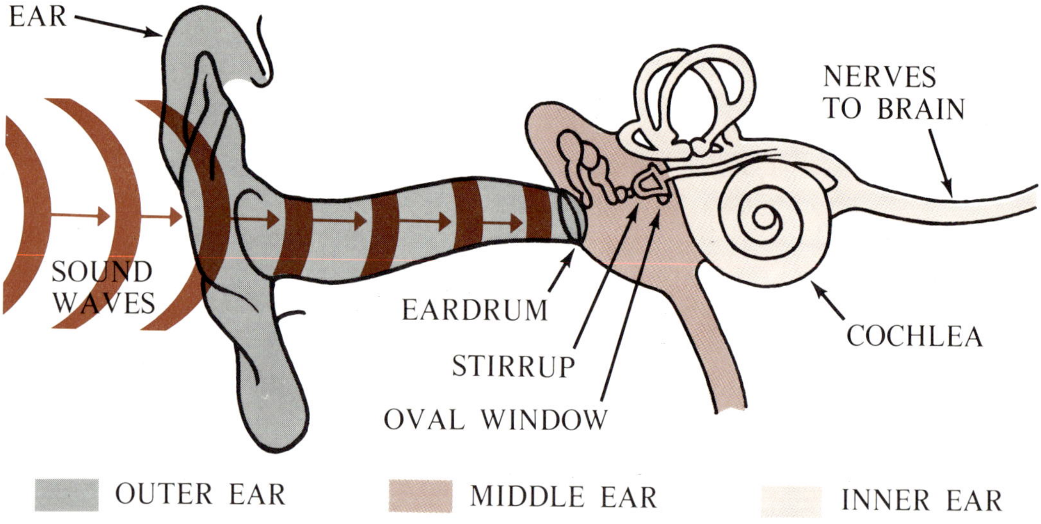


**13.9** Anatomy of human ear

**13.10** A ripple tank is used to study wave motion. The light shines down on the pan of water, and the waves produce shadows on the white cardboard upon the floor below.

*Norman D. Anderson*

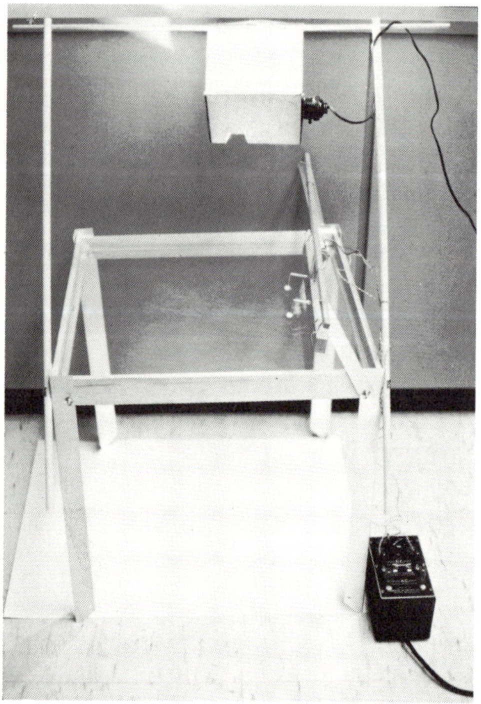

by two sources, the sound waves move through the air toward each other. Since each wave is a disturbance of the air molecules, when the waves meet they will affect the same particles of air. If an area of compression from one wave and an area of rarefaction from the other wave reach the same point at the same time, each will cancel out the other, and no movement of the air molecules will take place. Therefore, no sound will be heard at this point. We call the areas in which no movement takes place **nodes** (nōd).

But if areas of compression from both waves reach the same point at the same time, the movement of the air molecules is increased. The result of this is an increase in the loudness of the sound. These points are called **antinodes** (an′ ti nōd).

A ripple tank like the one in Figure 13.10 is often used in laboratories to study wave motion. When a vibrating object touches the water in the tank, waves are formed on the surface of the water. If two objects a few inches apart and vibrating at the same frequency touch the surface of the water, two sets of waves are produced. When the waves cross each other, many nodes and antinodes are made. Picture, if you can, the movement of these waves. As a compression of one wave moves ahead, it meets the rarefaction of the other. This point of meeting is *always in the same place*. Because of this, the node remains at the same location as the waves pass by it. The waves thus seem to remain stationary and for this reason they are called **standing waves.**

You can easily hear the effect of the interference of two different sound waves produced by a tuning fork.

## Interfering with Sound Waves

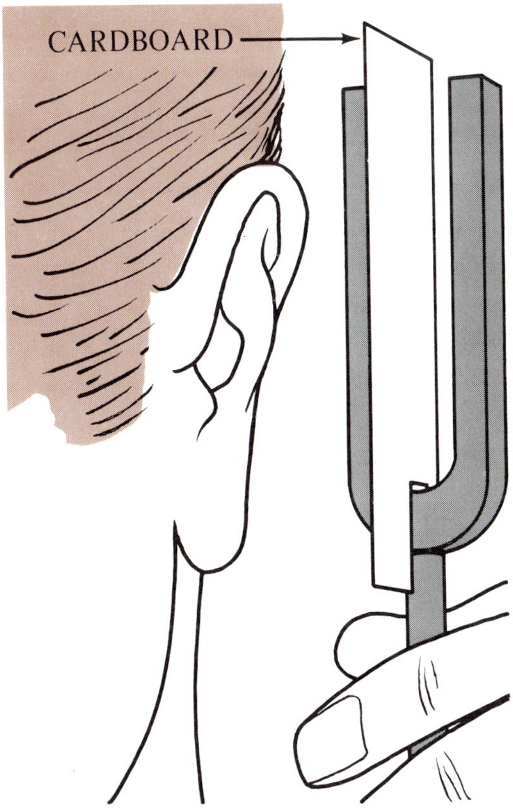


**MATERIALS:**

A tuning fork, a small piece of cardboard

**PROCEDURE:**

Strike the tuning fork on the rubber heel of your shoe or on the heel of your hand, and hold it close to your ear, as shown in the diagram. Slowly rotate it until you can hear no sound. Rotate it again until you hear the sound. In which position was the fork when you could not hear the note?

In the cardboard cut a notch slightly larger than one arm of the tuning fork. Again set the fork into motion, but this time shield one arm of the fork with the cardboard, as shown in the diagram. Hold the fork close to your ear, as shown in the diagram. Can you hear the sound? Without changing your position, remove the cardboard shield. What happens to the loudness of the sound?

Can you explain why the cardboard shield allowed you to hear the sound as long as it was in position?

In the activity above, the tuning fork produced two separate sound waves. The first was produced as the arms of the fork moved outward, causing a compression that moved away from the fork. The second wave was created as the arms moved *inward.* This wave moves at right angles to the first, as if it were produced at a point midway between the arms.

The only difference between these two waves is that they are exactly out of phase with each other. That is, as the compression of one is being created, a rarefaction of the other is also being produced. Where these waves overlap, the rarefaction of one cancels out the compression of the other, and a node occurs.

### Have You Learned?

On a sheet of paper list the numbers for the questions below. By each number write *T* if the statement is true and *F* if false.

1. Sound travels through matter in the form of longitudinal waves.
2. Vibrating objects always cause sound.
3. Sound vibrations are carried directly to the brain through the ear.
4. A node is a point at which two sounds cancel each other, and no sound is heard.
5. If the area of compression from one sound meets the area of compression from another sound, an antinode is produced.
6. The cochlea and stirrup are parts of the ear.
7. A wave that does not move is called a standing wave.
8. As the arms of a tuning fork move outward, an area of compression is formed between the arms of the fork.
9. All sounds can be heard.
10. The two waves produced by a tuning fork may cancel each other.

## 4. Properties of Sound

**ARE YOU READY?**

Look up the following words if you are not sure of their meanings:

amplitude; compression; cycle; frequency; pendulum.

If you were asked to describe a noise, you probably would mention two characteristics—its loudness and its **pitch.** You might use such phrases as "a loud, low rumble" to describe thunder, or "a soft, high whine" to describe the noise of an electric motor.

### Loudness of a Sound

The loudness of a noise depends a great deal upon the ability of a person to hear well. Since each person hears sounds differently, the scientist has developed a better term to use when he measures the amount of sound energy. This is **intensity** (in ten′ sə ti).

Intensity is a measure of the energy of a given wave. Therefore, it is determined by the *amplitude* of the wave. You will recall from Section 1 of this chapter that the amplitude of a wave is a measure of the maximum distance a single particle is moved from its normal position. The more coils of the spring you compressed, the more energy you put into the wave and the higher the amplitude of the wave.

The units used to measure the intensity of sound waves are called **decibels** (des′ ə bel). A sound with enough energy to be barely heard by normal human ears under average conditions is said to have an

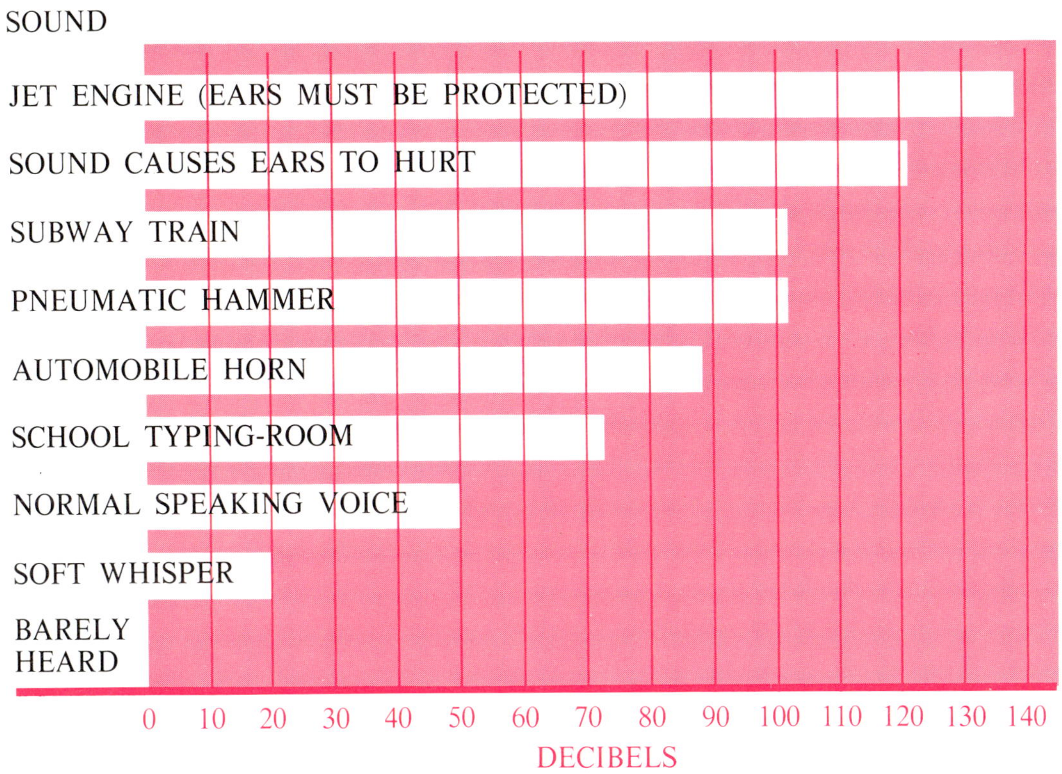


**13.11** The intensity of sound waves, measured in decibels

intensity of 0 decibels. A sound with 10 times this much energy will be rated at 10 decibels. A sound that is measured at 20 decibels *does not have twice* as much energy as a 10-decibel sound, however. It has 10 times as much energy as a 10-decibel sound, or 100 times as much energy as a 0-decibel sound. The intensity of a 30-decibel sound is 10 times greater than a 20-decibel sound, which makes it 1,000 times more intense than a 0-decibel sound. From this can you figure out how much energy a 40-decibel sound has? A 50-decibel sound? A 100-decibel sound?

If all other characteristics of the wave remain the same, an increase in the amplitude of a wave will result in an increase in the loudness of the sound. The harder you strike a drum, the farther you move the particles of the drumhead and the louder the sound.

You know from experience that the closer you are to the source of a noise, the louder it seems, even though the amplitude of the waves remains the same. This is because at a distance a smaller portion of the wave actually strikes your eardrum.

Imagine a bell that is hit. The sound waves spread out in a series of circles like the ripples on a pond. The energy of the hit spreads out as waves as it moves away from the source of the sound. At a distance of 20 meters from the bell, the energy wave is spread over four times as much area as it was at 10 meters from the bell. Therefore, only ¼ as much energy falls on your eardrum, and the loudness is only $\frac{1}{4}$ as great. At 40 meters, the noise will be only $^1/_{16}$ as loud as it would be at 10 meters.

## Pitch of Sound

The property of sound known as pitch depends upon the frequency of the wave. Since sound waves are caused by the vibration of some object, the frequency of a wave is equal to the number of times the object vibrates in a given length of time. It is a measure of the number of complete waves that strike your ears each second.

Sounds with a low pitch, such as the growl of a dog or a bass note on a piano, have low frequencies. A high-pitched sound, such as the squeak of chalk on the blackboard, is the result of a high-frequency vibration.

One complete vibration is called a cycle. A tuning fork that vibrates at 256 cycles per second produces a sound of the pitch or frequency close to that produced by the piano key called "middle C." Another tuning fork, vibrating twice as fast (512 cycles per second) produces a sound with a much higher pitch. This is the C an octave (8 notes) above middle C. A piano is tuned to a slightly higher frequency. A piano's middle C is about 262 cps.

Each tuning fork, each string of a piano, and almost every other object tend to vibrate at a certain number of cycles per second. Perhaps you have noticed that sometimes you can start a swing to vibrate back and forth by a series of small pushes. By shifting your weight back and forth at just the right time, the swing can be made to go very high. If, on the other hand, you do not shift your weight in time with the natural frequency of the swing, you cannot build up the motion of the swing.

### Investigating the Frequency of a Swing

**MATERIALS:**

A long string with a weight tied to the end, a watch with a sweep-second hand

**PROCEDURE:**

Tie the string from an overhead support so that it is free to swing. Pull the weight to one side, and release it. Count the number of cycles per minute this pendulum makes. Make the amplitude of the vibration smaller. Does this affect the frequency?

Now shorten the pendulum string until it is about one-half as long as before. Does this affect the frequency of the swing?

The natural frequency of a swing depends upon the length of the swing itself. By trial-and-error experimenting you discover what this frequency is. You lean forward in the swing just as the swing starts forward, and back as the swing moves back. The result of this motion is to increase the amplitude of the swing, using only small forces. When two objects move together like this, we say that they (in this case, the swing and you) are **resonating** (rez′ ə nāt).

To get a better understanding of how this works, try the following experiment.

## Observing the Movements of Two Pendulums

**MATERIALS:**

A meterstick, two pieces of string of the same length, two heavy weights (such as two large bolts)

**PROCEDURE:**

Construct two pendulums as you did in the activity on page 416, tying both to the same meterstick, about 20 cm. apart. Be certain that the lengths of the two pendulums are exactly the same. Have two friends hold the stick securely by each end. After the pendulums have come completely to rest, start *one* of them swinging. Describe the action of the second pendulum.

In this experiment you saw an example of resonance. The swinging pendulum caused small vibrations in the meterstick that were then transmitted to the second pendulum. Since these vibrations were the same as the natural frequency of the second pendulum, it too began to move. What would happen if the pendulums were of different lengths? Try it and see.

Resonating objects are common. Perhaps you have heard a rattle in your family's car that can be heard only at certain speeds. The loose part vibrates violently only when the vibrations of the motor match its natural frequency. A group of marching soldiers may cause a bridge to sway dangerously if the natural frequency of the bridge happens to equal the frequency of their marching. It is common for groups of marchers to "break step" before crossing a bridge.

Resonance also may be observed in musical instruments. The following activity will demonstrate this.

**13.12** Resonating tuning fork

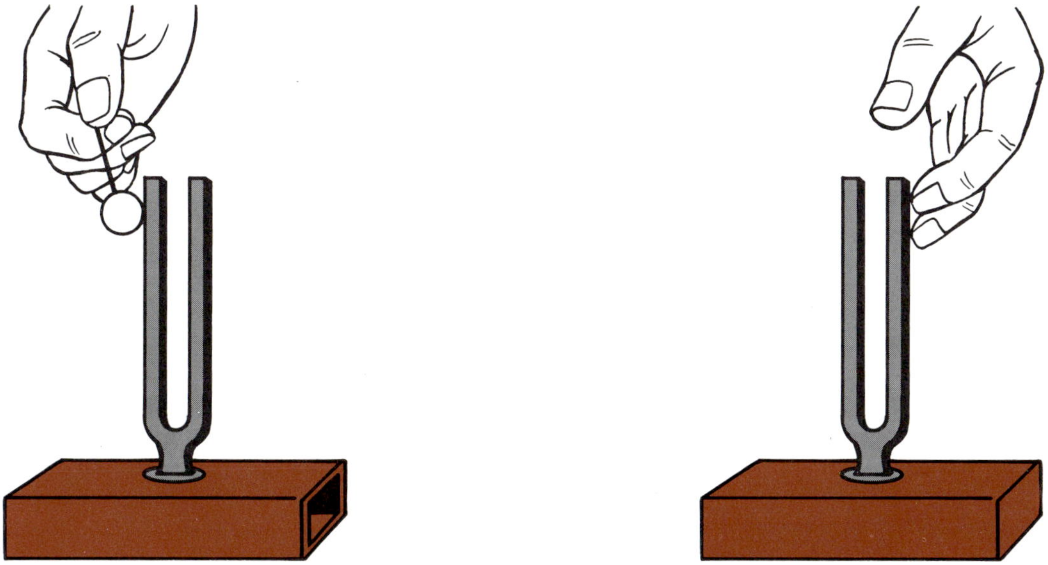

## Resonating Tuning Forks

**MATERIALS:**

Two resonance boxes with large tuning forks attached

**PROCEDURE:**

Place the resonance boxes as shown in the diagram, with their mouths opposite each other. Strike one tuning fork sharply with a rubber hammer. Gently touch the second fork. Can you feel it vibrate? Can you explain what happened?

A vibrating tuning fork may cause the string of a musical instrument to begin vibrating if the string has been tuned to the fork. Can you demonstrate this?

### Have You Learned?

Write on a sheet of paper the word that best completes the statement.

1. The scientist uses the term _____ to describe the loudness of a sound.
2. The loudness of a sound depends upon the energy or _____ of the wave.
3. Pitch depends upon the _____ of the sound wave.
4. If you increase the length of a pendulum, you _____ the frequency of its swing.
5. If two objects are vibrating at the same frequency, we say that they are _____.
6. The units used to describe the intensity of a sound are called _____.
7. A sound 10 meters away from you will be only ____ as loud as it would be if you were 5 meters away from it.
8. One complete vibration of a wave is one _____.
9. The musical note called "middle C" is caused by a tuning fork vibrating at 256 cps. The C above middle C vibrates at _____ cps.
10. If a piano string is tuned to a certain tuning fork and the fork is struck, the string will probably _____.

## 5. Music or Noise?

> **ARE YOU READY?**
>
> Look up the following words if you are not sure of their meanings:
>
> amplitude; antinode; clarinet; cycle; density; natural frequency; node; octave; pitch; rarefaction.

What is the difference between notes played on a piano and the sound of a bursting firecracker? Both create sound waves in the air, yet we identify one as music and the other as noise.

### Loudness and Pitch of Musical Sounds

While there would be some disagreement among different people, most of us agree that sounds produced by an object that vibrates regularly are generally pleasant. Such objects produce sound waves that are all the same length and of the same frequency. A sound that we would describe as noise is made of waves that vibrate irregularly.

Like all other sounds, musical sounds differ from each other in loudness and in pitch. Loudness, as you have already learned, is determined by the amplitude of the sound wave and is a measure of the energy of the wave.

Pitch depends upon the frequency of the wave, and is measured in the number of complete cycles of the wave per second—the greater the frequency, the higher the pitch. The frequencies of the sounds in two octaves are shown in Figure 13.13 on page 420. Notice that the frequency of a note in the upper octave is exactly twice that of the same note in the lower octave. What would be the frequency of the note in the next higher octave?

### Another Difference Between Musical Sounds

Loudness and pitch are not the only characteristics of musical sounds. With very little training, most of us can tell the difference between notes played on various instruments. For example, middle C played on a piano sounds very much different from middle C played on a clarinet. Yet the frequency of the sounds is the same. This difference is known as **quality.**

Differences in quality occur because all parts of an object may not vibrate at the same time. For example, if you pluck the string of a violin, the entire string vibrates. The tone that it produces is called a **fundamental,** and is caused by the natural frequency of the string. However, a bowed violin string may vibrate in several segments, as shown in Figure 13.14 on page 421. The quality of this sound depends upon the number of segments that are vibrating.

Objects that are forced to vibrate in segments produce notes that are called **overtones.** If a violin string vibrates in two segments, a *first overtone* sound wave will be produced. The frequency of this first overtone will be exactly twice the frequency of the fundamental tone. A *second overtone* may be created, caused by the vibration of the string in three segments. The frequency of this overtone will be *three* times the frequency of the fundamental. Half-a-dozen or more overtones, sounded with a fundamental tone, produce

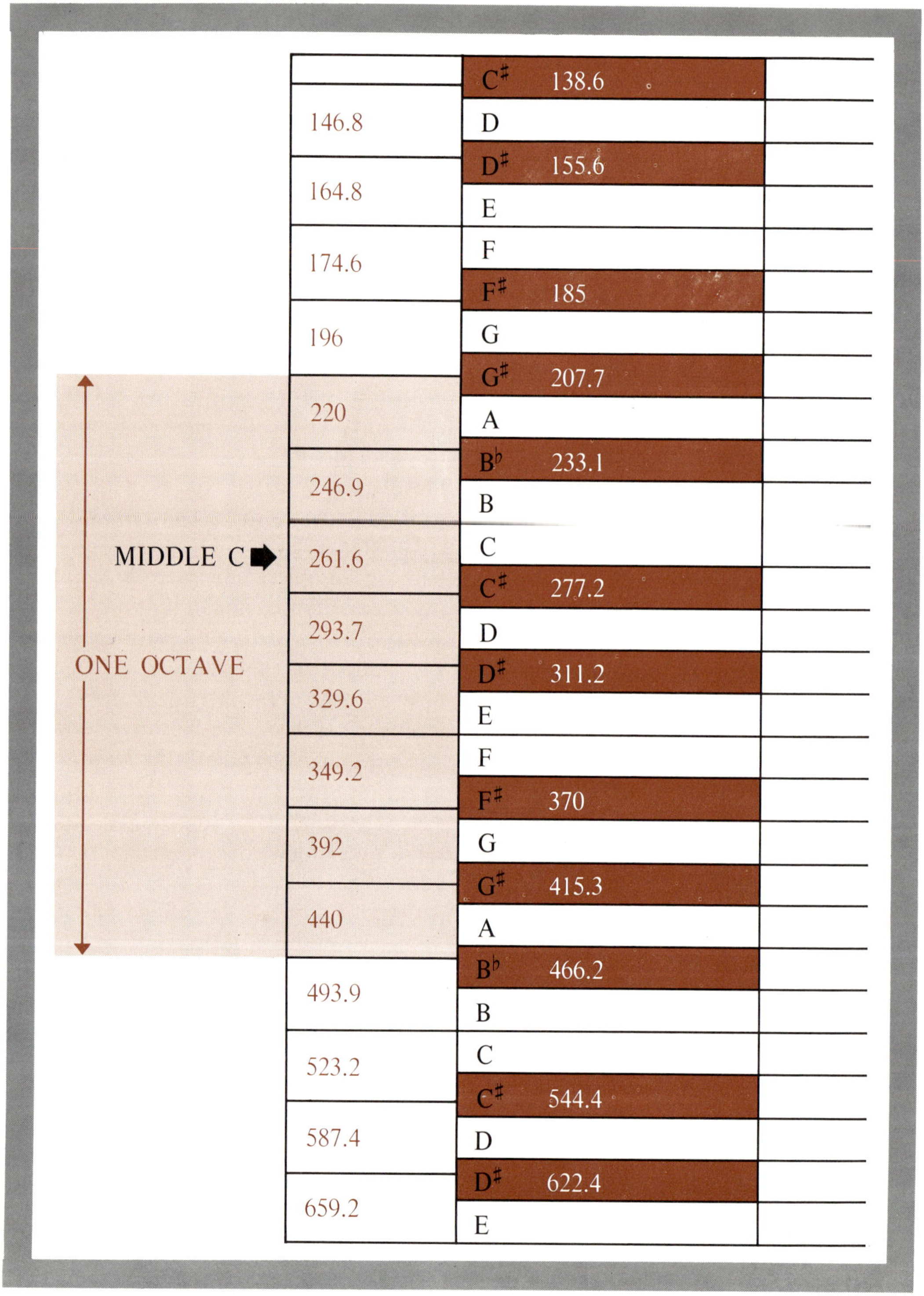


**13.13** The vibrations of notes of different pitches

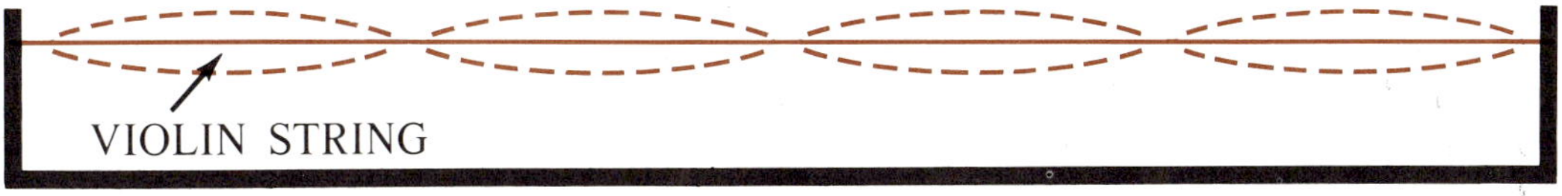


**13.14** The vibration of a music string

a sound with a certain quality. Without realizing it, we listen for characteristic overtone patterns in music and can thereby identify the sound as being from a violin, from a trombone, or from a human voice.

## Factors Affecting Pitch

But the most important characteristic of a musical sound is its pitch, and pitch is controlled by the natural frequency of the vibrating object. Look at the strings of a piano. Some are thick and heavy, while others are thin. Some are long, and others short. At one end of each string is a pin with which the piano tuner tightens or loosens each string (Figure 13.15 below).

The natural frequency of a string depends partly on its density and thickness. The thick, heavy strings vibrate more slowly than do the light, thin strings. Since the frequency of these strings is low, the pitch of the sound they produce is also low.

A long string has a lower frequency than it would if it were shortened, and therefore produces a note that is pitched

**13.15** With a tuning wrench the piano tuner adjusts pitch by increasing or decreasing the tension of each string.

*J. W. McDonald*

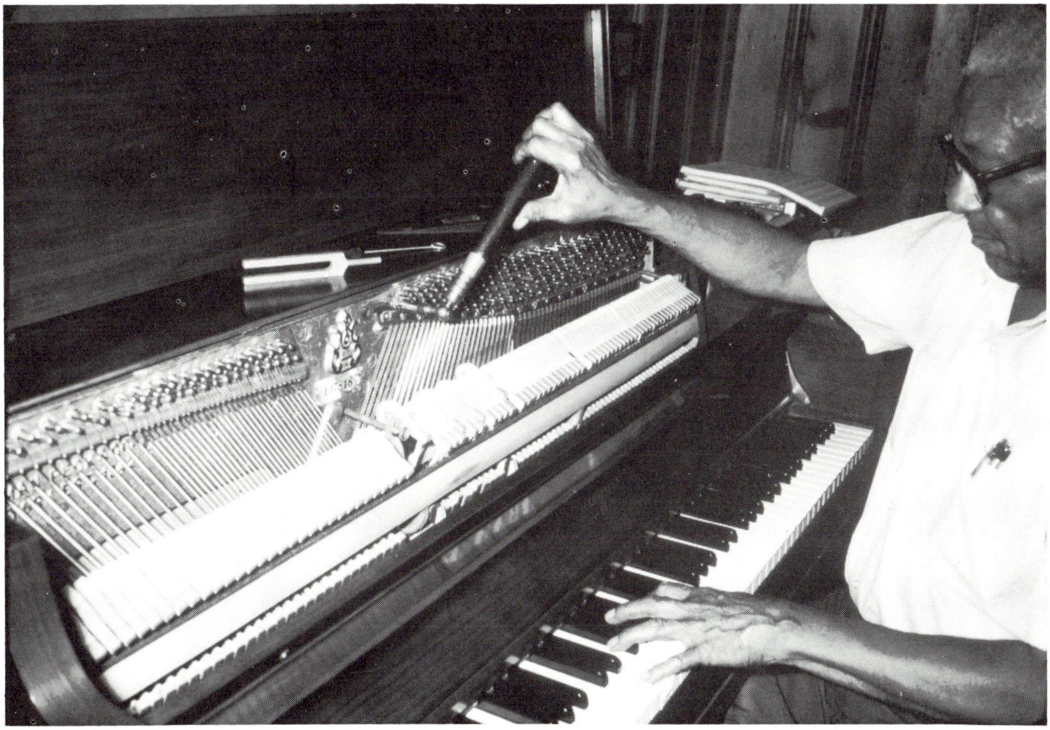

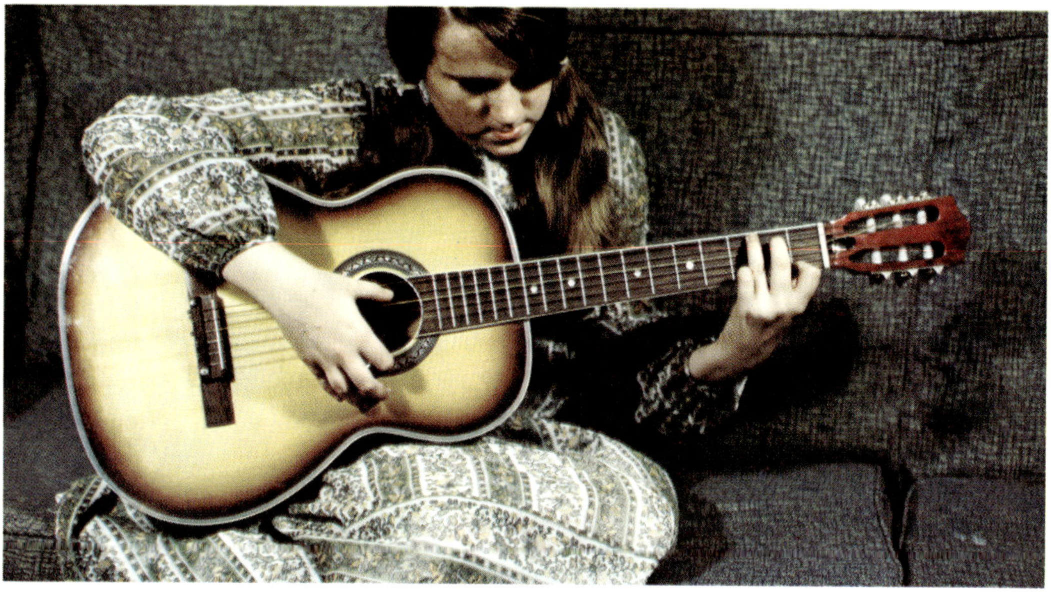

J. W. McDonald

**13.16** By pressing the strings upon the frets of the fingerboard, a guitarist shortens and thus raises the pitch of the strings.

lower. A violinist shortens the length of the strings of his instrument by pressing the string down with his finger. The closer his left hand is to the bow, the higher the pitch of the music he plays.

The tighter a string is stretched, the faster it vibrates. This increased frequency raises the pitch of the sound it produces. Stringed instruments are tuned by increasing or decreasing the **tension** (ten′ shən) of the strings (Figure 13.16 above).

When air is in a container, it has a natural frequency of vibration that depends upon the *length* of the column of air.

## Making Vibrating Columns of Air

**MATERIALS:**

Five bottles of the same shape (like those that soft drinks come in), a container of water

**PROCEDURE:**

Pour different amounts of water into each bottle, leaving one completely empty. Blow across the mouth of each bottle, so as to produce a musical note.

Arrange the bottles in order of their pitch, with the lowest on your left and the highest on your right. How does the length of the column of air compare with the pitch of the sound produced by it?

The waves produced in an air column are standing waves, similar to those discussed in Section 3 of this chapter. In a container that is closed at one end, the air near the sealed end cannot vibrate. Therefore, a node is formed at this point. At the open end, the air expands and escapes. This rarefaction creates an antinode. Thus, the longer the column of air, the longer the wave that can fit inside it.

If the column is open at both ends, antinodes will occur at each end. But still, the length of the column determines the wave length of the sound wave. In this way, it also determines the pitch.

All wind instruments are constructed on these principles. Look closely at a few of these types of instruments, and see if you can see how the length of the column of air is changed to produce different notes. Also try to determine how the air is made to vibrate in each instrument.

## Have You Learned?

Select the word from Column B that best answers each question in Column A. (Do not write in your book.)

*Column A*

1. Loudness of a sound is determined by what characteristic?
2. The pitch of a sound depends upon what characteristic?
3. We can tell the difference among various musical instruments by what characteristic of their sounds?
4. The tone produced by a string vibrating as a whole at its natural frequency is known as what?
5. Notes produced by objects vibrating in segments are called what?

6.-7. Pitch is controlled by what two characteristics of a string?

8. The natural frequency of a column of air depends upon what characteristic?
9. If a column of air is enclosed in a tube open at only one end, what is formed at the closed end?
10. If a string is tightened, what characteristic of its tone increases?

*Column B*

a. amplitude
b. antinode
c. frequency
d. fundamental
e. length
f. node
g. overtones
h. pitch
i. quality
j. thickness

## REVIEW QUESTIONS

1. How do transverse waves differ from longitudinal waves?
2. In describing the frequency of a wave, the words "vibration" and "cycle" are both used. Explain what these words mean and how they can be used to mean the same thing.
3. (A) A source of energy produces waves that have a frequency of 100 vps and a length of 3 meters. Calculate the velocity of the waves.
   (B) A wave has a velocity of 20 meters per second and a frequency of 5 vps. Calculate the length of this wave

4. Explain why you see the lightning flash before you hear the thunder.
5. If you stood 700 meters from a large building and shouted, how long would it take the echo to reach you? Explain how you got your answer.
6. Explain the difference between the elasticity and the density of a substance.
7. If two identical sounds are produced and their waves meet at a certain point, either a node or an antinode may be produced. How can you tell which is produced? Explain your answer.
8. Explain why, if you hold a vibrating tuning fork in exactly the right position, you cannot hear it.
9. Discuss the difference between the pitch and the intensity of a sound.
10. Explain why a middle-C tuning fork will cause a properly tuned middle-C string of a piano to vibrate.

## CAN YOU FIND OUT?

*It may be necessary to use encyclopedias or other reference books in answering the following questions.*

1. The speed of sound through air increases as the density of the air becomes less. Why will sound not travel well through a near vacuum, where the density of the air is nearly zero?
2. Does sound travel faster through air near the surface of the earth or through air several miles above the earth? Why?
3. What is "sonic boom"? What causes it? Why is it becoming a serious problem?
4. Select five different types of musical instruments, and describe how the sound of each can be changed.

## REFERENCES FOR ADDITIONAL STUDY

ALL ABOUT SOUND AND ULTRASONICS by Ira Freeman. Random House, Inc.
A well-illustrated account of present uses of sound and future applications

EXPERIMENTS WITH SOUND by Nelson Beeler. Thomas Y. Crowell Company.
Covers sources of sound, speed, measurements, uses, and ultrasonic sound

NOISE POLLUTION by Charles Lavaroni and Patrick A. O'Donnel. Addison-Wesley Publishing Co., Inc.
Gives background information on noise pollution and contains 23 student activities on sound and hearing

SOUND AND HEARING by S. S. Stevens, Fred Warshofsky and the Editors of Time-Life Books, A Division of Time Inc.
One book of the Life Science Library—describes various aspects of sound energy and hearing with short descriptions and many, many colored photographs

CHAPTER **14**

# Light

ALMOST DAILY we use instruments that help us see more clearly, instruments that help us look at tiny objects, instruments that help us study distant things, or instruments that record what we see. The development and manufacture of these instruments, as well as their proper use, depends upon the knowledge that scientists have been able to gain about light.

## 1. Sources of Light

**ARE YOU READY?**

Look up the following words if you are not sure of their meanings:

interior; light ray; model (scientific); nervous system.

Like sound, light can be defined in terms of the effect that it has on certain parts of the human nervous system. The true nature of light energy is much more complicated than heat and sound energy, and scientists are just beginning to understand it.

### Light-producing Objects

Some of the objects in your environment produce light. The sun, a burning candle, and a burning light bulb are all examples of **luminous** (lü′ mə nəs) (light-producing) objects.

Many objects are luminous only when they are hot. A bar of iron will glow only after it has been heated to a temperature above 800° C. The thin wires inside a light bulb may be more than 3,000° C. Our main source of light is the sun, whose interior temperature has been estimated to be 15 million degrees Celsius. Objects that give off light because of high temperature are called **incandescent.**

Not all luminous objects are incandescent. Touch a fluorescent tube and you will find that it is cool, even though it may have been on for some time. Perhaps you have seen insects called *lightning bugs* or *fireflies* that produce their own "cold light." Or perhaps you have seen a special kind of paint that glows in the dark.

But how do we see nonluminous objects? Have you ever been in total darkness

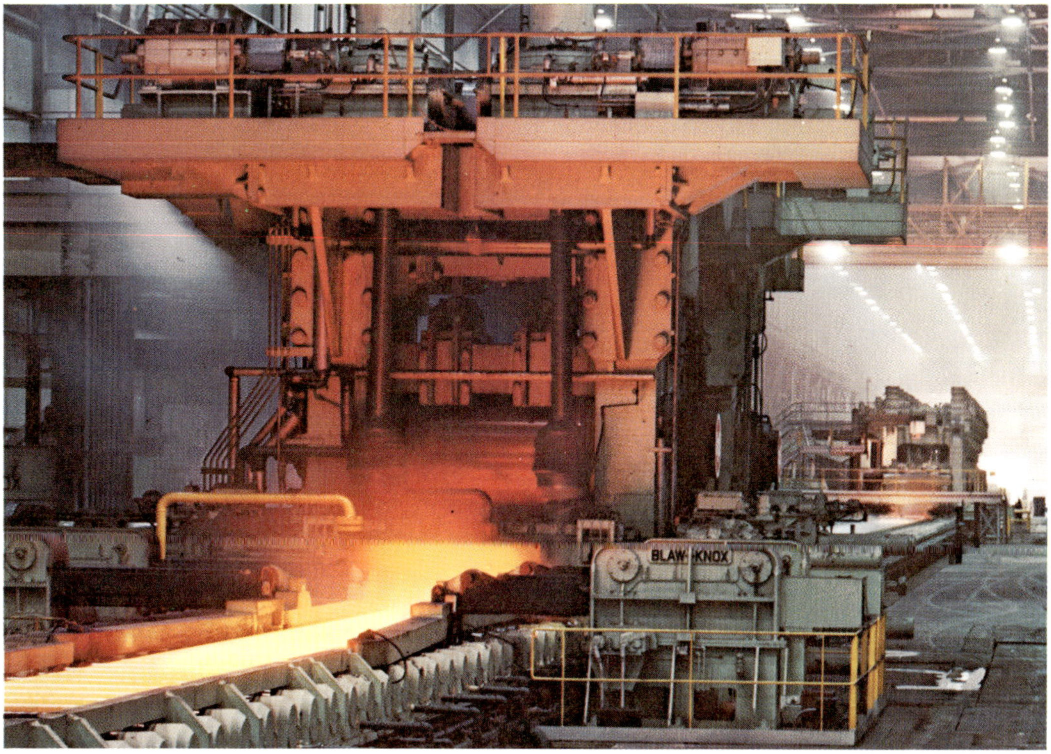


United States Steel Corporation

**14.1** Glowing steel in a rolling mill

—deep inside a cave, perhaps, where no light at all could be seen? Perhaps someone turned on a flashlight, and you could see again. You could see not only the luminous, incandescent bulb of the flashlight, but you could also see a portion of the nonluminous wall.

We see nonluminous objects by the **reflection** (ri flek′ shən) of light from luminous bodies. Look around you now. The light from the sun or from electric lights is striking many nonluminous objects. This light bounces off these objects and strikes your eyes.

## Light Travels in Straight Lines

Light appears to travel in straight lines from its source, as shown in Figure 14.2 on page 427. You can demonstrate this for yourself.

### Observing the Path of Light

**MATERIALS:**

Two small pieces of cardboard and a candle

**PROCEDURE:**

Punch small holes near the center of each piece of cardboard. Light the candle, and place it about 1 meter away from you. Have a friend hold one piece of cardboard about 30 cm from the candle, as shown in the diagram. Holding the second piece of cardboard to your eye, try to find a position from which you can see the candle flame through both holes. If you were to draw a line from the candle through both holes to your eye, would it be a straight line? (See Figure 14.3 below.)

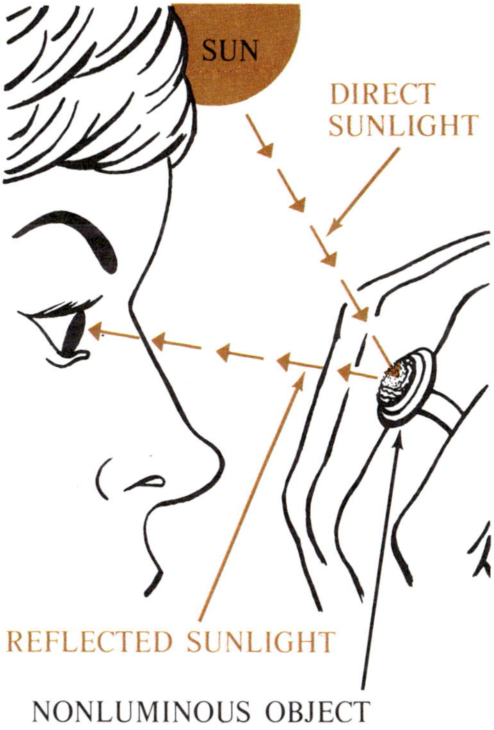


**14.2** Light striking a nonluminous object

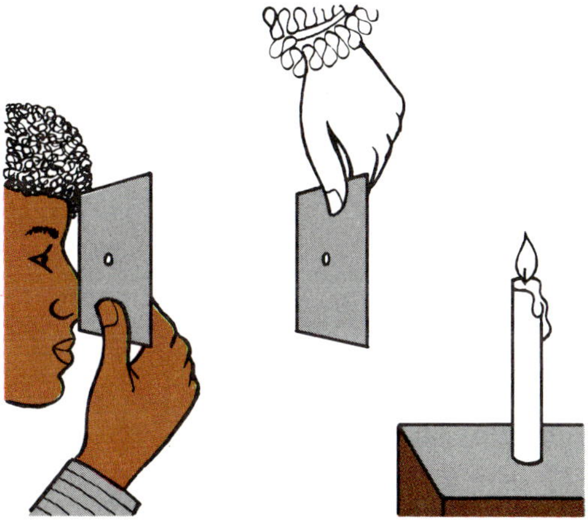

**14.3** Observing the Path of Light

From experiments such as this we assume that light rays travel only in straight lines. Under normal conditions this would appear to be true. However, the direction of light can easily be changed and scientists have taken advantage of this characteristic to make use of light energy.

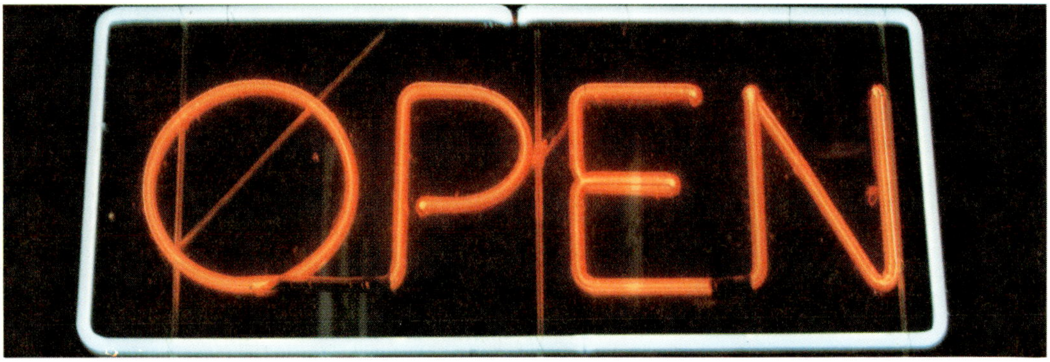


*Norman D. Anderson*

**14.4** A neon sign (See page 311.)

In much of the discussion that follows, we will speak of "light rays." You should understand that the idea of a ray is a mental model that is used to help us understand the behavior of light. Light probably does not travel in rays. A beam of light, such as is thrown by a flashlight, is considered to be made up of many, many rays.

### Have You Learned?

On a sheet of paper list the numbers for the questions below. By each number write *T* if the statement is true and *F* if false.

1. A luminous object is one that produces light.
2. A lightning bug (firefly) can be considered to be an incandescent object.
3. All luminous objects are incandescent.
4. All incandescent objects are luminous.
5. We can see nonluminous objects only by reflection of light from luminous bodies.
6. Light travels in the form of rays that are about the size of pencils.
7. Light rays appear to travel in straight lines.
8. The direction of light cannot be changed.
9. The sun is an incandescent object.
10. A flashlight is an incandescent object.

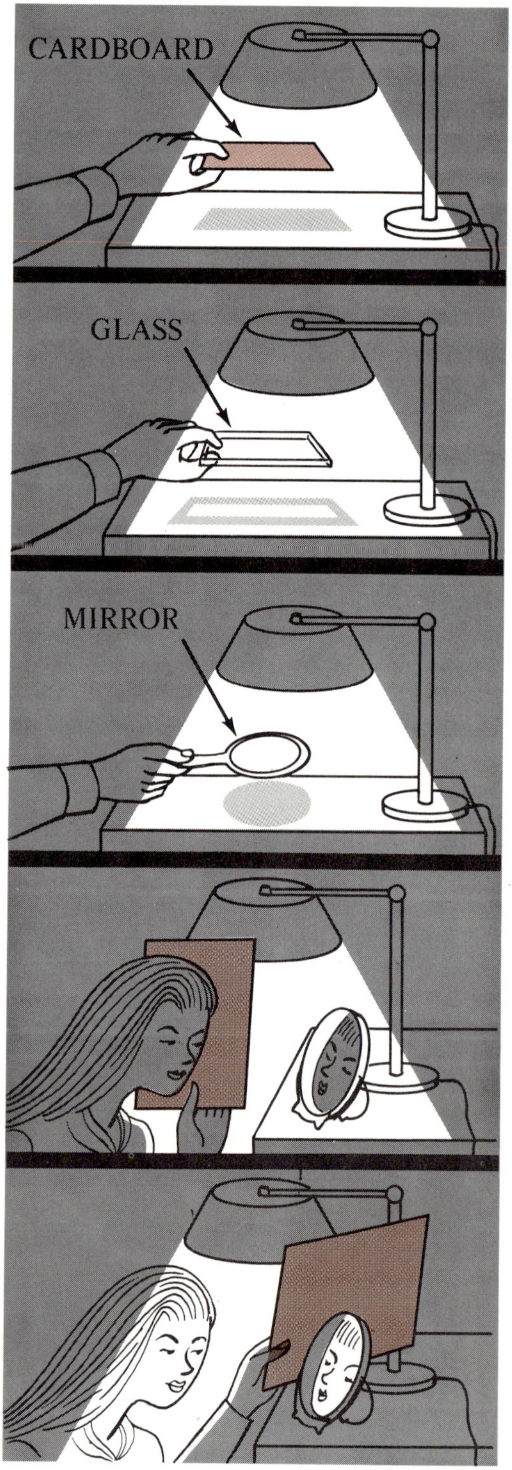


**14.5** Observing the Reflection of Light (See page 429.)

## 2. Reflection of Light

> **ARE YOU READY?**
>
> Look up the following words if you are not sure of their meanings:
>
> image; nonluminous; reflect; reflection; shadow.

One of the most useful characteristics of light is its ability to be reflected. Like an echo of a sound, light energy will bounce off many types of surfaces. Without this characteristic, nonluminous objects would be invisible.

Light is unable to pass through certain objects, such as cardboard. Such objects are said to be **opaque** (ō pāk′). Opaque objects cast shadows, and all of the light that strikes them is either absorbed or reflected.

### Observing the Reflection of Light

**MATERIALS:**

A darkened room, an electric lamp or similar light source, a piece of cardboard, a small piece of plain glass (such as is used in windows), a small hand mirror

**PROCEDURE:**

Hold the cardboard close to the table or floor and as directly under the light source as possible. Slowly move the cardboard upward toward the lamp. Describe the changes that take place in the shadow formed by the cardboard. (Figure 14.5 page 428)

Repeat the procedure, using the piece of glass in place of the cardboard. Can you see any shadow? If so, how does it differ from the shadow thrown by the cardboard in the first step?

Repeat the procedure again, this time using the mirror to cast the shadow. How does this differ from the shadows you observed before? Is the shadow cast by the mirror more like the shadow from the cardboard or from that of the plain glass?

Place the mirror on the table or floor so that you can see your reflection in it. First, hold the cardboard so that it blocks the light that falls on your face. Then move it so that it blocks the light that falls on the mirror. In which position can you see your face in the mirror more clearly? Can you explain why this is true?

You saw that when the cardboard was held some distance from the table, its shadow was not distinct. Figure 14.6 on page 430 shows why this happens. Since light comes from all parts of the light bulb, the light rays from one edge of the bulb pass on both sides of the cardboard, and overlap the shadow caused by rays from the opposite edge of the bulb. Only in the center of the shadow is there an area in which practically no light reaches the table.

A piece of glass is **transparent.** That is, light will pass through it without casting a shadow. If your piece of glass was highly transparent, it reflected very little light

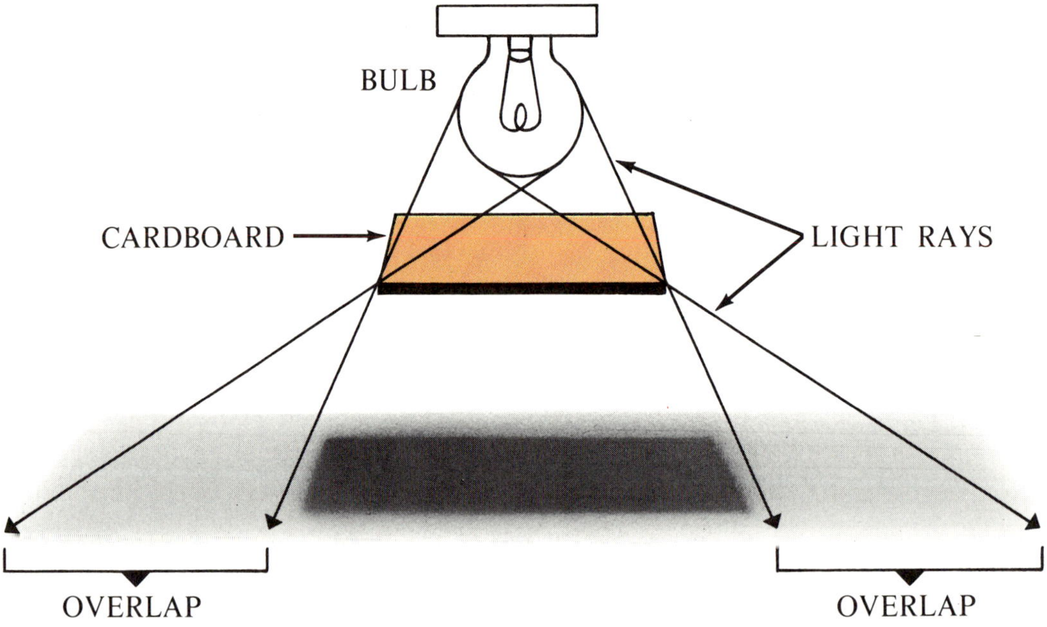


**14.6** Observing shadows cast by cardboard.

and was difficult to see even though the light shone directly on it. When you looked at an object through the glass, you could see it clearly.

Some objects will allow some light to pass through them, but some of it is **diffused** (di fūz′) or spread out. In addition, some of the light will also be reflected. This is called **translucence** (trans lü′ səns). Frosted glass is an example of a translucent material. Objects cannot be seen clearly through translucent glass.

## Mirrors

We can learn a great deal about the behavior of light by experimenting with a mirror. As you noticed in the activity above, the mirror is opaque. It reflects light differently than did the cardboard, however, since you can see your reflection in it. Look at the mirror and the piece of cardboard carefully. What differences do you see?

When light strikes the rough surface of an opaque object, it is diffused, or reflected in all directions, as shown in Figure 14.7.

**14.7** Light on smooth and rough surfaces

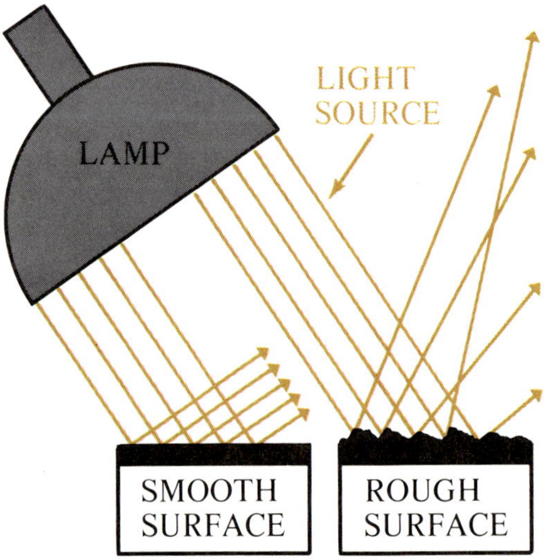

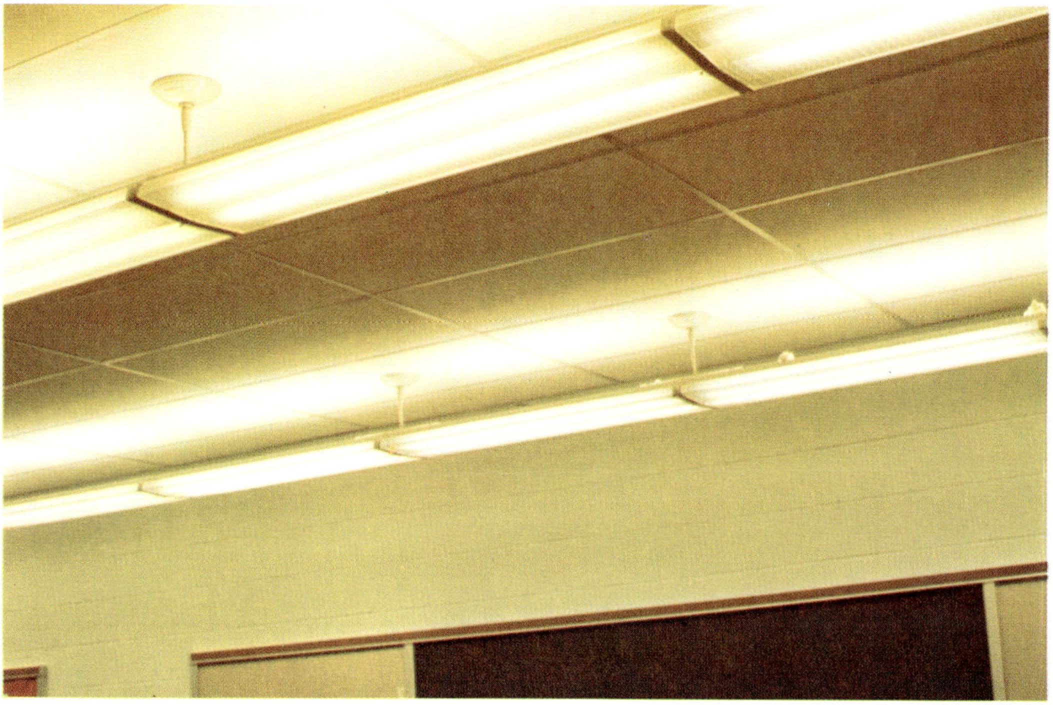

Walter R. Brown

**14.8** The diffusing shades below these fluorescent tubes are *translucent*.

This diffusion of reflected light accounts for the fact that you can see objects that are not struck directly by light rays. The light from the sun or from some other luminous object strikes the ground and particles of dust in the air and is reflected in all directions. Thus, we can see some light reflected from objects that are in a heavy shadow.

Figure 14.7 also shows light rays striking a very smooth surface, such as a mirror. Notice that all of the rays reflect from the mirror at the same angle. Because of this we are able to see **images** (im′ ij) reflected from the mirror. The image is what you see when you look in a mirror.

The following activity will help you to understand the behavior of light reflected from a smooth surface.

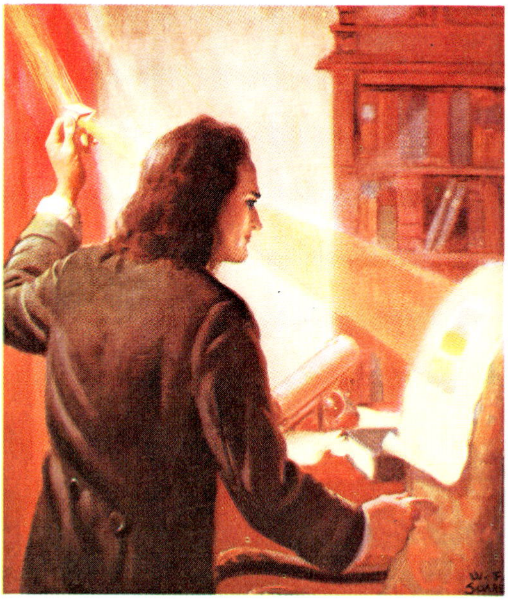

Bausch & Lomb

**14.9** Sir Isaac Newton and the prism

## Watching Reflected Light from a Mirror

**MATERIALS:**

A small flat mirror, two pencils, a sheet of paper, a protractor, a small ruler

**PROCEDURE:**

Support the mirror by leaning it against something in such a way that it is vertical. Position yourself so that you can see into the mirror but cannot see your own image. Place one pencil on the tabletop, and move it around until you can see its image in the mirror. Does the image of the pencil seem to be behind the mirror?

Lay the paper in front of the mirror, and place the second pencil against the mirror so as to cover the image of the first pencil. Mark the paper at this point. Also mark the paper to show where the base of the mirror is resting. Now lay the ruler down on the paper so that it indicates the direction from the pencil at the mirror to your eye, and mark this line. Also mark the line from the mirror to the pencil whose image you have been observing.

Construct a line that is perpendicular to the mirror and through the point at which the pencil touched the base of the mirror. Your diagram should look something like the one shown in Figure 14.11. Measure the two angles. Does angle R equal angle I?

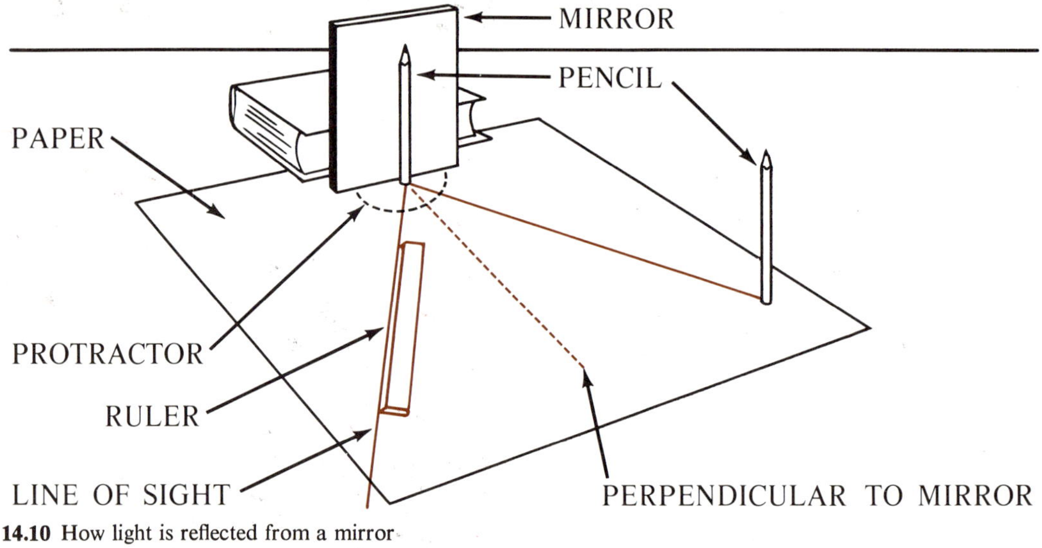


**14.10** How light is reflected from a mirror

Repeating the experiment several times will show you that the angle formed by the line from the pencil to the mirror and the perpendicular line, called the **angle of incidence** (in′ sə dəns), is always equal to the angle formed by the line from the image and the perpendicular **(angle of reflection)**. Try changing the position of the pencil and of your eye, and see if this is not true.

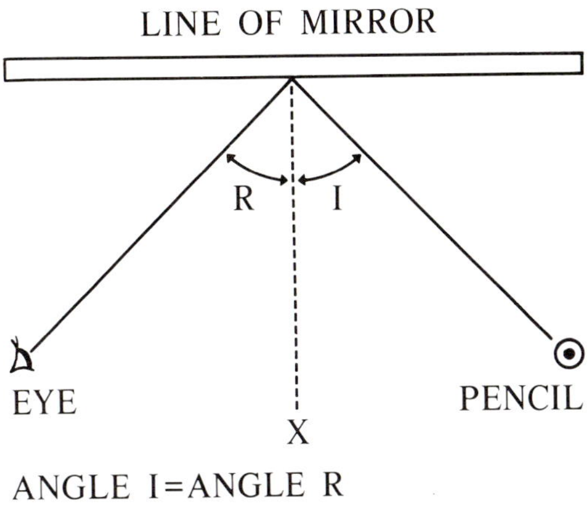


**14.11** Angle of incidence equals angle of reflection.

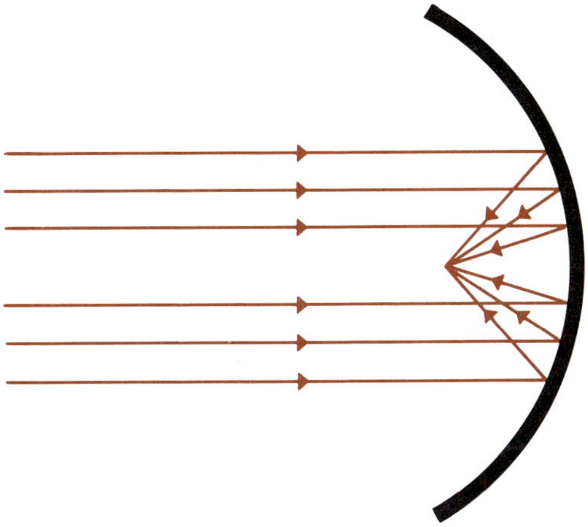

**14.12** Light reflected by a concave mirror

## Three Kinds of Mirrors

The mirror used in the activity on page 432 was a **plane** (plān) mirror. That is, it was flat. In a plane mirror, all of the light is reflected in the same direction.

In a **concave** (kon kāv′) mirror, which is curved inward, the light rays will be **focused** (fō′ kəs) at a certain point. Figure 14.12 makes this clear. Notice that the angle of incidence and the angle of reflection *for each light ray* are always equal.

By concentrating the light in this way, a spot of very bright light can be created. Since some light energy is transformed to heat energy when it strikes something, a "sun oven" can be easily constructed. By placing the object to be cooked at the focus point of a concave mirror, the sun's energy can be used directly (Figure 14.13).

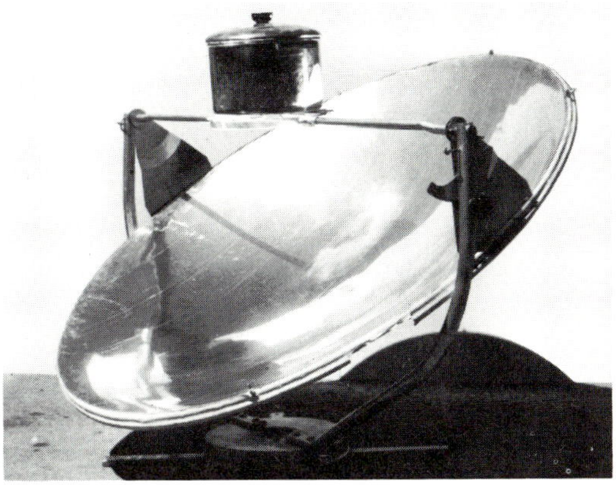

**14.13** A solar oven uses a concave mirror.

In a searchlight, the reverse situation occurs. The light source is placed at the point of focus in front of a concave mirror, and a beam of light is reflected away from the light, as shown in Figure 14.14.

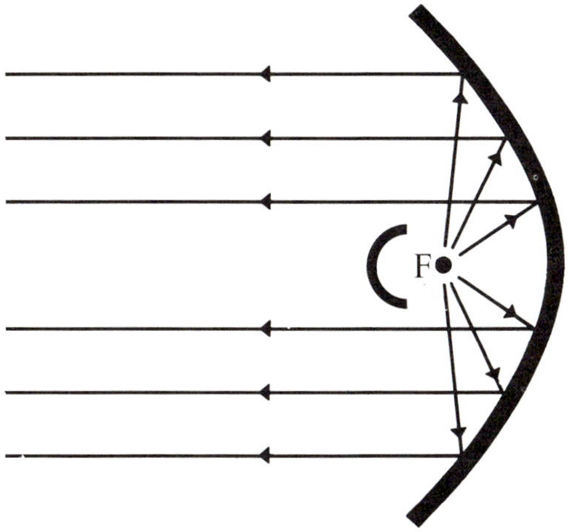


**14.14** Searchlight (F is the focal point.)

Figure 14.15 on page 434 shows what happens if light strikes a **convex** (kon veks′) mirror. Notice that the angle of incidence and the angle of reflection for each light ray are still equal. However, the shape of the mirror causes the light to be reflected in many directions.

## Have You Learned?

Select the word from Column B that best completes each statement in Column A. (Do not write in your book.)

| *Column A* | *Column B* |
|---|---|
| 1. A piece of cardboard throws a shadow because it is _____. | a. incidence |
| | b. concave |
| | c. diffused |
| | d. opaque |
| | e. image |
| 2. If light passes through an object in such a way that other objects may be seen clearly, we say that it is _____. | f. focused |
| | g. convex |
| | h. plane |
| | i. translucent |
| | j. reflection |
| | k. transparent |

3. A frosted light bulb will allow light to pass through it, but you cannot see the wires inside. This type of bulb is _____.
4. If light strikes a rough surface, the reflected light is _____ and no image is formed.
5.-6. The angle of _____ equals the angle of _____.
7. A mirror that is not curved is called a(n) _____ mirror.
8.-9. A mirror that is curved inward is called a(n) _____ mirror, and light reflected from it is _____ at a certain point.
10. In a searchlight the light is reflected from a(n) _____ mirror.
11. If you looked at yourself in a mirror that is slightly _____, you would appear to be much taller and wider than you actually are.

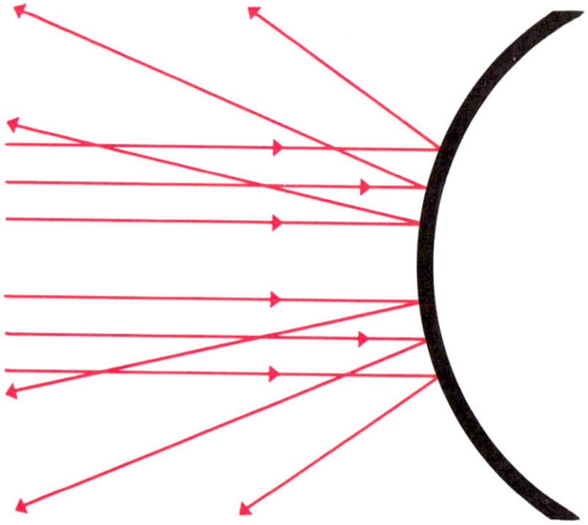

**14.15** Light reflected by a convex mirror

## 3. The Bending of Light

**ARE YOU READY?**

Look up the following words if you are not sure of their meanings:

beam of light; concave; convex; image; lens; ray of light; transparent.

Have you ever looked into a swimming pool and seen an object that looked as if it were only a few centimeters below the surface? But when you reached for it, you found that it was far beyond your reach. Or have you seen, in a glass of water, a drinking straw that looked bent? Then you found that when you took it out of the glass, the straw was really straight. Do you realize that the boy in Figure 14.16 on page 435 can see the fish, even though the dock is directly between the two of them?

### Viewing Objects Through Water and Lenses

From these observations, it is apparent that light does not always travel in straight

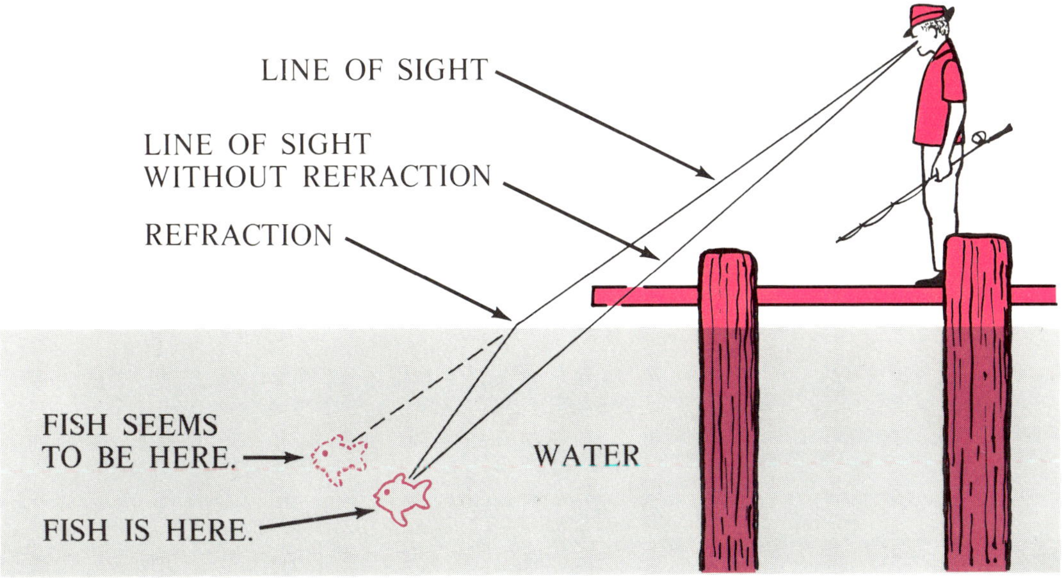


**14.16** The bending of light

lines. In almost every case where light passes from one substance to another at an angle, it will be bent.

The reason for the bending of light in these cases is that light does not travel through all substances at the same speed. To understand this effect, look at the drawing in Figure 14.17. It represents a beam of light composed of several light rays. As the first ray enters the piece of glass, it slows down. The other rays continue at their normal rate of speed until each reaches the surface of the glass. This slowing down of each ray in the beam in turn results in a bending of the beam. Can you explain why there is no bending if the entire beam strikes the surface of the glass at a right angle?

If the angle at which light strikes the surface of the new medium is greater than a certain amount, all of the light will be reflected and none of the light will pass through to the new medium. Because of this **internal reflection,** the diver in the diagram on page 436 cannot see the boy in the boat unless he moves more nearly under him.

The bending of light as it passes from one medium to another is called **refraction** (ri frak′ shən). We use curved pieces of glass or other transparent materials to make light bend as we want it to.

**14.17** Light is refracted by the glass block.

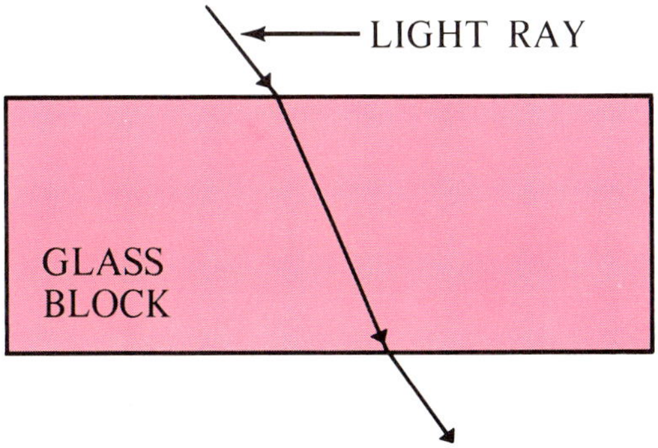

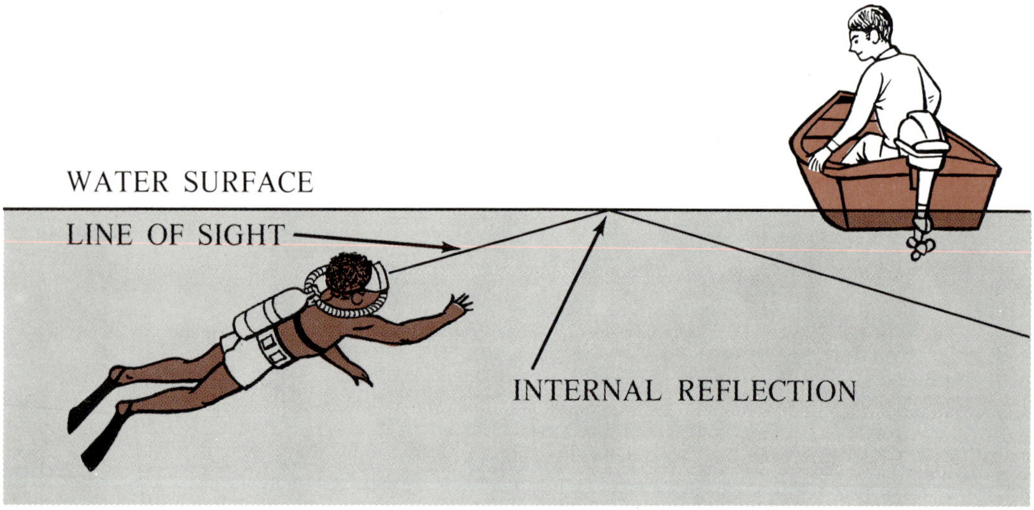


**14.18** Does the swimmer see the boy in the boat? Does the boy in the boat see the swimmer?

## Experimenting with Lenses

**MATERIALS:**

Several lenses (magnifying glasses), a source of light (such as a small candle), a yardstick or meterstick, a sheet of blank paper

**PROCEDURE:**

Select any one of the lenses that are available to you. Take it into the bright sunlight. Place a sheet of paper on the ground and hold the lens between the paper and the sun. Move the lens back and forth until you find the point at which the light from the sun forms the smallest spot possible. Measure the distance between the lens and the paper. Record this distance, and call it the **focal** (fō′ kəl) **length** of the lens.

Another way to find the focal length of your lens is to stand across the room from a brightly lighted window. Move your lens back and forth until you are able to focus a clear image of the window on the wall. Measure this distance. Does it agree closely with the distance you measured before?

Now take your lens into a darkened room. Place a lighted candle on a tabletop and lay the meterstick down so that its end touches the candle. Hold the lens at a point along the meterstick that is exactly four times the focal length of the lens. Hold the paper so that you can see a clear image of the candle projected on it.

Describe the image that you see. Is it right side up or **inverted** (in vėrt′)? Is it in color or in black-and-white? Is it larger or smaller than the real candle flame?

Move the lens toward the candle flame. Stop when the lens is at a distance from the flame that is equal to three times the focal length of the lens. Describe the image that you see. Is it larger than before?

Move the lens to a distance from the candle that is equal to twice the focal length of the lens. Describe the image. How does its size compare with the size of the real flame?

Move the lens to a distance from the candle that is equal to about 1½ times the focal length of the lens. Is the image larger or smaller than the actual candle flame?

Repeat the activity, using different lenses. Do all lenses have the same focal lengths? Do the images produced by each of the lenses differ at all?

Look carefully at the lenses you used in the activity. Probably most of them are convex lenses, thicker in the middle than they are on the edges. How does the shape of a convex lens compare with the shape of the convex mirror described in Section 2?

## How Lenses Refract Light

The light rays coming from a distant light source may be thought of as being *parallel* to each other. Since the edges of a convex lens are at a greater angle than the center of the lens, the light rays that pass through the edges are bent a great deal. Those rays that pass through the center of the lens are not bent at all. As shown in Figure 14.19, the **convex lens** causes the parallel light rays from a distant object to focus at a certain point. The distance between the lens and the point of focus is the focal length of the lens. For distant sources of light, the focal length of a particular lens will always be the same.

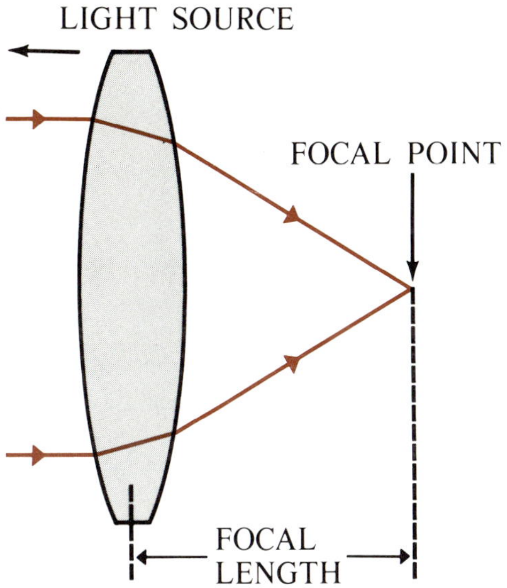


**14.19** How is light focused by a convex lens?

**14.20** Compare the size and location of the object on the left of the lens and its image on the right.

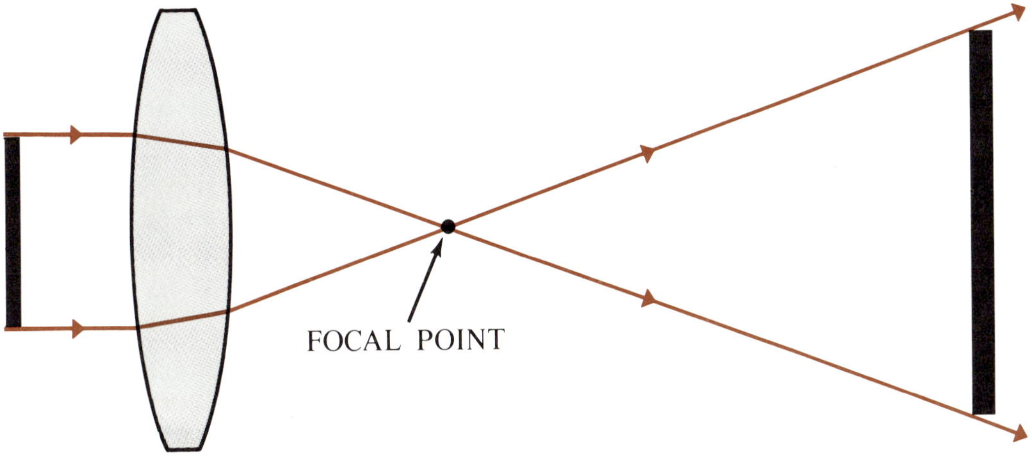

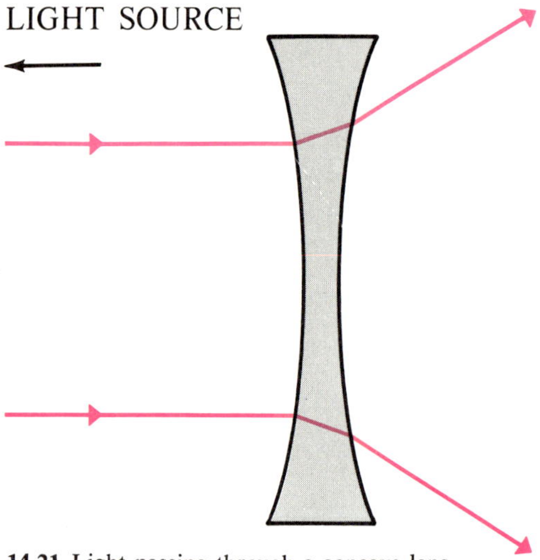


**14.21** Light passing through a concave lens

Figure 14.20 on page 437 shows what happens to the rays of light from an object that is close to the lens. Notice that when the object is close to the lens, the image is large and far beyond the focus point. When the object is moved farther away from the lens, the image is formed closer to the focus point and is smaller. The actual sizes of these distances and images depend upon the size and shape of the lens.

From what you have learned so far about the refraction of light, you should be able to guess what will happen to light as it passes through a *concave* lens. As shown in Figure 14.21, the **concave lens** causes the light to *spread outward.* Since the light is not focused at any point, an image cannot be formed on a screen.

## Have You Learned?

Select the answer that best completes each statement. (Do not write in your book.)

1. When light passes from one substance to another at an angle, it will usually _____ (be bent; continue in a straight line).
2. When light enters a piece of glass from the air, its speed _____ (increases; decreases).
3. Light that bounces off the surface of an object is said to be _____ (reflected; refracted).
4. If a piece of paper is placed at the focus of a convex lens, _____ (an image; a spot) will be formed.
5. A lens in which the edges are thinner than the center is said to be a _____ (convex; concave) lens.
6. When light passes through a concave lens, it is _____ (focused; spread out).
7. If light passes from one substance to another at right angles to the surface, it will _____ (be bent; continue in a straight line).
8. The bending of light as it passes from one substance to another is called _____ (reflection; refraction).
9. A convex lens causes light rays to be _____ (focused; spread out).
10. The focal length of two different-sized lenses will most likely be _____ (different; the same).

## 4. What Is Light?

> **ARE YOU READY?**
>
> Look up the following words if you are not sure of their meanings:
>
> angle of incidence; angle of reflection; frequency (of waves); interference; nodes (of waves); wavelength.

The ancient philosophers had observed that light seemed to travel in straight lines, that it reflected from smooth surfaces, and that it was bent when it passed from one medium to another. Some of these early scientists assumed that particles were given off by luminous objects and that these particles traveled to the eye. Others guessed that the eye itself gave off particles that traveled to the objects being seen and bounced back to the eye. These ideas of the nature of light were accepted until the mid-seventeenth century.

### Early Theories About Light

About 1675 Sir Isaac Newton tried to expand upon the theories of the earlier investigators. He assumed that light was indeed particles, or **corpuscles** (kôr′ pəs əl), as he called them. Like tiny balls traveling at very high speeds, light corpuscles would travel in straight lines. Since particles such as those he imagined could not bend around an object, a shadow would be formed. Like a thrown ball, light bounced off solid surfaces according to the law that states that the angle of incidence equals the angle of reflection. Newton's Corpuscular Theory explained the refraction of light by assuming that the molecules of the medium through which the light traveled attracted the light particles. Newton thought that as the light approached a denser medium, it was attracted by the particles of that medium, and its speed increased. This, he guessed, would cause a bending (refraction) toward the denser medium.

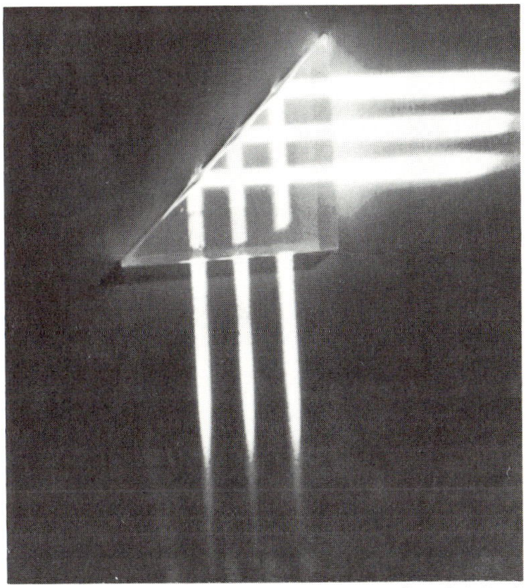

*Bausch & Lomb*

**14.22** Rays of light reflected by a prism

Newton's theory was widely accepted, in spite of the fact that it did not answer several important questions. For example, Newton himself had discovered that when light was refracted through a triangular piece of glass, called a **prism** (priz′ əm), it broke up into bands of red, orange, yellow, green, blue, and violet light. Yet his Corpuscular Theory could not explain why the red portions of light should be refracted less than the other portions. Likewise, he failed to explain the fact that two beams of light could cross each other, as shown in the photograph above, without the particles' hitting each other.

Across the English Channel from Newton, a Dutch physicist was developing another theory of the nature of light. In 1678 Christian Huyghens (hī′ gəns) suggested that light was really a form of wave energy. He explained the differing amounts of refraction of the various colors of light by suggesting that each had a different wavelength from the others. He also demonstrated that it was possible for waves of energy to cross each other without disturbance to either.

## More Research on Light

But Huyghens's ideas were not widely accepted. His theory, like Newton's, left too many questions unanswered. If light traveled in waves, like sound, why did it cast shadows? Sound waves, after all, are capable of going around obstacles placed in their path. And how did light waves travel through space? What medium was there between the sun and the earth that would conduct waves of energy?

Many experiments have been performed in attempts to answer these questions. In 1801 another English physicist, Thomas Young, answered the first. He shone two narrow beams of light on a screen so that they overlapped. Instead of the overlapped areas being brighter, as would be the case if light consisted of particles, a series of dark bands appeared. Young reasoned that the dark areas were nodes, caused by the interference of one wave by the other.

This discovery allowed him to measure the wavelength of the light waves, and he found them to be surprisingly short—averaging about $5 \times 10^{-5}$ (0.00005) centimeters! This extremely small measurement explained shadows very nicely. In order for a wave to bend around an object, the wavelength must be larger than the object itself. It has since been demonstrated that light waves will *not* pass around objects that are smaller than the figure given above.

## Modern Theories About Light

It now seems that light acts as if it were both particles and waves. A **photon** (fō′ ton), as the particle of light is called, is a bundle of energy. Light is produced and it is absorbed as photons, and the amount of energy of the individual photon depends upon the *frequency* of the light wave. How-

**14.23** Young's experiment

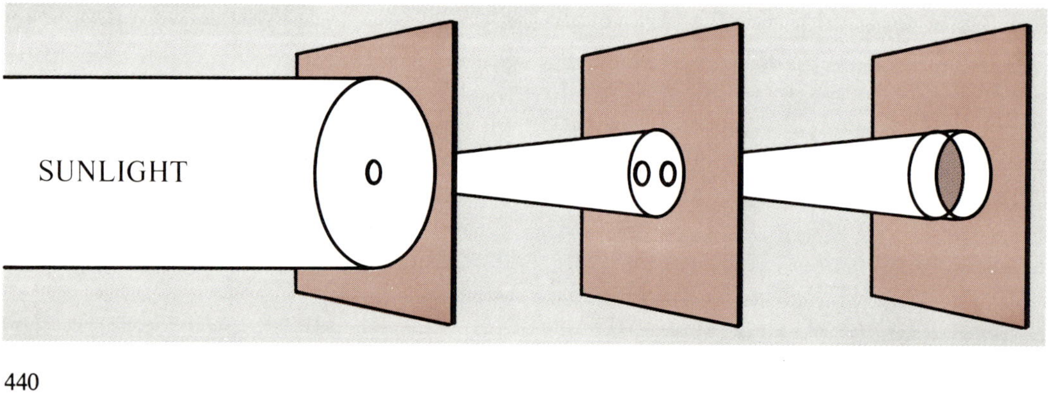

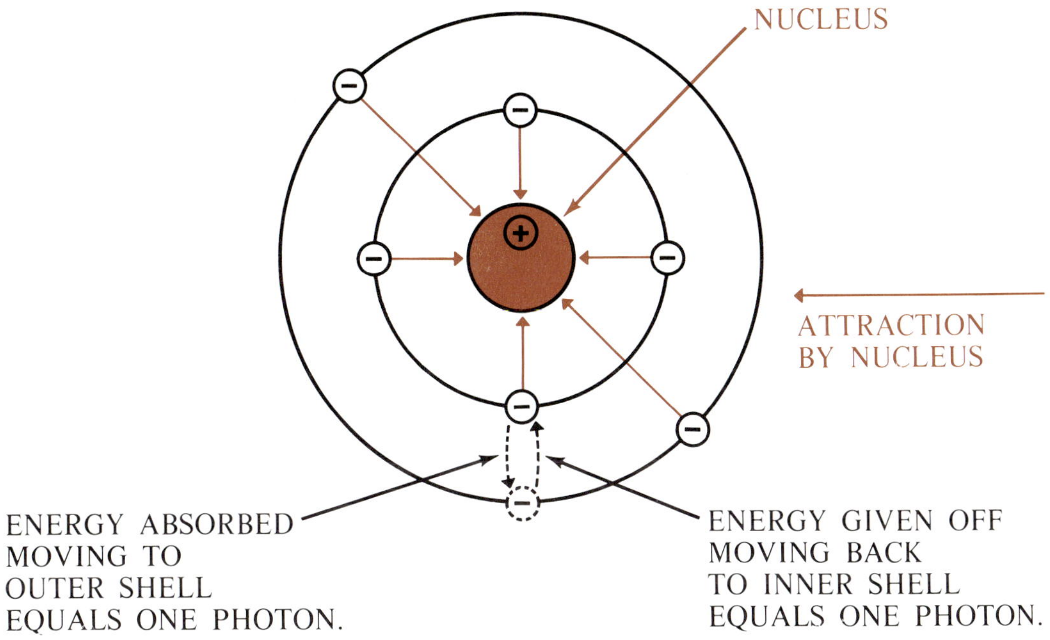


**14.24** As electrons move from one shell to another, energy is either absorbed or emitted.

ever, the photons of light energy travel in the form of waves.

It is theorized that light is produced by the movement of electrons from one orbit to another. You will recall from your study of chemistry that electrons circle around the nucleus of the atom in certain paths. Since the nucleus contains protons, which are positively charged, the negatively-charged electrons are attracted toward the center. Therefore, if an electron is moved from one shell to another that is farther away from the nucleus, a great deal of energy is required. If an electron "falls" back toward the nucleus from an outer shell, this energy will be released. The amount of energy that is absorbed by the process of lifting the electron to an outer shell is a photon. The same amount of energy is suddenly given off when the electron moves back to its original shell. In this way, energy is released *only* in certain amounts—photons.

So, for over 300 years scientists have argued and experimented, and still the question with which we began this section —What is light?—cannot be answered. As we have seen in other cases, a simple model does not seem to fit all situations. When working with certain types of phenomena, the scientist must think of light as waves of energy. But when he deals with other types of phenomena, he must consider it to be photons or "bundles" of energy, with some of the characteristics of particles. Meanwhile, hundreds of scientists continue to study the problem, and perhaps someday soon they will be able to give us a better answer.

### Have You Learned?

Answer the following questions, using brief complete sentences:

1. When Newton shone a light beam through a prism, what happened?
2. What discovery did Young make that contributed to the current theory of light?
3. If light travels in energy waves, why does it cast a shadow? Why don't sound waves also cast "shadows"?
4. What is a photon?
5. How are photons thought to originate?

## 5. How We See

**ARE YOU READY?**

Look up the following words if you are not sure of their meanings:

electrical impulse; focal length; focus; image; nerves; refracted.

You probably acquire more information about your environment through the sense of sight than through all the other senses combined. Sight allows you to sense things great distances away, while taste and touch require that you come in direct contact with an object.

### The Human Eye

The only nerves in the human body that are able to detect light energy lie in the back of the eye. The sensitive ends of these nerves form a thin layer called the **retina** (ret′ ə nə). These light receptors are of two types. Near the center of the retina, directly behind the lens of the eye, almost all of the nerves are shaped like tiny **cones.** The cones are capable of sensing various colors of light. Near the outer edges, the retina is composed largely of nerve endings known as **rods,** which are very sensitive to dim light. When trying to see something in very poor light, it sometimes helps if you do not look directly at the object. By looking to one side, you cause the light from the object to fall on the rods, and it is seen more clearly.

As light enters the eye, it passes through a transparent, protective covering, called the **cornea** (kôr′ ni ə), and the lens. Behind the cornea and the lens is a pocket of liquid—the **aqueous humor** (ā′ kwi əs hū′ mər). The amount of light that enters the lens is controlled by the colored **iris** (ī′ ris). When exposed to bright light, muscles cause the iris to expand, closing the **pupil** (pū′ pəl) and allowing only a small amount of light to pass through. After passing through the lens, the light must pass through a liquid that fills the entire eyeball, the **vitreous** (vit′ ri əs) **humor.**

The speed of light through the cornea, the aqueous humor, the lens, and the vitreous humor is almost exactly the same. Therefore, as the light enters the cornea, it is refracted. This causes an image to be formed on the retina, as shown in the diagram on page 443. Notice that this image is upside down, just like the images studied in Section 3.

The light stimulates the nerves of the retina, and nerve impulses travel to the brain. Through experience we have learned to interpret these impulses, which are electrical energy, as "sight." Can you explain why we do not see objects upside down, since this is the position of the image on the retina?

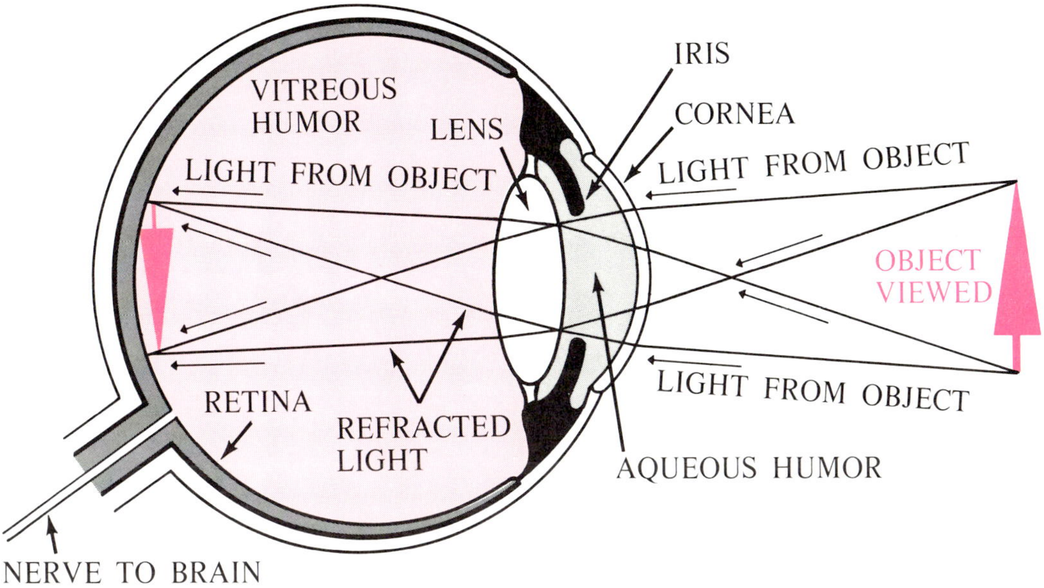


**14.25** The human eye has a lens that can change shape. Do we see things upside down?

## Making a Model Eye

**MATERIALS:**

A round flask, a convex lens, a candle, various clear liquids, white tempera paint or scouring powder, a piece of black construction paper

**PROCEDURE:**

The round flask will take the place of the *eyeball*. Brush half of it with thin paint or scouring powder mixed with a little water. If these are not available, tape a small square of plain, thin paper to one side of the flask. This white surface represents the *retina* upon which the image is formed. Fill the flask with water to take the place of the eye's *vitreous humor*. (See Figure 14.26 page 444.)

Cut a small round hole about 5 mm in diameter in the center of the sheet of construction paper. The opaque paper takes the place of the eye's *iris*, and the hole represents the *pupil*. Tape or hold the *lens* behind the hole in the paper, and place it in front of the flask, opposite the "retina."

Place the lighted candle a few meters away, and turn off the lights. Can you move the lens to throw an image onto the retina? You can see this better if you stand *behind* the flask, as shown in the diagram.

Describe the image. How does it compare with the image thrown by the lens alone? What happens to the image if the water is removed from the flask? Does the substitution of some other clear liquid, such as alcohol or syrup, change the image in any way? Can you explain these observations?

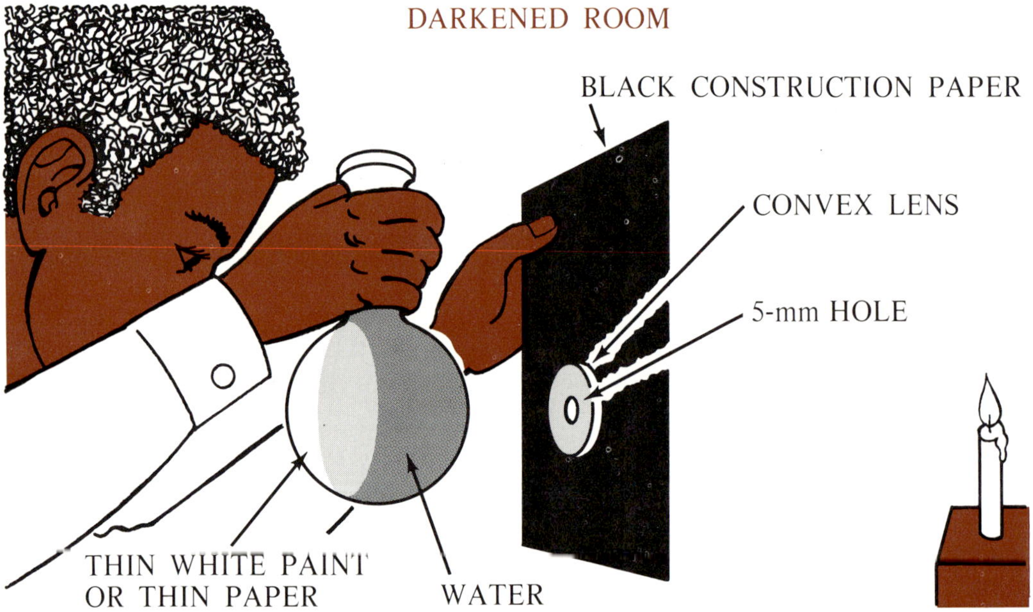


**14.26** Making a Model Eye

The material of the lens is a little denser than that of the other materials through which the light passes. However, an eye without a lens would still focus an image on the retina. The function of the lens is to change the focal length of the eye. This is done through changes in the thickness of the lens itself.

When looking at an object that is some distance from you, the muscles that control the lens of the eye are relaxed. As the object moves closer to you, the muscles around the lens tighten. This causes the lens to become thicker, which focuses the image on the retina.

Not everyone's eyes function perfectly. Some people can focus their eyes on distant objects but cannot make the adjustment for nearby objects. The cause of this farsightedness is a lens that is not curved

**14.27** Nearsightedness and farsightedness

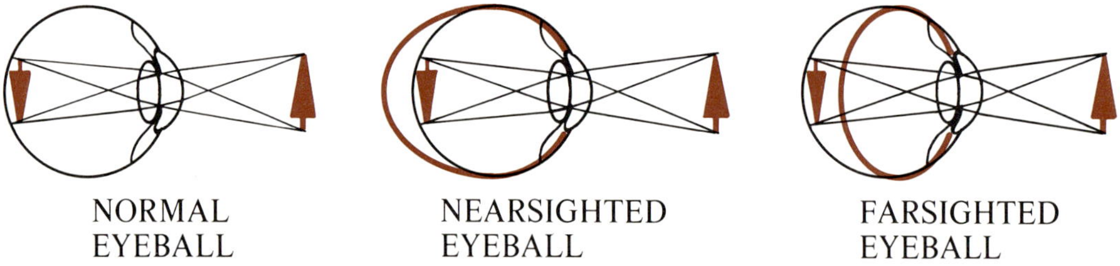

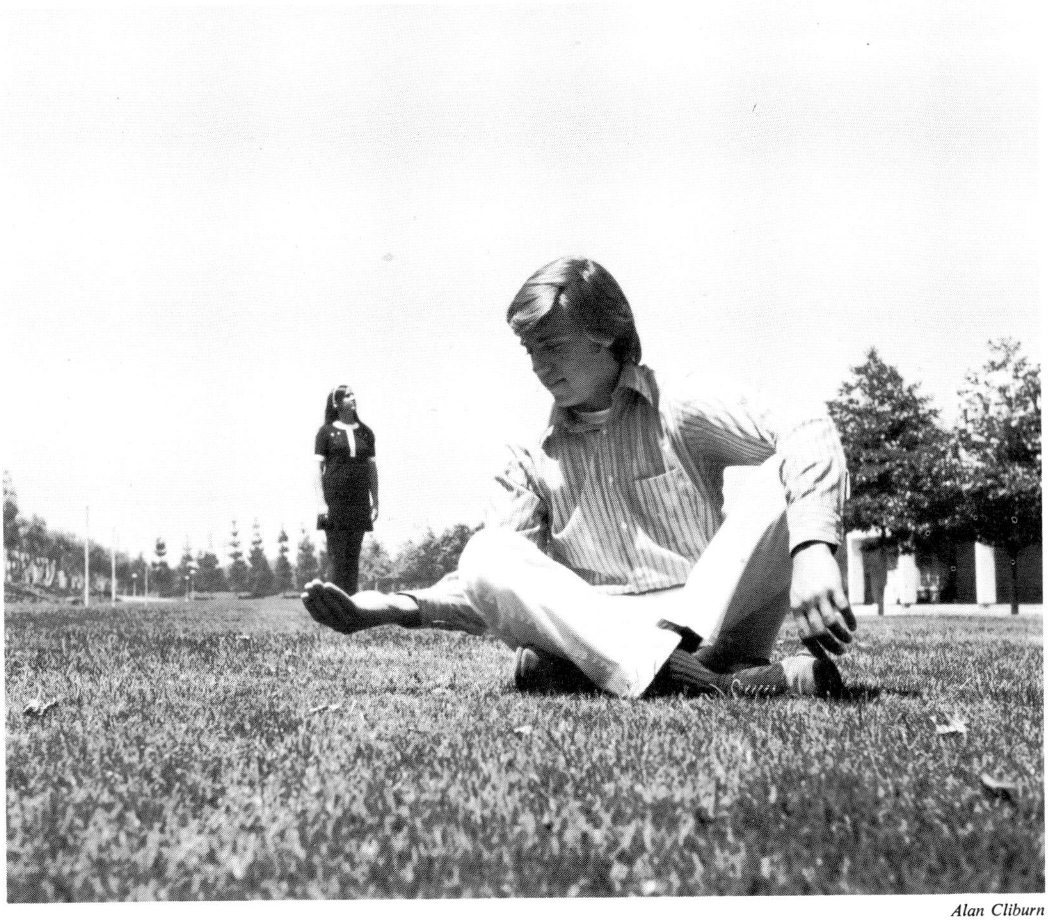

*Alan Cliburn*

**14.28** The human eye can be deceived.

enough, when in a relaxed condition, to focus the image directly on the retina. Instead, the focal point is somewhere behind the retina, as shown in Figure 14.27 on page 444. By placing a convex lens in front of the eye, the incoming light is refracted so that it is focused properly.

The opposite situation exists when the lens is curved too much. Since the image is focused at a point in front of the retina, the nearsighted person cannot see distant objects clearly. To correct this deficiency, a concave lens is used.

## Interpreting What You See Through Your Eyes

Your ability to see is largely learned through experience. Newborn babies are often unable to control the movement of their eyes. However, as the muscles develop, they quickly learn to move both eyes together and to focus on nearby objects. But throughout your life you must learn to interpret the electrical impulses that reach your brain.

Your judgment of distance is a good

example. Babies will reach for objects that are far away, such as the moon, because they have not yet learned to judge distance. You can easily estimate distances of objects that are not more than a few meters from you, because each of your two eyes sees a slightly different object. Within 2 meters these different images allow you to see depth. Perhaps you have seen stereo pictures, taken from slightly different positions. Although each picture is viewed with separate eyes, you seem to see a single picture that has depth.

Beyond 2 meters each eye sees essentially the same image and cannot, therefore, actually see the depth. Look at the photograph on page 445. You know, from experience, that the girl is farther away than the boy, because of his size. What other clues do you use to judge distance?

By taking into consideration the clues a person normally uses to judge size and distance, it is quite easy to create a situation that fools us. Look at Figure 14.29 below. This is an example of an optical illusion. You cannot make a model of it in wood or clay.

Scientists must constantly guard against observations that are not accurate. Instead of trusting their ability of observation, they will always use measuring instruments that cannot be fooled.

**14.29** Will your brain accept what your eye sees here?

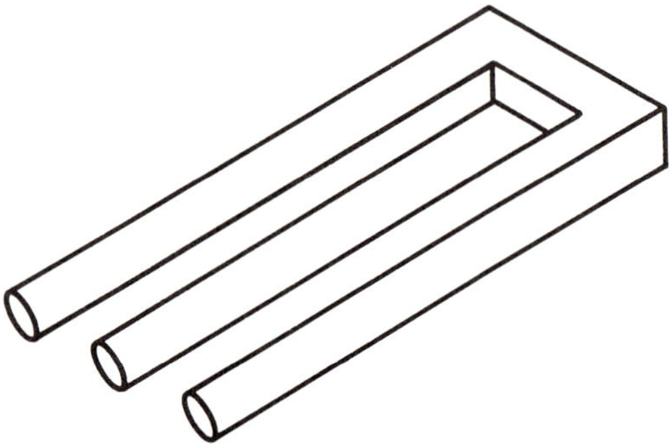

## Drawing Optical Illusions

It is easy to make drawings that will fool our eyes. Try these two on your friends.

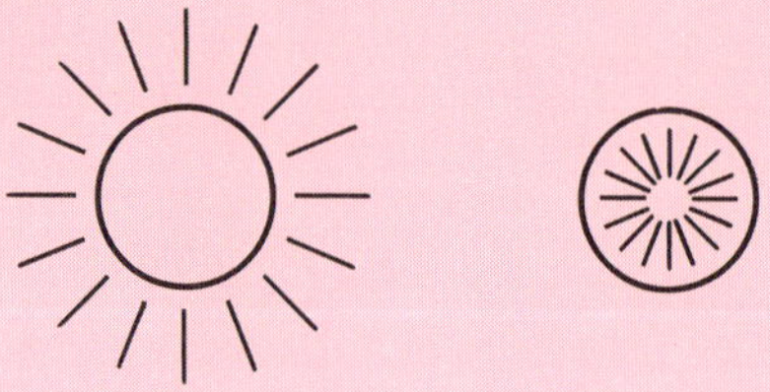

1. Draw two circles of equal size, using quarters as guides. Around one, draw several lines running from the outside edge of the circle away from the center, like the rays of a drawing of the sun. On the other circle draw lines running from the edge in toward the center of the circle. This second circle will look smaller to most people.

2. Draw two lines of equal length. On each end of one line draw two lines looking like arrow points. On the other, draw two lines running in the opposite direction, like the feathers of an arrow, on each end of the line. The second line will usually look longer to most people.

In both of these optical illusions, the lines running out from the object draw our eyes outward, making the object look larger. Lines running in toward the center of the object make us look toward the center, and make the object look smaller. Can you devise other drawings that will fool your eyes?

### Have You Learned?

On a sheet of paper list letters *A* through *G*, and by each letter write the name of the part of the eye as indicated in the diagram below.

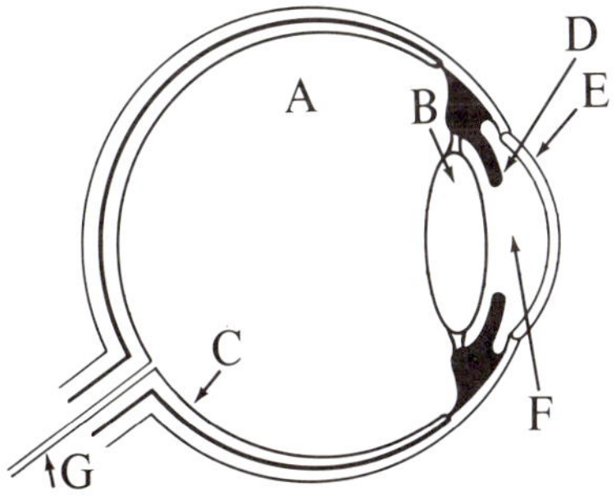


## 6. Measuring Light

**ARE YOU READY?**

Look up the following words if you are not sure of their meanings:

instantaneous; rotate; vacuum; watt.

Because scientists realize that their own observations are not always accurate, the ability to take accurate measurements is an important part of science. Many of the earliest scientists recognized this and tried to develop methods of measuring light. First, they tackled the problem of measuring the speed of light.

Galileo was one who did not accept the ancient suggestion that the speed of light was **infinite** (in′ fə nit). Early in the seventeenth century, he tried to measure its speed by flashing a light to a friend who stood on a hill about a mile away. As soon as the friend saw Galileo's light, he flashed a signal in return. Needless to say, Galileo's experiment was a failure.

### Roemer's Discoveries

Only a few years later, about 1676, a Danish scientist named Ole Roemer (rā′ mər) did succeed in making a rough measurement of the speed of light. Roemer realized that light must travel very rapidly and that the distances Galileo had tried to use were, therefore, much too short.

Roemer was an astronomer and was engaged in studying the movement of one of the moons of the planet Jupiter. He had measured the time that it took this moon to move across the face of the planet. Then he made an exciting discovery. He found that the time between the instant that the moon appeared from the planet's shadow on one side to the instant that it disappeared into the shadow on the opposite side was not always the same! If he took measurements exactly six months apart, he found that this difference in time was 16 minutes.

Roemer knew that the speed of this moon would not change in such a regular pattern. He also realized that one of his measurements was taken at the time of the year when the earth was on the *same side* of the sun as Jupiter and that the second measurement had been made when the earth was on the *opposite side* of the sun from Jupiter (Figure 14.30 on page 448). He also knew that the diameter of the earth's orbit was $299.2 \times 10^6$ kilometers.

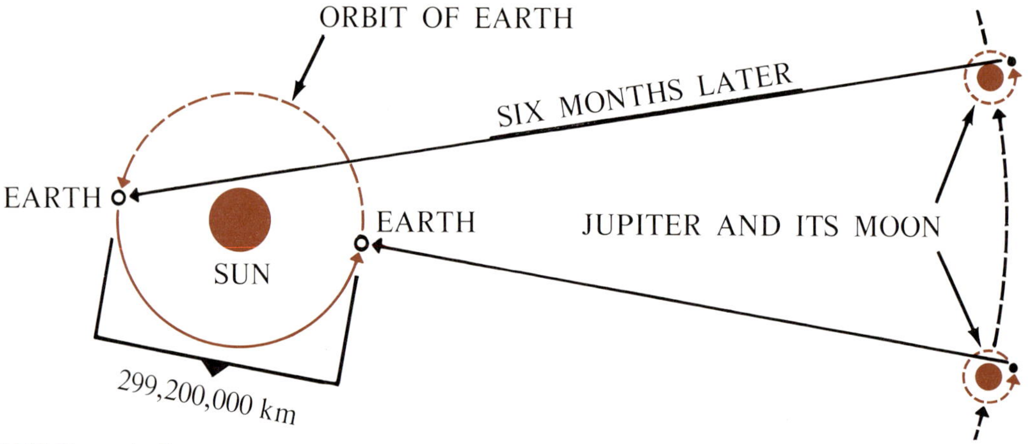


**14.30** Roemer's discovery

Knowing these things, Roemer reasoned that the 16-minute difference in his time measurements must be the length of time that it took the light to cross the additional 299.2 million km. Using these figures, he was able to calculate that the speed of light was about 311,670 km per second.

Other astromers used Roemer's methods and discovered more accurate ways of timing light. By 1729 a figure of 305,300 km per second was accepted as the speed of light through a vacuum.

It wasn't until the middle of the nineteenth century that scientists became sufficiently skilled at building machines to be able to measure the speed of light using the method that Galileo used. The first successful attempt was made in 1849 by a French physicist named Fizeau (fē zō). He flashed a light through a notch in a wheel. The light traveled a distance of 8 km, struck a mirror, and reflected back to the wheel. By spinning the wheel in such a way that the reflected beam of light passed through the second notch, Fizeau arrived at a figure for the speed of light that was not so accurate as those of the astronomers. But he showed later investigators a method that proved very accurate.

During the early part of the twentieth century, an American physicist, Albert Michelson, experimented with a slightly different technique. He used an eight-sided disk, with a mirror on each face that he rotated rapidly. He bounced a beam of light from one face of the disk, to a mirror set up 35.4 km away, and caught the reflected beam in the next mirror. He found that he had to rotate the disk at 530 revolutions per second. Thus, the light traveled the 30.8 km from the disk to the stationary mirror and back in $\frac{1}{8}$ of $^{1}/_{530}$ of a second. From this he calculated the speed of light as being 300,192 km per second. (See Figure 14.31 page 449.)

But the search continues for a more accurate answer to the question of how fast light travels. Recently, precise timing devices, using vibrations of molecules, have been developed. The currently accepted figure for the speed of light in a vacuum is 2,9979 $\times$ $10^5$ km per second.

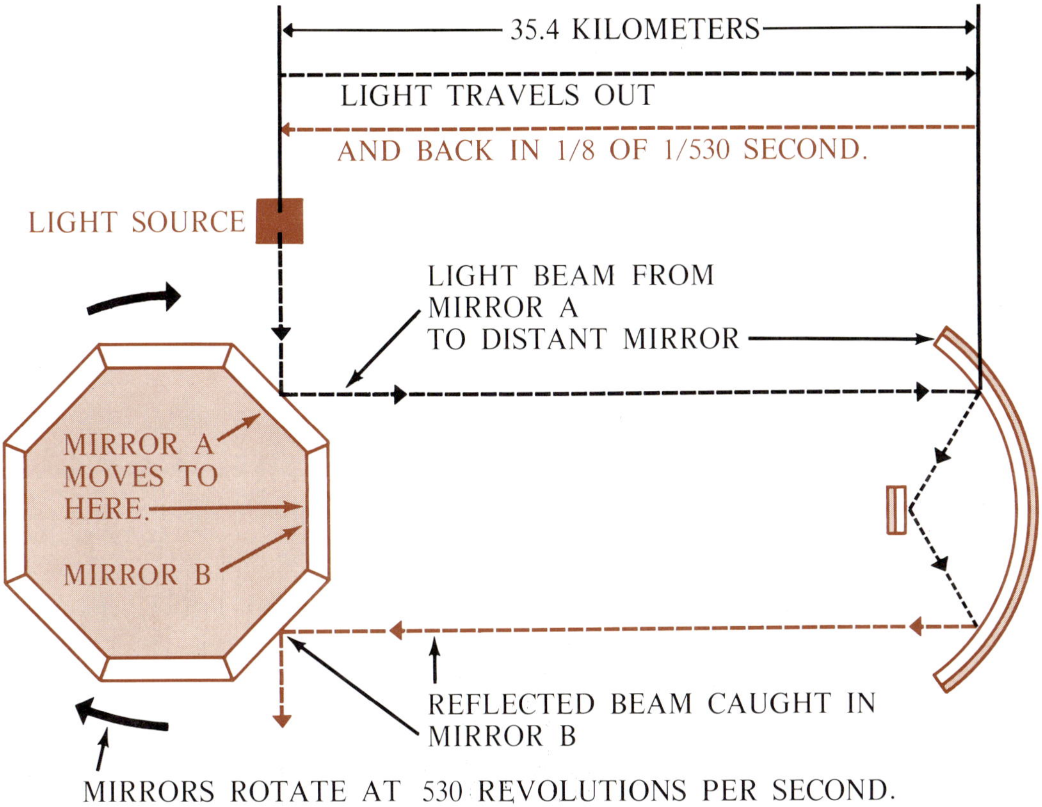


**14.31** Michelson's experiment

## Intensity of Light

Another measurement of light that is important to us is the amount of light at a certain place. The amount of light being produced by a light source can be measured by comparing it with the light produced by a **standard** source. The unit used is called a **candle**, because originally the standard light source was a candle made in a special way. Now the **candlepower** of a light source is measured by comparing it with a light bulb of a known candlepower. Most of the light bulbs normally used in our homes would be rated at about 100 candlepower.

Generally, we are not concerned with the intensity of the light produced by a source. Instead we would be more likely to be interested in the amount of **illumination** (i lü′ mə nā′ shən) or amount of light falling on a certain surface some distance from the source. Like sound, the farther away you are from the source of energy waves, the less the amount of energy that reaches you. If the light source is moved twice as far away from you, only one-fourth as much light falls on the book you are reading. Therefore, the distance between the source and the place at which you want to measure the illumination is very important. The unit used for the measurement of illumination is the **foot-candle**, which is the illumination produced by a 1-candlepower source on a surface one foot-away. It is not helpful at this time to use the metric system for measuring illumination. The units are *phots* and *luxes*.

A 100-watt bulb, such as those used in your home, produces about 130 candles of light. At a distance of one foot, the intensity would be 130 footcandles. At two feet, the intensity of this lamp would be only ¼ as much, or 32½ footcandles. At three feet, the intensity would be $^1/_9$ as great, or about 14.4 footcandles. To calculate the illumination of a light source you simply divide the candlepower of the source by the square of the distance. This result is the **Law of the Inverse Square.**

One instrument used to measure the candlepower of a light bulb (see below) uses this law.

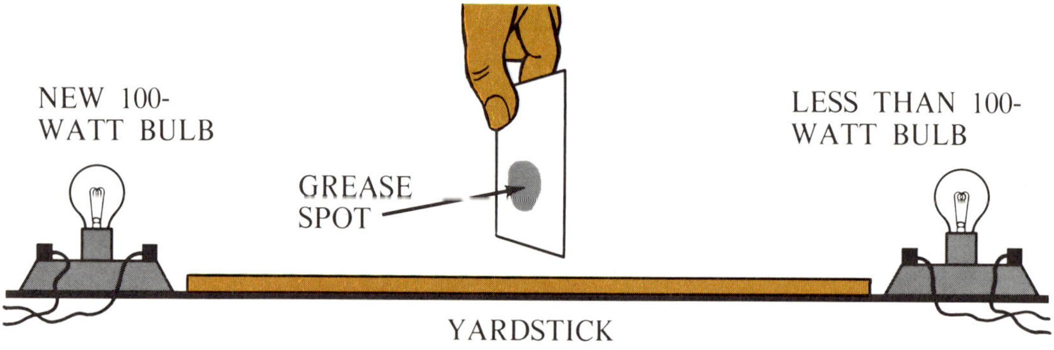


**14.32** Using a photometer to estimate candlepower

## Using a Photometer to Estimate Candlepower

**MATERIALS:**

A yardstick, a small piece of thin paper, a few drops of liquid cooking oil, a new 100-watt light bulb in an unshaded socket, a smaller light bulb in a socket

**PROCEDURE:**

Place the drop of oil near the center of the paper, and allow it to soak in thoroughly. Hold the paper between you and a light source. The grease spot looks lighter than the rest of the paper because the oil transmits light better than the unsaturated paper. Now hold the paper away from the light. The grease spot looks darker than the rest of the paper because the oil reflects less light than does the rest of the paper.

Place one light bulb at each end of the yardstick, and hold the paper between the two, near the center of the stick, as shown in the diagram. Look at the grease spot from one side of the paper, and then from the other. Which bulb is illuminating the paper more?

Slowly move the paper away from the brighter light, until the spot seems to disappear. At this point the illumination of the one light is equal to the illumination of the other. Note the distance from the paper to each lamp.

Your **photometer** (fō tom′ ə tər) showed that the illumination of the two bulbs was equal. Since the illumination of a light source is the candlepower of the source divided by the distance away from the source, the formula below may be used.

Assuming that the candlepower of a 100-watt bulb is 130, can you calculate the candlepower of the unknown bulb?

$$\frac{\text{Candlepower of lamp \#1}}{(\text{Distance of lamp \#1 from paper})^2} = \frac{\text{Candlepower of lamp \#2}}{(\text{Distance of lamp \#2 from paper})^2}$$

In our daily life we rarely need to calculate the candlepower of a luminous source. More often we are concerned with the illumination at a given place. To measure this, we might use a favorite instrument of photographers, the light meter.

The light meter, shown in the photograph below, contains a **photoelectric cell.** Like the photoelectric cells that are often found in automatic doors, the ones in the light meters change light energy into electric energy. A meter measures the strength of the electric current produced. The dial of the meter may be marked in such a way that the footcandles are read directly. Cameras are now being made with photoelectric cells built into them. In some of these cameras, the electric current produced by the photoelectric cell is used to open or close the shutter automatically to suit the light conditions.

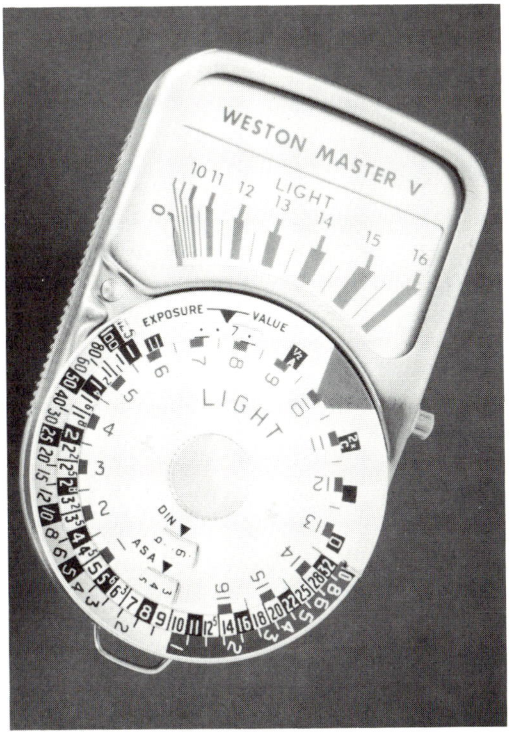


*Weston Instruments, Inc.*

**14.33** A light meter

## Have You Learned?

Answer the following questions using brief complete sentences.

1. Approximately how fast does light travel?
2. Define the terms *candle* and *footcandle*.
3. If a light bulb produces 100 candles of light, how much light would fall on a spot 5 feet away?
4. What is the difference between *candlepower* and *illumination*?
5. Suppose that you are using a photometer. The candlepower of the control bulb is 100. The illumination on the grease spot becomes equal when it is one foot away from the control bulb and two feet away from the lamp being tested. What is the candlepower of the new lamp?

## 7. Using Light

> **ARE YOU READY?**
>
> Look up the following words if you are not sure of their meanings:
>
> camera; convex; focal length; focus; inverted; microscope; telescope.

Light is one form of energy that we use almost every minute that we are awake. Perhaps you have spent a few moments in an entirely lightless place such as a deep cave. If so, you realize how strange it seems to be without any light at all.

In addition to the ways your body uses light, scientists have developed many instruments that help us use light more effectively. The use of eyeglasses to help many of us see better has already been discussed.

### Cameras

A camera is a common instrument that allows us to record scenes. It is very similar to the human eye in many of its parts. A convex lens causes the image to be focused at the back of the camera. As in the human eye, this image is inverted. The amount of light that is allowed to enter the lens is

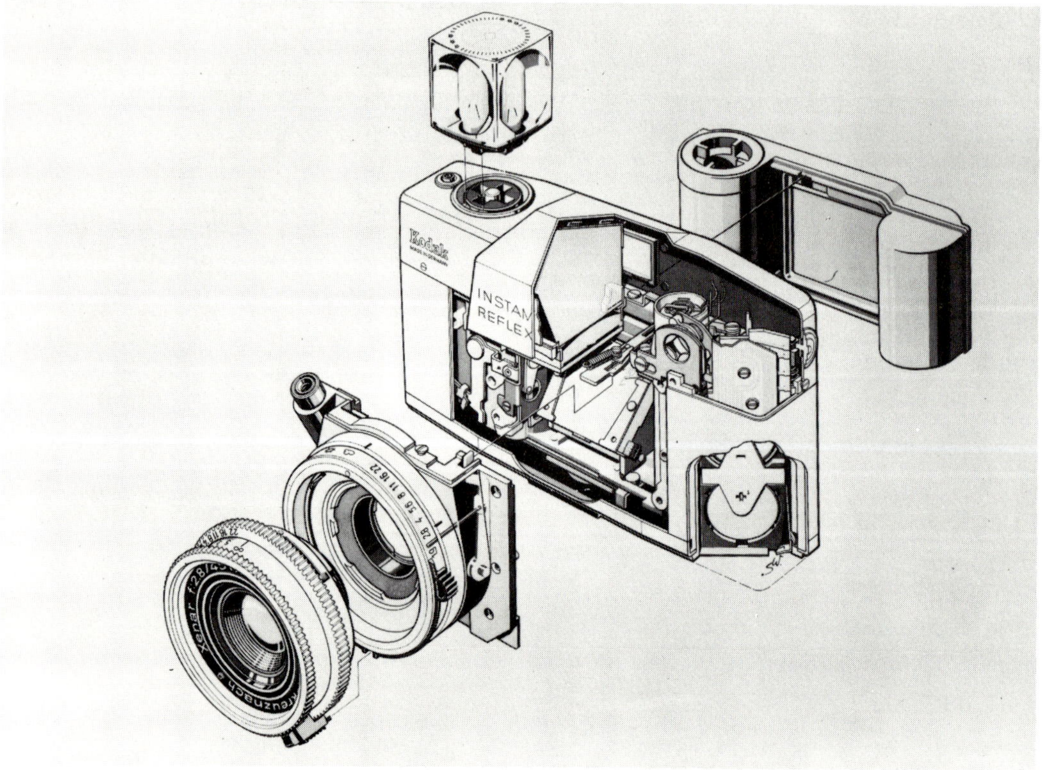


*Reproduced with the permission of Eastman Kodak Company*

**14.34** The mechanical components of a camera

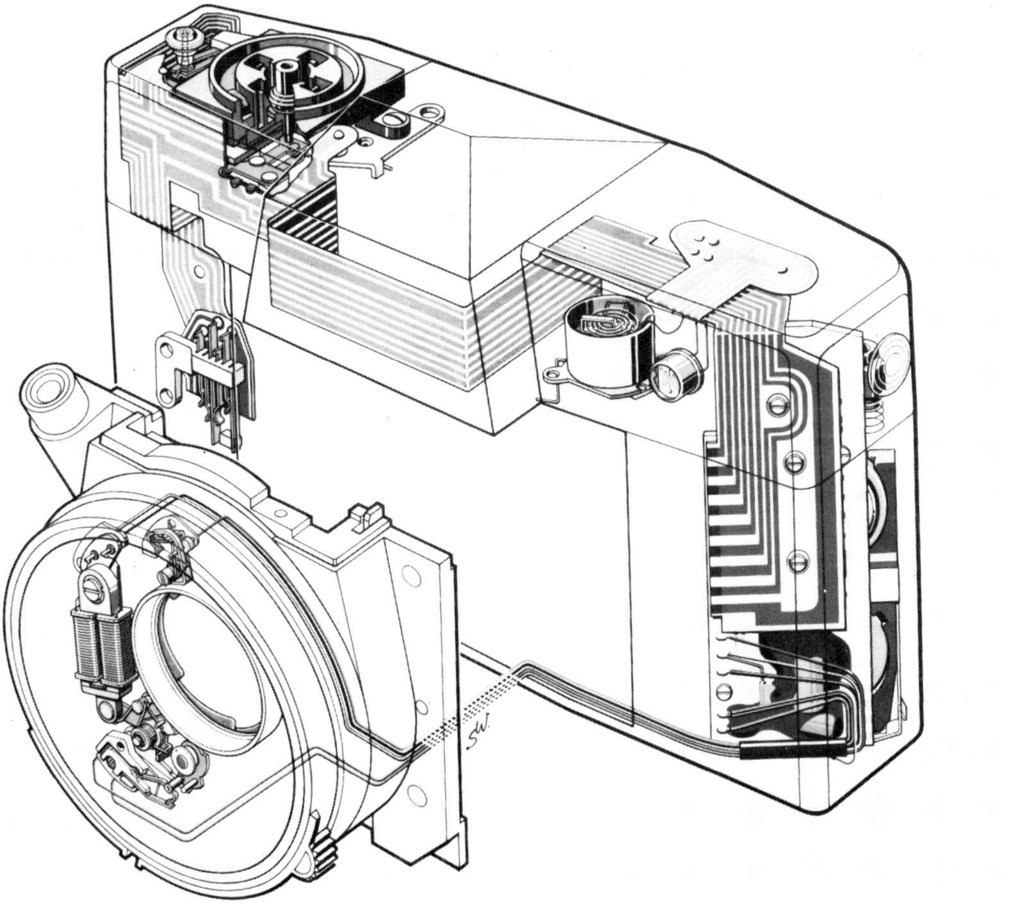


Reproduced with the permission of Eastman Kodak Company

**14.35** The electrical circuits of a camera

controlled by the *diaphragm* (Figure 14.36 page 454). What part of the eye does this?

The presence of film is, of course, the major difference between the camera and the eye. As the camera lens is opened, the light focuses on the film. A chemical compound on the film, generally made of silver bromide, captures electrons when exposed to light, and the molecules of silver turn black. As the film is developed, all unexposed silver bromide is washed off, leaving a dark "negative" of silver molecules.

## Magnifying Objects with a Microscope

In Section 3 of this chapter you studied the focal length of several convex lenses. Use these same lenses for the following activity.

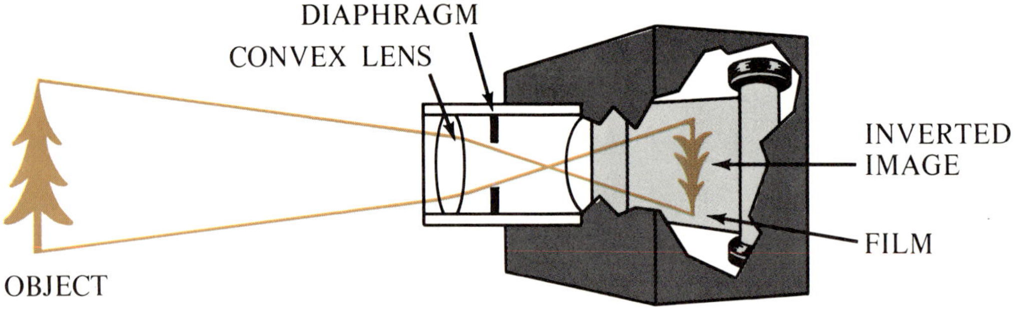


**14.36** This looks like an eye. Notice that the image on the film is inverted.

## Using Lenses to Magnify

**MATERIALS:**

Several convex lenses (such as those used in the activity on page 436), a yardstick or meterstick, a source of light

**PROCEDURE:**

Measure the focal length of each lens, as you did in the activity in Section 3. Hold each lens between your eye and this page, and move the lens back and forth until the print is in focus.

Which lens seems to produce the largest **magnification** (mag′ nə fə kā′ shən)? How does the focal length of this lens compare with the focal length of the other lenses?

Which lens seems to produce the least magnification? How does its focal length compare with the focal length of the other lenses?

Can you make a general statement about the relationship between the focal length of a lens and its power of magnification? What happens when you combine two lenses? Can you increase the magnification in this way?

Your school may have a **compound microscope** (kom′ pound mī′ krə skōp) such as the one shown in the photograph on page 455. A microscope like this one will contain two convex lenses, as shown in the diagram on page 455. The one at the lower end of the tube is called the objective lens. As the tube is moved up and down, the objective lens focuses on the tiny object below it, and forms an image within the tube. The upper lens, called the eyepiece, is focused on the image formed by the objective lens. What your eye sees is a magnified image of the image formed by the objective lens. Since this first image is larger than the object being viewed, the result is that you see a highly magnified image. You can calculate the number of magnifications by multiplying the number of magnifications of the objective lens by the number of magnifications of the eyepiece. These usually are marked on the lenses of the microscope. For example, a 10× eyepiece and a 43× objective lens will magnify things 430 times. Some compound microscopes produce magnifications of 1,000 times the actual size of the object.

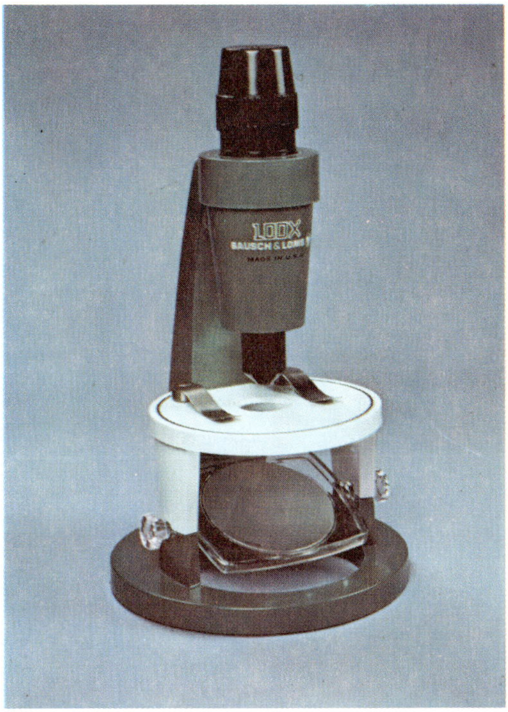


*Bausch & Lomb*

**14.37** A compound microscope

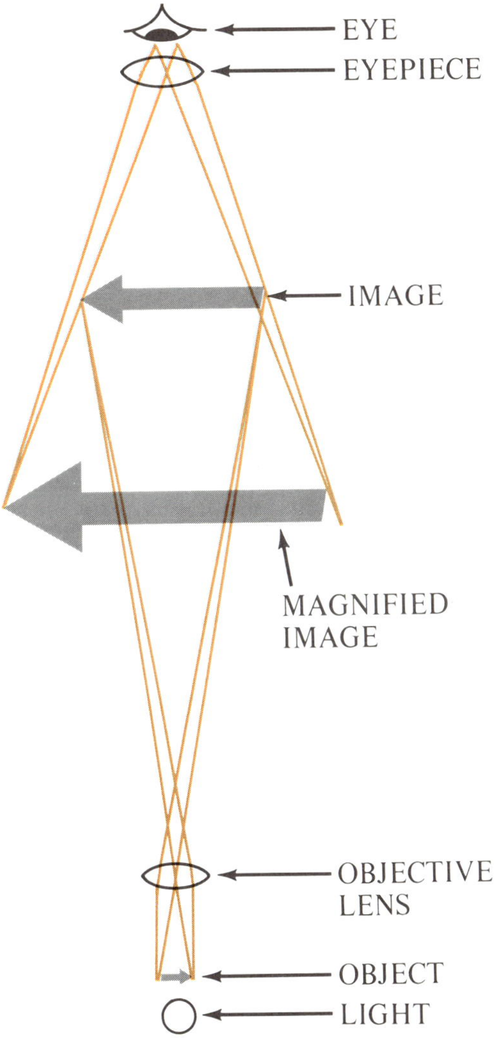


**14.38** Diagram of a compound microscope

## Viewing Distant Objects with Telescopes

One kind of telescope may contain two or more convex lenses, as the microscope does. Such telescopes work in exactly the same way as the microscope does. The major difference is that the focal length of the objective lens is much longer in the telescope than in the microscope.

Since large lenses are difficult and expensive to make, telescopes using lenses are rarely more than 15 centimeters in diameter. For larger telescopes, such as the one 508 centimeters in diameter shown in the photograph on page 456, a huge concave *mirror* is used instead of lenses. The light enters the tube and is focused by the curved mirror into a small, flat mirror as shown in Figure 14.40. This flat mirror reflects the light to the side, where it is viewed or photographed through an eyepiece containing a small, convex lens.

The image produced by a telescope is upside down. If we want to use such an instrument to look at distant objects on the earth, as with a spyglass or binoculars,

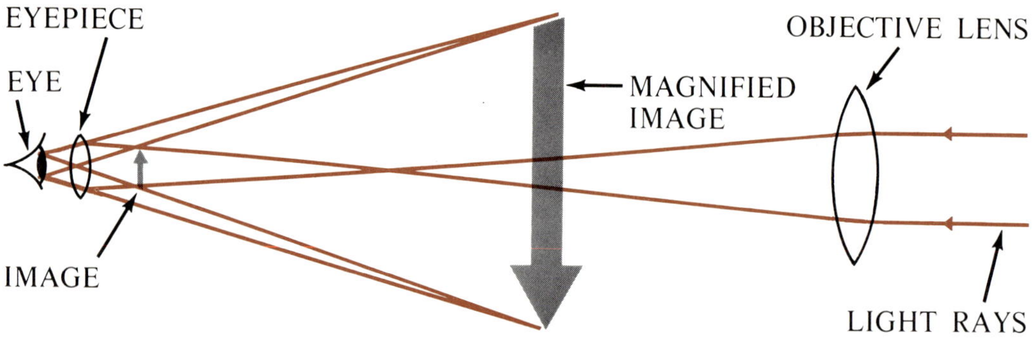


**14.39** Refracting telescope

it is necessary to add extra lenses that will turn the image back to its normal position.

### Have You Learned?

Answer the following questions, using brief complete sentences:

1. What part of a camera controls the amount of light entering the lens?
2. What is the major difference between the camera and the eye?
3. What kind of lenses does a compound microscope contain?
4. Which is the objective lens in a compound microscope?
5. Is the focal length of the objective lens of a telescope shorter or longer than that of a microscope?
6. What type of telescope uses a mirror?

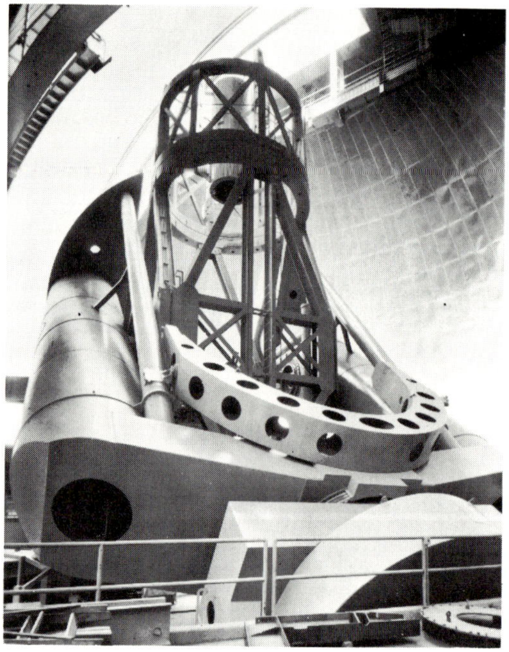

*Photo Researchers, Inc.*

**14.41** The 508-cm Hale reflecting telescope at Mount Wilson and Palomar Observatories

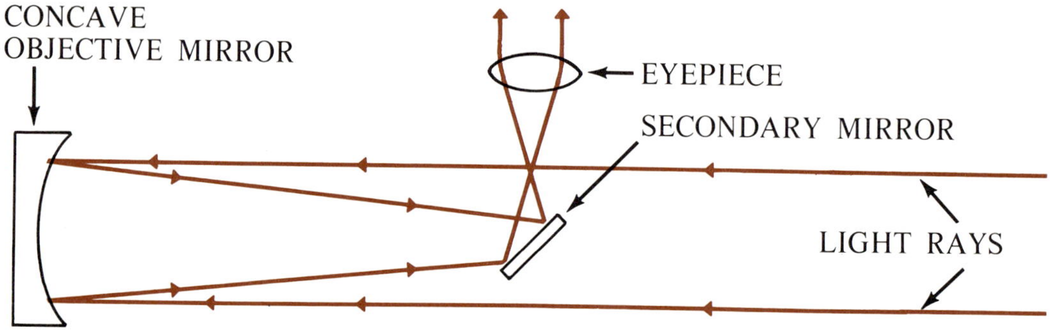


**14.40** Reflecting telescope

## REVIEW QUESTIONS

1. What is the major difference between a luminous object and a nonluminous one? Give five examples of each.
2. What is a light ray? Why do scientists use this term?
3. What is the difference between the terms "plain mirror" and "plane mirror?"
4. Should a light over a mirror be placed so that it will shine on your face or on the mirror? Explain.
5. The edges of most shadows will be gray rather than black like the center of the shadow. Explain why.
6. Explain the diffusion of light from a rough surface in terms of the angle of incidence and the angle of reflection of the light rays.
7. If a man is fishing with a spear he will not aim directly at the fish. Will he aim below or above where the fish appears to be? Explain.
8. Explain the difference between reflection and refraction.
9. Describe the different images that are formed by a convex lens when the reflecting surface is placed outside the focal length of the lens. Explain why each is formed.
10. Compare the theories of the nature of light developed by Newton and Huyghens with the currently accepted theory.
11. Compare light waves with sound waves. Which are larger? Why do light waves cast shadows while sound waves do not?
12. The image formed on the retina of the eye is inverted (upside down). Explain how it is that we can see things right side up.
13. Briefly describe the experiments that tried to measure the speed of light.

## CAN YOU FIND OUT?

*It may be necessary to use encyclopedias or other reference books in answering the following questions:*

1. Different types of metals become incandescent at different temperatures. Can you find out what these are for several common metals? Does the color of the glowing metal depend upon temperature?
2. Explain how a "solar oven" works. Are these being used in any way? What are the advantages and disadvantages of these ovens?
3. What are some uses of convex and concave lenses? Explain why one is used instead of the other in each case.
4. How does the average length of a light wave ($5 \times 10^{-5}$ cm.) compare with other forms of wave energy?
5. What optical illusions, other than those in this chapter, can you find? Explain why each fools your eyes.
6. How does a Polaroid camera develop film within the camera?
7. What is meant by the "resolving power" of a telescope?

## REFERENCES FOR ADDITIONAL STUDY

THE AMATEUR PHOTOGRAPHER'S HANDBOOK (Eighth Edition) by Aaron Sussman. Thomas Y. Crowell Company.
An excellent resource book that covers all phases of photography, including color photography

EXPERIMENTS IN VISUAL SCIENCE: FOR HOME AND SCHOOL by James R. Gregg. The Ronald Press Company.
An introduction to the science of optics, including 39 experiments on light

LIGHT AND VISION by Conrad Mueller and the Editors of Time-Life Books, A Division of Time Inc.
One book of the LIFE Science Library—has many colored photographs and interesting accounts of light phenomena and how we see

YOU AND YOUR CAMERA by Lou Jacobs, Jr. Lothrop, Lee & Shepard Company.
A helpful guide to taking better pictures, with major attention given to 35 mm and reflex cameras, and cameras using cartridge film

CHAPTER 15

# Light Waves: Visible and Invisible

OUR WORLD is full of color. Everywhere you look you see colors—unless you happen to be one of those rare people who cannot see colors at all.

You have already learned that light apparently travels in the form of energy waves. You know that there are many types of invisible energy waves such as radio and TV waves that also travel through the air. How are light waves different from these other energy waves? How are they similar?

## 1. The Nature of Color

**ARE YOU READY?**

Look up the following words if you are not sure of their meanings:

frequency; illumination; luminous; opaque; prism; refraction; translucent; transparent; wavelength.

During the year 1666 an important experiment was performed in England. A thin beam of sunlight was allowed to pass through a triangular piece of glass. But instead of the single, narrow beam of white light that had entered the prism, a broad rainbow of color was seen.

This was not the first time that this experiment had been performed. But what made this experiment so important was the presence of a certain man—Sir Isaac Newton. Newton reasoned that the prism had broken the sunlight up into its various parts, and therefore white light was actually composed of six colors mixed together. To test this idea, he placed another prism in the beam of colored light and changed the rainbow back into a beam of ordinary light.

The rainbow that Newton worked with is now called a **spectrum** (spek′ trəm). Look carefully at Figure 15.1 on the opposite page. As you can see, the beam of light enters the prism and is refracted by it. A spectrum of bands of red, orange, yellow, green, blue, and violet light are formed. Notice that the red band is formed by light that is refracted the *least*, the violet band is formed by light that is refracted the *most*, and the other colors fall between these two. Recalling what you learned about refraction in Section 3 of Chapter 14, can you figure out which color of light is slowed the most when it passes through the prism?

The difference between the waves of different colored light is their frequency and their wavelength. In Section 1 of Chapter 13 you learned that the speed of a wave can be calculated by multiplying the length of the wave by the frequency of the wave. But we know that the various colors of light travel at the same speed. Therefore, if the wave of one color has a

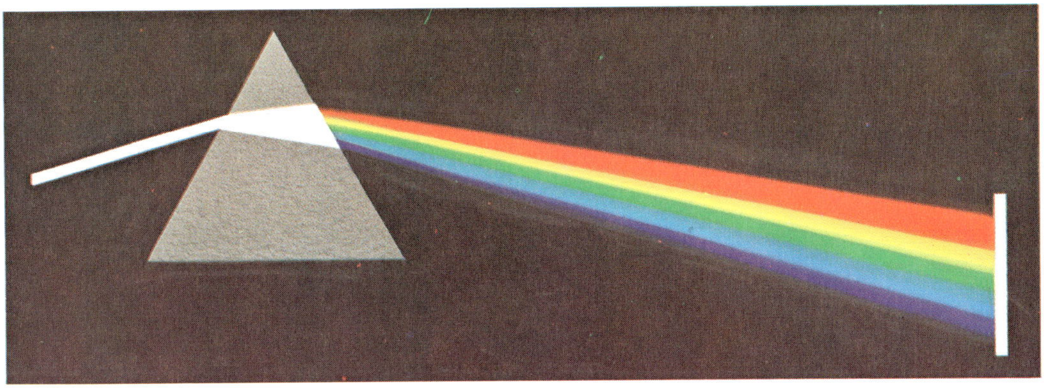

**15.1** Prism and spectrum

*longer* wavelength than the wave of another color, it must have a *lower frequency*. And this is exactly what has been found. The wavelength of red light is about twice as long as the wave of violet light. And the frequency of the red waves is only half that of the violet light.

## Why Are Some Objects Colored?

What causes an object to be a certain color? The color of luminous objects depends upon their temperature, since temperature determines the wavelength and the frequency of the light being produced. The temperature of a glowing substance can be estimated by the color of the light coming from it. This is one way astronomers have for determining the temperature of the stars. An expert can judge the temperature of the steel in a blast furnace by its color.

Sometimes we see a transparent or translucent object, such as glass or thin paper, that appears to be colored. White light enters the object, but only colored light emerges from the other side. In this case, the object is able to transmit only certain frequencies of light, and the other frequencies are absorbed. For example, white light strikes a red glass filter. All of the light frequencies except those near the red end of the spectrum are absorbed by the glass. Only red light rays come through

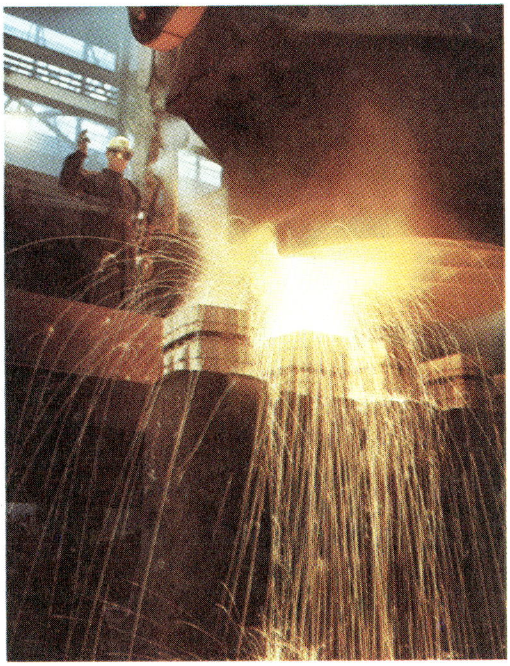

*Bethlehem Steel Corporation*

**15.2** The color of luminous objects depends upon their temperature.

the filter, and the glass appears to us to be red (Figure 15.4 page 462).

We can see an opaque object because the light is reflected from its surface. If all frequencies of light are reflected equally well, the object appears to be white. If all of the frequencies are absorbed except red, which is reflected, we see the object as being colored red. What color do you think an opaque object would be if *none* of the light were reflected? (Figure 15.5 page 462)

## Experimenting with Colored Light

**MATERIALS:**

A flashlight, red, blue, yellow, green cellophane, a package of construction paper of various colors

**PROCEDURE:**

In a dark room, hold the red cellophane sheet over the flashlight, and look around you. The things around you are being illuminated by only red light rays. Look at a white sheet of paper. What color is it? Can you explain why?

Look at each sheet in the multicolored package of construction paper. Can you explain why each sheet appears to be the color that you see? Repeat this experiment, using the other colors of cellophane that you have.

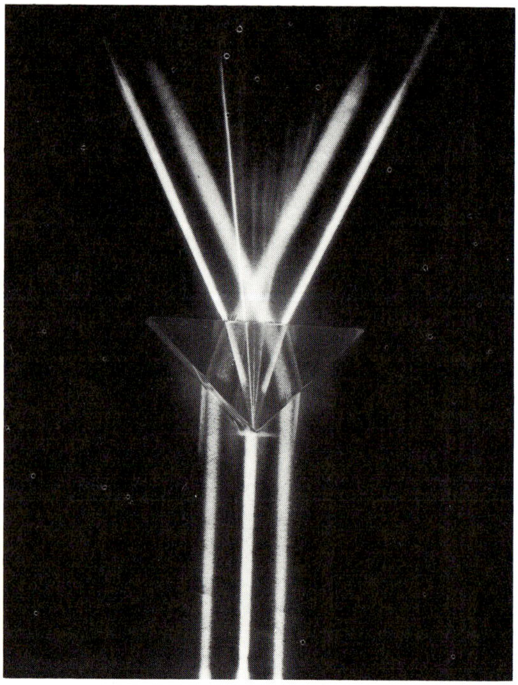

A glass prism breaks up white light into a rainbow, but what causes the rainbow that you often see during a rain shower? Figure 15.6 on page 463 explains this phenomenon.

White light, generally coming from behind you, strikes raindrops in the clouds. The drop of water acts like a tiny prism, refracting the light. If the angle between the sun, the raindrops, and your eye is exactly right, the light will be reflected by the inside of the drop. It will again be refracted as it leaves the water and enters the air. The result is a spectrum, with the red band nearest the earth and the violet band at the top.

**15.3** Light rays and a prism

*Bausch & Lomb*

## Have You Learned?

On a sheet of paper list the numbers for the questions below. By each number write *T* if the statement is true and *F* if false.

1. Newton was the first man to make a prism.
2. Red light is refracted more than violet light when it passes through a prism.
3. If a beam of light has a longer wavelength than another beam, it must also have a lower frequency.
4. The color of a luminous object depends largely upon its temperature.
5. If a piece of glass is red, we know that only the red light is passing through it.
6. If a piece of construction paper is red, we know that only red light is being absorbed.
7. If a piece of cardboard is white, we know that no light is being reflected from it.
8. If we see a rainbow, we know that there are water droplets in the air.
9. Red light has a wavelength that is longer than the wavelength of violet light.
10. A rainbow is a spectrum.

## 2. Mixing Colors

**ARE YOU READY?**

Look up the following words if you are not sure of their meanings:

absorb; prism; reflect; spectrum.

You have already learned that if you direct a beam of white light through a prism the light is broken up into several colors. You know also that if you recombine these colors, the single beam of light will be *white*. On the other hand, you may have learned that if several colors of paints are mixed they produce the color black. How can we explain this surprising observation?

### Adding Light

The color of a beam of light is determined by the length of the waves present. Therefore, when we mix light beams of different colors, we are really adding different wavelengths to the total. If we add wavelengths from all parts of the spectrum, we will produce white light.

By experimentation, it has been discovered that it is not necessary to combine all six colors of the spectrum to produce white light. Figure 15.7 on page 463 shows what would happen if red, green, and blue beams of light were to be projected onto a white surface and allowed to overlap. Where all three blended, white light is produced. Can you explain why? Because of their ability to produce white light when mixed together, red, green, and blue light are called the **primary light colors.**

Notice in Figure 15.7 that three other colors are also produced. Where green light and blue light overlap, a blue-green color called **cyan** (sī′ an) is produced. Where red light and green light mix, yellow is the result. And where red light and blue light combine, a purplish **magenta** (mə jen′ tə) is seen.

These three colors—cyan, magenta, and yellow—are said to be **complementary** (kom′ plə men′ tə ri) to the primary colors of light opposite each one in Figure 15.7

on page 463. Can you guess what the resulting color would be if you were to mix a beam of cyan-colored light with a beam of red-colored light? Or a yellow beam with one colored blue? To answer these questions you will have to remember that each complementary color is made by the combination of *two* primary colors.

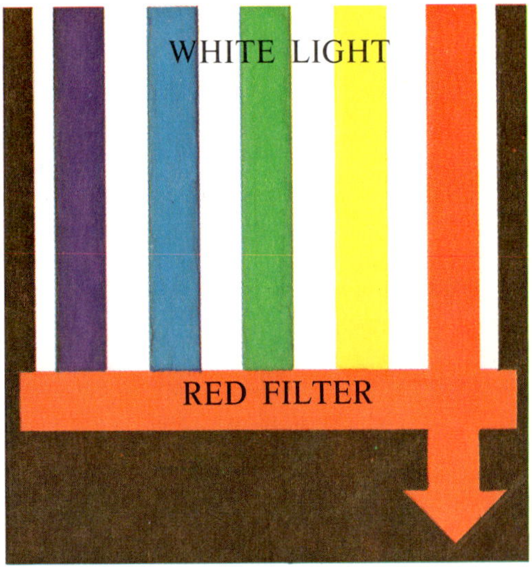


**15.4** Red light passes through a red filter.

## Subtracting Light

Now perhaps you can understand why an opaque object appears to be colored. If white light falls on a piece of colored construction paper, it is clear that the paper is absorbing, or *subtracting*, some of the wavelengths of the white light. If the paper is blue, we know that it is not reflecting light from the red end of the spectrum. From this, can you guess what color would result if you mixed paint from *all* parts of the spectrum together?

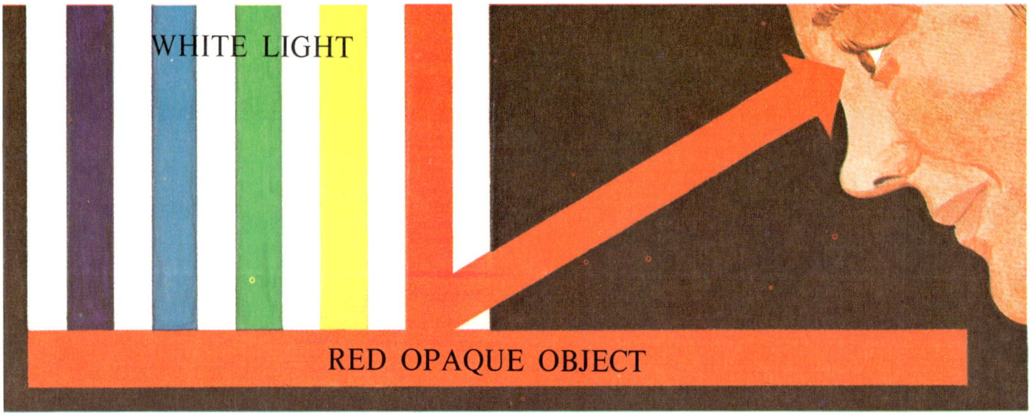


**15.5** Red light is reflected from red objects.

Because colored paints subtract certain wavelengths of light, the mixing of different colors of paint is more complicated than the mixing of colored light. Blue paint, for example, absorbs almost all of the red, orange, and yellow wavelengths. It reflects most of the blue, as we can see from its color. But blue paint also reflects some of the violet and green light that strikes it. This explains the results we get when we mix two colors of paints.

The **primary paint colors** are red, yellow, and blue. From these three colors, an artist can make a mixture that will be any

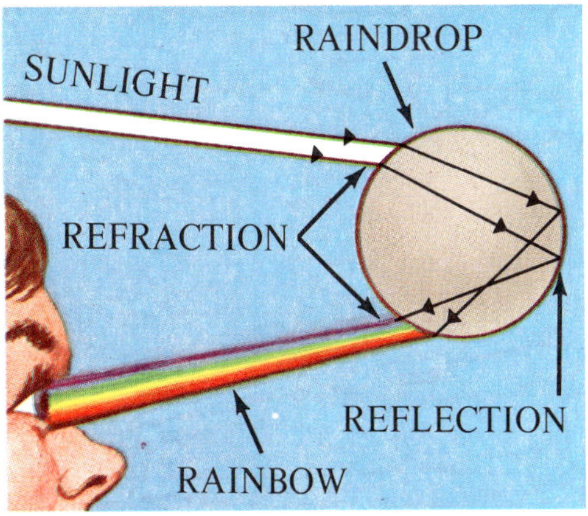


**15.6** Rainbows are formed when sunlight is refracted by billions of raindrops.

color that he wants. Figure 15.8 shows how this is possible.

This is a circular spectrum. We can use it when we want to determine which colors are absorbed and which are reflected by a colored paint. Assume that the colored paint reflects the color that you see *plus* some of the colors on either side of it. The three colors on the opposite side of the diagram are all absorbed.

For example, a red paint will reflect mostly red wavelengths of light and some of the violet and orange light. It will absorb almost all of the blue, green, and yellow light that strikes it. On the other hand, yellow paint reflects yellow, orange, and green light and absorbs blue, violet, and red light.

Using this information, can you predict what color will be produced if red paint is mixed with blue paint? To do this, first list the colors that will be reflected by each paint. Red reflects violet, red, and orange, while blue reflects green, blue, and violet. Then list the colors that each paint will absorb. Red absorbs yellow, green, and blue, while blue paint absorbs red, orange,

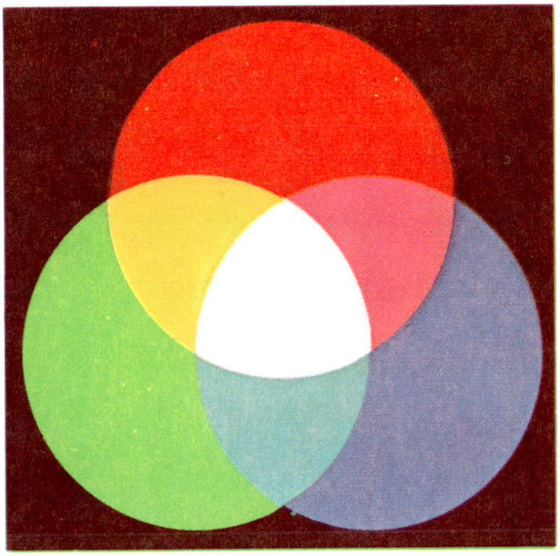

**15.7** What color is produced by adding red, green, and blue light (in the right intensity)?

and yellow. Subtracting the absorbed colors from the reflected colors, we find that violet is the only color that is left.

Reflected = violet, red, orange, green, blue
Absorbed = red, orange, green, blue, yellow

Can you use this method to predict what color will be formed if we mix yellow and blue? Or yellow and red?

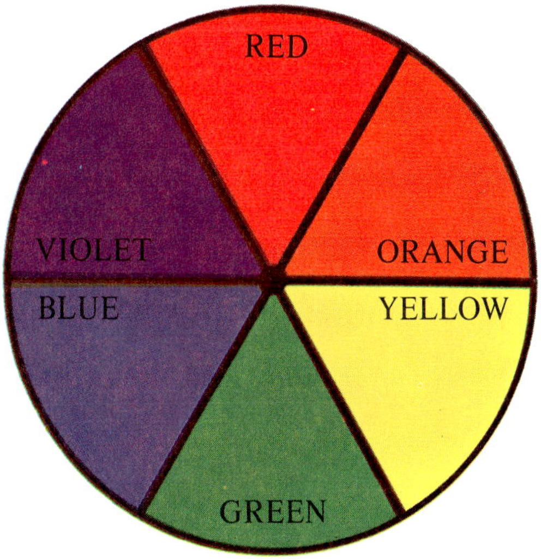


**15.8** Do you see what orange is?

### Have You Learned?

Answer the following questions, using short complete sentences.

1. What are the primary light colors? Why are they so named?
2. What are the three complementary light colors? Why are they so named?
3. What are the primary paint colors? Why are they so named?
4. When yellow paint is mixed with blue, what color results? Why?
5. In mixing paints, how is black produced? Why?

## 3. Seeing Color

**ARE YOU READY?**

Look up the following words if you are not sure of their meanings:

complementary colors;
cones (of the eye); retina; spectrum.

As you have probably guessed by now, color cannot be considered to be a characteristic of an object. If we were to be very scientific when we described a substance, we would say that it was able to reflect certain wavelengths of light energy. The property that we call color depends upon the effect that these wavelengths have on the light receptors in the retina.

Scientists do not fully understand how we see color. The theory accepted by the majority of scientists is based on the idea that the cones of the eye are of three types. One of these is sensitive to light waves from the shorter end of the spectrum. Therefore, these cones respond to blue light more than to light of any other color. Another type of cone responds to light from the green portion of the spectrum, which is composed of waves with medium wavelengths. The remainder of the light-sensitive cones respond primarily to the longer, or red, waves.

By referring to Figure 15.7 you can understand that if all three types of receptors are stimulated equally, our brain interprets the light as being white. If blue and red wavelengths enter our eyes, we see what we call *magenta.*

Recent research has indicated that the theory presented here may be much too simple. It now appears that the brain is capable of comparing the long wavelengths that it receives with the shorter wavelengths, and of "seeing" colors that are not really there.

This misinterpretation by the brain should not surprise you, since you know that the stimulation of sight received by the brain is in the form of electrical impulses. Like a computer the brain interprets the electric signals that it receives from the eyes. If we can provide it with false signals, it will produce false answers.

### Observing Colors That Are Not There

**MATERIALS:**

This book, open to page 466, Figure 15.10, a piece of white paper, bright sunlight

**PROCEDURE:**

On page 466 is a picture of the American flag. It is black, yellow and blue. Take this book into bright sunlight. Stare at the flag steadily for at least thirty seconds. Then cover the book page with the sheet of white paper, and stare at the white surface. What do you see? Do you continue to see the flag that you had looked at? What are the colors of the **afterimage?**

What is the relationship of the colors of the afterimage to those in Figure 15.10?

---

The cause of the phenomenon that you have observed is **retinal fatigue** (ret′ ə nəl fə tēg′). As you stare at the blue diagram, a portion of the cones of your retina receive light waves from the blue part of the spectrum. The rest of your retina receives all lengths of waves from the white paper around the diagram. After a period of time, the cones receiving only the blue light become "tired," probably because the supply of a certain chemical is used up by these nerve cells. When you cover the blue diagram and look at the white surface, the cones that are tired do not respond to the blue wavelengths striking them. However, the other cones in the area of the retina covered by the diagram's image are not tired, and they respond. Therefore, you see an area the size and shape of the diagram but colored with the complementary color of the actual color of the diagram.

## Color Blindness

Many people will be unable to see all colors equally well. This is due to an **inherited** (in her′ it) defect in the color-sensitive nerves. About 7 percent of the men and 1 percent of the women in the world are born with such a defect (Figure 15.9).

This color blindness takes several forms. Some people see all of the waves from the shorter end of the spectrum as blue. Others see all of the longer waves as yellow. In these cases, the cones that are supposed to be stimulated by certain wavelengths do not function well. Occasionally, a person will be born with cones that are not stimulated by any of the different wavelengths. These people will be unable to distinguish any color, seeing light in various shades of gray.

### Have You Learned?

On a sheet of paper list the numbers for the questions below. By each number write *T* if the statement is true and *F* if false.

1. Scientists do not fully understand how we see color.
2. Color is sensed by the cones of the eye.
3. The light-sensitive parts of the eye respond to all wavelengths of light equally well.
4. The brain can be fooled into seeing colors that are not really there.
5. All people see color equally well.

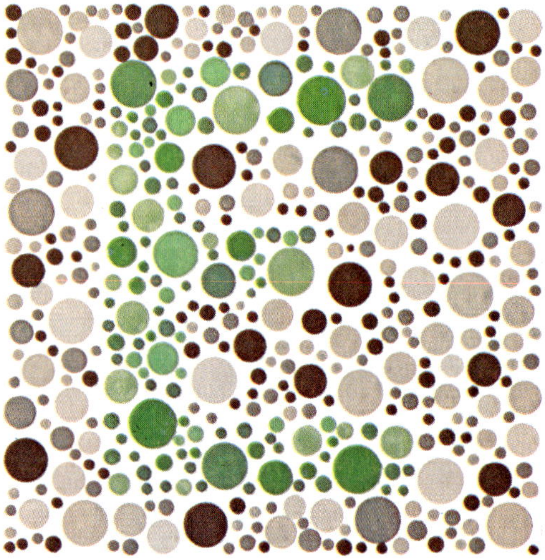

**15.9** What letter of the alphabet do you see?

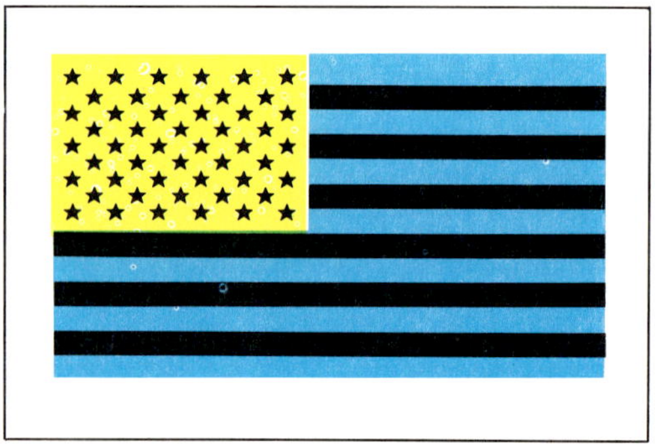

**15.10** Observing colors that are not there (pages 464-465)

## 4. Putting Rainbows to Work

**ARE YOU READY?**

Look up the following words if you are not sure of their meanings:

absorb; complementary colors; fluorescent lamp; incandescent lamp; luminous; negative (in photography); spectra; telescope.

Scientists have found many valuable uses for the spectrum. One of the most important research instruments is called the **spectroscope** (spek′ trə skōp). It consists of a prism, which produces a spectrum, and a small telescope that is used to look at the spectrum.

A number of important studies can be made using the spectroscope. For some of these, a device for measuring the spectrum is added. Therefore, this instrument is called a **spectrometer** (spek trom′ i tər). If photographs are taken, the instrument is known as a **spectrograph** (spek′ trə graf′). In each of these the scientist is able to observe the spectrum produced by the prism.

### Making a Simple Spectroscope

**MATERIALS:**

A one-inch square **diffraction** (di frak′ shən) **grating,** which your teacher can obtain for you, a shoe box, two double-edged razor blades, transparent tape

**PROCEDURE:**

In one end of the shoe box, cut a hole about 1 centimeter in diameter. Tape the diffraction grating over the hole so that the lines on it are *vertical.* In the end of the shoe box opposite the diffraction grating and *directly across* from it, cut a narrow, vertical slit. Tape one razor blade to the box so that its edge lies vertically along the middle of the slit. Tape the second razor blade on the other side of the slit so that the two blades make a slit that is 1 mm wide.

To use your spectroscope, simply put the top on the box, and look at some light source. To do this, sight through the slit between the two razor blades. Like a prism, the grating breaks up the light into its colors. Can you see a different pattern of light between two different light sources, such as an incandescent lamp and a fluorescent lamp? Do different-colored neon lights produce different patterns?

## Spectra of the Elements

The usefulness of the spectroscope by scientists lies in the fact that each element produces a certain type of spectrum when it is heated. You have seen this phenomenon in the bursting of fireworks, where different elements are used to produce a wide range of colors. **Strontium** (stron′ shi əm) is used to produce red. Sodium is used for yellow, and the greens are produced by copper. You have already learned that these different colored lights have different wavelengths. By use of the spectroscope, these differing wavelengths of light can be carefully measured and studied.

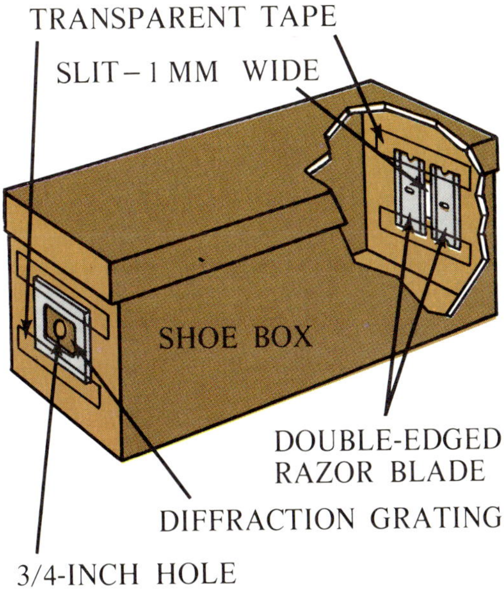

**15.11** Making a simple spectroscope

When an element is heated, it will become incandescent above a certain temperature. If the light from this source is directed through a prism, a spectrum will be formed. But since only certain wavelengths of light are produced by an incandescent element in the gaseous form, only certain colors will be seen. Figure 15.12 on this page shows the spectra for several elements, as seen through a spectroscope. These are known as **bright line spectra** (spek′ trə), since the spectra

**15.12** Bright-line and dark-line (also called absorption) spectra

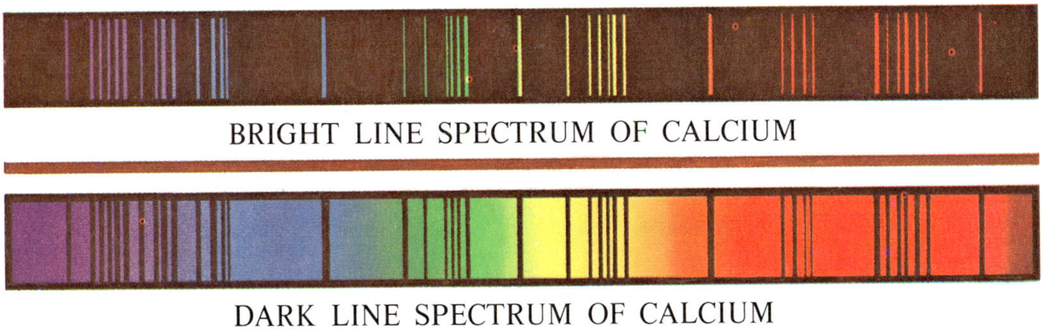

formed by single elements contain a great deal of dark space with only a few bright lines of color scattered throughout certain portions of it. In this way, the spectroscope "fingerprints" each element. By comparing the bright line spectrum of an unknown element with the pattern produced by known elements, chemists can identify any element they wish. Even the elements that make up compounds can be sorted out and identified.

If a white light passes through a gas and then through the spectroscope, a spectrum like the lower band in Figure 15.12 on page 467 will be formed. Compare this with the bright line spectrum. Notice that the black lines in this spectrum correspond closely with the lines of color in the bright line spectrum. The explanation for this is that apparently the elements in the gas through which the white light passes absorb the same wavelengths of light that the elements would produce if the gas had been incandescent. These are called **absorption** (ab sôrp′ shən) **spectra** and are used in the same way as bright line spectra.

The advantage of the absorption spectra is, of course, that the elements being studied do not have to be incandescent. Astronomers have made good use of absorption spectra to study the elements found in the atmospheres of various planets.

## Color Photographs

The scientists' knowledge of the nature of colored light allows us to take and print colored photographs. Actually, as you may know, there are two types of color film. One of these is used to produce colored slides, while the other is used to produce colored prints of our pictures. Both of these types of film are about the same and can be discussed together.

Color film that is used in cameras is made of three light-sensitive layers. Each of these film layers has been treated with special silver compounds that absorb *only* certain wavelengths of light. The first records only the blue light, the second is sensitive only to the green light, while the third layer responds only to red light.

Light enters the camera and is focused on the film. As it passes through the first layer, almost all of the blue light is absorbed and makes a chemical change in the silver salt molecules that it touches. A yellow filter is usually placed beneath this film layer to absorb any blue light that may pass through. Then the light, minus the blue wavelengths, strikes the second layer of film. Here the green wavelengths are absorbed by silver salts and make a chemical change in the salts. Now only the red wavelengths of light remain. These enter the third layer of film and affect the silver molecules there. Any excess light is absorbed by the black backing of the film.

During the developing process, a three-layered *negative* is produced. At first, images that reflected blue light into the camera are seen as dark images on the blue-sensitive layer. These areas are clear on the other two layers. Can you explain why?

In a similar way, green light produces dark images on *only* the green-sensitive layer. And red light creates dark images *only* on the red-sensitive layer.

At the same time, the three-layered negative is dyed. But the film is not dyed blue, green, and red. Instead it is dyed with the *complementary colors* of these primary colors. And it is the clear areas of each layer, not the dark areas, that receive the dye. The clear areas of the blue-sensitive layer are dyed yellow. The clear areas of the green-sensitive layer are colored with magenta dye. And the red-sensitive layer receives cyan-colored dye on its clear areas. After this is completed, the dark silver areas are washed clear, leaving a transparent area on each negative layer that corresponds with the image formed by the various colors of light.

In the printer or in the slide projector, white light is shone through all three of the dyed layers. Let's imagine that light passes through a certain area of the negative. At the first layer it strikes yellow dye, and the blue wavelengths are absorbed. It then passes through the magenta dye, which absorbs the greens. The only light that reaches the third layer of the negative is red light, and at this particular spot the red-sensitive layer is clear. Therefore, a beam of red light passes through the negative and onto the print paper or screen.

In a similar way, where the yellow dye overlaps the cyan dye, a green image is produced. The light passing through both cyan and magenta dye is seen as blue. What conditions produce white areas on a color print? Black areas? Look at color negatives and prints, and see if you can identify spots that are similar to those described above.

## Color Printing

The printing industry also uses the knowledge of color discovered by the scientist. The best quality of color printing uses only four colors of inks—yellow, magenta, cyan, and black.

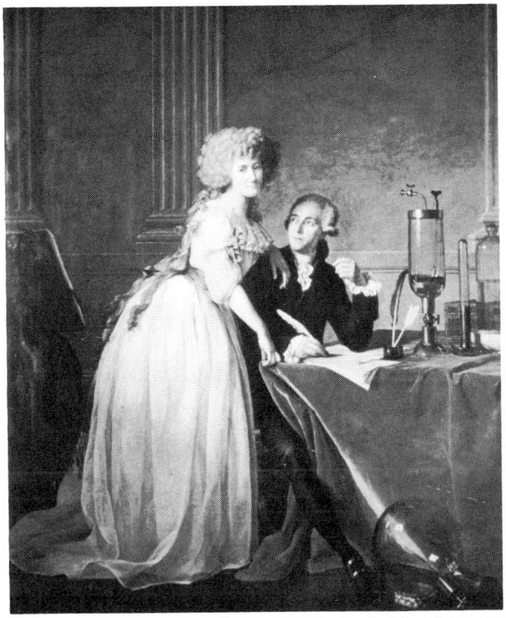

*Courtesy of The Rockefeller University*

**15.13** Compare this black-and-white picture with the color picture on page 152.

The first step in the four-color printing process is the taking of four photographs of the page to be printed. First, a red filter is used to absorb all of the wavelengths of light from the red end of the spectrum. This produces a "cyan negative" that shows dark areas wherever red is not present. A second photograph is taken, this time using a green filter. This "magenta negative" is dark in the areas where green light is absent. A third photograph through a blue filter produces a "yellow negative," and a final photograph without filters fills in the black areas.

A separate metal plate for each negative is then etched. The cyan negative allows the red areas of the photograph to be etched out, leaving the cyan images raised enough to catch the ink. The other negatives are used in the same way to produce plates that will print the magenta, yellow, and black portions of the page to complete the image.

The raised portions of each plate are coated with the proper color of ink. The paper passes under each plate in turn. First the cyan-colored portions of the page are printed and the ink allowed to dry. Next the yellow ink is placed on the paper, then the magenta, and finally the black. Can you explain what colors will appear on the page where each combination of two of these inks overlap?

### Have You Learned?

Select the answer that best completes each statement. (Do not write in your book.)

An instrument called a (1) _____ (microscope; spectroscope) is used to study spectra. The principle of this instrument lies in the fact that when an element is heated it produces light of a certain (2) _____ (wavelength; speed). If light from an incandescent element is directed through a prism, a (3) _____ (bright line; absorption) spectrum is formed. This helps chemists (4) _____ (combine; identify) elements.

Color film for cameras has (5) _____ (three; two) light-sensitive layers. When colored light strikes these film layers it causes (6) _____ (black-and-white; colored) images to be formed. A color negative is composed of (7) _____ (single; several) layers. Where cyan dye overlaps yellow dye on a negative, a (8) _____ (green; red) color is seen.

In printing color pictures only four colors of ink are required. These are black, (9) _____ (yellow, magenta, and cyan; red, blue, and green).

## 5. Above and Below the Spectrum

**ARE YOU READY?**

Look up the following words if you are not sure of their meanings:

gamma ray; RADAR; transverse wave; X ray.

You have learned about some other types of transverse waves of energy that are of different wavelengths than light. Some of these, such as radio and television waves, are many times longer than the red end of the light spectrum. Other transverse waves, such as X rays and gamma rays, are shorter than the violet wavelengths.

### Energy in the Form of Waves

Light energy travels in the form of waves. As you have learned, the length of the light wave determines the color of the light. You know that we see light because our eyes contain nerves that are sensitive to these lengths of energy waves.

In spite of the tremendous differences in wavelength of these energy waves, they all travel through a vacuum or through air at the same speed—about $3 \times 10^{10}$ cm per second (speed of light). The reason for this unexpected and interesting relationship between these different forms of energy is that all of them are apparently produced in the same way. Each is the result of the acceleration of a charged particle—an electron, atom, or molecule.

You will remember from Chapter 3 that acceleration means *any* change in speed or direction. Thus, energy waves may be given off when a particle speeds up, slows down, or is forced in a new direction. The waves produced by this acceleration have both electrical properties and magnetic properties. Because of this, all of these energy waves are classified together as **electromagnetic** (i lek′ trō mag net′ ik) waves.

Imagine a particle that is being accelerated in a certain pattern. For example, an electron in a radio antenna is made to move in one direction for a short period of time, then is stopped and forced to move in the opposite direction. With each change in direction electromagnetic waves will be created. These waves will travel away from the moving electron at a speed of $3 \times 10^{10}$ cm per second through the air.

You know that the frequency times the wavelength equals the velocity of a wave. Since the velocity of all electromagnetic waves is the same ($3 \times 10^{10}$ cm per second), the *frequency* of the change in direction of the electron will determine the *length* of the wave. The slower the frequency, the longer the waves will be.

It is possible to arrange all of these forms of energy into a single chart, according to the wavelength and the frequency of the waves. This chart is called the **electromagnetic spectrum** and is shown in Figure 15.15.

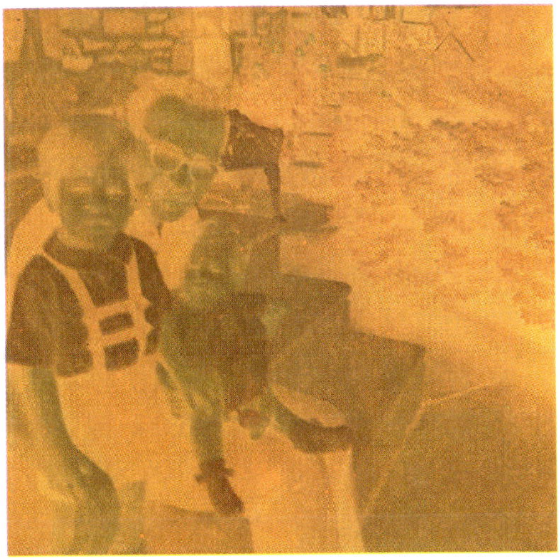

**15.14** One type of color film (negative)

## The Electromagnetic Spectrum

Notice that visible light makes up a very small portion of this spectrum, ranging from a wavelength of $75 \times 10^{-6}$ (0.000075) cm at the red end down to waves of only $40 \times 10^{-6}$ (0.000040) cm at

**15.15** Electromagnetic spectrum

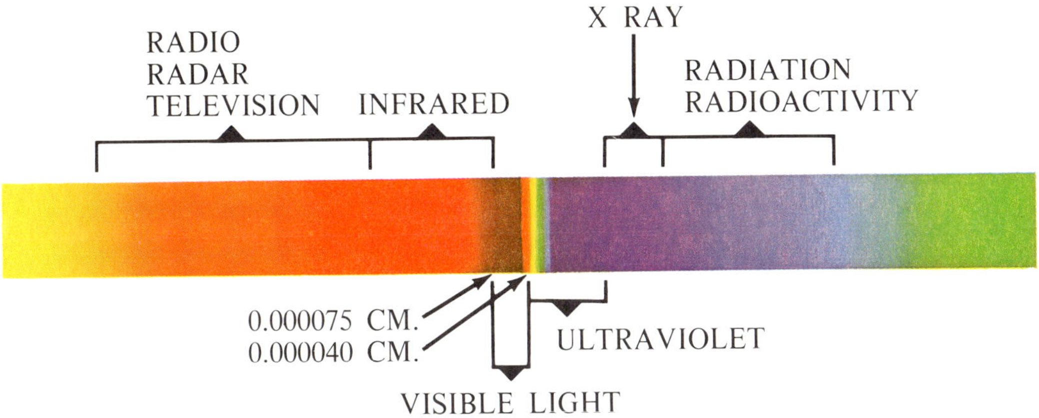

the violet end. Immediately below the visible spectrum is an area of **ultraviolet** energy, whose waves may be as short as $10^{-6}$ cm. Below this are the X rays and the radiation produced by radioactivity.

Longer than the red light is an area of **infrared** energy, with waves as long as $^1/_{10}$ cm. Longer still are the RADAR, television, and radio wavelengths.

The various wavelengths listed in this chart are not important enough to be memorized. They are used here to show that scientists now think that *all* forms of electromagnetic wave energy are similar. The primary difference among them is that each form of electromagnetic energy has a different frequency and wavelength.

### Have You Learned?

Select the answer that best completes each statement. (Do not write in your book.)

1. _____ (Radio; X-ray) waves are shorter than light waves.

2. All waves shown on the electromagnetic spectrum are _____ (longitudinal; transverse).

3. _____ (Some; All) waves in the electromagnetic spectrum travel at $3 \times 10^{10}$ cm per second.

4. The waves of ultraviolet light are _____ (longer; shorter) than the visible light waves.

5. The primary difference among the various forms of energy making up the electromagnetic spectrum is their _____ (frequency; speed).

## 6. Lasers and Masers

**ARE YOU READY?**

Look up the following words if you are not sure of their meanings:

amplification; elevated; emission; retina; stimulated.

In 1951 a new way of amplifying radio waves was being discussed in scientific journals. By 1954 an American scientist, Charles H. Townes, and his co-workers, built the first **maser** (mā′ zər). The name of the device stands for *m*icrowave *a*mplification by *s*timulated *e*mission of *r*adiation. The maser led Townes and Arthur Schawlow to investigate optical masers that would produce a narrow beam of high-intensity light. They published an article in 1958 describing how this could be done. By 1960 Theodore Maiman had built and demonstrated the first **laser** (lā′ zər) (*l*ight *a*mplification by *s*timulated *e*mission of *r*adiation).

### How the Laser Works

The maser and laser are based on the same scientific principles. In the case of the laser, a burst of very, very bright light in the form of a narrow beam can be produced. This light is said to be **coherent** (kō hēr′ ənt) light because it consists of a single definite frequency moving in a single direction. This is in contrast to the light produced by a light bulb, which is made up of many frequencies and traveling in many directions. The light from a light bulb is said to be **incoherent** (in′ kō hēr′ ənt). What evidence do you have that sunlight is made up of many different frequencies and therefore incoherent?

In one type of laser a ruby crystal in the shape of a cylinder is used to produce a beam of coherent light. One end of the cylinder is silvered so that it acts as a mirror. The other end is only partially silvered so that some of the light produced in the crystal can pass through it. A flash tube that produces bright flashes of light is wrapped around the ruby rod. The energy of these light flashes causes electrons in chromium atoms in the ruby to move into outer orbits. These atoms with electrons in elevated orbits are said to be *excited.* In time, when electrons fall back into empty inner orbits, energy is given off.

The light energy produced when an electron moves back to an inner orbit causes electrons in other excited atoms to move back into lower orbits. This chain reaction is called *stimulated emission.* The light produced this way is the same color and travels in the same direction as the light causing the emission. Light traveling along the axis of the ruby rod bounces off the silvered ends. But as the light travels back and forth through the rod, other stimulated emissions occur and the intensity of the beam increases. When the intensity reaches a certain level, part of the light passes through the partly silvered end of the rod to form the laser beam.

In addition to crystal lasers, such as the one using a ruby rod, lasers using tubes of gas and small blocks of semiconductor material have been developed. Although they operate in much the same way, each type has its advantages. For example, a gas laser, although less powerful than crystal lasers, can produce a continuous beam instead of short bursts of energy. The nature of the light produced by gas lasers is well suited for use in communications.

## How Lasers Are Used

Many applications of lasers have been developed since their invention just a few years ago. A laser beam can be used as a source of intense heat, producing temperatures of 5,500° C and higher in a small area. Laser beams are used in medicine to burn away diseased tissue and correct an eye condition called "detached retina." They also are used in the same way as RADAR to find distances between two objects. Lasers are involved in producing special photographs called **holograms** (hol′ ə gram). A hologram gives a three-dimensional image of an object and, besides being fascinating to look at, represents an important new research tool for many fields of science.

Lasers have played an important role in the space program. On man's first trip to the moon, Astronaut Neil Armstrong placed a specially designed laser reflector on the moon's surface. Scientists then fired pulses of laser light through the huge telescopes at Lick Observatory in California and McDonald Observatory in Texas. It wasn't long before they were able to detect the signals being reflected off the moon's surface. Laser beams of course travel at the speed of light. Can you estimate how long it would take a laser pulse to reach the moon some 400,000 kilometers away and to return?

Once the distances from the two observatories to a spot on the moon are known, it is possible to find accurately how far apart the two observatories are. This information will be useful to map makers and in answering such questions as whether the continents are slowly drifting apart.

## Have You Learned?

Select the answer that best completes each statement. (Do not write in your book.)

1. Light of a single wavelength and moving in a single direction is called _____ (coherent; incoherent) light.
2. A continuous beam of light is produced in a _____ (crystal; gas) laser.
3. A laser beam travels at the speed of _____ (light; sound).
4. The light produced from a _____ (gas; crystal) laser can be used in communications.
5. Temperatures up to ____ (5,500° C; 15,500° C) can be produced from a laser beam.

## REVIEW QUESTIONS

1. Explain why if the wave of one color of light has a longer wavelength than that of another color of light, the first will also have a lower frequency.
2. If you take a red piece of paper into a dark room and shine a violet light on it, what color will you see? Explain why.
3. Explain how a rainbow is formed.
4. If you mix all colors of light together, white light is produced. If you mix all colors of paint together, black is produced. Explain why this is so.
5. Explain the currently accepted theory of how we see color.
6. What is retinal fatigue?
7. Explain the difference between—
   a. spectroscope, spectrometer, and spectrograph;
   b. bright line spectrum and absorption spectrum.
8. Explain how color photographs are produced.
9. Explain how colored pictures can be printed in books.
10. What is the electromagnetic spectrum? Why is it important?
11. Describe how a laser works and tell some of the ways it is used.

## CAN YOU FIND OUT?

*It may be necessary to use encyclopedias or other reference books in answering the following questions.*

1. What are the frequencies and wavelengths of the colors of the rainbow?
2. What recent experiments have been done to discover how we see color? Can all animals see color? How do scientists know this?
3. What is color blindness? Can it be dangerous? Can it be of any advantage for a person to be color blind?
4. How are spectroscopes used by astronomers?
5. How do Polaroid cameras produce colored photographs?
6. Can you find out more about how lasers operate, different types of lasers, and how they are used?

## REFERENCES FOR ADDITIONAL STUDY

THE ART AND SCIENCE OF COLOR by Hal Hellman. McGraw-Hill Book Company.
Covers the science of light and color as well as the interesting effects and applications

COLOR IN YOUR LIFE by Irving Adler. The John Day Company, Inc.
Covers a broad range of topics—reflection, refraction, absorption, diffraction, color mixing, color printing, and photography

LIGHT AND COLOR by Harold Highland. Grosset & Dunlap, Inc.
Covers most phases of the science of light and contains directions for doing many simple activities

MASERS AND LASERS by H. Arthur Klein. J. B. Lippincott Company.
Describes how lasers operate and some of their uses

# *Workshop... Unit VI*

**Determing the Speed of Sound.** One way to measure the speed of sound is to go outdoors on a still day and measure the time between when you see something happen and when you hear it. For example, place a bass drummer at one end of a football field and have an observer with a stopwatch at the other end of the field. Measure the length of time between when the observer sees the drum being hit and when he hears it. You may also wish to use a starting pistol. In this case, measure the time between when you see the puff of smoke and hear the report. If you know the distance between the source of the sound and the observer and the time it takes for the sound to travel this distance, can you calculate the speed of sound in meters per second? In the case of races where the starter is at one end of the track and the timers are at the other end, should the timers start their watches when they see the puff of smoke or when they hear the bang? Explain what difference this would make (Figure W6.1).

**Finding the Speed of Sound with a Tuning Fork.** Place a piece of glass tubing about 2.5 cm in diameter and 60 cm long in a tall beaker or jug of water as shown in Figure W6.2. Hold a vibrating tuning fork over the top of the glass tubing, and move the glass tubing up and down until the loudest sound is produced. When the sound is loudest, the column of air inside of the glass tubing is in resonance with the tuning fork. Measure the distance from the top of the glass tubing to the level of the water, which is the length of the resonating column of air.

The wavelength of the sound produced by the tuning fork is found by multiplying the length of the resonating column of air times four. For example, if the column is 30 cm long, the wavelength of the sound is 120 cm ($30 \times 4$).

Once the frequency and wavelength of a sound are known, the speed can be calculated using the formula, speed = wavelength $\times$ frequency (number of vibrations per second). To see how this works, imagine that the tuning fork we are using vibrates 256 times per second and that the resonance occurs when the column of air is 30 cm high. We have seen that the wavelength is 1.2 meter (length of the column of air times 4). We can find the speed by multiplying the wavelength times the frequency ($1.2 \times 256 = 307.2$ m per second). How does this value compare with the speed of sound at room temperature?

Practice finding the speed of sound with this method, using tuning forks of varying

**W6.1** This is one way you can measure the speed of sound with a stopwatch.

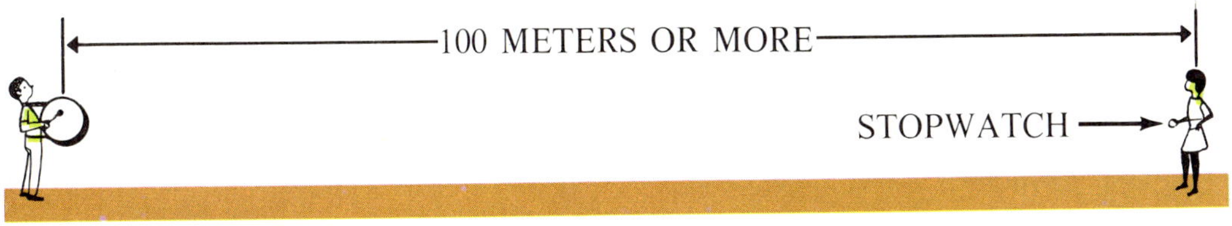

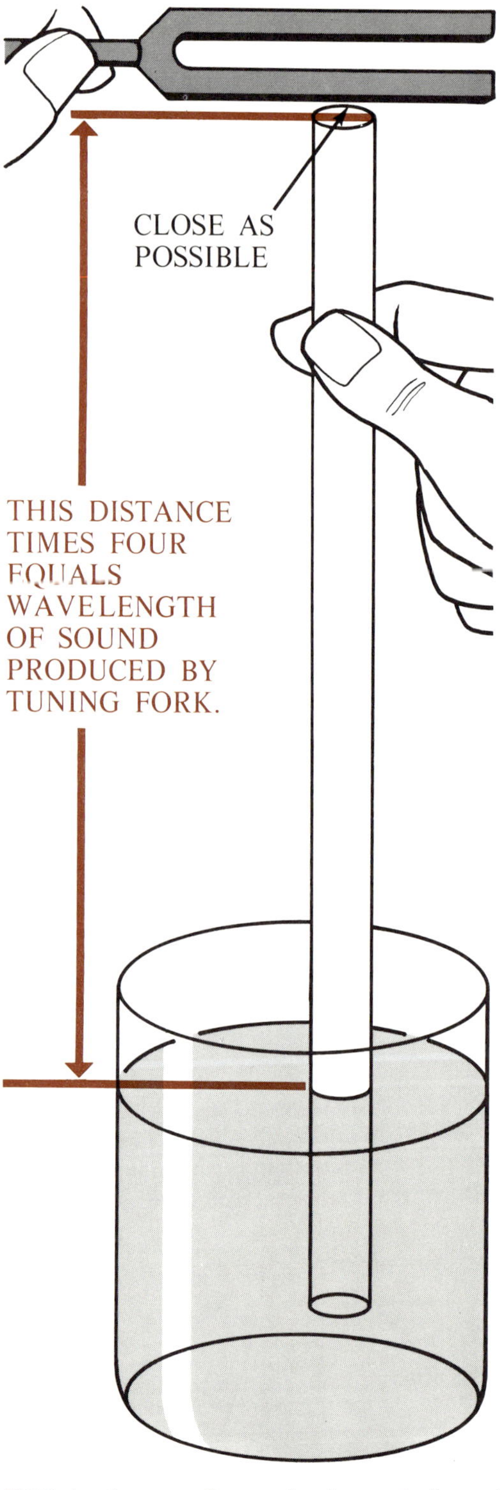


**W6.2** Another way of measuring the speed of sound

pitches. Can you figure out a way to use this method to determine the pitch of an unmarked tuning fork?

**Studying Reflection and Refraction.** Fill a large aquarium with water, and add a few drops of food coloring or milk. This will make it easier to see a beam of light passing through the water. Place a large flat mirror in the bottom of the aquarium as shown in Figure W6.3. Position a slide projector above the aquarium as shown. To make a narrower beam, place a cardboard slide with a half-inch hole in the projector.

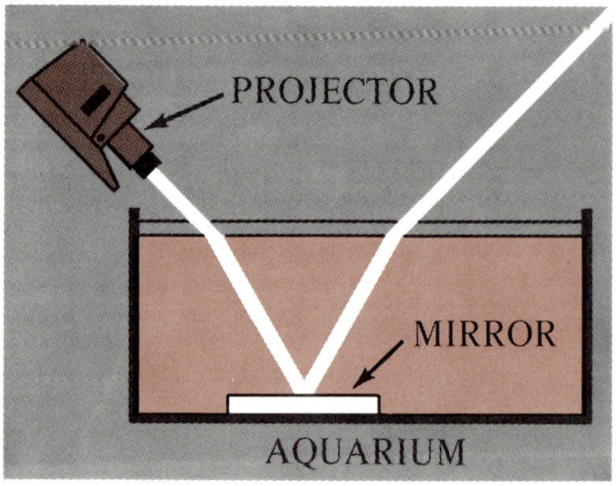


**W6.3** Reflection and refraction made visible

Use a grease pencil to trace on the side of the aquarium the path of the light beam. Which way is the light beam refracted when it enters the water? Can you explain why it is bent in this direction? Is the angle between the incoming light beam and the mirror equal to the angle between the mirror and the light beam leaving the mirror? Change the position of the projector so it is higher above the aquarium. Are the two angles between the light beam and the mirror still equal? Which way is the light beam refracted as it leaves the water?

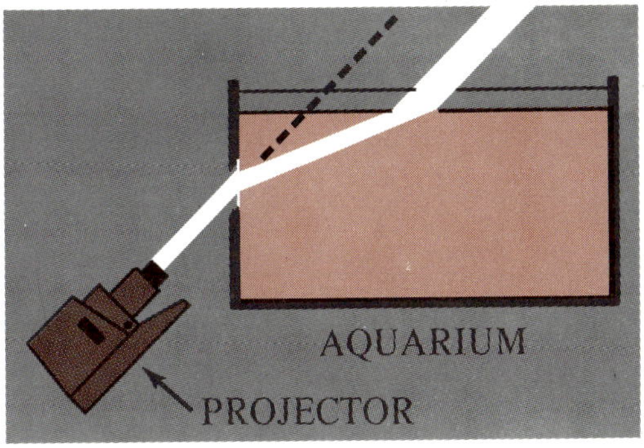


**W6.4** Try to explain what you see.

Place the projector so that it shines upward through the water (Figure W6.4). Explain why the light beam does not travel straight through the water.

**Making a Pinhole Camera.** An inexpensive pinhole camera can be made using a one-pound coffee can or, if a can is not available, a box about 15 cm long can be used. In the bottom of the can make a hole about 2 cm across. Paste a piece of black construction paper over the hole, and use a Number 10 needle to make a small hole in the black paper. This small hole should be as close to the center of the can as possible. Use tape and a piece of black paper to make a flap to cover the pinhole (Figure W6.5).

In a darkroom, tape a piece of photographic film on the inside of the lid of the can, and place the lid on the can. The can must be light-tight when the film is inside. In the case of a plastic lid, paint it with dull-black paint. (Painting the inside of the can with black paint will help cut down reflection inside the can when the exposure is being made.)

Take your pinhole camera outdoors on a sunny day. Place it on a post or other sturdy object while making the exposure. The exposure is made by lifting the flap and allowing light to pass through the pinhole and strike the film. Since the length of the exposure will depend on the size of the pinhole, the brightness of the day, and the kind of film you are using, you will have to experiment to find the proper exposure time. Start out by making exposures for about 30 seconds, then 1 minute, and then 2 minutes and compare your results.

The film must be removed from the pinhole camera in a darkroom. You can develop your negative following the procedures described in the Workshop at the end of Unit III.

**W6.5** Have a contest with your pinhole cameras.

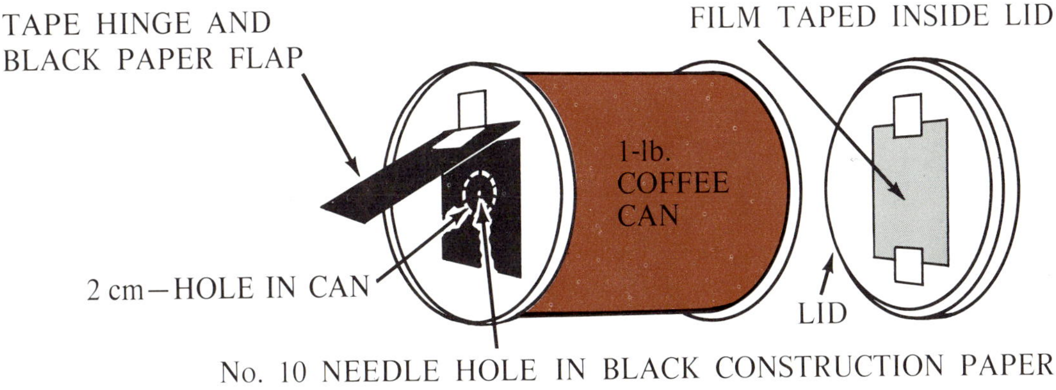

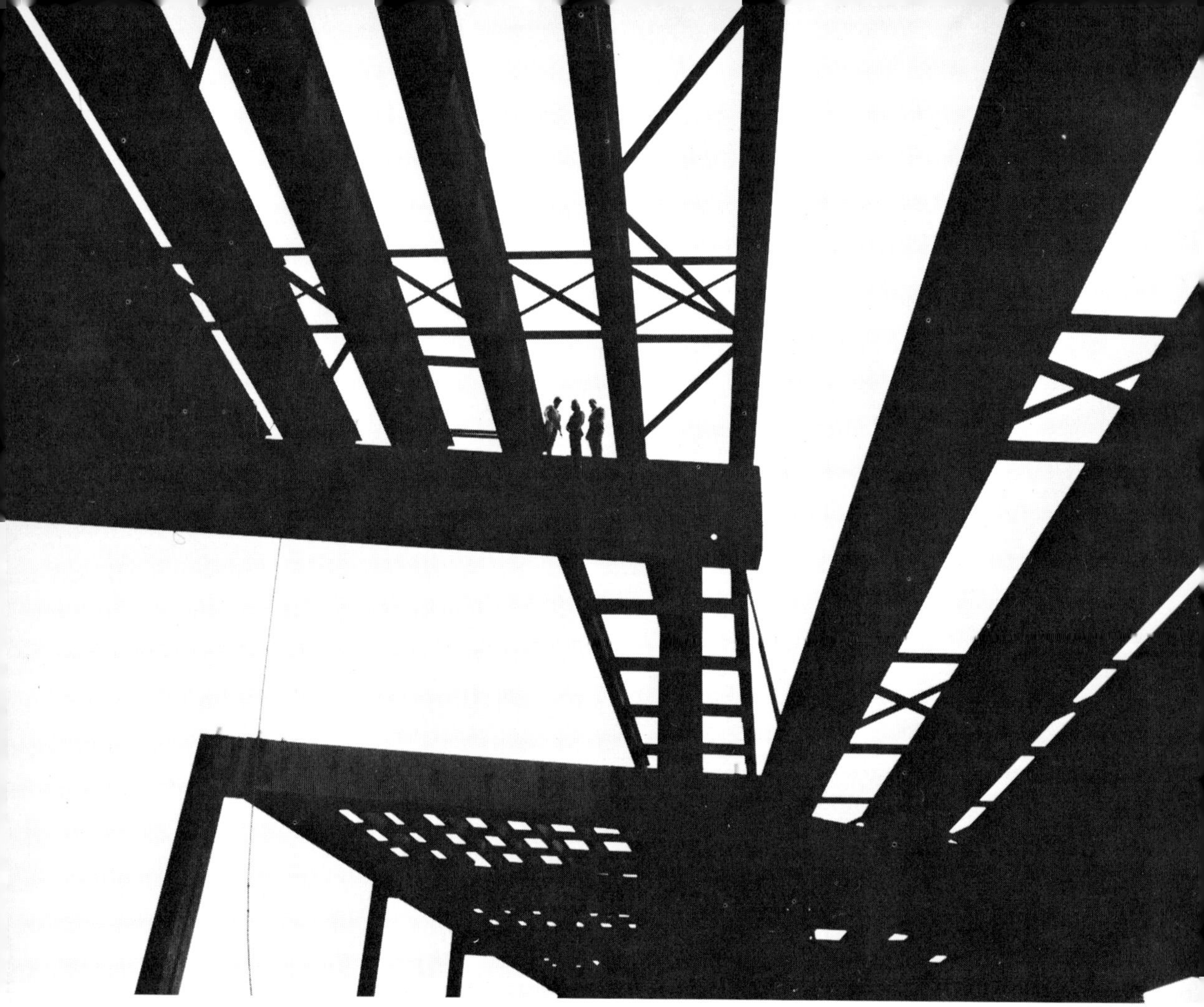

# unit VII

## careers: putting it together

Ellis Herwig/Stock, Boston

CHAPTER 16

# Your Future in Science

WITHIN THE NEXT few years you will be faced with the need for earning a living. School will be behind you, and the world of work will lie ahead. Which of the thousands and thousands of job opportunities will you choose?

At first it may seem that you will be able to choose any career you want. And you do have an almost unlimited choice. But the choice you make after you finish school may be limited by the choices you make while you are still in high school.

During the next few years you will have to make many decisions—about what courses to take and about how much you learn while taking these courses. Making these decisions wisely is a difficult job. It requires that you know a lot about the type of job you may want to choose later. It also requires that you know a lot about yourself.

## 1. The Need For Physical Scientists

**ARE YOU READY?**

Look up the following words if you are not sure of their meanings:

engineer; environment; pollution; prediction research; technology.

As you have seen as you studied this book, there are many different kinds of physical scientists. There are also many different kinds of jobs in technology. The men and women who earn their living with their knowledge of physical science are very valuable members of our society. They are also well paid for their skill.

**MAKING A JOB SURVEY**

Try to list all of the jobs that you can think of that require some knowledge of physical science. Discuss your list with your friends and make one large list. You may also wish to check the want ads in a city newspaper for ideas. How many jobs can you think of?

### Forecasting Future Opportunities

It is difficult for anyone to predict with any accuracy how many scientists, engineers, and technologists we will need in the future. If we could, your choices would be much easier to make.

There are many reasons why the attempts to make such predictions go wrong so often. The number of jobs in any field depends upon the health of the economy in general, and this is difficult to predict. Many of the jobs in science-related fields depend upon the action of the federal government in its attempt to solve national problems. And it is impossible to predict what kind of scientific breakthroughs will occur. Then it is difficult to predict what effect these will have on the types of physical science jobs that will be available in a few years.

During the past few generations, the number of people working in science-related jobs has increased greatly. Since 1930 the number of scientists and engineers in the United States has nearly doubled. In 1903 there were only three industrial research labs in this country. Today there are more than 3,000. During the 1960s the number of people graduating from college with degrees in physical science, engineering, or mathematics increased by 50%. And thousands of more people went into physical science jobs that require less than a college degree.

The growth in scientific knowledge constantly creates new jobs. One estimate says that 90% of all the scientists *who ever lived* are alive today! In other words, there are more job opportunities in science now than there have been in the whole history of the world put together.

Because of this rapid growth in scientific knowledge, however, it is impossible for anyone to say what types of jobs in physical science will be open in several years. That is when you will be ready to go to work. Therefore, when you make a choice about your education, it is important that you avoid making a decision that might prevent you from going into a new field later on.

**16.1** A group of scientists looks like any other group of people. Scientists often hold international meetings in order to exchange ideas. Communication and discussion are necessary in science.

*Wide World*

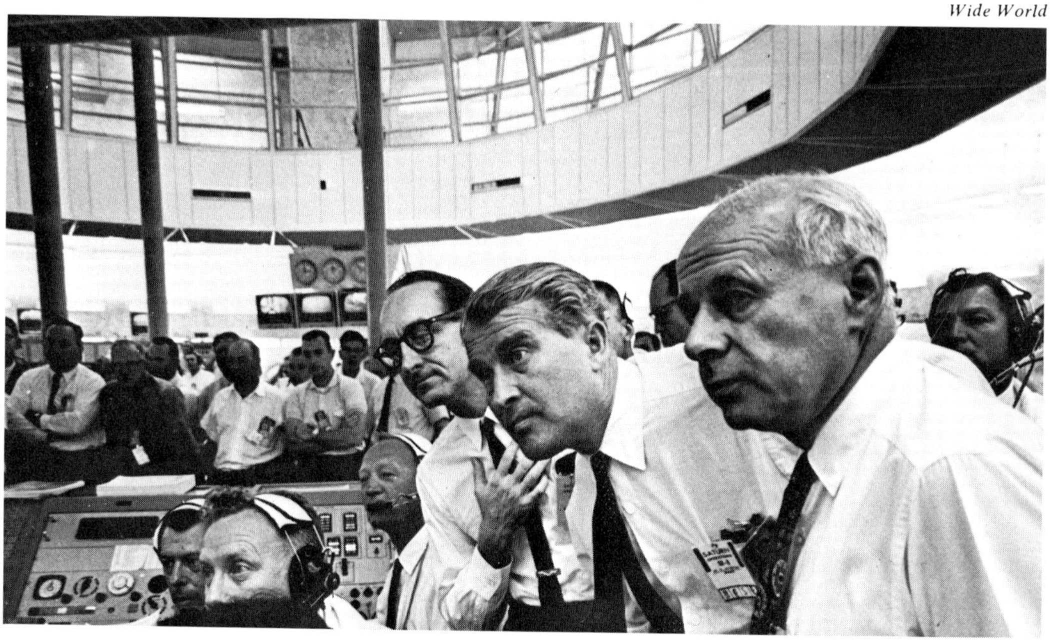

## Making Decisions

Many students make a mistake when they decide not to take advanced courses in high school. They decide too quickly upon a course that will prevent them from taking other courses later. Or they take courses that will not help them go to college. They make up their minds that they do not want more education after high school.

Science and mathematics courses in high school are good springboards to a wide variety of job opportunities. A knowledge of these subjects may not seem to be of much use to people in certain professions. But an understanding of the important ideas of science and mathematics certainly *is an advantage* in most jobs. And taking these courses often gives you the chance to go into jobs that you never expected to enter.

The number of jobs available in any field varies with many factors, of course. The need for people trained in one branch of science may be high one year and then suddenly drop. Statistics on employment of recent college graduates show that students trained in non-science fields have more trouble finding jobs than do students who have taken science and mathematics courses. Not all science students become research scientists, but most of them find jobs in professions related to science.

## Solving Our Environmental Crisis

Some students seem to have decided to stay away from science because of the crisis with our environment. They may feel that science and technology are responsible for the damage that our surroundings have suffered. What these students fail to realize is that the only hope people have of saving

**16.2** Environmentalists should have a very broad understanding of many sciences. This scientist is advising a farmer how best to take advantage of the contours of his land in plowing it.

*Grant Heilman*

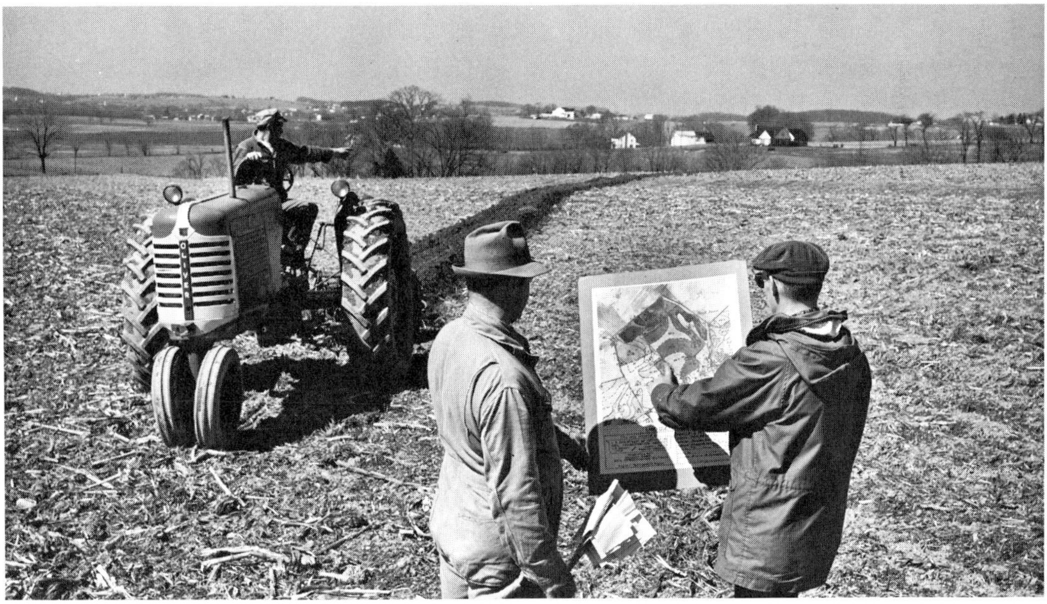

the environment lies in more and better understanding of science and more intelligent use of technology. Part of our environmental problems will be solved in the future by men and women who are well trained in science and mathematics.

For example, our pollution of water by chemical and human wastes probably will not be corrected by cutting back on either manufacturing or population. Instead, it will be solved by new methods of treating these wastes so that they will not damage the environment. Our energy shortage will not be totally solved by cutting back on our use of energy. It will be solved by the discovery of how to use different sources of energy. These solutions will be found by the scientists and engineers of the future.

Even the people who are not working toward the discovery of new knowledge need to have a strong background in science. Much of our present environmental crisis was caused by poor decisions by government officials and by those who run the industries. It is therefore necessary that these types of jobs be filled in the future by people who know something about science and how it affects people.

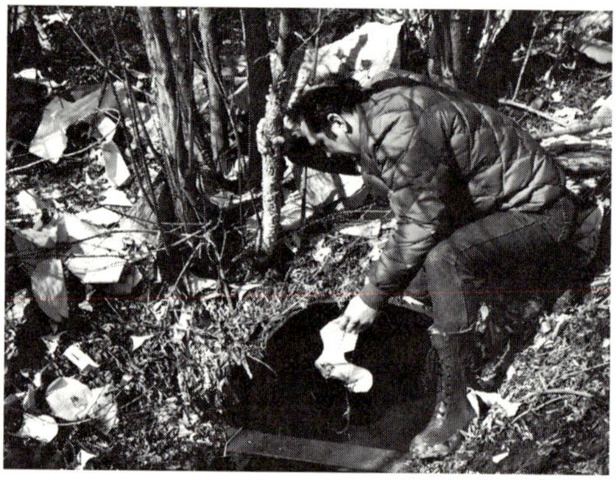

*Grant Heilman*

**16.3** This scientist is checking a polluted spring.

## Know Yourself

The first step you should take in making intelligent decisions about your future career is to learn as much as possible about yourself. You have certain abilities, skills, and interests. You should consider these before you make any decision that will affect how you live for the rest of your life. You also need to consider the amount and kind of education you can afford. And it is necessary for you to look at the educational opportunities that are available to you in your community.

**STUDYING YOURSELF**

On a sheet of paper write down an honest statement about yourself. How good a student are you? Do you do well in your science classes and mathematics courses? Do you seem to have the ability to go to college? Re-read the paragraphs in Chapter 1 on scientific attitudes. How many of these do you have?

On another sheet of paper write a statement about the interests you have developed. Do you like to work with your hands better than you like to work with people? Do you like to explain things to other people? What subjects in school have you found to be the most interesting and why?

If you need help in answering these questions, talk to your teacher and to your guidance counselor. How do abilities and interests match up with various kinds of jobs in science?

Now it is time to start looking at the possible jobs that are available to you. As you read through the next sections of this book, think about how you might fit into each of the jobs described. Ask yourself what courses in school would be of help to you in preparing for these jobs.

**HAVE YOU LEARNED?**

On a sheet of paper list the number for the questions below. By each number write *T* if the statement is true and *F* if false.

1. It is difficult to predict exactly how many people with training in physical science will be needed in future jobs.
2. There are about the same number of scientists and engineers today as there were in 1930.
3. What you do in high school has little effect on what you can do later.
4. College students who take science courses have less trouble finding jobs than do students trained in the non-science fields.
5. Women and men with training in science are needed to help solve the environmental crisis.

## 2. Professional Engineers and Scientists

**ARE YOU READY?**

Look up the following words if you are not sure of their meanings:

chemistry; electronic; engineer; industry; objectively; observer; physics; research; self-discipline; theoretical.

In the last section you were asked to make lists of your abilities and interests. Look at these lists again. What kind of a person are you? Do you have the ability, skill, and self-discipline to be a good student? Can you reason accurately and objectively? Do you read well? Can you write and speak in such a way that other people understand what you are trying to say? Do you feel comfortable working with mathematics?

Do you like to know how things work? Are you a careful observer? Are you open to new ideas and do you find new ideas exciting? If your answer to most of these questions is "yes," perhaps you should think about being a professional engineer or scientist.

### The Engineer

The job of the engineer is to turn the discoveries of the scientist into something useful. People trained in various fields of engineering design and build our water–supply systems, sewage systems, and power plants. They develop ways of manufacturing everything we use. They build our roads, cars, and spacecraft. And they are responsible for providing the raw materials for all of these.

There are more than a million engineers working in the United States at the present time. More than half of these work in manufacturing industries. They help design and make our electrical equipment, airplanes, and cars. Another large group of engineers are employed by construction companies and public utilities. The federal and state governments employ many thousands of engineers in such varied programs as agriculture, transportation, space exploration, and national defense.

There are more than 25 different branches of engineering from which the student may choose. A few of these special fields are discussed below.

**Automotive–aerospace engineers** are specialists in cars and trucks, airplanes, and spacecraft. Engineers with special types of training work on all phases of these machines from the first designs through production and final testing. The largest employer of aerospace engineers at the present time are those companies that make airplanes. But there is also a need for people who have knowledge and skills that can be used in space and missile programs.

**Agricultural engineers** are concerned with developing ways to produce and handle farm products more efficiently. They design and build machinery and buildings for use on the farm. They also design and build the equipment that makes the products used by the farmer and the equipment that is used to process the products of the farm. The wise use of water, soil, and energy is also the job of the agricultural engineer.

**Chemical engineers** do a wide variety of jobs. These are the people who design the machinery and plants that manufacture chemicals and chemical products. Other engineers work at discovering new, more efficient ways to manufacture these products. Solving the pollution problems sometimes caused by chemical manufac-

**16.4** Thousands of engineers are hired by the automotive industry to plan, develop, and test its many products.

*Ford Motor Company*

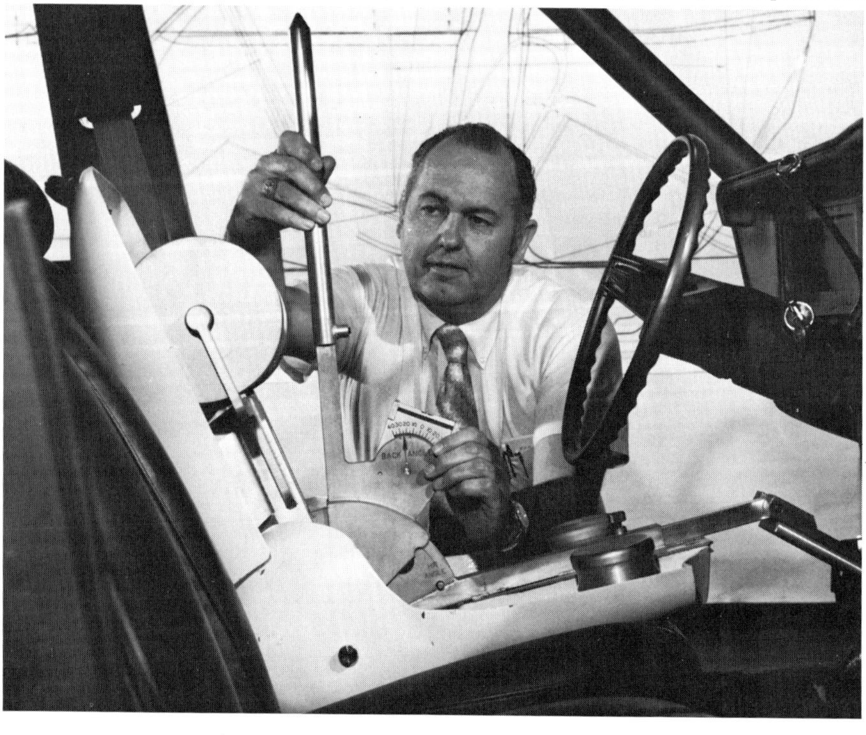

turing is also a job of the chemical engineer.

**Civil engineers** design and oversee the building of roads, bridges, and tunnels. They also work on the construction of large buildings. Some civil engineers specialize in the building of sewage and water systems. There are many other branches of this type of engineering.

**Electrical engineers** work on the design and production of all types of electrical and electronic equipment. These products include everything from television and radar to computers and spacecraft. Electrical engineers are also concerned with the production and distribution of electric power. This is the largest branch of the engineering profession.

**Mechanical engineers** work with machines. They are concerned with producing and using power. Any machine that you see was designed and built by people with training in mechanical engineering.

Almost all of the jobs in engineering require at least four years of college and a **bachelor's degree.** Usually, the first two years are spent studying basic science subjects, such as chemistry, physics, mathematics, English, and the social sciences. During the last two years, the future engineer studies their special field.

Some engineering jobs require a **master's degree,** which normally takes another year or two of specialized training. A few of the more technical engineering jobs need people who have **doctor's degrees,** which takes another two or three years of school beyond the master's degree.

**16.5** Electrical and electronic engineers are always in demand. Note the wide-angle-lens distortion.

*Ellis Herwig/Stock, Boston*

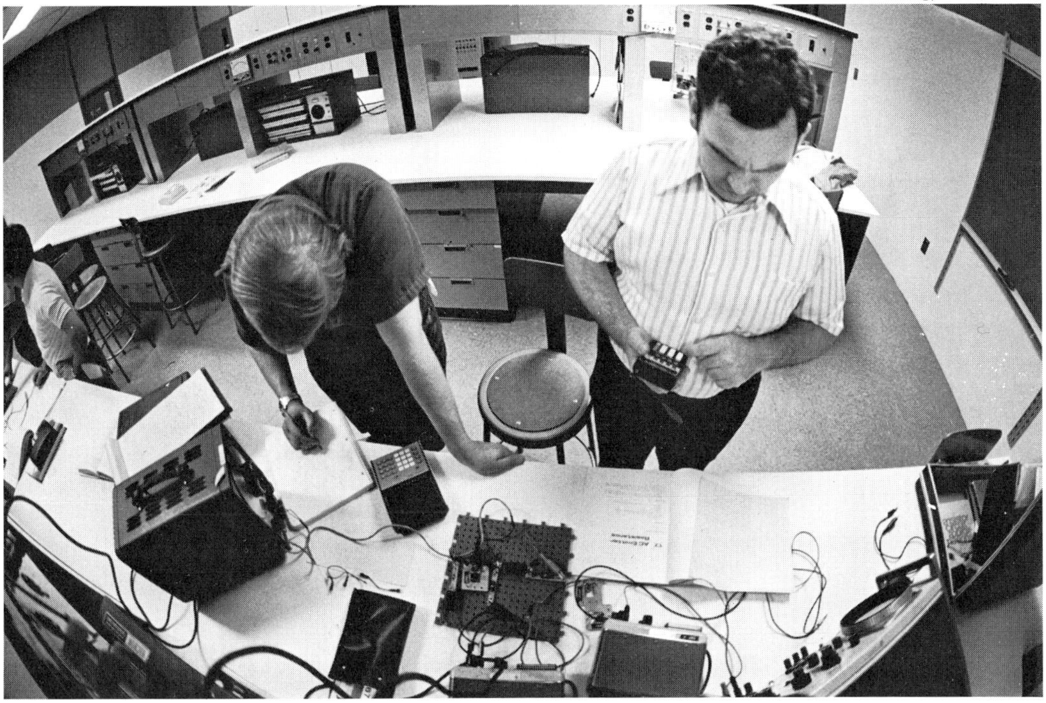

## The Physical Scientist

It is often difficult to separate the work of the engineer from the work of the scientist. Many scientists work at discovering new knowledge, but many others try to find ways to apply knowledge to the development of new processes and products. Because of this, the training of the scientist and the engineer is, in some fields, very similar.

The major branches of physical science are chemistry and physics. Each of these is divided into the special fields that you learned about as you read this book. For example, some chemists specialize in chemical compounds that contain carbon. Do you know what they are called?

People who have college degrees in one of these specialties can work in many types of jobs. Many physical scientists work for the federal government or one of the state governments. But most physical scientists earn their living by working in industry.

Nearly three-fourths of the physical scientists in the United States are chemists. About half of the chemists work in chemical manufacturing. About one-third of the people who have degrees in physics work for electrical industries, while others work for aerospace, instrument, and chemical companies.

As in the case of engineers a professional chemist or physicist must have at least a four-year bachelor's degree. During the first two years of college work, the future scientist usually studies English, the social sciences, mathematics, and sciences. The last two years are spent largely in studying more specialized science subjects.

Advanced degrees—the master's and doctor's degrees—are usually required for the person who wants to do research in physical science. A student interested in a career in basic research should plan on two to five years of study beyond his bachelor's degree.

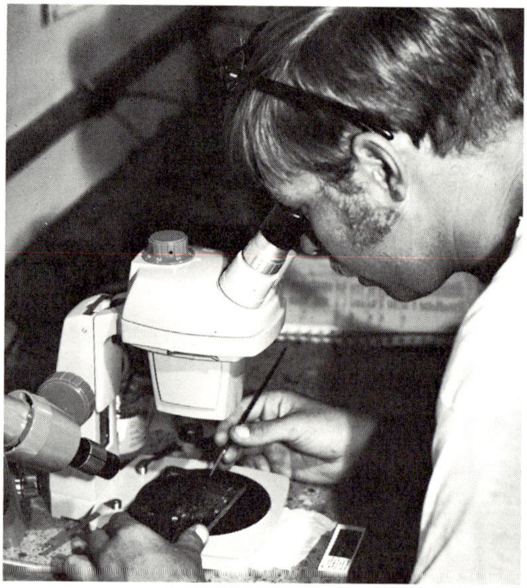

*Grant Heilman*

**16.6** Here a physical scientist is using a microscope. Life scientists are not the only people who use them. They are useful tools.

## Mathematicians

Mathematics is one of the most basic of the sciences. Without the work of the mathematician, the engineer and the physical scientist would not be able to make much progress. It surprises some people to learn that there are more mathematicians in this country than there are physicists.

The work of the mathematician may be divided into two categories. **Theoretical mathematicians** search for new knowledge. **Applied mathematicians** try to use their knowledge in practical ways.

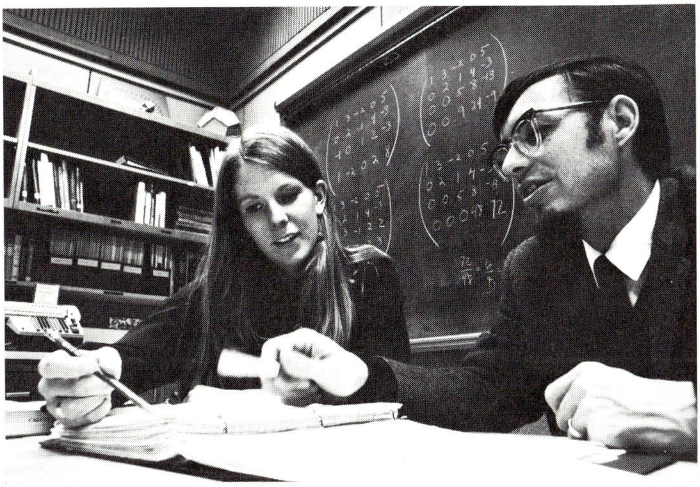

**16.7** Mathematicians are essential as teachers, scientific researchers, astronomers, economists, engineers, and many other occupations.

*Van Bucher/Photo Researchers, Inc.*

All types of industries employ people trained in mathematics. Government agencies at all levels also employ mathematicians. These jobs require at least a bachelor's degree and research positions often require doctor's degrees.

## Teaching

Many people with degrees in mathematics, physics, chemistry, or engineering earn their livings as teachers. To teach in schools below the college level requires at least a bachelor's degree. College teaching usually requires master's or doctor's degrees.

## Is It Worth It?

Spending four to nine years in college is expensive. The person who wants to be an engineer or a scientist must be able to pay fees and buy books. You must also buy food and pay for a place to live. In addition, you must give up the salary that you might have earned during those years.

A recent study has shown that people with bachelor's degrees can expect, on the average, to earn nearly *twice* as much money during their lifetimes as those who do not go beyond high school! Four years of extra study could be worth as much as a *half-million* dollars to a person with the right ability, interests, and skills. And a doctor's degree is worth, on the average, almost another $300,000.

In addition, of course, a college education will allow you to do the kind of work you want to do. Is it worth it?

**HAVE YOU LEARNED?**

1. What is the basic difference between the work of the scientist and the work of the engineer?
2. Name several branches of engineering.
3. Name two main branches of physical science.
4. Most of the physical scientists in the United States have specialized in what field?
5. Why are mathematicians so important to physical scientists and engineers?

## 3. You Don't Have to Go to College

**ARE YOU READY?**

Look up the following words if you are not sure of their meanings:

aerospace; computer; drafting; engineer; nuclear energy; scientist; technician.

From reading the last section, you may have gotten the idea that people who can't go to college are not able to work in physical science or engineering. This is not true!

In the United States, the number of people working as engineering and science technicians is large. It is more than double the number of people working as scientists. The number of technicians is almost as large as the number of engineers.

Technicians are needed to assist and support the work of almost every scientist and engineer. They work in drafting plans, as mathematics aids, writers, and artists. They help make tools, machines, and electronic equipment. They assemble everything from experimental telephones to spacecraft. Most of the actual laboratory work done in chemical research is done by technicians rather than by chemists.

Besides the technicians hundreds of thousands of men and women also work as clerks, typists, salespeople, and on other jobs that are related to the physical sciences. You can see that there are many jobs in physical science that do not require a college degree. All of these jobs, however, require an understanding of science and mathematics.

Let's take a look at a number of industries that employ people who know something about physical science. These are just samples of the many jobs that are available, of course, but they will give you an idea of the opportunities open to people who like physical science.

### Mining

The mining industry is one of our smaller industries. It includes the removal from the earth of such things as coal, oil, natural gas, and metals. Many scientists and engineers are needed to find, extract, and process these necessary resources. Many more skilled people are used to help in these important jobs.

In addition to hiring people to actually dig the ore or drill the wells, this industry needs people who have skills such as drafting, metal working, typing, and the like. All of these workers must know something about the physical science they deal with. Many of these jobs require some training beyond high school.

**16.8** Mining engineers and technicians

*Paolo Koch/Rapho/Photo Researchers, Inc.*

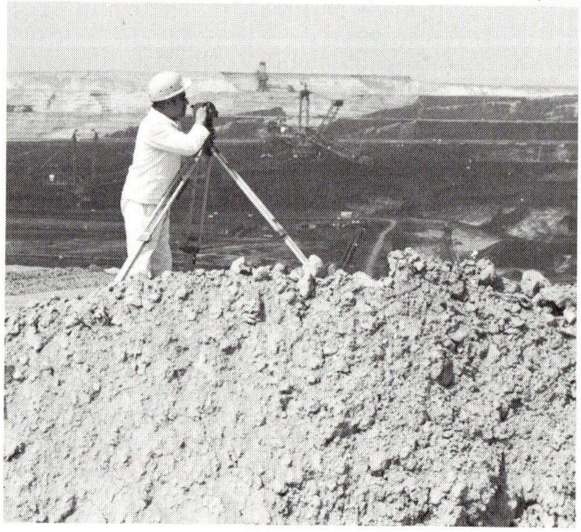

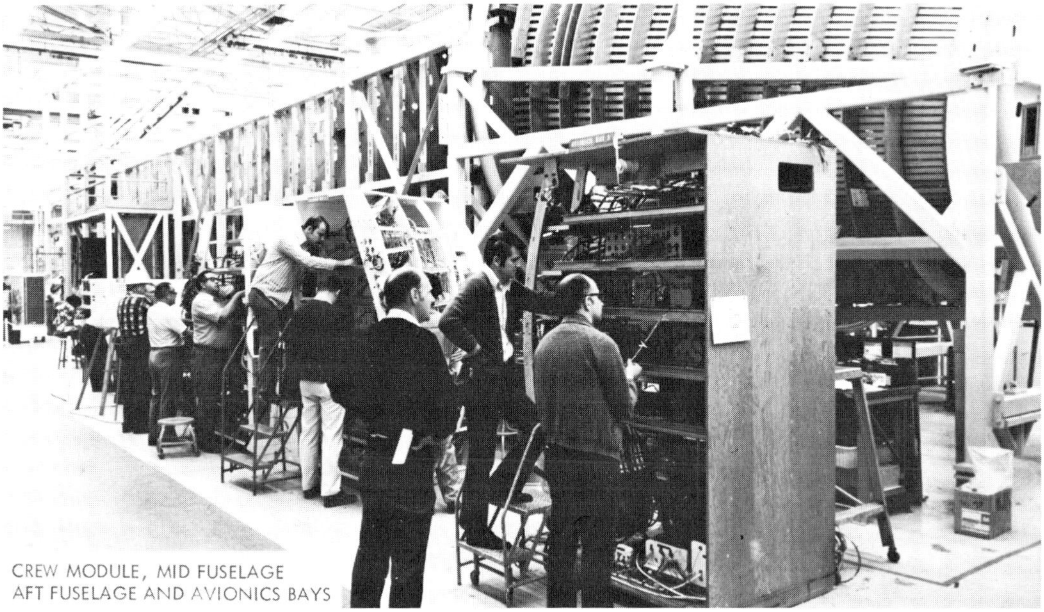


*NASA*

**16.9** Engineers and technicians are at work wiring and piping the aft and mid-fuselage sections of a space shuttle orbiter. This spacecraft is being built by Rockwell in Downey, California.

## Automotive–Aerospace Industry

Taken together, the industries that design and build automobiles, the numerous kinds of trucks and tractors, airplanes, missiles, and spacecraft make up one of our largest industries. Technicians with the proper knowledge and skill may work with scientists and engineers in designing automobiles, trucks, airplanes, rockets, and spacecraft. Or they may do the mathematical calculations that help the engineers to estimate the stress that will be on an aircraft or the cost of building the machine.

Electricians, chemical technicians, and inspectors in the aerospace field are highly paid and in short supply. Mechanics, machinists, and metal workers of all types also are needed as well as writers, artists, draftspeople and salespeople.

Most of the jobs in the automotive-aerospace industry require a high degree of skill. Many of the companies that make parts for the industry have training programs, whereas others need people who have learned their skills in school. All of these workers profit a great deal by having learned something about physical science and mathematics.

## Nuclear Energy Industry

An important group of industries has grown up around nuclear energy. Peaceful uses of this valuable type of energy, as well as military uses, continue to be studied. Nuclear energy industries need workers at all levels–from the experienced research scientist to the people skilled in the various crafts.

Present uses of nuclear energy include

the production of electricity, the propulsion of ships, the preparation of foods, and its uses in various types of health programs. Research is now being done to try to find ways to use nuclear energy in the recovery of gas and oil, in the safe production of electricity, and in the propulsion of spacecraft.

Technical help is needed in all of these industries. Electronics, chemical, and other types of scientific technicians are used in drafting and the use of the various radiation monitoring instruments. Mechanics, machinists, plumbers, and pipefitters who have a basic knowledge of physical science are also needed.

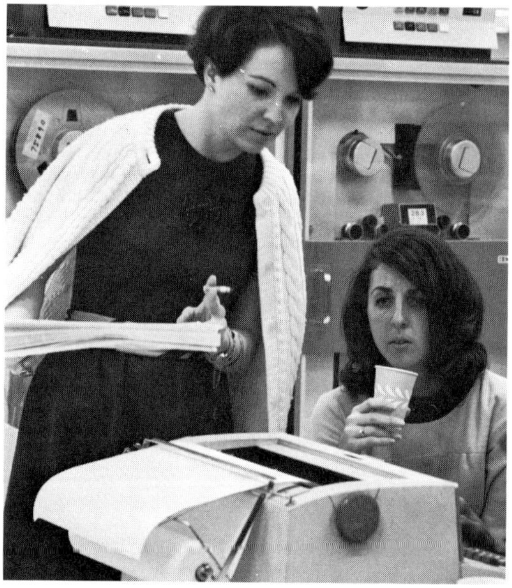

*Photo courtesy of IBM*

**16.10** The design, manufacture, and use of computers offer employment to thousands of science-oriented people.

### Chemical Manufacturing

More than a half million Americans are employed by the companies that make chemicals, plastics, synthetic fibers, and synthetic rubber. This is one of the fastest growing industries in the country today, primarily because of the research activities of these companies.

Approximately 100,000 of the people employed by the chemical industry are scientists, engineers, and technicians. The technicians assist the chemists and chemical engineers in the laboratory where the research is being done. Or they assist in the manufacturing plant where the quality of the product is being tested. Many of these technicians perform laboratory experiments for the scientists and engineers and then write reports of the results.

The education of these technicians is varied. Because their work is so technical, most of them are graduates of technical institutes or junior colleges. Their studies must include adequate mathematics, physical science, and English.

### Computers, and Duplicating and Other Office Machines

The companies in this type of industry make and sell all types of office machines, including typewriters, adding machines, scales, and computers. Two-thirds of the employees in this industry work at making computers or their parts. The rapid growth of the use of computers is shown by the fact that up to 1945 there were no computers produced in this country.

In such a new industry as this, there are many opportunities for research scientists and engineers. As in other industries, these researchers must have the help of many people trained in technical subjects—skilled craftspeople who understand basic science and mathematics. One out of every ten people employed in this industry is a technician.

Most of these technicians in the computer and office machines industry are electronics specialists. They help the scientists and engineers who are trying to develop new products. They test and inspect the equipment that the companies produce. Some computer technologists do the complicated assembly work, which is an important part of the industry. Others specialize in programming computers or in repairing them.

Other types of technicians also find work in this industry. These include people who are trained in chemistry, photography, drafting, and mathematics.

## Air Conditioning and Refrigeration

The industry that specializes in controlling the temperature of our environment is important. Technically-trained people are used at all levels of the business. Technicians assist scientists in the search for new ways to control heat. They work with engineers in designing new heating, cooling, or refrigeration systems. Other technicians test equipment that has been manufactured. Others work with the salespeople to determine the needs of customers. Others supervise the installation of the equipment.

At a less technical level, this industry employs over a hundred thousand mechanics who install and repair the furnaces and cooling units. High school courses in mathematics, physics, and industrial arts are helpful to people looking for jobs of this type.

## It Takes More Training

The work of technicians, regardless of the type of industry they work for, requires more training than a person can get in the

**16.11** If you have gaps in your learning background, you can get special training on the job. On the chalkboard you can see that it is helpful if you learn some mathematics.

*General Motors Corporation*

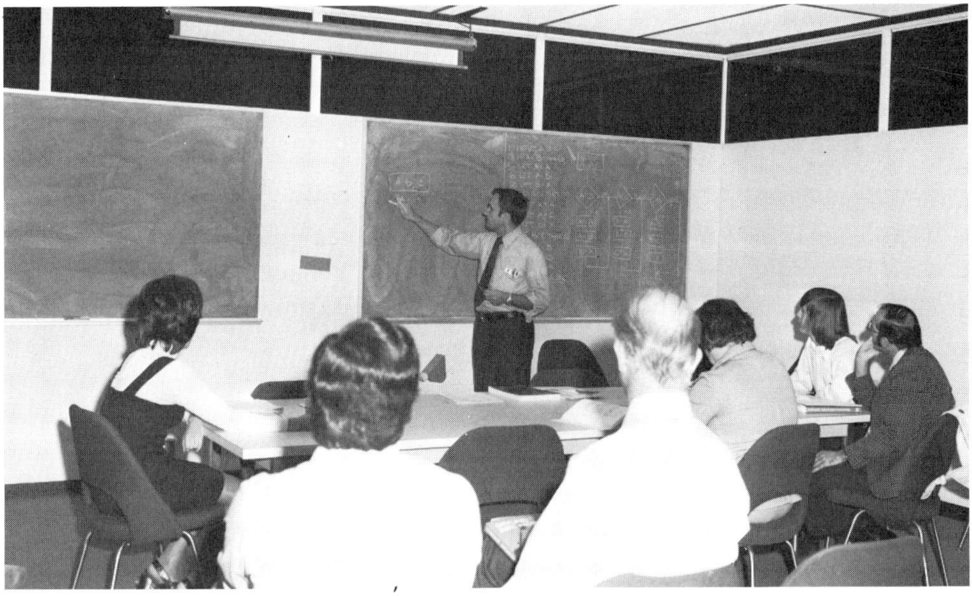

usual high school. The same is true for any skilled craftsperson. Some types of jobs are learned within a company. Other technical jobs require that you go to school for a year or two after you have graduated from high school. A variety of technical institutes, community colleges, vocational technical schools, and colleges offer courses that will help you get one of these technical jobs. The Armed Forces is another place to get the technical training you want.

In general, in order to go on to a school offering courses in technical fields, you must have a high school diploma. Or you must be able to pass a test that shows that you have the ability to do advanced work. A high school student who is interested in a career in technology must get a good background in all of the sciences, in mathematics, and in English.

## Is It Worth It?

We often hear students in junior and senior high schools talking about dropping out. At age 15 or 16 many students find jobs that pay what seems to them to be good wages.

"Why should I stay in school?" they ask. "I'm making a good salary working now. I don't make anything while I go to school. If they would pay me a salary, I would finish high school."

This sounds logical. But let's look at the facts. The graph to the right shows that students *are* being paid to finish high school! They won't receive their pay checks until sometime in the future. But the time they spend in school will be paid for by higher earnings once they take a job.

As you can see from this graph, the more education you have, the higher your lifetime income will be. These are averages, of course. Everyone can name someone who quit school in the third grade and made a million dollars before age twenty. But these people are the exceptions.

On the average, the person who finishes high school can expect to make about one-third more money than will the person who quits after the eighth grade. No one knows exactly how much this will be, but it certainly will be more than $100,000 difference. Four years spent studying in high school is worth, on the average, $25,000 per year or more!

Technical training, which usually requires several years of schooling beyond high school, also pays well. A few years ago, one study of the starting salaries of technicians showed that they received salaries that were 25% higher than the starting salaries of unskilled workers. Many skilled craftspeople started to work at even higher salaries.

**16.12** Set long-term goals—not short ones.

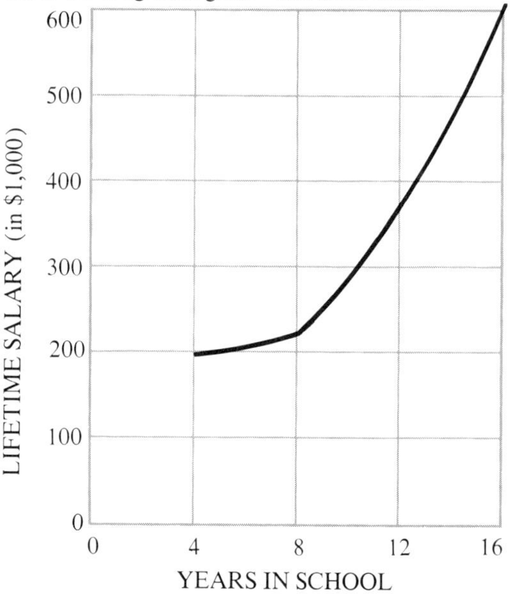

Yes, education pays. Not only are the starting salaries of people trained in science and mathematics high, but their futures are almost unlimited. Many technicians learn more about their jobs and are promoted to even higher paying jobs. Some go back to school and eventually become scientists and engineers. Others go into sales work. Still others become managers and supervisors in their industries.

**HAVE YOU LEARNED?**

On a sheet of paper list the numbers for the questions below. By each number write *T* if the statement is true and *F* if false.

1. Everyone who works in physical science jobs has a college degree.
2. There are more technicians in the United States than there are scientists.
3. The aerospace industry is one of this country's largest.
4. Everyone who works in nuclear energy has a college degree.
5. There are more computers in the United States now than there were 20 years ago.
6. It usually pays to stay in school.

## REVIEW QUESTIONS

1. Briefly describe the differences between technology and science.
2. Why is it difficult to make accurate predictions about the number of scientists, engineers, and technologists we will need in the future?
3. What has been the general trend in job opportunities in science-related fields during the past few decades?
4. Discuss the value of science courses to people who do not become scientists or engineers.
5. Why does solving our environmental crisis depend upon our having a great number of people with training in science?
6. What are some of the differences between science and engineering?
7. Briefly describe the job of the aerospace engineer, the agricultural engineer, the chemical engineer, the civil engineer, the electrical engineer, and the mechanical engineer.
8. What are usually the differences in time required to get a bachelor's degree, a master's degree, and a doctor's degree?
9. What does the future physical scientist study while in college?
10. What is the difference between a theoretical mathematician and an applied mathematician?
11. What are the differences in salaries of people who have bachelor's degrees and people who do not go on to further education after high school?
12. How is the work of technologists important in scientific discovery and engineering projects?
13. Choose one type of industry (mining, aerospace, nuclear energy, chemical manufacturing, computers and other office machines, or air conditioning and refrigeration) and discuss the types of technical jobs available in it.
14. What are some of the places a person can get technical training beyond high school?
15. What are the financial rewards of finishing high school?

## CAN YOU FIND OUT?

*It may be necessary to use an encyclopedia or other reference books in answering these questions.*

1. Which industries are expected to grow the most during the next ten years?

2. In what industries and for what age groups is the unemployment rate the highest?
3. What college or university nearest you offers degrees in engineering? What type of student are they looking for?
4. What college or university nearest you offers degrees in physics and chemistry? What type of student are they looking for?
5. How do the beginning salaries of engineers and scientists compare?
6. What is a biomedical engineer? A ceramic engineer? An industrial engineer?
7. What do physicians and dentists have to understand about physical science?
8. What kind of physical science does the environmentalist need to know?
9. How do the starting salaries of science and engineering technologists compare with those of other jobs in your part of the country?
10. What schools near you offer courses in technical fields? For which fields do they prepare students? What type of students are these schools looking for?
11. What opportunities for employment are there near your home for people skilled in the trades and crafts—carpentry, masonry, plumbing, electronics, and machine work?

## REFERENCES FOR ADDITIONAL STUDY

*Below are listed some of the many places you may write for more information about careers in science, engineering, and technology.*

Acoustical Society of America
335 East 45th Street
New York, NY 10017

American Chemical Society
Education Office
1155 16th Street, NW
Washington, DC 20036

American Institute of Physics
355 East 45th Street
New York, NY 10017

American Society for Metals
Metals Park, OH 44073

Dow Chemical Company
Barstow Building
2020 Dow Center
Midland, MI 48640

General Motors Corporation
Public Relations Staff
Room 1-101, General Motors Building
Detroit, MI 48202

International Business Machines Corporation
Armonk, NY 10504

The Mathematical Association of America
1225 Connecticut Avenue, NW
Washington, DC 20036

National Aeronautics and Space Administration
Counseling and Career Guidance Officer
Code FE, Educational Program Division
Office of Public Affairs
Washington, DC 20546

Society for Technical Communication
Suite 421
1010 Vermont Avenue, NW
Washington, DC 20005

Technical Education Research Centers
44 Brattle Street
Cambridge, MA 02138

U.S. Department of Labor
Bureau of Labor Statistics
Washington, DC 20212

U.S. Office of Education and Training
Smithsonian Institution
Washington, DC 20560

# USING THE METRIC SYSTEM

| Units | Equivalents |
|---|---|
| LENGTH | |
| meter (m) | 39.37 inches |
| millimeter (mm) | 0.04 inch; 0.001 meter; 0.1 centimeter |
| centimeter (cm) | 0.4 inch; 0.01 meter; 10 millimeters |
| kilometer (km) | 0.6 mile; 1,000 meters |
| MASS (weight) | |
| gram (g) | 0.035 ounce |
| milligram (mg) | 0.001 gram |
| kilogram (kg) | 2.2 pounds; 1,000 grams |
| metric ton (t) | 2,200 pounds; 1,000 kilograms |
| VOLUME | |
| liter (l) | 1.06 quart |
| milliliter (ml) | 0.001 liter; 1 cubic centimeter (cc or $cm^3$) |

**Approximate Conversion of English Measures to Metric Measures**

| When You Know | Multiply by | To Find |
|---|---|---|
| LENGTH | | |
| inches (in) | 2.54 | centimeters (cm) |
| feet (ft) | 30 | centimeters (cm) |
| | 0.3 | meters (m) |
| miles (mi) | 1.6 | kilometers (km) |
| AREA | | |
| square inches ($in^2$) | 6.5 | square centimeters ($cm^2$) |
| square miles ($mi^2$) | 2.6 | square kilometers ($km^2$) |
| WEIGHT (mass) | | |
| ounces (oz) | 28 | grams (g) |
| pounds (lb) | 0.45 | kilograms (kg) |
| short tons (2,000 lb) | 0.9 | metric tons (t) |
| VOLUME | | |
| teaspoons (tsp) | 5 | milliliters (ml) |
| fluid ounces (fl oz) | 30 | milliliters (ml) |
| quarts (qt) | 0.95 | liters (l) |
| gallons (gal) | 3.8 | liters (l) |
| cubic feet ($ft^3$) | 0.03 | cubic meters ($m^3$) |
| TEMPERATURE | | |
| Fahrenheit degrees (°F) | subtract 32 then multiply by 5/9 | Celsius (°C) (Centigrade) |

**Approximate Conversion of Metric Measures to English Measures**

| When You Know | Multiply by | To Find |
|---|---|---|
| LENGTH | | |
| millimeters (mm) | 0.04 | inches (in) |
| centimeters (cm) | 0.4 | inches (in) |
| meters (m) | 3.3 | feet (ft) |
| kilometers (km) | 0.6 | miles (mi) |
| AREA | | |
| square centimeters ($cm^2$) | 0.16 | square inches ($in^2$) |
| square meters ($m^2$) | 1.2 | square yards ($yd^2$) |
| square kilometers ($km^2$) | 0.4 | square miles ($mi^2$) |
| MASS (weight) | | |
| grams (g) | 0.035 | ounces (oz) |
| kilograms (kg) | 2.2 | pounds (lb) |
| metric tons (1,000 kg) | 1.1 | short tons (2,000 lb) |
| VOLUME | | |
| milliliters (ml) | 0.03 | fluid ounces (fl oz) |
| liters (l) | 1.06 | quarts (qt) |
| cubic meters ($m^3$) | 35 | cubic feet ($ft^3$) |
| TEMPERATURE | | |
| Celsius degrees (°C) | multiply by 9/5 then add 32 | Fahrenheit (°F) |

# glossary

**absolute temperature scale** the temperature scale having at the lower end *absolute zero*, the temperature at which molecular motion ceases, and on which 273° is the freezing point of water and 373° is the boiling point of water at sea level

**absorption spectrum** (ab sôrp′ shən spek′ trəm) a spectrum having dark lines caused by light energy of these wavelengths being absorbed by material between the light source and the observer

**acceleration** (ak sel′ ər a′ shən) change in the speed or direction of an object

**acid** (as′ id) a substance that produces hydronium ions in water solution; tastes sour and turns blue litmus paper red

**adhesion** (ad ′hē′ zhən) the attractive force between unlike molecules

**alcohols** (al′ kə hôl) a group of carbon compounds that contain one or more hydroxyl (OH) groups

**aldehydes** (al′ də hīd′) a group of carbon compounds that contain a −CHO group

**alkaline** (al′ ka līn) descriptive of compounds that are bases or have properties of bases

**alloy** (al′ oi) a mixture of two or more metals that are dissolved together as liquids and cooled to the solid state

**Pronunciation Key** The pronunciation of each word included in this glossary can be found in the parentheses after the word. The pronunciation follows the key* listed below. The accent (′) indicates primary stress. A lighter accent (′) indicates secondary stress.

| | | | | | |
|---|---|---|---|---|---|
| a | hat, cap | f | fat, if | p | paper, cup |
| ā | age, face | g | go, bag | r | run, try |
| ã | care, air | h | he, how | s | say, yes |
| ä | father, far | i | it, pin | sh | she, rush |
| b | bad, rob | ī | ice, five | t | tell, it |
| ch | child, much | j | jam, enjoy | th | thin, both |
| d | did, red | k | kind, seek | ᴛʜ | then, smooth |
| e | let, best | l | land, coal | u | cup, butter |
| ē | equal, see | m | me, am | u̇ | full, put |
| ėr | term, learn | n | no, in | ü | rule, move |
| ə | *represents:* | ng | long, bring | ū | use, music |
| a | in about | o | hot, rock | v | very, save |
| e | in taken | ō | open, go | w | will, woman |
| i | in pencil | ô | order, all | y | young, yet |
| o | in lemon | oi | oil, voice | z | zero, breeze |
| u | in circus | ou | house, out | zh | measure, seizure |

*From THORNDIKE-BARNHART ADVANCED JUNIOR DICTIONARY by E. L. Thorndike and Clarence L. Barnhart. Copyright © 1968 by Scott, Foresman and Company.

**alpha particle** (al′ fə pär′ tə kəl) composed of two protons and two neutrons and given off during the decomposition of some radioactive materials; a stream of these particles is called *alpha rays.*

**alternating current** (ôl′ tər nāt ing kėr′ ənt) an electrical current that reverses direction at regular intervals; abbreviated A.C. or a.c.

**amino acid** (ə mē′ nō) organic acids that are the basic building blocks of proteins

**ammeter** (am′ mē′ tər) an instrument used to measure electrical current or amperage

**ampere** (am′ pēr) a unit used to measure the amount of electrical current; also called an *amp* and the amount of current in a circuit is called the *amperage*

**amplitude** (am′ plə tüd) the size or strength of a quantity; in the case of waves, the height of the wave from its midpoint

**analog computer** (an′ ə lôg′ kəm püt′ ər) a type of computer used to solve a specific kind of problem

**angle of incidence** (ang′ gəl in′ sə dəns) the angle formed by a light ray and a perpendicular to the surface of a mirror or other object

**angle of reflection** (ang′ gəl ri flek′ shən) the angle formed by a reflected light ray and a perpendicular to the surface of the reflecting surface

**anode** (an′ ōd) the element of a vacuum tube that is positively charged and to which electrons are attracted; called the *plate*

**atom** (at′ əm) the smallest particle of an element; composed of protons, electrons, and neutrons

**atomic number** (ə tom′ ik) the number of protons in the nuclei of atoms of an element; also indicates the number of electrons an atom has

**atomic pile** one type of nuclear reactor

**atomic weight** the weight of an atom compared to the isotope of carbon that has an atomic weight of 12; also called the *atomic mass*

**base** (bās) a compound that produces hydroxyl (OH) ions in solution; turns red litmus paper blue

**battery** (bat′ ər i) two or more cells connected to produce an electrical current

**beta particle** (bā′ tə) fast-moving electrons given off during the decomposition of some radioactive materials; a stream of these particles is called *beta rays.*

**betatron** (bā′ tə tron′) a device used to bombard atomic nuclei with beta particles

**biochemist** (bī′ ō kem′ ist) a scientist who specializes in the chemistry of living things

**biology** (bī ol′ ə ji) the science of living things

**bond** the attractive force that holds two or more atoms together

**breeder reactor** (brēd′ ər ri ak′ tər) a nuclear reactor in which fissionable material is produced

**bright line spectrum** a spectrum having bright lines (against a dark background) that is produced when an element is heated and viewed through a spectroscope

**buoyancy** (boi′ ən si) the ability to float in a liquid or gas, or the upward force on an object in a liquid or gas

**Caloric Theory** (kə lôr′ ik thē′ ə ri) the theory that heat was a substance called *caloric* and that it flowed from one substance to another

**calorie** (kal′ ə ri) the amount of heat required to raise the temperature of one gram of water one degree Celsius; equal to $^1/_{1,000}$ of a large Calorie used to measure the heat content of food

**capillary action** (kap′ ə ler′ i ak′ shən) the rise of a liquid in a small tube, caused by the adhesive force between the liquid and the walls of the tube and the surface tension of the liquid

**carbohydrate** (kär′ bō hī′ drāt) a group of compounds found in foods, containing the elements carbon, hydrogen, and oxygen

**carbon dating** (kär′ bən) a method used to estimate the age of the remains of living things by measuring the amount of $C^{14}$ they contain

**catalyst** (kat′ ə list) a substance that affects the rate of a chemical reaction but is not changed in composition at the end of the reaction

**cathode** (kath′ ōd) the element in a vacuum tube that gives off electrons

**cathode rays** a flow of electrons in a vacuum tube

**cellulose** (sel′ ū lōs) a polysaccharide found in plants

**Celsius** (sel′ sē əs) a temperature scale having 0° as the freezing point of water and 100° as the boiling point of water at sea level; abbreviated C.; also called the *Centigrade temperature scale*

**center of gravity** the point in an object about which the object's mass is evenly distributed

**centigrade** (sen′ tə grād) see Celsius

**centimeter** (sen′ tə mē′ tər) a unit of length in the metric system equal to $^1/_{100}$ meter or about two-fifths of an inch

**chain reaction** the fission of a radioactive material in which the disintegration of one atom produces neutrons that cause other atoms to disintegrate

**charge** (chärj) the amount of electricity present on an object

**chemical change** (kem′ ə kəl) a change that involves the formation of new substances during a chemical reaction

**chemical energy** the energy released or used up during a chemical reaction

**chemical property** the quality of a substance that determines how it reacts with other substances

**chemistry** (kem′ is tri) the science that deals with the composition of matter and the changes in its composition, such as those that occur during a chemical reaction

**chlorophyll** (klô′ rə fil) the green pigment in plants that is necessary for photosynthesis

**chromatography** (krō′ mə tog′ rə fē) a method of separating different substances by their being absorbed at various rates by filter paper or other materials

**circuit** (sėr′ kit) a pathway or closed loop through which electricity flows, including a source and wires connecting the source to devices that use electricity

**coefficient of linear expansion** (kō′ ə fish′ ənt lin′ i ər eks pan′ shən) a numerical quantity equal to the amount a substance will increase in length for each degree of temperature increase

**coherent light** (kō hēr′ ənt) light in which the high and low points of the waves are all in step, as in a laser beam

**cohesion** (kō hē′ zhən) the attractive force between molecules of the same kind

**combustion** (kəm bus′ chən) a chemical reaction involving the combination of oxygen with a substance, which usually produces heat and light

**complementary colors** (kom′ plə men′ tə ri) two colors, such as yellow and blue, that when mixed in the right proportion, produce white

**compound** (kom′ pound) a chemical combination of two or more elements, having properties different from those of the elements of which it is composed

**compression** (kəm presh′ ən) the decrease in volume that occurs when pressure is applied to an object; the part of a longitudinal wave in which the particles are packed more closely together than is normal

**concave** (kon kāv′) descriptive of a shape like that of the inside of a hollow ball or a spoon

**conduction** (kən duk′ shən) the process by which energy, such as heat, sound, and electricity, is transmitted by a material called a *conductor* from one place to another

**conservation of energy** (kon′ sər vā′ shən) the principle that energy can be changed from one form to another but cannot be created or destroyed, except in nuclear reactions

**conservation of matter** the principle that matter can be changed from one form to another but cannot be created or destroyed, except in nuclear reactions

**control rod** a rod-shaped piece of metal that absorbs neutrons and is used to control the rate of reaction in a nuclear reactor

**convection** (kən vek′ shən) the movement of hot material through a gas or liquid

**convex** (kon veks′) descriptive of a shape like that of the outside of a ball or a spoon

**coolant** (kül′ ənt) substance used to conduct heat, such as water in a car radiator or nuclear reactor

**corpuscle** (kôr′ pəs əl) a small particle, such as that proposed by one theory of light

**coulomb** (kü lom′) an electrical charge of $6.28 \times 10^{18}$ electrons

**covalence** (kō vā′ ləns) the combining power of an atom that shares electrons with one or more other atoms

**covalent bonds** (kō vā′ lənt) the attractive force between atoms that share one or more pairs of electrons

**critical mass** (krit′ ə kəl) the smallest amount of fissionable material that will keep a chain reaction going without an outside source of neutrons

**cryogenics** (krī′ ō jen′ iks) the study of very low temperatures and their effects on materials

**cubic centimeter** (kū′ bik) a unit of volume equal to the space enclosed in a cube one centimeter on each side; abbreviated cc.

**curie** (kūr′ i) a unit of radioactivity equal to the amount of material that undergoes $3.7 \times 10^{10}$ disintegrations per second; equal to 1,000 *millicuries*

**cyan** (sī′ an) a blue-green color produced when green light and blue light are added to each other

**cycle** (sī′ kəl) a series of events that occur in the same order and are repeated regularly; for example, the movement of electrons back and forth in a conductor or the movement of a tuning fork

**cyclotron** (sī′ klə tron) a device used to bombard the nuclei of atoms

**data** (dā′ tə) information collected during an experiment or while making observations

**decibel** (des′ ə bel) a unit used to measure the loudness of sound

**declination** (dek′ lə nā′ shən) the difference between the direction a compass points and true north

**decomposition reaction** (dē′ kom pə zish′ ən ri ak′ shən) a chemical reaction in which a compound is broken down into simpler compounds or elements

**density** (den′ sə ti) the amount of material in a given volume; the ratio of the mass of a substance to its volume

**diffusion** (di fū′ zhən) the mixing of molecules or atoms as a result of their motion; the movement of light through a translucent material or the reflection of light by a rough surface

**digital computer** (dij′ ə təl) the most common type of computer, which operates with numbers expressed as digits in the decimal, binary, or other number system

**diode** (dī′ ōd) a device that contains two electrodes and conducts electricity in one direction; a type of vacuum tube

**direct current** an electrical current that flows in one direction; abbreviated D.C. or d.c.

**disaccharide** (dī sak′ ə rīd) a double sugar having the general formula of $C_{12}H_{22}O_{11}$

**disintegration series** (dis in′ tə grā′ shən sēr′ iz) a series of steps through which a radioactive substance goes as it breaks down into simpler substances

**domain** (dō mān′) the region in a ferromagnetic material in which the atoms are so arranged that a magnetic field is thereby produced

**double replacement reaction** a reaction between two compounds in which atoms or radicals in one compound change places with the atoms or radicals in the other compound

**electric meter** a device that measures electricity

**electrical energy** a kind of energy composed of electrons

**electrolyte** (i lek′ trə līt) a compound that when placed in water conducts electricity

**electromagnetic spectrum** (i lek′ trō mag net′ ik) the range of frequencies of electromagnetic radiations, including television and radio waves, light, X rays, and gamma rays

**electromagnetic waves** kinds of energy having both electrical and magnetic properties, such as light and radio waves

**electromotive force** (i lek′ trə mō′ tiv fôrs) the force that causes electricity to move; abbreviated emf

**electron** (i lek′ tron) a negatively-charged particle found in the shells of atoms and in static and current electricity

**electronics** (i lek′ tron′ iks) the study of electrons and their use in various devices such as radio, television, RADAR, and computers

**electroscope** (i lek′ trə skōp) an instrument used to detect small charges of electricity

**element** (el′ ə mənt) a substance that cannot be broken down into a simpler substance by ordinary chemical means; a high-resistant conductor that produces heat in electrical appliances such as toasters and irons; one of the parts in a vacuum tube, such as the cathode or grid

**energy** (en′ ər ji) the ability to do work

**enzyme** (en′ zīm) a catalyst contained in a living thing

**equation** (i kwā′ zhən) in chemistry, an expression using symbols that indicates the elements or compounds that react and the products that are formed. In mathematics, a statement that two quantities are equal

**erg** (ėrg) a unit of energy

**esters** (es′ tər) a group of carbon compounds, many of which have the odor of ripe fruit, that are produced by the reaction between an alcohol and an acid

**ethers** (ē′ thər) a group of carbon compounds that have two carbon chains connected by an oxygen atom, such as diethyl ether, $CH_3CH_2OCH_2CH_3$, which is used as an anesthetic

**evaporate** (i vap′ ə rāt) to change from a liquid to a gas

**exponent** (eks pō′ nənt) a number placed above and to the right of another number, which tells how many times the base is to be multiplied by itself; for example, three is the exponent in $10^3$, which equals $10 \times 10 \times 10$ or 1,000.

**Fahrenheit** (far′ ən hīt) a temperature scale on which the freezing point of water is 32° and the boiling point of water at sea level is 212°; abbreviated F.

**fallout** radioactive materials in the atmosphere produced by a nuclear explosion

**fermentation** (fėr′ men tā′ shən) a chemical reaction in which certain carbohydrates are changed, such as sugar being changed to alcohol or cider to vinegar

**ferromagnetic** (fer′ ō mag net′ ik) materials, such as iron and nickel, that are attracted by a magnet

**fission** (fish′ ən) the splitting of atomic nuclei, which is accompanied by the release of energy

**flame test** a method used to identify certain elements that give off a characteristic color when heated in a flame

**flammable** (flam′ ə bəl) any material that is easily set on fire

**fluorescence** (flü′ ə res′ əns) the property that some materials have of giving off radiation when they are exposed to radiation from another source

**focal length** (fō′ kəl) the distance from the center of a lens or curved mirror to the point where a parallel beam of light is brought together

**footcandle** a unit of illumination produced by a one candlepower source shining on a surface one foot away

**force** a push or pull

**formula** (fôr′ mū lə) a mathematical equation for a certain relationship, such as $D = M/V$ that indicates the relationship of mass and volume to density; in chemistry, an expression using the symbols for the elements to represent a compound or molecule, such as $H_2O$ or NaCl

**frequency** (frē′ kwən si) the number of vibrations per second or the number of waves that pass a given point each second

**fundamental** (fun′ də men′ təl) the sound, or tone, produced when the entire string vibrates on a musical instrument

**fusion** (fū′ zhən) the process by which atomic nuclei of light-weight elements combine to form the nucleus of a heavier atom and in so doing release large amounts of energy

**galvanometer** (gal′ və nom′ ə tər) an instrument used to measure small electrical currents

**gamma rays** (gam′ ə) high-energy radiation given off during the disintegration of some radioactive materials

**Geiger counter** (gī′ gər) an instrument used to detect and measure radioactivity

**gram** (gram) a unit of mass in the metric system equal to 0.0353 of an ounce

**gravitational attraction** (grav′ ə tā′ shən əl ə trak′ shən) the attraction of all objects in the universe by all other objects; in the case of the earth, the pull of the earth which causes objects to have weight

**grid** (grid) the screen or parallel wires in a vacuum tube used to control the flow of electrons from the cathode to the anode

**grounded** an electrical circuit which is connected to the ground or to a large common conductor such as the frame of an automobile or airplane

**half-life** the length of time it takes for half of the atoms of a certain amount of a radioactive material to disintegrate

**horsepower** (hôrs′ pou′ ər) a unit of power used to measure the rate at which work is done; equal to 550 foot-pounds per second or 746 watts

**hydrocarbons** (hī′ drō kär′ bən) compounds containing only the elements carbon and hydrogen

**hydronium ion** (hī drō′ ni əm) a combination of a hydrogen ion and a water molecule that acids form in water solution; $H_3O^+$

**hypothesis** (hī poth′ ə sis) a proposed explanation based on the available data

**illumination** (i lü′ mə nā′ shən) the amount of light striking a surface

**image** (im′ ij) a picture projected on a surface by a lens or mirror or what is observed by the eye through a lens or in a mirror

**incandescent** (in′ kən des′ ənt) refers to objects that are heated to high temperature and give off light

**inclined plane** one of the simple machines consisting of a flat surface slanting upward, such as a ramp

**incoherent light** (in′ kō hēr′ ənt) light in which the high and low points of the waves are not in phase with each other, as in sunlight

**induced magnetism** (in düs′ mag′ nə tiz əm) the effect of a magnetic field on a nonmagnetized piece of iron, resulting in its acting as a magnet

**inert elements** (in ėrt′) the elements, such as neon and argon, that do not combine chemically with other elements under ordinary conditions

**inertia** (in ėr′ shə) the characteristic of matter at rest to remain at rest and matter in motion to stay in motion unless acted upon by an outside force

**infinite** (in′ fə nit) without limit

**infrared** (in′ frə red′) the invisible radiation with a wavelength slightly longer than red light, which is sensed as heat

**inorganic chemistry** (in′ ôr gan′ ik) the chemistry of all the elements except carbon; sometimes used to designate the chemistry of nonliving materials

**in-phase** describes two or more events that

occur with the same frequency and at the same time, such as tuning forks that produce the same pitch that are set into vibration at the same time

**insoluble** (in sol′ ū bəl) describes something that does not dissolve

**insulated** (in′ sə lāt′) covered with a material that prevents or reduces the passage of electricity, heat, or sound

**ionization** (ī′ ən ə zā′ shən) the process by which charged particles, called *ions*, are produced from molecules and atoms

**isomers** (ī′ sə mər) two or more molecules that contain the same number and kinds of atoms but in which the atoms are arranged differently

**isotopes** (ī′ sə tōp) atoms of an element that have different atomic weights because they contain differing numbers of neutrons

**Kelvin scale** (kel′ vən skāl) another name for the Absolute temperature scale

**ketones** (kē′ tōn) a group of carbon compounds made up of two hydrocarbon groups connected by a $-\overset{\overset{O}{/\!/}}{C}-$ group

**kilo-** (kē′ lō) a prefix used in the metric system to indicate 1,000; for example, *kilocalorie*, *kilocycle*, *kilogram*, *kilometer*, and *kilowatt*

**kinetic energy** (ki net′ ik) the energy of a body in motion

**laser** (lā′ zər) a device that generates and amplifies light waves in a narrow and very intense beam of light

**latent heat** (lā′ tənt) the heat absorbed or given off when a substance changes state, such as the heat required to melt ice or boil water

**lines of force** in the case of magnetism, the lines between two unlike poles, which can be demonstrated with iron filings; in electricity, the path a positive charge follows in going from a plus to minus pole

**liter** (lē′ tər) a unit of volume in the metric system; slightly larger than a liquid quart

**longitudinal waves** (lon′ jə tü′ də nəl) waves, such as sound waves, in which the particles of the medium through which the energy travels, move back and forth in the same direction that the wave is moving

**luminous** (lü′ mə nəs) lighted up or illuminated; giving off light

**magenta** (mə jen′ tə) a deep purplish red color produced when red and blue light are added to each other

**magnetic field** (mag net′ ik) the space around a magnet in which magnetic effects, such as the deflection of a compass needle or the pull on iron filings, are observable

**magnetohydrodynamics** (mag nē′ tō hī′ drō dī nam′ iks) the science dealing with matter in the plasma state

**magnification** (mag′ nə fə kā′ shən) the apparent enlargement of an object when viewed through a lens or in a curved mirror

**maser** (mā′ zər) a device that generates and amplifies electromagnetic waves

**mass** (mas) the amount of matter in an object, which is always the same regardless of the location of the object

**matter** (mat′ ər) anything that has mass and occupies space

**mechanical advantage** (mə kan′ ə kəl ad van′ tij) the ratio of the force exerted by a machine to the force applied

**mechanical energy** the energy of moving objects and that found in machines

**medium** (mē′ di əm) the substance in which something occurs, such as the material through which sound or light travels

**megacycles** (meg′ ə sī′ kəl) one million cycles; abbreviated mc.

**meters** (mē′ tər) the unit of length in the metric system, equal to about 39.37 inches; also, devices used to measure the amount of something, such as the flow of water or electricity

**meterstick** a measuring stick that is one meter long

**metric system** (met′ rik) a system of weights and measures using grams, meters, and liters as units

**milligram** (mil′ ə gram) a unit equal to $^1/_{1,000}$ of a gram; abbreviated mg.

**millimeter** (mil′ ə mē′ tər) a unit of length equal to $^1/_{1,000}$ of a meter, or 0.03937 inch; abbreviated mm.

**mixture** (miks′ chər) two or more materials that are intermingled with each other, but are not combined chemically

**model** (mod′ əl) a way of explaining something not directly observable; also, objects used to represent something else, such as colored balls used to represent atoms or planets in the solar system

**moderator** (mod′ ər ā′ tər) a material, such as graphite or water, used in a nuclear reactor to slow down neutrons so they are more readily absorbed by atoms of the fuel

**modulated** (moj′ ů lāt) waves that are changed by alternation of the height of the wave (*amplitude modulation* or AM) or the frequency of the wave (*frequency modulation* or FM)

**molecule** (mol′ ə kūl) the smallest particle of a substance that has all the chemical properties of the substance; usually composed of two or more atoms held together by covalent bonds

**momentum** (mō men′ təm) the tendency of an object to keep moving; equal to an object's mass times its velocity

**monosaccharide** (mon′ ə sak′ ə rīd) a group of simple sugars whose molecules may contain four, five, or six carbon atoms

**mutation** (mū tā′ shən) a sudden change in the characteristics of an animal or plant; that is, the offspring has one or more characteristics different from its parents.

**negative** (neg′ ə tiv) the type of electrical charge carried by the electron; also used to describe an object or an atom that has more electrons than protons, such as a negative electrode or a negative ion

**neutralization** (nü′ trə li zā′ shən) a type of chemical reaction in which an acid reacts with a base to form a salt and water

**neutralize** (nü′ trə līz′) in electricity, to remove an electrical charge; in chemistry, to add an acid and base together

**neutrino** (nü trē′ nō) a particle with no electrical charge and zero rest mass that is emitted along with beta particles during the decomposition of some radioactive substances

**neutron** (nü′ tron) a neutral particle found in the nucleus of all atoms except the isotope of hydrogen that has an atomic weight of one; weighs about the same as the proton

**Nobel Prize** (nō bel′ prīz) a prize given to honor outstanding scientific contributions in chemistry, physics, and medicine or physiology

**node** (nōd) in a vibrating string or other object, the part that has little or no motion

**nuclear energy** (nü′ kli ər) the energy produced as the result of fission or fusion of atomic nuclei

**nuclear reactor** a device, in which nuclear fission takes place, that is used as a source of power and to manufacture radioactive materials; also called an atomic reactor or atomic pile

**nucleus** (nü′ kli əs) the central part or core of an atom; the plural of which is *nuclei*

**ohm** (ōm) a unit used to measure the resistance of a material to a flow of electricity

**Ohm's Law** states the relationship of resistance in ohms to current in amps and the electromotive force in volts; Resistance = EMF/Current.

**opaque** (ō pāk′) materials that do not transmit light or forms of radiation

**organic chemistry** (ôr gan′ ik) the chemistry of carbon compounds

**oscilloscope** (ə sil′ ə skōp′) an instrument containing a cathode ray tube, which is used to study sound, alternating currents, and other kinds of vibrations

**overtone** (ō′ vər tōn′) sound waves produced when an object such as a string or cord is forced to vibrate in segments

**parallel circuit** (par′ ə lel) a circuit containing two or more branches through which the current may flow

**particle accelerator** (pär′ tə kəl) a device used to bombard atomic nuclei with neutrons, alpha particles, and other particles

**Pascal's Law** (pas kal′) states that the pressure applied to an enclosed liquid acts equally in all directions.

**permeable** (pėr′ mi ə bəl) a description of solids that allow the passage of liquids and gases

**pH scale** a scale ranging from 0 to 14 used to indicate how acidic or basic a substance is, with seven being neutral, values less than 7 indicating an acid, and values greater than 7 indicating a base

**phenomenon** (fə nom′ ə non) a natural happening that can be explained on a scientific basis

**phlogiston theory** (flō jis′ tən thē′ ə ri) a theory that stated that a substance called *phlogiston* escaped when a substance was burned or rusted

**photoelectric cell** (fō′ tō i lek′ trik) a device that changes light to electricity

**photometer** (fō tom′ ə tər) an instrument used for measuring the intensity of light

**photosynthesis** (fō′ tō sin′ thə sis) the process in green plants in which the energy of sunlight is used to manufacture sugar from carbon dioxide and water

**photon** (fō′ ton) a package or bundle of light energy

**physical change** (fiz′ ə kəl) changes, such as changes in state, that do not involve any changes in the chemical composition of a substance

**physical properties** characteristics of a substance, such as color, mass, volume, or density, which do not involve a chemical change

**physical science** the branches of science dealing with such nonliving things as matter and energy

**physics** (fiz′ iks) the branch of science dealing with the study of matter and different forms of energy, such as electricity and light

**physiology** (fiz′ i ol′ ə ji) the branch of science that deals with the function of the various parts of a living organism

**piezoelectric effect** (pī ē′ zō i lek′ trik) the production of very small electrical currents when pressure is applied to certain kinds of crystals

**pitch** (pich) the property of a sound determined by its frequency

**plane mirror** a flat mirror

**plasma** (plaz′ mə) a fourth state of matter composed of charged particles at very high temperatures

**polarity** (pō lar′ ə ti) the state or direction of a magnetic field

**pole** (pōl) a point from which a magnetic or electrical field appears to come

**polymerization** (pə lim′ ər i zā′ shən) the process by which *polymers*, or giant molecules, are formed by the combining of smaller molecules

**polysaccharide** (pol′ i sak′ ə rīd) any one of the carbohydrates, such as starch and cellulose, that are made of many saccharide groups

**porosity** (pô ros′ ə ti) the physical property of a solid that is able to absorb or to allow liquids and gases to pass through

**positive charge** (pos′ ə tiv) a type of charge carried by the proton; also used to describe an object or atom that has more protons than electrons, such as a positive electrode or a positive ion

**potential energy** (pə ten′ shəl) stored energy that is able to do work because of an object's position or chemical condition

**power** (pou′ ər) a measure of the amount of work done in a given time

**pressure** (presh′ ər) the amount of force acting on a unit area of surface such as 1 kilogram of force per square centimeter

**primary colors** (prī′ mer′ i) the three colors of light: red, green, and blue, which can produce all other colors when mixed in the proper combination

**prism** (priz′ əm) a triangular piece of glass that separates white light into the colors of the spectrum

**protein** (prō′ tēn) a group of large complex compounds whose large molecules are composed of many amino acid molecules; contain the elements carbon, hydrogen, oxygen, nitrogen, and frequently sulfur and phosphorus

**proton** (prō′ ton) a positively-charged particle found in the nucleus of the atom

**quality** (kwol′ ə ti) the property of a musical tone that distinguishes it from another tone having the same pitch and loudness

**RADAR** (rā′ där) an electronic system used to determine the location of an object by bouncing radio waves off it

**radiation** (rā′ di ā′ shən) the transfer of heat and other forms of energy through space; also, the particles and rays given off during the disintegration of a radioactive material

**radical** (rad′ ə kəl) a group of atoms that stay together or act as a single unit, during a chemical reaction

**radioactive** (rā′ di ō ak′ tiv) descriptive of materials that disintegrate naturally and emit alpha, beta, or gamma radiation

**radioautograph** (rā′ di ō ô′ tə graf′) a picture or exposed negative made by exposing a photographic negative to the radiations given off by some radioactive material

**radioisotope** (rā′ di ō ī′ sə tōp) a radioactive isotope of an element

**ratio** (rā′ shi ō) the relationship between two numbers, expressed as the quotient resulting from the division of the first number by the second

**reaction** (ri ak′ shən) a process by which one or more new substances is formed; a chemical change; also, the changes that take place in the nucleus of the atom; in physics, a force equal to and in the opposite direction of an applied force

**reactor** (ri ak′ tər) see nuclear reactor.

**reflection** (ri flek′ shən) the change in direction of objects or energy, such as light and sound, when they strike a substance, but do not pass through it

**refraction** (ri frak′ shən) the bending of light rays when they pass obliquely from one substance into another or through a medium of varying density

**refrigerant** (ri frij′ ər ənt) the liquid or gas used in refrigerators as a cooling agent

**resonating** (rez′ ə nat ing) descriptive of a condition in which the natural frequency of vibration of an object, such as a tuning fork, or in an electrical system, such as a radio receiver, is matched in frequency to an outside source of vibration energy; results in a vibration of larger amplitude

**respiration** (res′ pə rā′ shən) the processes by which an animal, plant, or living cell secures oxygen from the air or water, distributes it, combines it with substances in the tissues, and gives off carbon dioxide

**roentgen** (rent′ gən) a unit used to measure the amount of X rays or gamma radiation absorbed by living things; the *milliroentgen* is equal to 1/1,000 of a roentgen

**science** (sī′ əns) the organized body of knowledge about the universe and the methods and attitudes related to the search for new knowledge

**scientific method** (sī′ ən tif′ ik meth′ əd) generally, the procedures used by scientists in their search for new knowledge and the testing of existing knowledge

**semiconductors** (sem′ i kən duk′ tər) materials that do not conduct electricity as well as metals but better than poor conductors such as glass and rubber; used in making transistors

**series circuit** (sēr′ iz) a circuit arranged like a loop so that electricity flows through all of the things in the circuit

**short circuit** a pathway through which electricity flows with very little resistance

**simple replacement reaction** a chemical reaction in which one or more atoms in a compound is replaced by another atom or atoms

**solar battery** (sō′ lər) a device that produces electricity by the action of sunlight on certain kinds of crystals

**solubility** (sol′ ū bil′ ə ti) the relative amount of a substance that will dissolve in another substance

**solution** (sə lü′ shən) a mixture of two substances in which the particles are uniformly distributed so that it cannot be separated by filtering or other mechanical means

**spectroscope** (spek′ trə skōp) an instrument that breaks light into colors of the spectrum and which is used to observe various kinds of spectra

**spectrum** (spek′ trəm) the band of colors formed when white light passes through a prism; also see *electromagnetic spectrum.*

**standard** (stan′ dərd) a unit used as the basis of a system of weights and measures, such as the meter in the metric system, or to describe certain conditions, such as *standard pressure* or *standard temperature*

**standing waves** do not seem to move since their nodes are stationary.

**starch** (stärch) a group of polysaccharides found in the seeds, tubers, and other parts of plants

**static electricity** (stat′ ik i lek′ tris′ ə ti) an accumulation of an electrical charge on a body; an electrical charge at rest

**Stellarator** (stel′ ər ā′ tər) a device used in research to investigate the possibility of controlling the fusion of atomic nuclei and using the energy produced for peaceful purposes

**step-down transformer** a transformer used to reduce the voltage of an alternating electrical current

**structural formula** (struk′ chər əl) a diagram that shows the number and kinds of atoms and their arrangement in a molecule

**superconductor** (sü′ pər kən duk′ tər) a substance with little or no electrical resistance, such as certain metals cooled to temperatures near absolute zero

**surface tension** (sėr′ fis ten′ shən) the property of a liquid to have an apparent skin on its surface, caused by the attraction of the molecules in the liquid for each other

**symbol** (sim′ bəl) a letter, abbreviation, or other sign used to represent a chemical element, a quantity, or a mathematical operation

**synchrotron** (sing′ krə tron′) a very powerful particle accelerator used to bombard atomic nuclei

**synthetic** (sin thet′ ik) descriptive of man-made things, such as *synthetic detergents* and *synthetic fibers*

**technology** (tek nol′ ə ji) the application of science to practical purposes

**thermocouple** (thėr′ mə kup′ əl) device consisting of the junction of two unlike metals in which an electrical current is induced when the junctions are maintained at different temperatures

**thermonuclear reaction** (thėr′ mō nü′ kli ər) a fusion reaction that occurs at very high temperatures; see fusion.

**thrust** forward force produced by a propellor, jet engine, or rocket

**trace elements** (trās) elements needed in only very small amounts by plants and animals

**tracer** (trās′ ər) a radioisotope, or "tagged" atom, used in tracing the path of a chemical or in other kinds of research

**transformer** (trans fôr′ mər) a device used to change voltage of an alternating current

**transistor** (tran zis′ tər) a small device that contains a semiconductor and which is used in place of a vacuum tube to control or amplify an electric current

**translucent** (trans lü′ sənt) a substance such as frosted glass that allows light to pass through, but diffuses the light so that objects cannot be clearly viewed

**transmit** (trans mit′) to send from one place to another, such as radio waves being sent by a *transmitter* or electricity on *transmission lines*

**transmutation** (trans′ mū tā′ shən) the process of changing one element into another

**transparent** (trans pãr′ ənt) able to transmit light so that an object can be seen clearly through it

**trial-and-error approach** an attempt to solve a problem by trying something and, if it doesn't work, trying something else without formulating a plan

**triode** (trī′ ōd) a vacuum tube with three elements—cathode, grid, and anode (plate)

**turbine** (tėr′ bən) a machine with blades that are turned by a stream of water, steam, or gas

**turbojet** (tėr′ bō jet′) a type of jet engine that contains a turbine that drives a compressor that compresses the air that the fuel is burned in

**turboprop** (tėr′ bō prop′) similar to a turbojet engine except that the turbine also drives a propellor that produces most of the engine's thrust

**ultraviolet** (ul′ trə vī′ ə lit) the invisible radiation with a wavelength slightly shorter than violet

**vacuum tube** (vak′ ū əm) a container from which the air has been removed and which contains two or more elements between which electrons are free to move

**valence** (vā′ ləns) the capacity of an atom of an element to combine with other atoms or groups of atoms

**vector** (vek′ tər) a quantity that has both direction and amount, such as a force or velocity

**velocity** (və los′ ə ti) the speed and direction of a moving object

**vestigial** (ves tij′ i əl) showing a trace of something that has gone

**vibration** (vī brā′ shən) back-and-forth motion

**vitamins** (vī′ tə min) any of the many organic substances produced by plants and necessary for the proper nutrition of man and other animals

**volt** (vōlt) unit used to measure electromotive force

**voltage** (vōl′ tij) the amount of electromotive force, measured in volts, that exists between two points

**voltmeter** (vōlt′ mē′ tər) instrument used to measure voltages between two points

**watt** (wot) a unit of electrical power equal to $^1/_{746}$ horsepower

**wavelength** the distance between a point on the top of one wave and the corresponding point on the top of the next wave

**work** energy transferred from one object to another; equal to the force times the distance the force moves

# index

Boldface numbers indicate illustrations.